Essential Neuroscience

Allan Siegel, Ph.D

Professor
Department of Neurology and Neurosciences
Department of Psychiatry
New Jersey Medical School
Newark, New Jersey

Hreday N. Sapru, Ph.D

Professor
Department of Neurological Surgery
Department of Neurology and Neurosciences
Department of Pharmacology and Physiology
New Jersey Medical School
Newark, New Jersey

Case Histories written by Heidi E. Siegel, M.D.

Essential Neuroscience

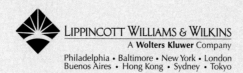

LIPPINCOTT WILLIAMS & WILKINS
A **Wolters Kluwer** Company

Philadelphia · Baltimore · New York · London
Buenos Aires · Hong Kong · Sydney · Tokyo

Editor: Betty Sun
Managing Editor: Elena Coler
Marketing Manager: Joe Schott
Illustrator: Anne Rains
Production Editor: Caroline Define
Compositor: Maryland Composition
Printer: R.R. Donnelley & Sons—Willard

Library of Congress Cataloging-in-Publication Data
Siegel, Allan, 1939–
    Essential neuroscience / Allan Siegel, Hreday N. Sapru ; case
histories written by Heidi E. Siegel.
        p. ; cm.
    ISBN 0–7817–5077–6 (pbk.)
    1. Neurosciences—Outlines, syllabi, etc. I. Sapru, Hreday N. II. Title.
    [DNLM: 1. Nervous System Physiology. 2. Mental Disorders—physiopathology.
3. Nervous System—anatomy & histology. 4. Nervous System Diseases. WL 102 S571e 2006]
RC343.6.S54 2006
612.8—dc22
                                                                        2005016237

05 06 07 08 09
1 2 3 4 5 6 7 8 9 10

This book is dedicated to our wives, Carla and Millie.

---

*"We have learned much from our teachers and from our colleagues
more than from our teachers, but from our students,
more than from them all."*

PREFACE

Over the past few decades, there has been a dramatic explosion of information in the field of neuroscience. This explosion of information has presented a great challenge to those of us who teach neuroscience in terms of synthesizing a coherent approach in which the diverse topics encompassed by neuroscience can be taught in a lucid and effective manner. We have attempted to meet this challenge by designing a book that considers all of the basic neuroscience topics to allow the students to focus on the essential concepts and facts intrinsic to any given topic without overwhelming them with distracting or confusing extraneous information. Consistent with this approach, each chapter begins with learning objectives followed by a discussion of the subject matter in a succinct yet informative manner. To present the material in an integrated fashion, sections on physiological and clinical considerations are included. At the end of each chapter, a clinical case is presented, which is followed by test questions that can also be used for USMLE preparation.

Recent developments in neuroscience have also been incorporated in the text. For example, in recent years, great strides have been made in the identification of neurotransmitter malfunction in several diseases. Therefore, a detailed chapter has been included on neurotransmitters and implications of their malfunctions in mental disorders. Similarly, genetic abnormalities involved in certain diseases (e.g., cystic fibrosis, schizophrenia, Huntington's chorea) have been briefly discussed. Malfunctions of the immune system in certain diseases (e.g., Lambert-Eaton syndrome, multiple sclerosis, myasthenia gravis) have also been discussed where applicable.

The genesis of this textbook evolved over the past 30 years, as a result of our efforts in teaching neuroscience to medical and graduate students in ways that would make learning the subject matter simple yet meaningful. After testing a variety of approaches, a building-blocks approach in the presentation of the subject matter evolved. Consistent with this approach, the book begins with analysis of the single neuron, which then expands to how neurons communicate with each other. Following discussion of the anatomy of the spinal cord and brain, the text continues with a detailed study of the sensory, motor, and integrative systems. This approach was deemed helpful by both students and faculty. Moreover, the building-blocks approach improved student performance on National Board and Neuroscience Shelf examinations.

The book consists of 28 chapters and a glossary. Chapters 1 through 4 (Overview of the Central Nervous System, Development of the Nervous System, Meninges and Cerebrospinal Fluid, and Blood Supply of the Central Nervous System) provide a background on and orientation in the structural organization of the brain and spinal cord. These chapters provide a basis for a more in-depth analysis of nervous system functions and clinical disorders.

Having provided the student with a basic understanding of the gross anatomy and general functions of the brain and spinal cord, the book then introduces a series of topics designed to provide an understanding of the basic elements of the nervous system and the role they play in neuronal communication. These topics are discussed in Chapters 5 through 8 (Histology of the Nervous System, Electrophysiology of Neu-rons, Synaptic Transmission, and Neurotransmit-ters). The basic physiological processes presented in these chapters prepare the student for further understanding of the varied functions of the nervous system in the subsequent sections. Chapters 9 through 13 (The Spinal Cord, Brainstem I: The Medulla, Brainstem II: Pons and Cerebellum, Brainstem III: The Midbrain, and The Forebrain) enable the student to examine the organization of the central nervous system in a systematic way. After learning about the key structures and functions at each level of the neuraxis of the central nervous system, the student will begin to develop an understanding of why damage to a given structure produces a particular constellation of deficits. Chapters 9 through 13 serve as a prerequisite for understanding the nature of cranial nerves (Chapter 14). Because of the importance of this chapter and the extent to which this material is tested on USMLE examinations, each cranial nerve is presented separately in terms of its structural and functional properties, as well as the deficits associated with its dysfunction.

At this point in the study of the nervous system, the student has now developed a basic knowledge of the anatomical organization of the central nervous system and its physiology and neurochemistry. Consequently, the student is now ready to study the sensory, motor, and integrative systems that require the knowledge accumulated thus far. The next section of the book includes Chapters 15 through 18 (Somatosensory System, Visual System, Auditory and Vestibular Systems, and Olfaction and Taste) and discusses anatomical and physiological properties of sensory systems.

The next section of the text turns to the study of motor systems, which includes the study of upper and lower motor neurons, basal ganglia, and the cerebellum (Chapters 19 to 21). These chapters examine, in an integrated manner, the anatomical, physiological, and neurochemical bases for normal movement and movement disorders associated with the cerebral cortex, basal ganglia, cerebellum, brainstem, and spinal cord.

The final section of the text (Chapters 22 to 28) concerns a variety of functions of the nervous system characterized by higher levels of complexity. These chapters include analyses of the functions of the autonomic nervous system, visceral processes, sleep, and wakefulness (Chapters 22 to 25). In addition, an analysis of the structure, functions, and dysfunctions of the cerebral cortex is provided in Chapter 26. Chapter 27 reviews vascular syndromes of the brainstem. This chapter was placed towards the end of the book because, at this time, the student would have a better understanding and appreciation of brainstem syndromes than if it had been presented earlier in the text. Vascular syndromes of the brainstem constitute an important review for the student on a topic that is heavily tested on USMLE examinations. The final chapter concerns behavioral disorders (Chapter 28) such as schizophrenia, depression, anxiety, and obsessive compulsion. These disorders have a clear relationship to abnormalities in neural and neurochemical functions and thus reflect an important component of neuroscience. These topics also receive attention on the USMLE.

The basic terms and concepts of neuroscience have been highlighted in bold script in each chapter and explained in an extensive glossary at the end of the book.

Although this text is primarily designed for medical students who study neuroscience, it can be used quite effectively by neurology residents, dental students, and graduate and undergraduate university students specializing in biological sciences.

Allan Siegel
Hreday N. Sapru

ACKNOWLEDGMENTS

The authors thank Dr. Leo Wolansky, Department of Radiology, New Jersey Medical School, for generously providing us with the MRIs and CT scans used in Chapter 27, and Dr. Lewis Baxter, University of Florida Medical School, Gainesville, for providing an MRI of a patient with obsessive-compulsive disorder shown in Chapter 28. The authors also thank Dr. Barbara Fadem, Department of Psychiatry, New Jersey Medical School, for her critique of Chapter 28. The authors appreciate the help, support, and guidance provided by Betty Sun, Elena Coler, and Dvora Konstant from Lippincott, Williams & Wilkins in the preparation of the book. We also thank Anne Rains for her excellent illustrations presented in the book.

CONTENTS

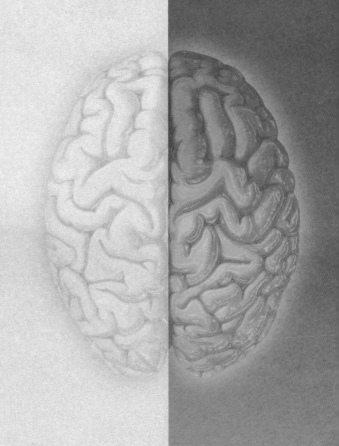

SECTION I

Gross Anatomy of the Brain

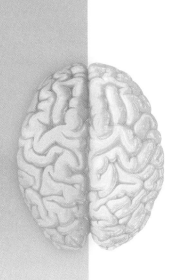

CHAPTER 1

OVERVIEW OF THE NERVOUS SYSTEM

OBJECTIVES

In this chapter, the student should:

1. Understand the basic language and terminology commonly used in neuroanatomy

2. Identify key regions and general functions within the cerebral cortex, including the precentral, prefrontal, postcentral, temporal, and occipital cortices

3. Identify the major functions of subcortical structures within the forebrain, including the ventricles of the brain, diencephalon, basal ganglia, and limbic system

4. Identify surface structures seen from ventral aspect of brainstem: the cerebral peduncles, pyramids, and inferior olivary nucleus; and from its dorsal surface: colliculi of midbrain and facial colliculus of pons

5. Identify cerebellum, including the attachments of cerebellum to the brainstem, and major lobes of the cerebellar cortex

GROSS ANATOMY OF THE BRAIN

Neuroscience is a composite of several disciplines including neuroanatomy, neurophysiology, neurology, neuropathology, neuropharmacology, behavioral sciences, and cell biology. An overview of the structural organization of the nervous system is helpful when beginning to study the neurosciences. However, first it would be useful to define some basic terms that will be essential for understanding the anatomy of the nervous system.

NEUROANATOMICAL TERMS

The spatial relationships of the brain and spinal cord usually are described by one or more of five paired terms: **medial–lateral**, **anterior–posterior**, **rostral–caudal**, **dorsal–ventral**, and **superior-inferior** (Fig. 1-1).

Medial–lateral: Medial means toward the median plane, and lateral means away from the median plane.

Anterior–posterior: Above the midbrain, anterior means toward the front of the brain, and posterior means toward the back of the brain. Below the midbrain, anterior means toward the ventral surface of the body, and posterior means toward the dorsal surface of the body.

Rostral–caudal: Above the midbrain, rostral means toward the front of the brain, and caudal means toward the back of the brain. Below the midbrain, rostral means toward the cerebral cortex, and caudal means toward the sacral end (or bottom) of the spinal cord.

Dorsal–ventral: Rostral to the midbrain, dorsal refers to the top of the brain, and ventral refers to the bottom of the brain. Caudal to the midbrain, dorsal means toward the posterior surface of the body, and ventral refers to the anterior surface of the body.

Superior–inferior: Both at positions above and below the midbrain, superior means toward the top of the cerebral cortex, and inferior means toward the bottom of the spinal cord.

Other terms commonly used in neuroanatomy are:

Ipsilateral–contralateral: Ipsilateral means on the same side with reference to a specific point; **contralateral** means on the opposite side.

Commissure and decussation: Commissure means a group of nerve fibers connecting one side of the brain with the other. Decussation means the crossing over of these nerve fibers.

Neuron: The anatomical and functional unit of the nervous system, which consists of a **nerve cell**

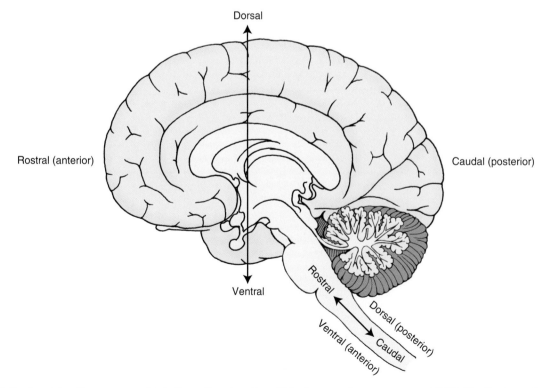

Figure 1–1 A variety of terms are used to indicate directionality within the central nervous system (CNS). The fixed axes for anatomical reference planes are superior–inferior and anterior–posterior. The other axes vary according to their location within the CNS.

body, **dendrites** (which receive signals from other neurons), and an **axon** (which transmits the signal to another neuron).

Nucleus: Refers to groups of neurons located in a specific region of the brain or spinal cord that generally have a similar appearance, receive information from similar sources, project their axons to similar targets, and share similar functions.

Tract: Many axons grouped together, which typically pass from a given nucleus to a common target region or to several regions.

White and gray matter: When examining the brain or spinal cord with the unaided eye, one can distinguish white or gray tissue. The region that appears white is called white matter, and the area that appears gray is called gray matter. The appearance of the white matter is due to the large number of **myelinated axons** (largely lipid membranes that wrap around the axons) that are present in this region. In contrast, the gray matter consists mainly of neuronal cell bodies (nuclei) and lacks myelinated axons.

Glial cells: These nonneural cells form the interstitial tissue of the nervous system. There are different types of glial cells, which include **astrocytes**, **oligodendroglia**, **microglia**, and **ependymal** and **choroid epithelial cells**. Details of the functions of each of these components are provided in Chapter 5.

Central and peripheral nervous systems: The **central nervous system (CNS)** includes the brain and spinal cord and is surrounded and protected by three connective tissue coverings called **meninges**. Within the CNS are fluid-filled spaces called ventricles. The bone of the skull and vertebral column surround the brain and spinal cord, respectively. The **peripheral nervous system (PNS)** consists of spinal and cranial nerves that are present outside the CNS.

Autonomic and somatic nervous systems: These are functional subdivisions of the nervous system (in contrast to the anatomical classifications described earlier). Both of these divisions are present in the CNS and PNS. The **autonomic nervous system** innervates smooth muscle and glands, whereas the **somatic nervous system** innervates mainly musculoskeletal structures and the sense organs of skin.

To understand the function of CNS structures, it is important to be able to identify and locate them in relation to one another. The many structures of the brain and spine may seem confusing in this initial overview, but knowing what they are is essential for developing a broader familiarity with neuroscience. It will not be necessary to memorize every structure and function in this introduction because the chapters that follow present these structures in greater detail.

We will begin with an examination of the major structures of the CNS, taking a topographical approach to the review of anatomical and functional relationships of structures in the cerebral cortex. Key structures will be identified as they appear in different views of the brain.

COMPONENTS OF THE CENTRAL NERVOUS SYSTEM

As we just indicated, the study of the CNS includes both the brain and spinal cord. This chapter provides an initial overview of these regions. A more detailed analysis of the structural and functional properties of the spinal cord is presented in Chapter 9 and is followed by a parallel morphological analysis of the structures contained within the **medulla, pons, midbrain,** and **forebrain** in subsequent chapters.

The **spinal cord** is a thin, cylinder-like structure with five regions that extend from its attachment to the brain downward. The most rostral region, which is closest to the brain, is the **cervical cord** and contains eight pairs of spinal nerves. Caudal to the cervical cord lies the **thoracic cord**, which contains 12 pairs of spinal nerves. Next is the **lumbar cord**, which contains five pairs of spinal nerves. The most caudal region, called the **sacral cord**, contains five pairs of spinal nerves; the caudal end of the spinal cord is called the **coccygeal region** and contains one pair of spinal nerves. In the cervical and lumbar regions, the spinal cord is enlarged because of the presence of greater numbers of nerve cell bodies and fiber tracts, which innervate the upper and lower limbs, respectively.

The brainstem, cerebellum, and cerebral hemispheres form the brain. The **brainstem** can be divided into three regions: the medulla, rostral to and continuous with the spinal cord; the pons, rostral to the medulla; and the midbrain, rostral to the pons and continuous with the diencephalon. The **cerebellum** is positioned like a tent dorsal to the pons and is attached to the brainstem by three massive fiber groups, or **peduncles**. The **cerebral hemispheres** contain the cerebral cortex, which covers the surface of the brain and is several millimeters thick, as well as deeper structures, including the **corpus callosum, diencephalon, basal ganglia, limbic structures,** and **internal capsule**.

CEREBRAL TOPOGRAPHY

One important aspect of the anatomical and functional organization of the CNS should be remembered throughout the study of neuroscience: for most **sensory** and **motor** functions, the left side of the brain functionally corresponds with the right side of the body. Thus, sensation from the left side of the body is consciously appreciated on the right side of the cerebral cortex. Similarly, motor control over the right arm and leg is controlled by neurons located on the left cerebral cortex.

LATERAL SURFACE OF THE BRAIN

Four lobes of the cerebral cortex—the **frontal**, **parietal**, and **temporal lobes** and a portion of the **occipital lobe**—can be identified on the lateral surface of the brain (Fig. 1-2). The lobes of the cerebral cortex integrate motor, sensory, autonomic, and intellectual processes and are organized along functional lines. For the most part, a fissure, called a **sulcus**, separates these lobes. In addition, pairs of **sulci** form the boundaries of ridges referred to as **gyri**.

The cortex consists of both cells and nerve fibers. The cellular components constitute the gray matter of cortex and lie superficial (i.e., toward the surface of the cortex) to the nerve fibers. As a general rule, the nerve fibers that comprise the white matter of the cortex pass between different regions of cortex, facilitating communication between the lobes of the cerebral cortex. In addition, large components of the white matter consist of fibers passing to and from the cortex to other regions of the CNS.

Frontal Lobe

The first step in identifying the main structures of the lateral surface of the brain is to locate the **central sulcus**, which serves as the posterior boundary

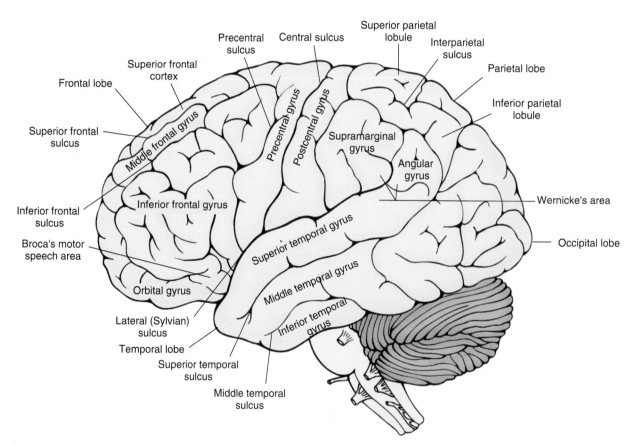

Figure 1–2 Lateral view of the cerebral cortex showing the principal gyri and sulci. Major structures include the central sulcus and the precentral (primary motor), premotor, and postcentral (primary somatosensory) gyri. Also note the gyri situated rostral to the premotor cortex, including the orbital gyri, which mediate higher order intellectual functions and contribute to the regulation of emotional behavior. Broca's motor speech area and Wernicke's area (for reception of speech) are important areas associated with speech. Of the three gyri comprising the temporal lobe, the superior temporal gyrus is important for auditory functions, and the inferior and middle temporal gyri mediate complex visual functions. Different aspects of the parietal lobe located just caudal to the primary somatosensory cortex integrate a variety of higher order sensory functions; the occipital lobe contains the primary receiving area for visual impulses.

of the frontal lobe (Fig. 1-2). This sulcus extends from near the longitudinal fissure (present along the midline but is not visible in the lateral view of the brain shown in Fig. 1-2) ventrally almost to the lateral cerebral sulcus (**Sylvian sulcus**). The frontal lobe, the largest of the cerebral lobes, extends from the central sulcus to the frontal pole of the brain. It extends inferiorly to the lateral sulcus. The frontal cortex also extends onto the medial surface of the brain, where it borders the **corpus callosum** inferiorly (see Fig. 1-3).

At the posterior aspect of the frontal lobe, the most prominent structure is the **precentral gyrus**, which is bounded posteriorly and anteriorly by the **central** and **precentral sulci**, respectively (Fig. 1-2). The function of the precentral gyrus is to integrate motor function signals from different regions of the brain. It serves as the primary motor cortex for control of contralateral voluntary movements. The neurons within the precentral gyrus are somatotopically organized. **Somatotopic** means that different parts of the precentral gyrus are associated with distinct parts of the body, both functionally and anatomically. The outputs from the precentral gyrus to the brainstem and contralateral spinal cord follow a similar functional arrangement. The region closest to the lateral (Sylvian) sulcus (the inferior part of the precentral gyrus) is associated with voluntary control over movements of the face and head. The neurons associated with motor control of the upper and lower limbs are found at progressively more dorsal and medial levels, respectively. The motor neurons associated with control over the lower limbs extend onto the medial surface of the hemisphere. When the parts of the body are drawn in terms of the degree of their cortical representation (i.e., in the form of a somatotopic arrangement), the resulting rather disproportionate figure that is depicted is frequently called a **homunculus** (see Chapters 19 and 26 for further discussion). The motor homunculus demonstrates how cell groups in the CNS associated with one part of the body relate anatomically to other cell groups associated with other parts of the body. In addition, the illustrative device shows the relative sizes of the populations of neurons associated with specific parts of the body.

Immediately rostral to the precentral gyrus is the **premotor cortex**, which extends from near the lateral fissure on to the medial surface of the brain; this region is referred to as the **supplementary motor area**. This cortex exercises control over movements associated with the contralateral side of the body by playing an important role in the initiation and sequencing of movements. Immediately anterior to the premotor cortex, three parallel gyri—the superior, middle, and inferior **frontal gyri**—are oriented in anterior–posterior positions (Fig. 1-2). Portions of these gyri are also involved in the integration of motor processes. For example, one part of the inferior frontal gyrus of the dominant (left) hemisphere is **Broca's "motor speech area"** and is important for the formulation of the motor components of speech. When damaged, the result is Broca's **aphasia** (or motor aphasia), a form of language impairment in which the patient has difficulty in naming objects and repeating words, while comprehension remains intact. Far rostral to this region, an area that includes inferior (orbital gyri), medial, and lateral aspects of the frontal lobe, called the **prefrontal cortex**, also plays important roles in the processing of intellectual and emotional events. Within the depths of the lateral (Sylvian) sulcus is a region of cortex called the **insula**, which can be seen only when the temporal lobe is pulled away from the rest of the cortex. It reflects a convergence of the temporal, parietal, and frontal cortices and has, at different times, been associated with the reception and integration of taste sensation, reception of viscerosensations, processing of pain sensations, and vestibular functions.

Parietal Lobe

The parietal lobe houses the functions that perceive and process **somatosensory** events. It extends posteriorly from the central sulcus to its border with the occipital lobe (Fig. 1-2). The parietal lobe contains the **postcentral gyri,** which has the **central sulcus** as its anterior border and the **postcentral sulcus** as its posterior border. The postcentral gyrus is the primary receiving area for **somesthetic** (i.e., kinesthetic and tactile) information from the periphery (trunk and extremities). Here, one side of the cerebral cortex receives information from the opposite side of the body. Like the motor cortex, the postcentral gyrus is somatotopically organized and can be depicted as having a sensory homunculus, which parallels that of the motor cortex.

The remainder of the parietal lobe can be divided roughly into two regions, a superior and an inferior parietal lobule, separated by an **interparietal sulcus**. The inferior parietal lobule consists of two gyri: the supramarginal and angular gyri. The **supramarginal gyrus** is just superior to the posterior extent of the lateral sulcus, and the **angular gyrus** is immediately posterior to the supramarginal gyrus and is often associated with the posterior extent of the superior temporal sulcus (Fig. 1-2). These regions receive input from auditory and visual cortices and are believed to perform complex perceptual discriminations and integrations. At the ventral aspect of these gyri and extending onto the adjoining part of the superior temporal gyrus is **Wernicke's area**. This region is essential for comprehension of spoken language. Lesions of this region produce another form of aphasia, Wernicke's aphasia (or sensory aphasia), which is characterized by impairment of comprehension and repetition, although speech remains fluent.

Occipital Lobe

Although a part of the **occipital lobe** lies on the lateral surface of the cortex, the larger component occupies a more prominent position on the medial surface of the hemisphere.

Temporal Lobe

The most important function of the temporal lobe is in the perception of auditory signals. Situated inferior to the lateral sulcus, the temporal lobe consists of superior, middle, and inferior temporal gyri. On the inner aspect of the superior surface of the **superior temporal gyrus** lie the transverse **gyri of Heschl** (not shown in Fig. 1-2), which constitute the primary auditory receiving area. The other regions of the temporal lobe are associated with visual discrimination and integration (see Chapter 26 for details).

MEDIAL SURFACE OF THE BRAIN

The principal structures on the medial aspect of the brain can be seen clearly after the hemispheres are divided in the **midsagittal** plane (Fig. 1-3). On the medial aspect of the cerebral cortex, the **occipital lobe** can be seen most clearly. It contains the primary visual receiving area, the visual cortex. The primary visual cortex is located inferior and superior to the **calcarine sulcus (calcarine fissure)**, a prominent sulcus formed on the medial surface that runs perpendicular into the **parieto-occipital sulcus**, which divides the occipital lobe from the parietal lobe (Fig. 1-3).

Moving more rostrally from the occipital lobe and situated immediately inferior to the precentral, postcentral, and premotor cortices is the **cingulate gyrus**. Its ventral border is the corpus callosum. The cingulate gyrus is generally considered part of the brain's limbic system, which is associated with emotional behavior, regulation of visceral processes, and learning (see Chapter 25).

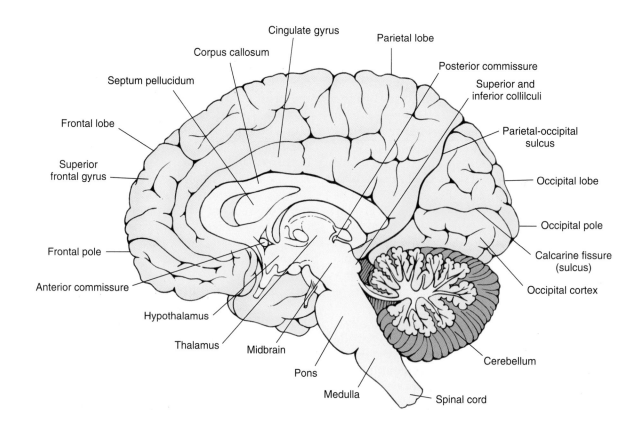

Figure 1–3 Midsagittal view of the brain. Visible are the structures situated on the medial aspect of the cortex, as well as subcortical areas, which include the corpus callosum, septum pellucidum, fornix, diencephalon, and brainstem structures.

Another prominent medial structure is the **corpus callosum**, a massive fiber pathway that permits communication between equivalent regions of the two hemispheres. The **septum pellucidum** lies immediately ventral to the corpus callosum and is most prominent anteriorly. It consists of two thin-walled membranes separated by a narrow cleft, forming a small cavity (cavum of septum pellucidum). It forms the medial walls of the lateral ventricles. The septum pellucidum is attached at its ventral border to the **fornix**.

The **fornix** is the major fiber system arising from the **hippocampal formation**, which lies buried deep within the medial aspect of the temporal lobe. It emerges from the hippocampal formation posteriorly and passes dorsomedially around the thalamus to occupy a medial position inferior to the corpus callosum but immediately superior to the thalamus. A basic function of the fornix is to transmit information from the hippocampal formation to the **septal area** and **hypothalamus**.

The **diencephalon** lies below the fornix and has two parts (Fig. 1-3). The **thalamus** is larger and responsible for relaying and integrating information to different regions of the cerebral cortex from a variety of structures associated with sensory, motor, autonomic, and emotional processes. The **hypothalamus**, the smaller structure, lies ventral and slightly anterior to the thalamus. Its roles include the regulation of a host of visceral functions, such as temperature, endocrine functions, and feeding, drinking, emotional, and sexual behaviors. The ventral aspect of the hypothalamus forms the base of the brain to which the pituitary gland is attached.

INFERIOR (VENTRAL) SURFACE OF THE CEREBRAL CORTEX

As part of our task in understanding the anatomical organization of the brain, it is useful to examine its arrangement from the inferior view.

The medial aspect of the anterior part of the prefrontal cortex contains a region called the **gyrus rectus** (Fig. 1-4). Lateral to the gyrus rectus lies a structure called the **olfactory bulb**, a brain structure that appears as a primitive form of cortex consisting of neuronal cell bodies, axons, and synaptic connections. The olfactory bulb receives information from the first (olfactory) cranial nerve and gives rise to a pathway called the **olfactory tract**. These fibers then divide into the medial and lateral olfactory branches (called **striae**). The lateral pathway conveys olfactory information to the temporal lobe and underlying limbic structures, whereas the medial olfactory stria projects to medial limbic structures and contralateral olfactory structures (via a fiber bundle called the **anterior commissure**; see Chapter 18).

POSTERIOR ASPECT OF THE CEREBRAL CORTEX: TEMPORAL AND OCCIPITAL LOBES

The **occipitotemporal gyrus** lies medial to the **inferior temporal gyrus** and is bound medially by the collateral sulcus. The **parahippocampal gyrus** lies medial to the **collateral sulcus**. There is a medial extension of the anterior end of the parahippocampal gyrus called the **uncus**. The **hippocampal formation** and **amygdala** (described below) are situated deep to the cortex of the parahippocampal gyrus and uncus (Figs. 1-4, 1-5, and 1-6). These structures have a very low threshold for induction of seizure activity and are frequently the focus of seizures in temporal lobe epilepsy.

FOREBRAIN STRUCTURES VISIBLE IN HORIZONTAL AND FRONTAL SECTIONS OF THE BRAIN

VENTRICLES

As shown in horizontal and frontal sections of the brain (Fig. 1-5), cavities present within each hemisphere are called **ventricles** and contain **cerebrospinal fluid** (CSF; see Chapter 3). In brief, CSF is secreted primarily from specialized **epithelial cells** found mainly on the roofs of the ventricles called the **choroid plexus**. CSF serves the CNS as a source of electrolytes, as a protective and supportive medium, and as a conduit for neuroactive and metabolic products. It also helps remove neuronal metabolic products from the brain.

The **lateral ventricle** is the cavity found throughout much of each cerebral hemisphere (Fig. 1-5). It consists of several continuous parts: an anterior horn, which is present at rostral levels deep in the frontal lobe; a posterior horn, which extends into the occipital lobe; an interconnecting body, which extends from the level of the **interventricular foramen** to the posterior horn; and, at the junction of the body and posterior horn, the inferior horn, which extends in ventral and anterior directions deep into the temporal lobe, ending near the amygdala (also referred to as amygdaloid complex) (Figs. 1-5 and 1-6).

Within the diencephalon, another cavity, called the **third ventricle**, can be identified. It lies along the midline of the diencephalon, and the walls are formed by the thalamus (dorsally) and the hypothalamus (ventrally). The third ventricle extends

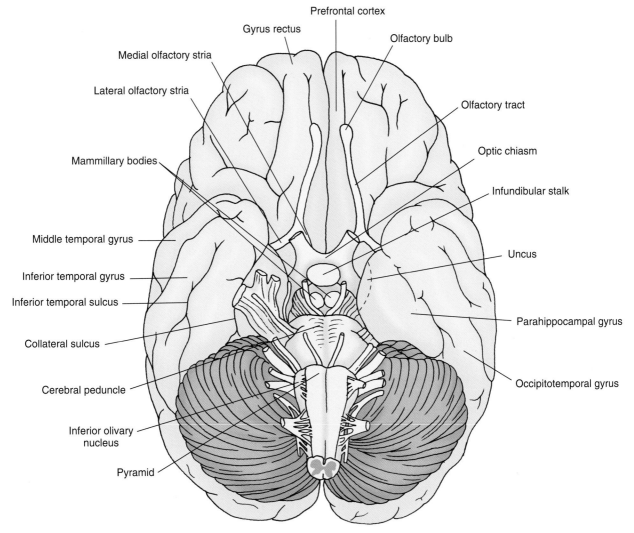

Figure 1–4 Inferior surface of the brain showing the principal gyri and sulci of the cerebral cortex. On the inferior surface, the midbrain, pons, parts of the cerebellum, and medulla can be clearly identified.

throughout the diencephalon and communicates anteriorly with the left and right lateral ventricles through the interventricular foramen. Posteriorly, at the level of the diencephalic–midbrain border, it is continuous with the **cerebral aqueduct**, which allows CSF to flow from the third ventricle to the **fourth ventricle** (Fig. 1-5), where it will exit the ventricular system through the lateral and median apertures into the subarachnoid space.

BASAL GANGLIA

The **basal ganglia** play an important role in motor integration processes. The most prominent structures of the basal ganglia are the **caudate nucleus**, **putamen**, and **globus pallidus** (Figs. 1-6 and 1-7). Two additional structures, the **subthalamic nucleus** and **substantia nigra**, are also included as part of the basal ganglia because of their anatomi-

cal and functional relationships with its other constituent parts (see Chapter 20).

The **caudate nucleus** is a large mass of cells that is most prominent at anterior levels of the forebrain adjacent to the anterior horn of the lateral ventricle and can be divided into three components (Fig. 1-8). The largest component, the head of the caudate, is found at anterior levels of the forebrain rostral to the diencephalon. As the nucleus extends caudally, it maintains its position adjacent to the body and inferior horn of the lateral ventricle but becomes progressively narrower at levels farther away from the head of the caudate. This narrow region of the caudate nucleus, distal to the head, is called the tail of the caudate nucleus. The region between the head and tail is referred to as the body of the caudate nucleus. The body and tail of the caudate nucleus are situated adjacent to the dorsolateral surface of the thalamus.

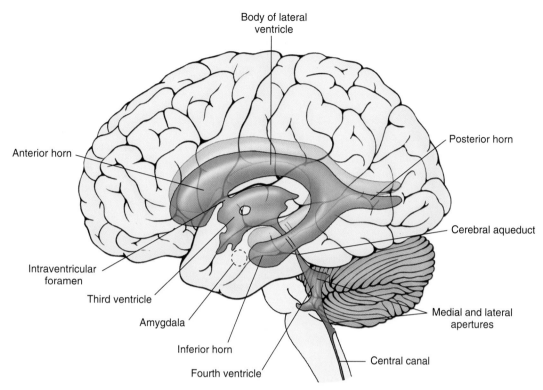

Body of lateral
ventricle

Anterior horn

Posterior horn

Cerebral aqueduct

Intraventricular
foramen

Third ventricle

Amygdala

Medial and lateral
apertures

Inferior horn

Central canal

Fourth ventricle

Figure 1–5 Lateral view of the positions and relationships of the ventricles of the brain. Note that the lateral ventricles are quite extensive, with different components (i.e., posterior, inferior, and anterior horns). The medial and lateral apertures represent the channels by which CSF can exit the brain (see Chapter 3 for details).

Figure 1–6 Horizontal section depicting internal forebrain structures after parts of the cerebral cortex have been dissected away. Visible are the caudate nucleus, thalamus, fornix, hippocampus, and amygdala. Note the shape and orientation of the hippocampal formation and its relationship to the amygdala, as well as the positions occupied by the globus pallidus and putamen, which lie lateral to the internal capsule, and the thalamus, which lies medial to the internal capsule.

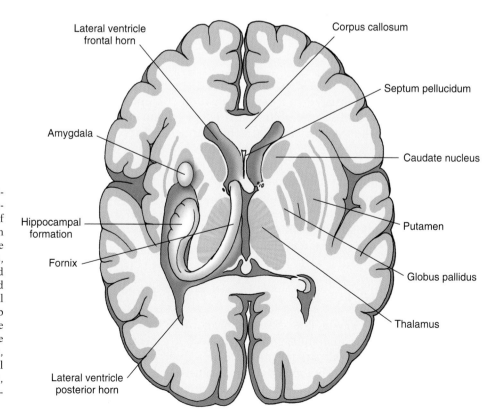

Lateral ventricle
frontal horn

Corpus callosum

Septum pellucidum

Amygdala

Caudate nucleus

Hippocampal
formation

Putamen

Fornix

Globus pallidus

Thalamus

Lateral ventricle
posterior horn

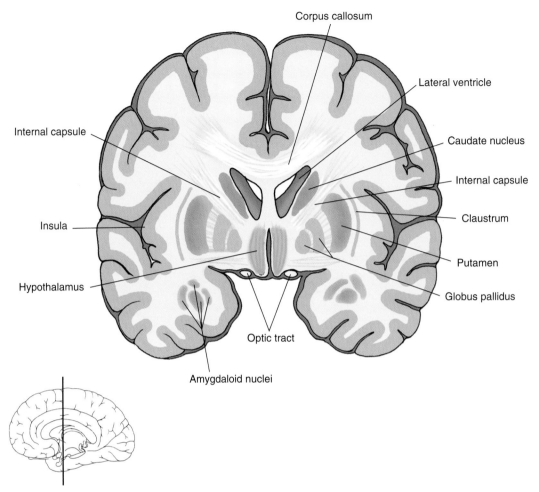

Figure 1–7 Frontal section taken through the level of the diencephalon. Note again the relationships of the caudate nucleus and diencephalon relative to those of the globus pallidus and putamen with respect to the position of the internal capsule. The level along the rostro-caudal axis of the brain at which the section was taken is shown in the sketch of the brain at the bottom of the figure.

The **putamen** is the largest component of the basal ganglia and is situated in a lateral position within the anterior half of the forebrain. It is bordered laterally by the external capsule, a thin band of white matter, and medially by the globus pallidus (Figs. 1-6 and 1-7).

The **globus pallidus** has both a lateral and medial segment. It lies immediately medial to the putamen and just lateral to the internal capsule, which is a massive fiber bundle that transmits information to and from the cerebral cortex to the forebrain, brainstem, and spinal cord (Figs. 1-6, 1-7, and 1-8).

DIENCEPHALON

As mentioned previously, the diencephalon includes principally the thalamus, situated dorsally, and the hypothalamus, situated ventrally. The medial border of the diencephalon is the third ventricle, and the lateral border is the internal capsule. The ventral border is the base of the brain, and the dorsal border is the roof of the thalamus. The diencephalon is generally considered to be bounded anteriorly by the **anterior commissure** (Fig. 1-3), which is a conspicuous fiber bundle containing many olfactory and temporal lobe fibers, and the **lamina terminalis** (not shown in Fig. 1-3), which is the rostral end of the third ventricle. The posterior limit of the diencephalon is the **posterior commissure**, a fiber bundle that crosses the midline between the diencephalon and midbrain.

LIMBIC STRUCTURES

Limbic structures serve important functions in the regulation of emotional behavior, short-term memory processes, and control of autonomic, other visceral, and hormonal functions usually associated with the hypothalamus. Several structures in the limbic system can be identified clearly in forebrain sections. Two of these structures, the **amygdala** and **hippocampus**, are situated within the tempo-

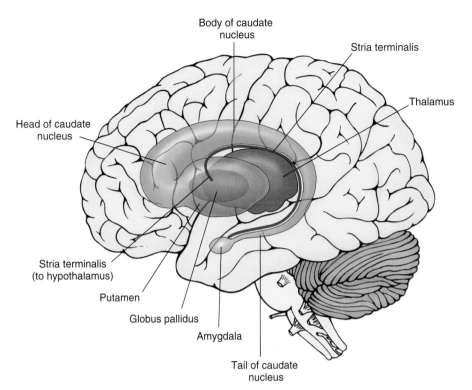

Body of caudate
nucleus

Stria terminalis

Thalamus

Head of caudate
nucleus

Stria terminalis
(to hypothalamus)

Putamen

Globus pallidus

Amygdala

Tail of caudate
nucleus

Figure 1–8 Schematic diagram illustrating the components of the caudate nucleus and their relationship to the thalamus, internal capsule, globus pallidus, putamen, and brainstem. Because of its anatomical proximity to the caudate nucleus, the stria terminalis, which represents a major efferent pathway of the amygdala to the hypothalamus, is included as well.

ral lobe (Fig. 1-6). The amygdala lies just anterior to the hippocampus. Both structures give rise to prominent fiber bundles that initially pass in a posterodorsal direction following the body of the lateral ventricle around the posterior aspect of the thalamus and then run anteriorly, following the inferior horn of the lateral ventricle.

The fiber bundle associated with the hippocampal formation is the fornix, which is situated just inferior to the corpus callosum (Fig. 1-3). The fiber system associated with the amygdala is the **stria terminalis** and is just ventromedial to the tail of the caudate nucleus (Fig. 1-8). The trajectory of the stria terminalis is parallel to that of the tail of the caudate nucleus. Both fiber bundles ultimately terminate within different regions of the hypothalamus (see Chapters 13, 24, and 25). Other components of the limbic system include the cingulate gyrus, the prefrontal cortex, and the septal area.

TOPOGRAPHY OF THE CEREBELLUM AND BRAINSTEM

CEREBELLUM

The cerebellum plays a vital role in the regulation and coordination of motor processes. It is attached to the brainstem by the cerebellar peduncles, three pairs of massive fiber bundles. One pair, the superior cerebellar peduncle, is attached rostrally to the

upper pons. Another pair, the inferior cerebellar peduncle, is attached to the dorsolateral surface of the upper medulla. The third pair, the middle cerebellar peduncle, is attached to the lateral aspect of the pons (Fig. 1-9A).

The cerebellum (see Chapter 21) contains bilaterally symmetrical hemispheres that are continuous with a midline structure, the **vermis**. The hemispheres are divided into three sections. The **anterior lobe** is located towards the midbrain. Extending posterior-inferiorly from the anterior lobe is the **posterior lobe**, the largest lobe of the cerebellum. The **flocculonodular lobe**, the smallest of the three lobes, is situated most inferiorly and is somewhat concealed by the posterior lobe. It is important to note that each of these lobes receives different kinds of inputs from the periphery and specific regions of the CNS. For example, the flocculonodular lobe primarily receives vestibular inputs, the anterior lobe receives inputs mainly from the spinal cord, and the posterior lobe is a major recipient of cortical inputs.

BRAINSTEM

Dorsal View of the Brainstem

Two pairs of protuberances at the level of the midbrain can be seen on the dorsal surface of the brainstem (Fig. 1-9B). The superior colliculus is more rostrally positioned and is associated with

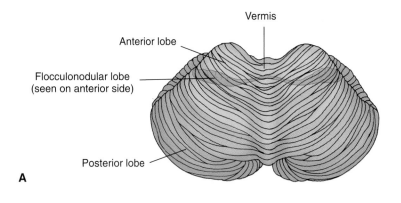

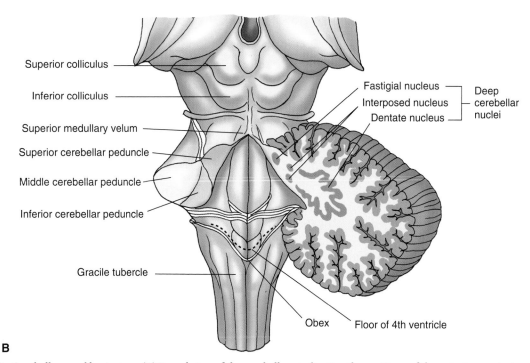

Figure 1–9 Cerebellum and brainstem. (A) Dorsal view of the cerebellum indicating the positions of the anterior, posterior, and flocculonodular lobes and the midline region called the vermis. (B) Dorsal view of the brainstem after removal of the cerebellum. The connections of the cerebellum to the brainstem are indicated by the presence of the inferior, middle, and superior cerebellar peduncles.

visual functions; the more caudally positioned inferior colliculus is associated with auditory processing. The dorsal surface of the pons and medulla form the floor of the fourth ventricle (Fig. 1-9B). The walls of the ventricle are formed by the **superior cerebellar peduncle**, and the roof of the fourth ventricle is formed by the **superior medullary velum**, which is attached to the superior cerebellar peduncle on each side.

In the caudal half of the medulla is the end of the fourth ventricle, the position at which the ventricle becomes progressively narrower and

ultimately continuous with the central canal that continues into and throughout the spinal cord. The position at which the fourth ventricle empties into the central canal is the **obex**. The part of the medulla that contains the fourth ventricle is the open medulla, and the part that contains the central canal is the closed medulla. On the dorsal surface of the caudal medulla are two protuberances, the **gracile** and **cuneate** tubercles. These contain relay and integrating neurons associated with ascending sensory fibers from the periphery to the medulla.

Ventral View of the Brainstem

Crus Cerebri

A massive fiber bundle passes from the cerebral hemispheres into lower regions of the brainstem and spinal cord at the level of the midbrain (Fig. 1-10). This fiber bundle is the **crus cerebri**, part of the descending complex of motor pathways that communicates signals from the cerebral cortex to the brainstem and spinal cord.

Pons and Medulla

The pons has two parts: a dorsal half, the **tegmentum**, and a ventral half, the **basilar region**. The basilar region forms the anterior bulge of the pons seen on a ventral view of the gross brain (Fig. 1-10). The tegmentum can only be seen on horizontal or cross sections of the brainstem (see Chapter 11). Several protuberances separated by a narrow fissure can be detected at the level of the medulla. Starting from the medial aspect, one protuberance, which passes in a rostral-caudal direction along the base of the brain, is called the **pyramid**. The axons contained within the pyramid originate in the cerebral cortex and thus represent a continuation of many of the same fiber bundles that contribute to the internal capsule and parts of the cerebral peduncle at the levels of the cerebral hemispheres and midbrain, respectively. In this manner, the pyramid serves as the conduit by which cortical signals pass to all levels of the spinal cord for the regulation of motor functions.

The pyramid can be followed caudally from the pons through most of the medulla. At the caudal end of the medulla, near its juncture with the spinal cord, the pyramid can no longer be easily seen from a ventral view. This is because most of the fibers contained within the pyramid pass in a dorsolateral course from the lower medulla to the contralateral side through a commissure, the pyramidal decussation. This pathway, referred to as the lateral **corticospinal tract**, descends to all levels of spinal cord (see Chapters 10 and 19). The **pyramidal (motor) decussation** is more clearly visible from a cross-sectional view of the caudal medulla. A small sulcus separates the pyramid from a more lateral protuberance, the olive. The olive is formed by the **inferior olivary nucleus**, a large nuclear mass present in the rostral half of the medulla (Fig. 1-10). The olive represents an important relay nucleus of the spinal cord and regions of the brainstem to the cerebellum.

Another important feature of the ventral surface of the brainstem is the roots of the cranial nerves; they will be discussed in detail in Chapter 14. These cranial nerves include the oculomotor (CN III) and trochlear (CN IV) nerves at the level of the midbrain, trigeminal (CN V), abducens (CN VI), and facial (CN VII) nerves at the level of the pons, and nerves IX through XII at the level of the medulla (not labeled in Fig. 1-10).

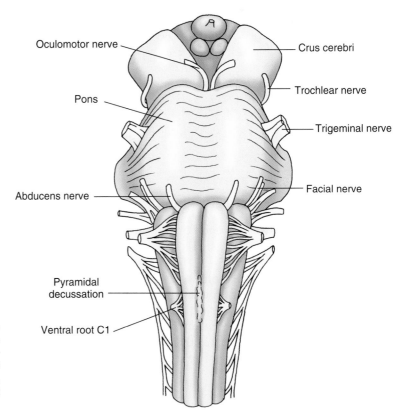

Figure 1–10 Ventral view of the brainstem. Note the positions of the cerebral peduncle, basilar part of the pons, pyramid, pyramidal decussation (situated immediately rostral to the cervical spinal cord), inferior olivary nucleus, which lies lateral to the pyramid, and root fibers of cranial nerves.

CLINICAL CASE

The following clinical case is intended to illustrate some of the basic neuroanatomical concepts presented in this chapter. You are not expected to diagnose the patient's condition or suggest any therapy or medical steps to be taken. Rather, we hope that this case and those that follow will demonstrate the very real clinical relevance of basic neuroscience information.

HISTORY

Saul is a 75-year-old man who recently learned from his internist that he had an irregular heartbeat. He was prescribed medication to regulate his heart rate and asked to return in a few days, but he was too frightened to fill the prescription or return for the appointment. One morning, 3 weeks after seeing his physician, he awoke and, upon attempting to get out of bed, was unable to move his left arm and leg. Using his right hand, he dialed 911. When the operator answered, he attempted to explain his problem, but his speech was so slurred that the operator could not understand him. The operator told him to remain on the line so that the call could be traced. An ambulance arrived shortly afterward, and Saul was taken to the nearest emergency room.

EXAMINATION

The emergency room staff noted Saul's irregular heartbeat. A neurologist arrived and confirmed that, although Saul's speech was quite slurred, much like that of an inebriated person, his sentences were grammatically correct and everything he attempted to say made logical sense. His blood alcohol level was zero. He could follow three-step commands and repeat statements, despite his slurred speech. When he tried to smile, his mouth drooped on the left side. But when he wrinkled his eyebrows, his forehead remained symmetric. His left arm was completely paralyzed, but he was able to wiggle his left leg minimally. Saul was admitted to the intensive care unit for treatment.

EXPLANATION

Saul's abnormal heartbeat is called **atrial fibrillation**, a rhythm characterized by irregularity and usually rapidity. It can cause strokes by dislodging small clots from the heart and causing them to travel as emboli to the cerebral blood vessels, causing occlusion.

Saul's condition is an example of a right frontal lobe cortical stroke involving the precentral gyrus or the primary motor cortex. The motor problems, including the slurred speech and arm and leg weakness, occurred because of involvement of these areas. This region is functionally organized as a homunculus, with representation of each region of the body in specific locations. The effects can be attributed mainly to occlusion of the middle cerebral artery (a branch of the internal carotid artery and a common location for emboli) because this artery subserves most of the affected region. However, the superior portion of this region is partially within the territory of the anterior cerebral artery. Clinically, this is demonstrated by the fact that the patient's leg is somewhat involved but not as extensively as his arm. Although there is weakness of the lower two thirds of the face, the forehead is not involved because of bilateral cortical innervation of this region. Because the majority of people are right-handed with left-sided cerebral dominance (the side where language originates), Saul's language disturbance is solely motor, and he is able to follow commands and construct sentences. Saul was transferred from the emergency room to another section of the hospital. After remaining in the hospital for approximately 4 weeks, he was sent to a nearby rehabilitation facility where he was able to regain most of his basic motor functions, including speech.

CHAPTER TEST

QUESTIONS

Choose the best answer for each question.

Questions 1 and 2

A 79-year-old woman is admitted to the emergency room after she was found unconscious in her apartment. After she regained consciousness, a neurologic examination indicated that she suffered a stroke with paralysis of the right arm and leg as well as loss of speech.

1. The most likely region affected by the stroke that could account for limb paralysis is:
   a. Prefrontal cortex
   b. Precentral gyrus
   c. Postcentral gyrus
   d. Superior temporal gyrus
   e. Parietal lobe

2. The loss of speech in this patient was due mainly to damage of:
   a. Superior frontal cortex
   b. Inferior temporal gyrus
   c. Inferior frontal gyrus

d. Occipital cortex

e. Medial aspect of parietal cortex

3. During routine surgery for appendicitis, a clot is released from the lung of a 75-year-old man, causing the patient to remain unconscious for a period of a week. Upon regaining consciousness, the patient finds that he is unable to maintain his balance and further displays tremors while attempting to produce a purposeful movement. In addition, the patient's movements are not smooth but jerky and lack coordination. The region affected most likely included the:

a. Spinal cord

b. Medulla

c. Pons

d. Midbrain

e. Cerebellum

4. A magnetic resonance image (MRI) scan taken of a 60-year-old woman revealed the presence of a tumor on the base of the brain that was situated just anterior to the pituitary and that impinged upon the adjoining neural tissue. A likely deficit resulting from this tumor includes:

a. Loss of movement of upper limbs

b. Speech impairment

c. Difficulties in breathing

d. Changes in emotionality

e. Loss of ability to experience pain

5. A 45-year-old man complained about having recurring headaches over a period of weeks. Subsequent tests revealed the presence of a tumor along the lateral wall of the anterior horn of the lateral ventricle, which did not produce hydrocephalus. One region that would be directly affected by the tumor is the:

a. Caudate nucleus

b. Putamen

c. Globus pallidus

d. Hippocampus

e. Cingulate gyrus

ANSWERS AND EXPLANATIONS

1. Answer: b

The primary motor cortex is located in the precentral gyrus, which is organized somatotopically. The functions of the upper and lower limbs are represented in different regions along the precentral gyrus. The postcentral gyrus represents a primary somesthetic receiving area for pain, temperature, pressure, kinesthetic, and tactile impulses from the periphery. Although the superior frontal gyrus contains certain groups of neurons (the supplementary and premotor motor areas) that also contribute to motor functions, it is not a primary motor area. The superior parietal lobule is associated with sensory discrimination processes and with the programming of signals to the premotor cortex. The posterior parietal cortex represents a region of sensorimotor integration and the organization of complex response patterns.

2. Answer: c

The posterior aspect of the inferior frontal gyrus contains a region called "Broca's motor speech" area. Lesions affecting this region produce motor aphasia, which is characterized by a loss of ability to express thoughts in a meaningful manner. The superior aspect of the frontal cortex is associated with movements of the lower limbs; the inferior temporal gyrus is associated with perceptual functions; the occipital cortex is associated with vision, and the medial aspect of the parietal lobe is associated with somatosensory functions involving the leg.

3. Answer: e

Although the spinal cord, medulla, pons, and midbrain play important roles in motor functions, the primary functions of the cerebellum include regulation of motor functions. Damage to parts of this structure causes a loss of balance, loss of coordination of movements, and tremors. Unlike the cerebellum, none of the other regions has a direct role in the regulation of these processes.

4. Answer: d

The optic nerve enters the brain at the level of the far anterior hypothalamus. Tumors of this region of the base of the brain frequently affect the hypothalamus, which plays an important role in the regulation of emotional behavior and autonomic functions. Such tumors would also likely affect visual functions. Movements of the limbs are affected by lesions of the internal capsule or precentral gyrus; speech impairment is affected by damage to the inferior frontal or superior temporal gyrus; breathing is affected by the lower brainstem; and pain is affected by parts of the brainstem, thalamus, and postcentral gyrus.

5. Answer: a

The head of the caudate nucleus is located adjacent to the lateral aspect of the anterior horn of the lateral ventricle. Therefore, a tumor in this region would include the head of the caudate nucleus. The putamen and globus pallidus lie lateral to the caudate nucleus at a position away from the lateral ventricle; the hippocampus lies adjacent to the inferior horn of the lateral ventricle, and the cingulate gyrus lies above the corpus callosum in a position not in proximity to the lateral ventricle.

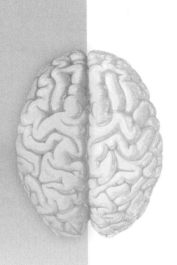

CHAPTER 2

DEVELOPMENT OF THE NERVOUS SYSTEM

OBJECTIVES

In this chapter, the student is expected to know:

1. The early aspects of brain development, including the formation of the primary brain vesicles

2. How the spinal cord and brainstem are formed

3. Where sensory, motor, and autonomic structures of the spinal cord and brainstem are situated relative to one another

4. The gross organization of the cerebellum and how it is formed

5. How forebrain structures, such as the diencephalon, basal ganglia, and limbic system, are formed

6. How the ventricular system of the brain is formed and organized

7. How congenital malformations associated with abnormal development may occur

EARLY ASPECTS OF DEVELOPMENT

The nervous system develops from **ectoderm**, the surface layer of embryonic tissue. By the third to fourth week of embryonic development, the **notochord**, of mesodermal origin, induces the development of the **neural plate (Fig. 2-1A)**. By the third to fourth week of embryonic development, there is a high rate of cell proliferation. As such, the anterior part of the **notochord** (of mesodermal

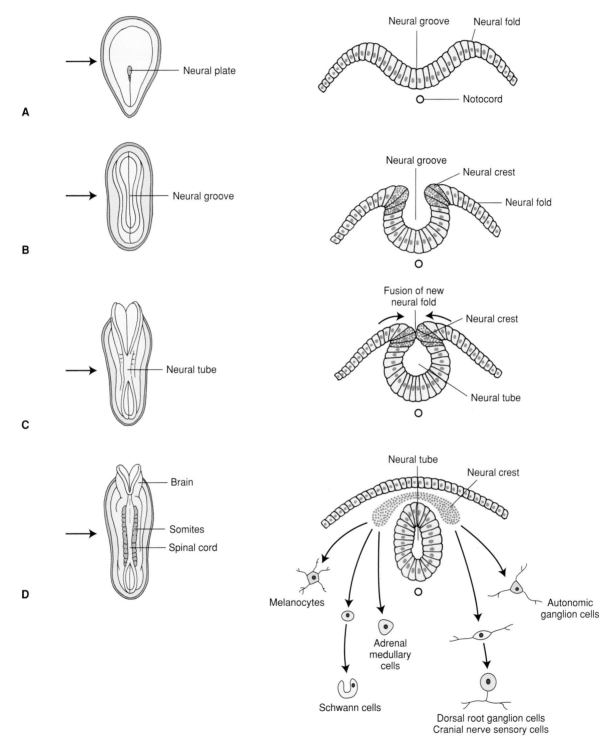

Figure 2–1 Early embryonic development of the central nervous system. Panels A-D depict early development (at the 3rd and 4th weeks of gestation) in which the neural plate (A), neural groove (B), and neural tube (C) are formed from the dorsal surface of the embryo. The left side of each panel depicts the developing embryo in a dorsal view, and the right side shows cross sections through the nervous system cut at the levels indicated by the arrows. Note also the cells formed from differentiated cells of the neural crest (D). (See text for details.)

origin) begins to thicken, and thus, the **neural plate** is formed by the third week of fetal life (Fig. 2-1A). The neural plate continues to thicken over the following week and expands laterally. As it expands, the faster growing lateral edges of the plate accumulate in a dorsal position as **neural folds** (Fig. 2-1B). As this plate grows and widens, it forms a shallow groove along its longitudinal axis known as the **neural groove** (Fig. 2-1B). The posterior end of the neural plate, which is narrower than the anterior end, will ultimately become the spinal cord, whereas the broader, anterior end will become the brain. As this plate grows and widens, the neural groove becomes deeper. In the process of its forming and deepening, some of the cells located in the lateral margin of the neural groove separate and migrate to a dorsal position to become the **neural crest** (Fig. 2-1B). As the embryo grows, the neural folds fuse along the midline, thus forming a **neural tube** (Fig. 2-1C).

Neural crest cells will differentiate into separate groups of neurons (Fig. 2-1D). One group differentiates into sensory neurons of cranial nerve (CN) ganglia (components of CN V, VII, IX, and X of the head region) and into the **dorsal root ganglia** (components of the body). A second group will differentiate into the autonomic ganglion cells (**postganglionic** neurons of the **paravertebral** and **prevertebral ganglia** of the sympathetic nervous system, as well as postganglionic neurons of the parasympathetic nervous system that are located in visceral organs; see Chapter 22). Other neural crest cells will become **chromaffin cells** (of the adrenal medulla), **Schwann cells** (that are critical for the formation of myelin in peripheral nerves), and **melanocytes**. In addition, groups of mesodermal cells located alongside the neural tube, called **somites**, will develop into skeletal muscle, vertebrae, and the dermal layer of the skin (Fig. 2-1D).

The anterior aspect of the neural plate develops subdivisions, which will initially form three brain vesicles and, ultimately, five brain vesicles. The three brain vesicles include the prosencephalon, mesencephalon, and rhombencephalon; caudal to these vesicles are cells from which the spinal cord will develop (Fig. 2-2A). The five vesicles derived from these vesicles are as follows: the rostral **prosencephalon (forebrain)**, which will later become the **telencephalon** and **diencephalon**, including the cells that will develop into the retina; the **mesencephalon**, which will form the **midbrain**; and the caudal **rhombencephalon (hindbrain)**, which will later form the **metencephalon (pons)** and **myelencephalon (medulla)** (Fig. 2-2B). When depicted in a lateral view, the flexures associated with each vesicle can be seen (Fig. 2-2C).

MORPHOGENESIS OF THE CENTRAL NERVOUS SYSTEM (SEE SUMMARY IN TABLE 2-1)

THE SPINAL CORD

The neural tube consists of three layers: an inner layer called the **ventricular layer**, which is in contact with the cavity of the neural tube; an intermediate layer called the **mantle layer**; and an outer layer called the **marginal layer** (Fig. 2-3A). The ventricular zone is the major proliferative layer and also the first layer of the forming neural tube to appear. The second layer to form is the marginal layer, followed by the mantle layer. Early in development, the wall of the neural canal becomes thickened, in part, by the formation of young or immature neurons that have yet to completely differentiate (sometimes called **neurocytes**) in the mantle layer. Because this layer contains the primary cell bodies of neurons, it will ultimately become the gray matter of the spinal cord. Axons associated with cells in the mantle layer will grow into the marginal layer.

The neural tube undergoes additional differentiation that can best be viewed in neural tube cross sections. During proliferation of immature neural cells, a pair of grooves appears at approximately the midpoints along the lateral margin of the neural canal. This groove, the **sulcus limitans** (Fig. 2-3A), is an important anatomical landmark with respect to later development of functional regions of the central nervous system (CNS). In essence, neural cells (**neurocytes**) accumulate in several locations in relation to the sulcus limitans. Neurocytes migrating dorsal to the sulcus limitans form the **alar plate**, whereas those migrating ventral to the sulcus limitans form the **basal plate** (Fig. 2-3A). Moreover, the developing cells that lie in an intermediate position adjacent to the sulcus limitans will become **autonomic** neurons. Thus, the alar and basal plates form the walls of the neural canal. The cells that lie along the dorsal midline are referred to as the **roof plate**, and cells that lie along the midline of the ventral aspect of the neural canal are known as the **floor plate** (Fig. 2-3A). The cells in the alar plate and the basal plate will contribute to sensory pathways and motor pathways, respectively (Fig. 2-3B).

The direction in which axons in the neural tube travel depends on the specific location of these cells within the mantle layer. Axons generally situated more ventrally within the mantle layer (i.e., the basal plate) will invade adjacent segments (called **somites**) that will constitute different regions of the body. They will become functionally

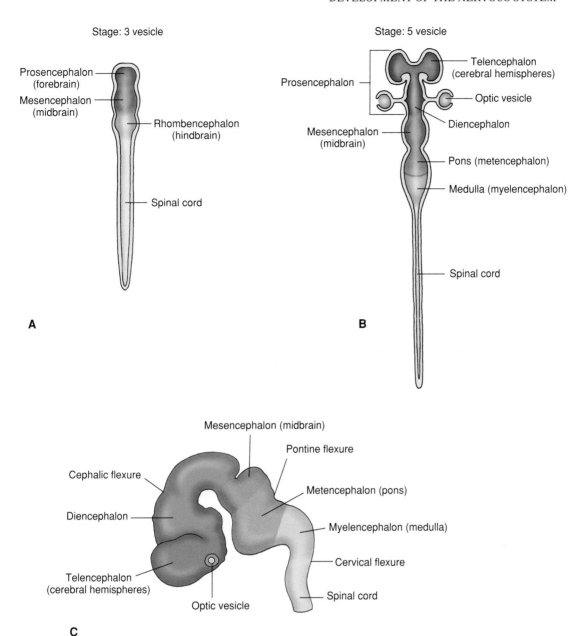

Figure 2–2 Formation of the vesicles of the brain. The figures depict the division of the forebrain vesicle into three (A) and five (B) vesicle stages to form the telencephalon and diencephalon (from the prosencephalon), as well as the formation of the midbrain, and the metencephalon and myelencephalon (from the hindbrain). These illustrations are dorsal views of the neural tube at the two different stages in which the flexures are not shown. Panel C depicts these stages in a lateral view. The flexures result from the proliferation of cells in the cerebral hemispheres and brainstem in the cranium, which is somewhat restricted in size. (See text for details.)

linked by nerve fibers from the mantle layer that will form the **ventral root** of the spinal cord (Fig. 2-3C). In so doing, these axons will develop into the motor neurons of the nervous system. Axons are initially found in the marginal layer growing toward rostral or caudal levels of the spinal cord or toward the brain. Some of the axons arise from spinal cord neuronal cell bodies in the gray matter; some arise from **dorsal root ganglion** cells, whose axons form the **dorsal root**; and a little later, some

will descend from the brain (Fig. 2-3C). Axons added rapidly during development become the characteristic outer white matter of the spinal cord (Fig. 2-3C). The developing spinal nerves contain the following functional components: **general somatic afferent (GSA), general somatic efferent (GSE), general visceral efferent (GVE),** and **general visceral afferent (GVA) neurons**. GSA neurons include those that transmit sensory impulses from the periphery to the brain. They transmit

Table 2–1 Differentiation of the Neural Tube During Its Development

Embryonic Derivative	Spinal Cord	Rhombencephalon (hindbrain), Myelencephalon (medulla), and Metencephalon (pons and cerebellum)	Mesencephalon (midbrain)	Prosencephalon (forebrain) (diencephalon and telencephalon)
Roof Plate	Region of posterior median septum	Superior medullary velum	Commissures of the superior and inferior colliculi	Choroid tela and choroid plexus of the lateral and third ventricles
Alar Plate	Dorsal gray columns	Sensory nuclei of CN V, VII, VIII, IX, X; cerebellum, deep pontine nuclei, inferior olivary nucleus, mesencephalic nucleus(CN V) [but displaced to midbrain]	Superior and inferior colliculi, red nucleus, substantia nigra, main sensory nucleus (CN V); some nuclei of reticular formation?	It has been suggested that diencephalon (thalamus and hypothalamus) telencephalic structures are derived from alar plate, but derivation is still unclear at this time
Basal Plate	Ventral gray columns; nucleus of CN XI	Motor nuclei of CN V, VI, VII, IX, X, XII; nuclei of reticular formation	Motor nuclei of CN III, IV; nuclei of reticular formation	—
Floor Plate	Region of ventral median fissure	—	—	—

such information as changes in temperature, noxious stimulation, touch, pressure, and information involving **proprioceptors** (i.e., stretch of a muscle, tendon, or bodily position). GSE fibers transmit signals from the CNS to skeletal muscle. GVE fibers, which originate close to the **sulcus limitans**, transmit autonomic signals from the CNS to smooth muscle and glands. GVA fibers originate from visceral structures and provide the CNS with information concerning their status.

An important feature in development of the spinal cord relates to the relative differences in the rates of growth of the spinal cord in comparison to the vertebral column. Although the growth rates for both during the first 3 months are approximately equivalent, there is a change in the succeeding 4 months. Specifically, during this latter period, the growth rate of the vertebral column is considerably more rapid than that of the spinal cord. Because of the differential rates of growth, at birth, the spinal cord does not fill the entire extent of the neural canal but, instead, reaches only as far as the third lumbar vertebra; the spinal cord reaches the second lumbar vertebra in the adult. This differential rate of growth also alters the orientation of nerve fibers that exit from the spinal cord. While nerve fibers that arise from more rostral levels of the spinal cord exit at approximately right angles, those exiting from more caudal levels become elongated and are oriented much more ventrally (see Chapter 9, Fig. 9-2).

THE BRAIN

Myelencephalon (Medulla)

Recall that the alar and basal plates of the mantle layer, which are separated by a shallow groove called the sulcus limitans, form the walls of the neural canal of the developing nervous system. Although the size of the neural canal remains relatively small in the developing spinal cord, this is not the case for the **brainstem**. In the part of the developing brainstem that contains the fourth ventricle, the roof plate expands greatly so that the alar plate becomes located lateral to the basal plate (Fig. 2-4, A and B).

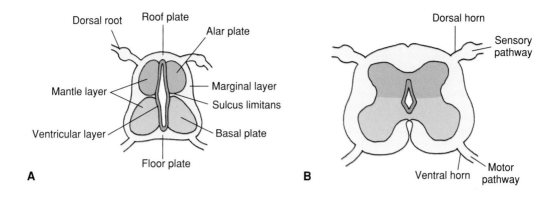

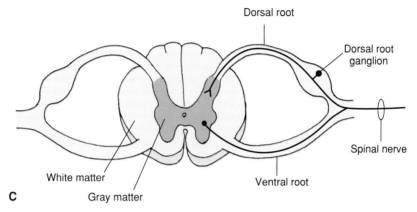

Figure 2–3 Development of the spinal cord: (A) early stage of development; (B) intermediate stage of development; and (C) late stage of development. Note also the positions of the alar, basal, and roof and floor plates as shown in panel A and the structures derived from them shown in panels B and C. (See text for details.)

Based on the previous discussion, we can say that structures associated with motor functions tend to lie medial to structures associated with sensory functions. More precisely, the motor and sensory neurons are arranged in columns that are oriented in a dorsomedial to ventrolateral fashion. The following descriptions illustrate this organization. Cranial nerve motor nuclei, which supply neurons to skeletal muscles of somite origin such as the hypoglossal nucleus, are classified as **GSE** fibers and lie near the midline (Fig. 2-4C). Cranial nerve motor nuclei, such as CN IX (glossopharyngeal) and CN X (vagus), also supply axons that innervate skeletal muscle derived from the pharyngeal arches. They lie in a column situated relatively more laterally but, nevertheless, medial to sensory neurons. Such neurons are classified as **special visceral efferent (SVE) neurons**.

Like the developing spinal cord, structures that mediate autonomic functions develop from neurocytes situated close to the sulcus limitans. Here, neurons that mediate autonomic functions are located in the general position between sensory and somatic motor structures. This column contains neurons that innervate visceral organs and glands and include components of CN VII (metencephalon, see next section), IX, and X (myelencephalon). These neurons are classified as **GVE neurons**.

Immediately lateral to the sulcus limitans lies the next column, which includes a class of sensory neurons referred to as **GVA** and **special visceral afferent (SVA) neurons**. GVA neurons are associated with autonomic functions (such as **baroreceptors**, which sense changes in blood pressure and heart rate) and receive visceral afferent information from CN IX and X associated with such processes as changes in blood pressure and functions of the body viscera. SVA neurons are concerned with components of CN VII, IX, and X that receive information from peripheral **chemoreceptors** (i.e., receptors that respond to changes in the chemical milieu of their environment).

Sensory functions that involve mainly sensory components of the trigeminal nerve lie in a column positioned further laterally within the medulla and are referred to as **GSA neurons**. The sensory column located most laterally concerns neurons that are associated with special senses.

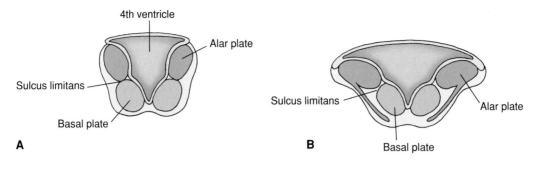

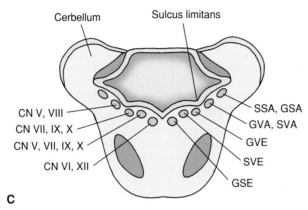

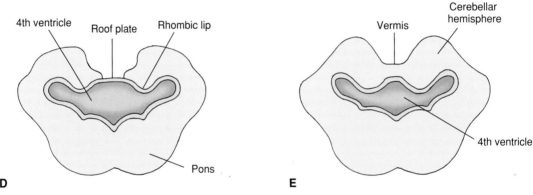

Figure 2–4 Development of the brainstem. Panels A-C depict the development of the lower brainstem. Arrows shown in panel A depict how the nuclear organization is transformed from the dorsal-to-ventral orientation in the spinal cord to a medial-to-lateral orientation shown in panels B and C. Panel C depicts how cranial nerve nuclei are organized in the brainstem in terms of their medial-to-lateral position. Here, it can be seen that motor nuclei (GSE, SVE) are situated medial to the sulcus limitans; sensory nuclei (SSA, GSA) are located lateral to the sulcus limitans; and autonomic nuclei (GVA, SVA, GVE) are found in the region adjoining the sulcus limitans. Panels D and E depict development of cerebellum. Note the development and formation of the cerebellum from the rhombic lips that become fused at the midline. (See text for details.)

Within the brainstem, these include **auditory** and **vestibular nuclei** of the eighth cranial nerve and are classified as special sensory afferent (SSA) neurons. A more detailed analysis of the structure and functions of cranial nerves is discussed in Chapter 14.

The size of the neural canal has now expanded greatly and will become the **fourth ventricle** (Fig. 2-4D). The roof plate also shows great expansion, as if it were stretched in a lateral plane to a position

where it becomes connected with the lateral aspect of the alar plate. Only the floor plate remains relatively fixed in its original position.

The walls of the cavity that will become the fourth ventricle include **mesenchymal** tissue that will become highly vascular. This tissue will become attached to the **ependymal wall** of the ventricle and will generate **pia mater** as well. This vascular tissue will also become relatively pronounced along the central portion of the roof of the ventricle where it invaginates into the developing ventricle and will become the **choroid plexus**. During later periods of development (i.e., months 4 and 5), a pair of foramina develops along the roof of the ventricle. The foramina come to be situated laterally and are called the lateral apertures or **Foramina of Luschka**. Another foramen becomes situated medially and is called the median aperture or **Foramen of Magendie**.

The marginal layer of the developing myelencephalon, like that of the spinal cord, contains considerable amounts of white matter. In particular, on the ventral aspect of the medulla, one can identify large groups of axons that arise from prominent cells of the cerebral cortex, called **pyramidal cells**, which are distributed to regions throughout the brainstem and spinal cord. At the level of the medulla, these nerve fibers are referred to as the **pyramids**. The lateral aspect of the medulla also contains fibers that are part of the marginal layer and, to some extent, represent an extension of the fibers contained in the marginal layer of the spinal cord. Thus, this aspect of the marginal layer contains such ascending systems from the spinal cord as the **spinocerebellar and spinothalamic pathways**.

Metencephalon

The metencephalon consists of two principal components: the **pons** and **cerebellum**. The pons contains two basic divisions: a dorsal region called the **tegmentum**, which is an extension of the myelencephalon, and a ventral region called the **basilar part** of the **pons**.

Pons

With respect to the tegmentum, the same principle applies to this region that was described earlier in attempting to understand the organization of the medulla. In general, developing neurons that lie within the basal plate tend to form the medial half of the tegmentum, whereas neurons that are part of the alar plate are more or less distributed throughout more lateral aspects of the tegmentum. In this manner, motor neurons, such as the nuclei of CN VI (GSE) and CN VII and V (SVE), are situated along a diagonal plane relatively medial to the planes in which sensory neurons, such as the lateral and superior vestibular nuclei or the spinal, main sensory or **mesencephalic nuclei** of CN V (GSA), are located. Additionally, autonomic nuclei of the pons (i.e., GVE neurons of CN VII) tend to lie in a diagonal plane somewhat interposed between the planes containing sensory and somatic motor neurons (Fig. 2-4C).

The basilar portion of the pons (Fig. 2-4D) is derived mainly from neurons migrating from the alar plate. The neurocytes that are found in this region give rise to axons that grow in a transverse direction, ultimately extending beyond the body of the pons to form a major peduncle of the cerebellum called the middle cerebellar peduncle. This pathway then becomes a major route by which information from the pons can enter the cerebellum. Other fiber bundles contained within the basilar portion of the pons include descending axons that originate from the cerebral cortex and that are destined to supply nuclei of the lower brainstem and spinal cord. Therefore, these neurons evolve as part of the development of the cerebral cortex, which is described later in this chapter.

Cerebellum

The **cerebellum** is derived from the dorsal aspect of the alar plate. Cells from the alar plate migrate further laterally and dorsally until they become situated dorsal and lateral to the lateral walls and lateral aspect of the roof of the developing fourth ventricle, respectively (Fig. 2-4D). As the medial aspect of the developing roof bends further medially, it thins out to form a narrow roof plate of the ventricle. This transitional region is referred to as the **rhombic lips** (Fig. 2-4D). As the rhombic lips proliferate, they extend over the roof plate, and cells from each side of the developing brain begin to approach each other. After 3 months of development, these groups of cells ultimately merge and fuse (Fig. 2-4E). The cells formed in the central region are referred to as the **vermis**, and those in the lateral region constitute the **cerebellar hemispheres**. The vermal region will display little additional growth; whereas, in contrast, the hemispheres will continue to expand considerably. At approximately the fourth month of development, fissures begin to develop with respect to the anterior lobe of cerebellum; and by the seventh month, other aspects of the cerebellar hemispheres are apparent.

Cellular development of the cerebellum occurs in a variety of ways. Some cell types, such as those found near the surface of the developing cerebellar cortex, migrate inward to form a granule cell layer. **Purkinje cells**, which also appear quite early, contribute to the development of the cerebellar cortex by forming a distinctive layer called the Purkinje cell layer just superficial to the granule cell layer. The outer layer contains mainly the axons of **granule cells**. These axons are called parallel fibers because they run parallel to the cortical surface. They remain in the superficial surface region of the cortex, in contrast to their cell bodies, which have migrated inward. Because of the paucity of cell bodies and extensive presence of fibers near the cortical surface, this layer is called the molecular layer. The neurons of the cerebellar cortex do not project out of the cerebellum. However, several of these cells can contact other cells, which show little migration from their original positions and remain close to the fourth ventricle. **Deep cerebellar nuclei** give rise to axons, which project out of the cerebellum by growing into portions of the brainstem and forebrain. For example, neurons of the developing dentate and interposed nuclei grow within a fiber bundle that later in development is called the **superior cerebellar peduncle**. This growth is directed toward the midbrain where fibers of the interposed nuclei reach the red nucleus (involved in motor functions); other fibers originating from the dentate nucleus extend beyond the midbrain into the lateral **thalamus** (see Chapters 13 and 26). Other fibers originating from the fastigial nucleus display a different trajectory in their growth patterns. Axons of these cells emerge from the cerebellum in bundles that pass close to the inferior cerebellar peduncle and reach the lower brainstem where they make synaptic connections with neurons of the reticular formation and vestibular nuclei of the pons and medulla.

Mesencephalon (Midbrain)

The midbrain can be divided into three general regions: a **tectal** region, located dorsally; a **tegmentum**, which is a continuation of the tegmentum of the pons and medulla and is located in an intermediate position; and a **peduncular region**, which is located in a ventral position (see Chapter 12).

The cavity of the midbrain vesicle, in contrast to the large size of the fourth ventricle found at the level of the upper medulla and pons, will continue to remain narrow and constitute a channel by which cerebrospinal fluid (CSF) can flow from the forebrain into the fourth ventricle. It is referred to as the cerebral aqueduct (**Aqueduct of Sylvius**).

Neurocytes developing from the basal plate at this level will differentiate into motor neurons (i.e., GSE) of CN III (oculomotor) and IV (trochlear) and parts of the tegmentum. Axons of CN III are directed in a ventral direction where they exit the brain in a medial position from its ventral surface. However, neurons associated with CN IV emerge from the brain on its dorsal surface and completely cross within the **superior medullary velum**, exiting the brain just inferior to the **inferior colliculus**. Other developing neurons from the basal plate will differentiate into parasympathetic nuclei of CN III (i.e., GVE). These neurons will serve as an important mechanism for reflexes involving both **pupillary constriction** and the accommodation reaction.

Neurocytes developing from the alar plate will differentiate into neurons of the tectum, which consists of both the superior and inferior colliculi. These neurons are associated with sensory processes; the **superior colliculus** is linked to the regulation of eye movements, and the inferior colliculus constitutes a relay in the ascending auditory pathway. Other neurocytes from the alar plate will differentiate into the **mesencephalic nucleus** of CN V and possibly into the substantia nigra and red nucleus.

The **peduncular region** of the midbrain is derived from the marginal layer of the basal plate and consists of fibers that arise from the cerebral cortex and that descend caudally to the midbrain, pons, medulla, and spinal cord.

Prosencephalon (Forebrain)

At approximately the fourth or fifth week of development, the most rostral of the primary brain vesicles, the prosencephalon (forebrain), begins to display selective changes. One change includes the formation of an optic vesicle at a ventral aspect of the anterior forebrain. The optic vesicle expands outward toward the overlying ectoderm, while its connection to the forebrain (called the optic stalk) becomes constricted. The fiber bundles thus formed are called the **optic nerves** anterior to the optic chiasm, whereas their continuation posterior to the chiasm is called the **optic tract**, which terminates in the diencephalon. The optic vesicle contributes to inductive interactions upon the overlying surface ectoderm to produce the **lens placode**, which will form the lens of the eye. The part of the forebrain that lies rostral to the optic vesicle will become the telencephalon (see Fig. 2-2C). In particular, the portion of the telencephalon that lies in a lateral position will form the cerebral hemispheres. The remaining part, which lies in a medial position, will become the **diencephalon**.

Diencephalon

The diencephalon appears as swellings of the lateral aspect of the neural canal. In this region, the canal originally had a large lumen. The lumen is diminished with the emergence of the swellings forming the **thalamus**, dorsally, and **hypothalamus**, ventrally (Fig. 2-5). The derivation of the diencephalon is somewhat controversial. However, it has been suggested that it develops mainly from the alar plate because the basal plate appears to be absent in this region. Likewise, the diencephalon does not appear to contain a floor plate but does retain a roof plate, which differentiates into **choroid plexus** after becoming attached to pia mater.

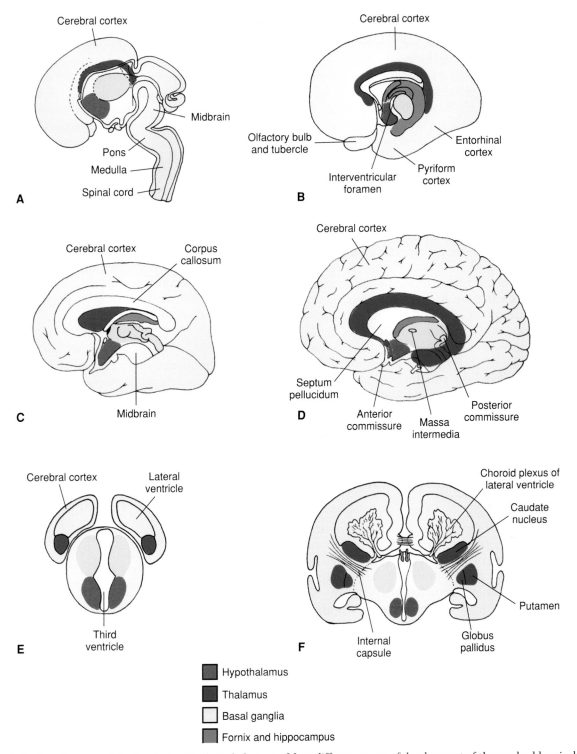

Figure 2–5 Development of the forebrain. (A-D) Medial views of four different stages of development of the cerebral hemispheres and their fusion with the diencephalon. Note the C-shaped arrangement of the telencephalic structures, including the hippocampus and fornix as well as the basal ganglia complex formed later in development. (E and F) Cross-sectional diagram taken from levels indicated in panels A and D illustrating how the cerebral hemispheres are formed at different stages of development. Note that, as shown in panel F, the choroid plexus develops from the roof of the ventricles.

The thalamus displays the greatest amount of growth and becomes the largest component of the diencephalon. The cells will differentiate into many cell groups, forming the varied nuclei of the thalamus. In fact, the rapid growth of the thalamus is such that a small bridge is often formed between the two sides called the **massa intermedia** (or interthalamic adhesion) (Fig. 2-5D).

As the walls of the third ventricle expand ventrally, they do so to a much smaller extent than at dorsal levels. This region will become the hypothalamus and will contain a smaller number of anatomically well-defined nuclei than the thalamus. However, other structures will become associated with the hypothalamus. These structures include the optic chiasm, which is formed at a rostral level of the hypothalamus and is the product of the growth of retinal fibers; rounded bodies called the **mammillary bodies**; the **tuber cinereum**; and the **infundibulum**; all of which are located on the ventral surface of the hypothalamus (see Chapter 24). The infundibulum gives rise to a pituitary stalk and neural **hypophysis** (posterior lobe of pituitary). The anterior lobe of the pituitary is derived from ectodermal diverticulum called **Rathke's pouch**, which is in contact with the infundibulum. Rathke's pouch ultimately develops into the anterior lobe of pituitary (adenohypophysis). The rostral limit of the third ventricle is formed by the **lamina terminalis**, in front of which lies the telencephalon.

Telencephalon

After the growth of the telencephalic vesicles from the dorsal aspect of the forebrain, primitive sac-like structures form within each cerebral hemisphere in the developing brain. These structures will become the lateral ventricles, which are continuous with the third ventricle through a small channel known as the **interventricular foramen (of Monro)** (Fig. 2-5B).

The cerebral cortex is formed by the continued growth of the cerebral hemispheres in both anterior and dorsal directions during the third and fourth months of development (see Fig. 2-2B). The anterior and dorsal expansion results in the formation of the frontal lobe. Expansion laterally and dorsally results in development of the parietal lobe, and growth in a posterior and ventral direction results in the development of the temporal and occipital lobes. As immature neurons within the cortex begin to differentiate, they form different cell groups. Much of the cerebral cortex contains six histologically distinct layers, which are present in higher vertebrates; this form of cortex is referred to as **neocortex**. One cell type that is formed, the pyramidal cell, gives rise to axons that

will grow out into other regions of cortex and form the internal capsule (see discussion in *Internal Capsule* section). Thus, this cell type constitutes the principal means by which the cerebral cortex communicates with other regions of the CNS, including the spinal cord. Other cell types are also formed; the most common is the granule cell, which receives input principally from different regions of the thalamus.

As the cerebral hemispheres display growth in rostral and dorsal directions, the roof plate becomes fused with pia mater, which contains tissue of vascular mesodermal origin to form the **choroid plexus** of the lateral ventricle (Fig. 2-5F). With continued growth, the choroid plexus becomes most extensive within the lateral ventricles. As the cerebral hemispheres continue to expand, the lateral ventricles also appear to be carried along with them, thus contributing to their continued growth and elongation.

Basal Ganglia

Major components of the basal ganglia, which include the caudate nucleus, **putamen**, and **globus pallidus**, are formed when immature neurons within the floor of the telencephalon and situated lateral to the interventricular foramen begin to proliferate. With continued growth of the basal ganglia, differentiation is noted. One group of cells, the **caudate nucleus**, comes to occupy a dorsomedial position. A second group of cells arise from the same general region but migrate ventrally to form the amygdaloid complex (see Chapter 1). Other groups of cells, the **lentiform or lenticular nucleus** (i.e., putamen and globus pallidus), display considerable growth and development and are displaced in a ventrolateral position relative to that of the caudate nucleus. The putamen assumes a position directly lateral to that of the globus pallidus (Fig. 2-5F).

The main body of the caudate nucleus (i.e., the region that will become the head and body of the caudate nucleus) displays little change from its original position, whereas the posterior aspect (i.e., the part that will become the tail of the caudate nucleus) becomes elongated by virtue of the growth of the hemisphere. The resulting effect is that the tail of the caudate follows the growth pattern of the lateral ventricle, which, in turn, is directed by the rapid growth of the cerebral hemispheres relative to that of the diencephalon. In this manner, the tail of the caudate is first pulled backward toward the occipital pole, then downward, and, finally, somewhat anteriorly together with the inferior horn of the lateral ventricle. The trajectories of both structures, therefore, basically follow the contour of the posterior aspect of the thalamus.

Internal Capsule

Neurons associated with the cerebral cortex give rise to axons that are directed caudally to the basal ganglia, thalamus, brainstem, and spinal cord. These developing neurons form the internal capsule and pass between the thalamus and the lentiform nucleus (i.e., globus pallidus and putamen) (Fig. 2-5F). Neurons associated with much of the frontal lobe contribute to the formation of the anterior limb of the internal capsule. Neurons located in portions of the cortical region that will develop into the precentral and postcentral gyri as well as other parts of the parietal lobe contribute to the formation of the posterior limb of the internal capsule. Those fibers situated in the temporal lobe are called the **sublenticular** component of the internal capsule. In addition, the internal capsule is also formed by fibers arising in the thalamus that grow toward the cerebral cortex and innervate different regions of the cortex.

Hippocampal Formation and Related Structures

The **hippocampal formation (archipallium)** arises from the medial surface of the telencephalic vesicle, and the **entorhinal** and **pyriform cortices (paleopallium)** arise from the ventral surface of the telencephalon and are further directed in a ventromedial direction where they become situated on the medial and ventral surfaces of the temporal lobe adjacent to the hippocampal formation in which the entorhinal cortex lies caudal to the pyriform cortex (Fig. 2-5B). With the growth of the temporal neocortex, the hippocampal formation is pulled in a caudal direction that follows the course of the inferior horn of the lateral ventricle. Axons of the hippocampal formation form a major pathway called the **fornix** that is directed in a dorsomedial direction to the level of the **anterior commissure**, at which point it then passes downward and caudally until it makes contact with hypothalamic nuclei (Fig. 2-5D). The anterior aspect of the forebrain becomes enlarged to form structures directly associated with olfactory functions, which include the olfactory bulb and a region located near the ventral surface of the anterior aspect of the forebrain called the **olfactory tubercle** and **paraolfactory region** (Fig. 2-5B).

Commissures

Several prominent **commissures** can be identified within the forebrain. These include the **corpus callosum** (Fig. 2-5C), **anterior commissure** (Fig. 2-5D), and the **posterior commissure** (Fig. 2-5D). The corpus callosum is the largest and most extensive of the commissures. It grows out of the dorsal aspect of the lamina terminalis and extends caudally beyond the level of the posterior aspect of the thalamus. The corpus callosum arises from pyramidal cells of the cerebral cortex and extensively connects **homotypical** regions of both sides of the brain.

The anterior commissure passes through the lamina terminalis and provides a connection between the temporal lobes, olfactory cortices, and olfactory bulbs on both sides of the brain. The posterior commissure is located on the border between the midbrain and diencephalon. The posterior commissure is located on the border between the midbrain and diencephalon and connects the **pretectal area** and neighboring nuclei on both sides of the rostral midbrain.

MYELINATION IN THE CENTRAL NERVOUS SYSTEM

Myelination within the CNS is essential for efficient and rapid transmission of signals. It begins at approximately the fourth month of fetal development at cervical levels of the spinal cord. But myelination within the spinal cord is not completed until after the first year of birth. In the brain, myelination begins at approximately the sixth month of gestation and is generally limited to the region of the basal ganglia. This is followed by myelination of ascending fiber systems, which extends into the postnatal period. The striking feature is that much of the brain remains unmyelinated at birth. For example, the **corticospinal tract** begins to become myelinated by the sixth month after birth and requires several years for myelination to be completed. Other regions of the brain may not be fully myelinated until the beginning of the second decade of life.

ABNORMALITIES IN DEVELOPMENT OF THE NERVOUS SYSTEM

SPINA BIFIDA

Spina bifida, called **myeloschisis**, occurs when the posterior neuropore fails to close. It is manifested by a failure of the vertebral canal to close, and spina bifida follows. Two types of spina bifida have been described: spina bifida occulta and spina bifida aperta (also called spina bifida cystica). **Spina bifida occulta** represents a simple defect of mesodermal origin in which one or more vertebrae fail to close (Fig. 2-6B). Here, there is no involvement of the meninges or the underlying spinal cord, and the overlying skin is closed. As a result, there may be improper development of the spinal cord, which can be detected by radiography. In general, there are few neurologic symptoms associated with this

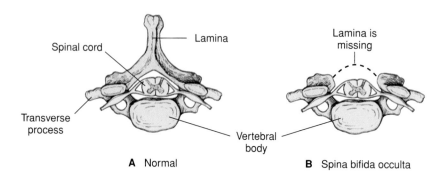

A Normal

B Spina bifida occulta

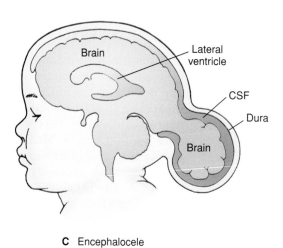

C Encephalocele

Figure 2–6 Examples of abnormalities in the development of the brain and spinal cord. (A) The normal arrangement of the vertebra and associated spinal cord. (B) Figure illustrates a given vertebra and the neural tube where the posterior arch failed to close. It is an example of spina bifida occulta. It is characterized by the absence of the vertebral lamina at a particular level or levels, the effect of which is to allow the meninges to be exposed. (C) An example of an encephalocele, a defect in the cranium in which there is an occipital herniation, causing a protrusion, in this case, of the meninges alone.

disorder except if there is bony compression of the exposed area of spinal cord or if there are fat deposits that form in the exposed region.

Spina bifida aperta involves the protrusion of either the meninges alone (called a **meningocele**) or spinal cord together with the meninges (called a **meningomyelocele**).

A **meningocele** is a condition that typically involves the lumbar and sacral portions of the spinal cord and is covered by the meninges and by overlying skin. There is little evidence of motor or sensory deficits, although this disorder may produce defects in the development of the vertebral column and lower aspect of the spinal cord (called **myelodysplasia**).

A **meningomyelocele** involves herniation of the spinal cord (or brainstem) and adjoining meninges through the defect in the vertebral column. This condition, which is much more common than meningocele, is not limited to a specific region of spinal cord. In fact, not only can it affect any of the regions of spinal cord, but it can also involve the brainstem as well. A meningomyelocele produces

much more severe deficits than a meningocele. In particular, it may produce symptoms characteristic of a partial or total transection of the cord, especially if it involves the cervical region. It may also involve hydrocephalus and its associated sensory, motor, and autonomic deficits.

A related disorder involving the brainstem and cerebellum is called the **Arnold-Chiari malformation.** Because the vertebral column grows faster than the spinal cord, the cerebellum and parts of the medulla are displaced and consequently pulled through the foramen magnum. This effect will block the flow of CSF that normally passes from the roof of the fourth ventricle to the cisterns, causing hydrocephalus (see Chapter 3 for description of CSF flow) and even syringomyelia (see next section).

SYRINGO(HYDRO)MYELIA

A developmental abnormality in the formation of the central canal is called **syringo(hydro)myelia.** In this condition, there is a cavitation filled with CSF in the region of the central canal, which damages the crossing fibers of the spinothalamic tract, the net effect of which is to cause segmental loss of pain and temperature (see Chapter 9). Clinically, children with this anomaly have motor dysfunction from interruption of the corticospinal tract, which travels through the spinal cord. A full diagnosis is often made by magnetic resonance imaging (**MRI**) of the lower spine. These children are often treated with surgical closure of the defect.

TETHERED CORD

This malformation involves the anchoring of the lowest part of the spinal cord to the sacrum. The disorder can result in sensory and motor deficits of the lower extremities as well as bladder difficulties, back pain, and scoliosis.

ENCEPHALOCELE

Encephalocele, which constitutes a failure of portions of the **anterior neuropore** to close, is manifested by the protrusion of a sac from the cranium consisting of portions of the meninges and CSF, glial tissue, and brain substance with or without the ventricles. This anomaly is rarely an isolated occurrence and is usually associated with abnormalities of the cerebral hemispheres, cerebellum, and midbrain. Similar malformations have been produced in animals experimentally from exposure to **teratogens** (a drug or agent taken by the mother during pregnancy that causes an abnormality in development) during early gestation. Clinical findings are variable and depend upon the extent and location of the sac; however, mental retardation and corticospinal tract dysfunction (such as weakness) are two of the most commonly encountered problems among children with this anomaly. Figure 2-6C depicts an example of an occipital encephalocele.

Cerebral malformations may also result in neonatal and infantile seizures, although many other factors may contribute to infantile seizures such as metabolic disorders, hypocalcemia, and injury in delivery. Seizures can be treated with antiepileptic drugs, but this approach can be a problem if the seizures are not associated with electroencephalographic discharges.

Neural tube defects can be detected by several methods, including ultrasound examination and amniocentesis. Amniocentesis is a procedure based on the assumption that α-fetoprotein, a principal component of fetal serum, leaks out into the amniotic fluid when the neural tube is not closed. This results in significantly elevated levels of this protein, which enables its detection.

DANDY-WALKER SYNDROME

This malformation appears to involve the congenital absence of the lateral apertures (of **Luschka**) and the median aperture (of **Magendie**), which, through lack of communication with the remainder of the ventricular system, can be one cause of hydrocephalus. As a result of this malformation, there is a partial or complete agenesis of the cerebellar vermis, in addition to cystic dilation of the posterior fossa communicating with the fourth ventricle. Other malformations may be found in approximately 68% of patients, the most common of which is the absence of a corpus callosum. There is a mnemonic for remembering the components of this syndrome: *Dandy-Walker syndrome: Dilated 4th ventricle, Water on the brain, Small vermis* (see also the explanations of the questions in Chapter 3 for hydrocephalus).

Clinically, the most common problem seen with this defect is **macrocephaly**, or an enlarged cranium. Other problems these children may have include vomiting, headaches, delayed acquisition of motor skills, breathing problems, truncal ataxia (a lack of coordination in the trunk), and cranial nerve problems. All of these symptoms and signs are a result of hydrocephalus, compression of portions of the posterior fossa, and absence of the cerebellar vermis. A definitive diagnosis is made with the use of a computed tomography (CT) scan or an MRI of the head. This condition may also be treated with surgery, which may include decompression of the cyst and the insertion of a shunt, which serves to redirect the CSF from the brain to another part of the body better able to absorb it, such as the peritoneum.

ANENCEPHALY

This anomaly consists of partial or complete absence of the brain with associated defects of the cranial vault and scalp. It occurs as a result of a severe failure of the anterior neuropore to close at the 21st to 26th day of gestation. Portions of the cranial bones may be absent, and the exposed tissue underneath becomes a fibrous mass containing degenerated neural and glial tissue. The cerebellum, brainstem, and spinal cord may be present but are often small and malformed. The eyes are well developed, but the optic nerves are usually absent. In addition, the pituitary gland and adrenal glands may be small or absent. Often, the arms are relatively large compared to the legs. This anomaly is not compatible with life.

HISTORY

Jimmy is a 4-month-old infant who was the product of a normal, full-term pregnancy. His parents thought that everything was fine until he developed spells upon awakening from sleep. These spells consisted of sudden, bilateral contractions of the muscles of the neck, trunk, and limbs occurring in clusters every 20 seconds for periods of 20 to 30 minutes. Each contraction lasted only a second or two and was often followed by a tonic contraction. The contractions involved flexion of the head, trunk, and limbs. He often cried between spells, and his parents noted some abnormal eye movements at these times, as well.

EXAMINATION

The pediatric neurologist reviewed videotape of the spells and examined the infant. Jimmy had just recently begun to smile, and his motor tone was diffusely somewhat diminished. An electroencephalogram (EEG) showed an irregular pattern of high voltage slow waves and epileptiform spikes called hypsarrhythmia. An MRI scan of Jimmy's brain showed several areas of ectopic cortical tissue in the superficial white matter of the left frontal lobe. His doctor started him on corticosteroids (to reduce possible brain swelling), and the episodes stopped.

EXPLANATION

The spells described are examples of infantile spasms, a type of seizure, usually first manifesting between the fourth and seventh month of life. They often occur in clusters and are abrupt contractions of the neck, trunk, and limb muscles. The most frequent type is flexor spasms, often called "Salaam spasms." Infantile spasms are most often seen as either part of a syndrome called West Syndrome or a triad of infantile spasms, mental retardation, and a chaotic pattern seen on the EEG called hypsarrhythmia. Infantile spasms are caused by many different problems including neonatal infections, anoxic-ischemic insults surrounding birth, cerebral malformations, diffuse brain damage, metabolic problems, and genetic problems. Developmental delay often accompanies the presence of infantile spasms.

A gray matter heterotopia is a type of migrational disorder where cells of the gray matter fail to reach their destination. This may be caused by a variety of toxic, metabolic, and infectious disorders. Migrational disorders may occur any time from the second month of gestation until the postnatal period.

CHAPTER TEST

QUESTIONS

Choose the best answer for each question.

Questions 1 and 2

Examination of a 2-month-old infant revealed that the anterior neuropore had failed to close. Later on, a number of severe deficits appeared.

1. The most likely deficits to be expected include:
   a. Loss of spinal reflexes
   b. Difficulty in swallowing
   c. Mental retardation
   d. Loss of tactile sensation
   e. Cardiovascular abnormalities

2. As the infant grows into childhood, the most likely region of the CNS to be affected is the:
   a. Hypothalamus
   b. Pontine tegmentum
   c. Medulla
   d. Cerebral cortex
   e. Globus pallidus

3. A young child is brought to the hospital for evaluation after displaying a series of major problems, including an enlarged cranium, cerebellar damage, and headaches, vomiting, an inability to learn and maintain acquisition of motor skills, and lack of coordination of the trunk. This disorder can best be described as:
   a. Meningomyelocele
   b. Dandy-Walker syndrome
   c. Anencephaly
   d. Spina bifida
   e. Tethered cord

4. During prenatal development, an abnormality occurs in which the neural crest cells fail to migrate properly. As a result, a number of different types of cells fail to develop, while others are preserved. Among the cell types listed below, which one would be preserved?
   a. Dorsal root ganglion
   b. Autonomic ganglion cells
   c. Chromaffin cells
   d. Ventral horn cells
   e. Schwann cells

5. The hypoglossal nucleus is derived from the:

   a. Roof plate
   b. Floor plate
   c. Alar plate
   d. Basal plate
   e. Neural crest cells

ANSWERS AND EXPLANATIONS

1. and 2. Answers: 1-c, 2-d

Failure of the anterior neuropore to close results in protrusion of the meninges, CSF, glia, and related brain tissue. This deficit is associated with considerable damage to the cerebral hemispheres, cerebellum, and midbrain. Damage to the cerebral hemispheres will invariably lead to mental retardation. The other choices for question 1 involve functions associated with structures linked to the lower brainstem or spinal cord. Concerning question 2, the cerebral cortex is the structure primarily affected by this disorder, whereas the other choices for that question appear to show little or no damage.

3. Answer: b

The symptoms described in this question are characteristic of the Dandy-Walker syndrome, which involves primarily hydrocephalus with loss of the cerebellar vermis. Recall again the mnemonic for the components of this syndrome: **D**ilated 4th ventricle, **W**ater on the brain, **S**mall vermis. The other choices involve developmental disorders, which affect the cerebral cortex and other regions of the brain (meningomyelocele and anencephaly), spinal cord, or sensory and motor deficits of the lower extremities (spina bifida and tethered cord); none of these other disorders would produce the symptoms described in this question.

4. Answer: d

The neural crest is formed from cells associated with the neural folds that become separated from the neural tube on its dorsal aspect. Dorsal root ganglion cells, autonomic ganglion cells, chromaffin cells, and Schwann cells are derived from the neural crest. Because neural crest cells become separated from the neural tube, those cells developing from the walls of the neural tube that include the alar, basal, and floor plates have no relationship with neural crest cells. The ventral horn cells are derived from the basal plate.

5. Answer: d

In the medulla, the brain tissue situated medial to the sulcus limitans is derived from the basal plate. The cranial nerve nuclei in this region relate to motor functions and include such motor nuclei as those of CN XII (hypoglossal nucleus), CN X, and CN IX (nucleus ambiguus). Cranial nerve nuclei situated lateral to the sulcus limitans relate to sensory functions. The roof and floor plates do not give rise to cranial nerve nuclei. The neural crest cells give rise to autonomic ganglia, cranial nerve sensory ganglia, Schwann cells, and cells of the suprarenal medulla.

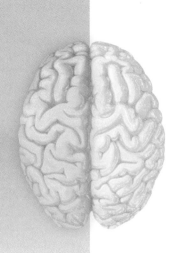

CHAPTER 3

MENINGES AND CEREBROSPINAL FLUID

OBJECTIVES

In this chapter, the student should learn:

1. The anatomy and function of the coverings of the brain and their relationship to venous sinuses and subarachnoid fluid spaces (cisterns)

2. The differences between the coverings of the spinal cord and the brain including anatomical features of the lumbar cistern and its importance in lumbar puncture

3. The ventricular system of the brain; anatomical and functional characteristics of choroid plexuses; the formation, composition, circulation, and function of the cerebrospinal fluid (CSF)

4. Role of arachnoid villi in the absorption of CSF into the venous sinuses and alteration of CSF in pathological conditions

5. The nature of the blood–brain and blood–CSF barriers

6. Disorders associated with the circulation and absorption of CSF

THE MENINGES

The tissues comprising the brain and spinal cord are very delicate and require special protection. This is provided by the bony cranial vault, the bony vertebral canal, and three layers of connective tissue membranes (dura, arachnoid, and pia mater). The arachnoid and pia are known as the **leptomeninges** ("lepto" means thin and fine in Greek). There are several differences in the meninges covering the brain and spinal cord, and accordingly, they are discussed separately. The meninges consist of fibroblasts and collagen fibrils. The amount of collagen varies in different meningeal layers. For example, the dura mater contains copious amounts of collagen fibrils, while the arachnoid mater has no collagen.

COVERINGS OF THE BRAIN

DURA MATER

The cranial dura mater (Fig. 3-1) is a tough, fibrous membrane consisting of two connective tissue layers: an external periosteal layer and an inner meningeal layer. These two layers are fused together except where the dural venous sinuses are located (e.g., superior sagittal sinus). The **periosteal** layer of the dura mater adheres to the inner surface of the skull bone and is highly vascular and innervated. There is no space between the dura and the cranium (Fig. 3-1B). Thus, the **cranial epidural space** is a potential space that becomes filled with a fluid only in pathological conditions. The cranial epidural space (when present) is located between the periosteal layer of the dura and the cranium. The **meningeal** layer of the dura is smooth and avascular and is lined by mesothelium (a single layer of squamous-like, flattened cells) on its inner surface. At the **foramen magnum** (a large opening at the base of the occipital bone through which the medulla is continuous with the spinal cord), the meningeal layer of the cranial dura joins the spinal dura.

Sheet-like processes, called **septa**, extend from the meningeal layer of the dura deep into the cranial cavity, forming freely communicating compartments. The function of these septa is to reduce or prevent displacement of the brain when the head moves. One of the septa, the **falx cerebri**, is vertically oriented, divides the cranium into two lateral compartments, and separates the two cerebral hemispheres. The **tentorium cerebelli** is attached dorsally to the falx cerebri in the midline and posteriorly to the ridges of the occipital bone. Its rostral edge is free and forms the boundary of the **tentorial notch** through which the midbrain traverses. The tentorium cerebelli forms a tent-like roof over the posterior cranial fossa. The occipital lobes lie on the dorsal surface of the tentorium cerebelli, while the dorsal surface of the cerebellum lies inferior to it. The **falx cerebelli** consists of a vertically oriented triangular projection into the posterior fossa. It separates partially the cerebellar hemispheres located in the posterior fossa.

The anterior part of the dura is supplied by the anterior meningeal arteries (which arise from the anterior ethmoidal branches of the ophthalmic arteries); the posterior part is supplied by the branches of the vertebral and occipital arteries; and the lateral aspect is supplied by the middle meningeal artery and its branches. Some of the branches of these vessels supply bones of the scalp. As a result of severe head injury, these vessels may become damaged, leading to a hematoma that can cause a variety of neurological deficits. The dura is drained by meningeal veins that travel parallel to the meningeal arteries. Further discussion of the vascular supply of the meninges is presented in Chapter 4.

ARACHNOID MATER

The location of arachnoid mater and the structures associated with it are shown in Figure 3-1. This membrane lies between the dura and pia mater. It is a delicate, avascular membrane and surrounds the brain loosely without projecting into sulci. The space between the arachnoid and pial membranes, called the **subarachnoid space**, is filled with **cerebrospinal fluid** (CSF). The formation and distribution of CSF are described later in this chapter. Fine strands of connective tissue, called **arachnoid trabeculae**, arise from the arachnoid, span the subarachnoid space, and then connect with the pia. These trabeculae help to keep the brain suspended within the meninges. At several places in the cranial cavity, the subarachnoid space is enlarged; these enlargements are called subarachnoid **cisterns**. The **cerebellomedullary cistern**, located between the medulla and the cerebellum, is the largest cistern and is accordingly called the **cisterna magna** (Fig. 3-1). To identify pathological processes, such as those caused by tumors in the brain, it is essential to use radiological procedures to visualize subarachnoid cisterns adjacent to the suspected site of the pathological process. For example, the **chiasmatic cistern** is located adjacent to the optic chiasm (Fig. 3-1), so to identify pathological processes adjacent to the optic chiasm, radiological visualization of the chiasmatic cistern may be necessary.

Small tufts of arachnoidal tissue, called arachnoid villi, project into the superior sagittal sinus

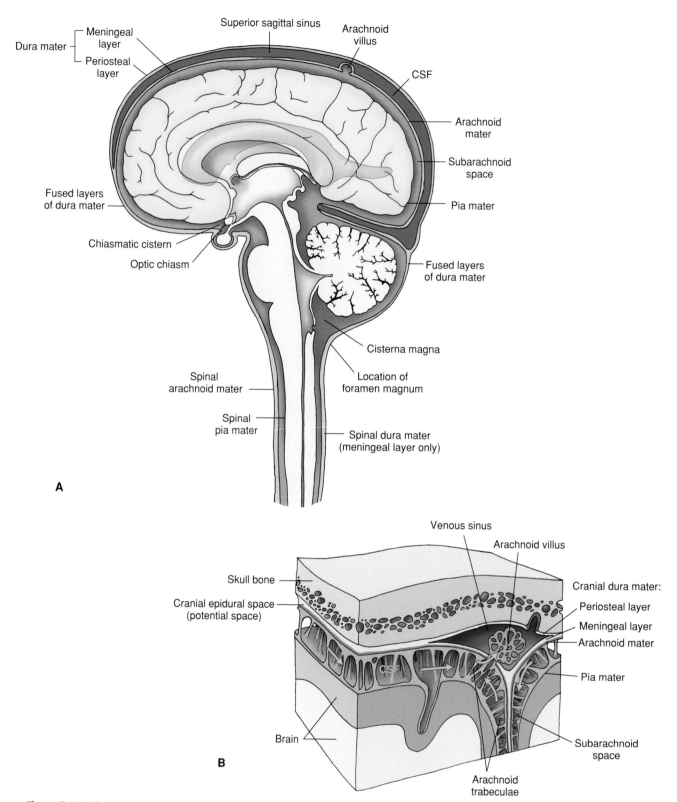

Figure 3–1 The coverings of the brain and spinal cord. (A) The brain and spinal cord are covered with three membranes: dura, arachnoid, and pia mater. The periosteal and meningeal layers of the dura are separate at the dural sinuses (e.g., superior sagittal sinus). At other places, the dura consists of fused periosteal and meningeal layers. The space between the arachnoid and pial membranes is called the subarachnoid space. The subarachnoid space is enlarged at some places (e.g., cisterna magna and chiasmatic cistern). Small tufts of arachnoidal tissue (arachnoid villi) project into the dural venous sinuses. Other structures are shown for orientation purposes. (B) Magnified view of the dura, arachnoid, and pia maters.

(Fig. 3-1) and other **dural sinuses**. Large aggregations of arachnoid villi are called **arachnoid granulations**. The arachnoid villi consist of a spongy tissue with many interconnecting small tubules and function as one-way valves. The CSF flows from the subarachnoid space into the dural venous sinuses through arachnoid villi, but the blood from the dural venous sinuses cannot flow back into the subarachnoid space via these villi. Normally, the pressure in the subarachnoid space is greater (about 200 mm H_2O) than that in the dural venous sinuses (about 80 mm H_2O); this pressure difference promotes the CSF flow into the dural venous sinuses through the fine tubules located in the arachnoid villi. However, even if the pressure in the dural venous sinuses exceeds that of the subarachnoid space, the blood from the dural sinuses does not flow back into the subarachnoid space because the tubules in the arachnoid villi collapse.

PIA MATER

The location of pia mater is shown in Figure 3-1. This membrane is the innermost layer of the meninges. It is tightly attached to the surface of the brain and projects into the fissures as well as sulci. Pia mater consists of small plexuses of blood vessels that are embedded in connective tissue and is externally covered with mesothelial cells (a single layer of flattened cells). When small branches of blood vessels penetrate the brain tissue, they carry with them a cuff of pia and arachnoid into the brain for a short distance creating a small space, called the **perivascular space**, around the vessel. This space is continuous with the subarachnoid space. It has been suggested that the perivascular space may serve as a channel for movement of CSF into the brain tissue, but its exact function has not been established with certainty.

COVERINGS OF THE SPINAL CORD

The conical-shaped caudal end of the spinal cord, known as the **conus medullaris**, is located at the caudal edge of the first or rostral edge of the second lumbar vertebra (Fig. 3-2). A thin filament enclosed in pia and consisting of ependymal cells and astrocytes (for the description of these cells, see Chapter 5) emerges from the conus medullaris. This filament is called the **filum terminale internum**. It extends from the conus medullaris and passes through the caudal end of the dural sac (which ends at the second sacral vertebra). At this level (S2), a caudal thin extension of the spinal dura, called the **coccygeal ligament (filum terminale externum)** surrounds the filum terminale. It emerges and anchors the dural sac to the vertebral canal.

The spinal cord is also covered by three membranes: the spinal dura, arachnoid, and pia mater (Fig. 3-2C). These coverings are generally similar to those of the brain. However, there are some differences. First, the spinal dura is single-layered and lacks the periosteal layer of the cranial dura. Second, the spinal epidural space is an actual space in which venous plexuses are located and is used clinically for the administration of epidural anesthesia to produce a paravertebral nerve block. (The cranial epidural space is a potential space that becomes filled with a fluid only in pathological conditions.) Third, the spinal epidural space is located between the meningeal layer of the dura (there is no periosteal layer) and the periosteum of the vertebra, whereas the cranial **epidural space** (when present) is located between the periosteal layer of the dura and the cranium.

SPINAL DURA MATER

The spinal dura mater consists of only the meningeal layer and lacks the periosteal layer of the cranial dura. Rostrally, the spinal dura joins the meningeal layer of the cranial dura (Fig. 3-1) at the margins of the foramen magnum. The spinal epidural space separates the spinal dura from the periosteum of the vertebra and is filled with fatty connective tissue and plexuses of veins. Caudally, the spinal dura ends at the level of the second sacral vertebra (Fig. 3-2A). As mentioned earlier, at this level, it becomes a thin extension (the coccygeal ligament or filum terminale externum) and serves to anchor the fluid-filled spinal dural sac to the base of the vertebral canal.

SPINAL ARACHNOID MATER

The spinal arachnoid mater invests the spinal cord and is connected to the dura via connective tissue trabeculae (Fig. 3-2C). Rostrally, it passes through the foramen magnum to join the cranial arachnoid, and caudally it surrounds the cauda equina. The **cauda equina** consists of a bundle of nerve roots of all the spinal nerves caudal to the second lumbar vertebra (Fig. 3-2B).

SPINAL PIA MATER

The spinal pia mater (Fig. 3-2C) is thicker compared with the cranial pia mater. It is a vascular membrane and projects into the ventral fissure of the spinal cord. At intervals, toothed ligaments of pial tissue, called **dentate ligaments**, extend from the lateral surfaces of the spinal cord; these ligaments serve to anchor the spinal cord to the arachnoid and the inner surface of the dura.

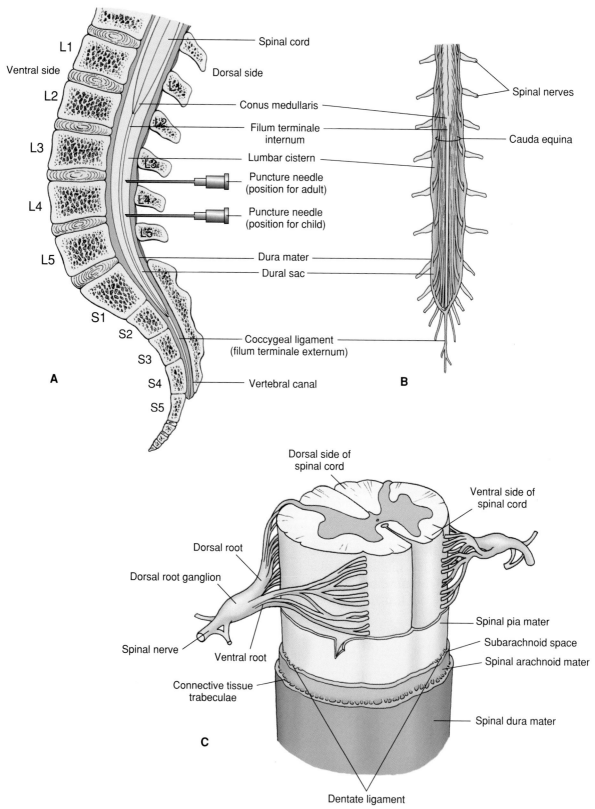

Figure 3–2 The spinal cord. (A) The lumbar cistern extends from the caudal end of the spinal cord (conus medullaris) to the second sacral vertebra (S2). The subarachnoid space (widest in this region) contains the filum terminale internum (a thin filament). (B) The subarachnoid space in the lumbar cistern also contains the cauda equina (a bundle of nerve roots of all the spinal nerves caudal to the second lumbar vertebra). (C) The three membranes of the spinal cord: the dura, arachnoid, and pia mater. The dorsal and ventral sides of the spinal cord, spinal nerves, the dorsal and ventral roots of the spinal nerves, and dorsal root ganglion are shown for orientation purposes.

LUMBAR CISTERN

The lumbar cistern extends from the caudal end of the spinal cord to the second sacral vertebra. The subarachnoid space (Fig. 3-2) is widest in this region and contains the filum terminale internum and nerve roots of the cauda equina. Because of the large size of the subarachnoid space and relative absence of neural structures, this space is most suitable for the withdrawal of CSF by lumbar puncture. This procedure is used to gain specific information about the cellular and chemical composition of the CSF in disorders such as meningitis. As noted earlier, the caudal end of the spinal cord in the normal adult is located at the caudal end of the first (L1) or rostral edge of the second (L2) lumbar vertebra. Therefore, a needle for lumbar puncture is usually inserted between the third and fourth lumbar vertebrae (L3-L4) in the adult patient.

In children, the caudal end of the spinal cord is usually located at the third lumbar vertebra (L3). Therefore, the needle for lumbar puncture is inserted at the L4-L5 level in children (Fig. 3-2A). Usually 5 to 15 mL of the CSF is removed during the lumbar puncture to perform the cell count, protein analysis, and microbiological studies. For the procedure of lumbar puncture, the patient is placed in a lateral recumbent position, and the CSF pressure is measured by a manometer. Normally, the CSF pressure is between 100 and 150 mm H_2O ($<$ 200 mm H_2O) in the adult person and between 60 and 150 mm H_2O ($<$ 180 mm H_2O) in young children and infants. If the intracranial pressure (ICP) is high, withdrawal of CSF is contraindicated because brain tissue may get herniated through the foramen magnum.

BRAIN VENTRICULAR SYSTEM

Four cavities, known as **ventricles**, are present in the brain (Fig. 3-3A), including two **lateral** ventricles and the **third** and **fourth** ventricles. Each lateral ventricle corresponds to the shape of the cerebral hemisphere in which it is located and consists of four basic components: the **anterior** (frontal) **horn** located in the frontal lobe, the **body** located in the parietal lobe, the **posterior** (occipital) **horn** located in the posterior lobe, and an **inferior horn** located more ventrally in the temporal lobe.

The two **lateral ventricles** are connected with the third ventricle through two short channels called the **interventricular foramina** or **foramina of Monro** (Fig. 3-3A). The **third ventricle** forms the medial surface of the thalamus and the hypothalamus (see Chapter 1). The floor of the third ventricle is formed by a portion of the hypothalamus. Anteriorly, a thin plate or wall, called the **organum vasculosum lamina terminalis** (OVLT) forms the anterior limit of the third ventricle (Fig. 3-3B). Thus, the third ventricle occupies the midline region of the diencephalon. The third ventricle is connected with the fourth ventricle via a narrow and relatively short channel, called the **cerebral aqueduct** (**aqueduct of Sylvius**) (Fig. 3-3A). The cerebral aqueduct traverses throughout the rostro-caudal extent of the mesencephalon (see Chapter 1).

The **fourth ventricle** is located posterior to the pons and upper half of the medulla and ventral to the cerebellum. Its floor is flat and rhomboid-shaped (sometimes referred to as rhomboid-fossa), and its roof is tent-shaped, with the peak of the tent (the fastigium) projecting into the cerebellum. The fourth ventricle communicates with the subarachnoid space via two lateral apertures, called the **foramina of Luschka**, and one medial aperture, the **foramen of Magendie** (Fig. 3-3A). At the caudal end of the fourth ventricle, a small **central canal** extends throughout the spinal cord but is patent only in the upper cervical segments.

THE CHOROID PLEXUS

A **choroid plexus**, which produces CSF, is present in each ventricle. In each lateral ventricle, the choroid plexus is located in the medial wall and extends from the tip of the inferior horn to the interventricular foramina (Fig. 3-3A). In the third and fourth ventricles, the choroid plexus is located in the roof (Fig. 3-3A). A choroid plexus consists of three layers of membranes: (1) an endothelial layer of the choroidal capillary wall, which has fenestrations (openings), (2) a pial membrane, and (3) a layer of choroidal epithelial cells that contain numerous mitochondria and have many basal infoldings and microvilli on the surface facing the inside of the ventricle. **Tight junctions** (see *Cerebrospinal Fluid Formation* section below) exist between adjacent choroidal epithelial cells.

CEREBROSPINAL FLUID

FORMATION

About 70% of the CSF present in the brain and spinal cord is produced by the choroid plexuses. The remaining 30% of CSF, which is secreted by the parenchyma of the brain, crosses the ependyma (a single layer of ciliated columnar epithelial cells lining the ventricular system) and enters the ventricles. The formation of CSF is an active process involving the enzyme carbonic anhydrase and specific transport mechanisms.

The formation of the CSF first involves filtration of the blood through the fenestrations of the en-

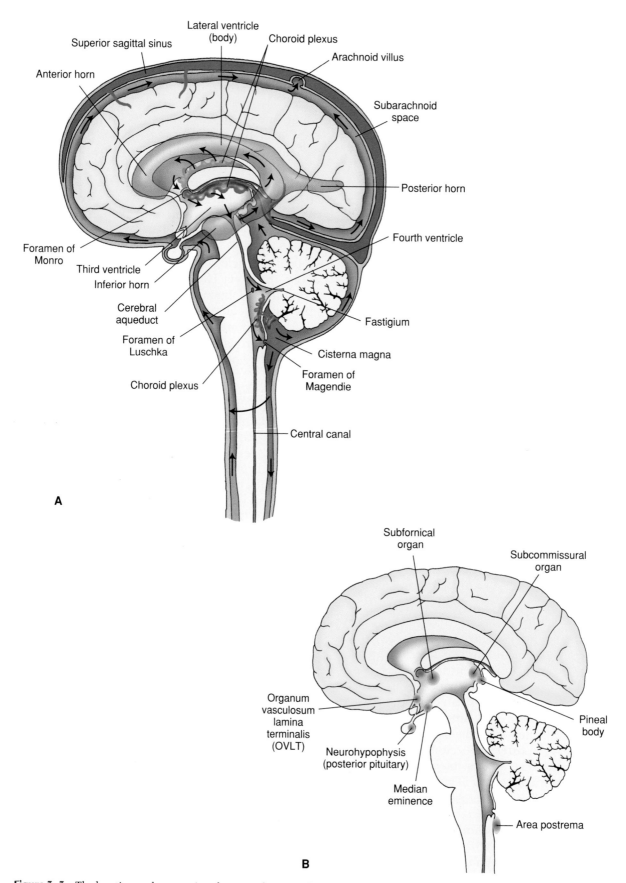

Figure 3–3 The location and connections between the ventricles of the brain. (A) Note the lateral ventricles (consisting of anterior, posterior, and inferior horns) and the third and fourth ventricles. Also, note the positioning of the choroid plexus. Black arrows indicate the flow of CSF. (B) The location of circumventricular organs.

dothelial cells that line the choroidal capillaries. However, the movement of peptides, proteins, and other larger molecules from this filtrate into the CSF is prevented by the tight junctions that exist in the neighboring epithelial cells that form the outer layer of the choroid plexus. Energy-dependent active transport mechanisms are present in the choroidal epithelium for transporting Na^+ and Mg^{2+} ions into the CSF and for removing K^+ and Ca^{2+} ions from the CSF. Water flows across the epithelium for maintaining the osmotic balance. Normally, the rate of formation of CSF is about 500 mL/day and the total volume of CSF is 90 to 140 mL, of which about 23 mL is in the ventricles, and the remaining is in the subarachnoid space.

CIRCULATION

The movement of CSF is pulsatile. It flows from the lateral ventricles into the third ventricle through the foramina of Monro (Fig. 3-3A; the direction of flow is indicated by arrows) where it mixes with more CSF. Then, it flows through the cerebral aqueduct (aqueduct of Sylvius) into the fourth ventricle, where additional CSF is secreted. The fluid leaves the ventricular system via the foramina of Luschka and Magendie and enters the **cerebellomedullary cistern (cisterna magna)**. The CSF then travels rostrally over the cerebral hemisphere where it enters the **arachnoid villi** (Fig. 3-1A). The arachnoid villi allow flow of CSF into the dural venous sinuses but do not allow flow in the opposite direction because the pressure in the subarachnoid space is higher (about 200 mm H_2O) compared with the pressure in the dural venous sinuses (about 80 mm H_2O). The CSF in the cerebellomedullary cistern also flows downward into the spinal subarachnoid space and then ascends along the ventral surface of the spinal cord into the basal part of the brain where it courses dorsally to empty into the dural sinuses (Fig. 3-1A).

FUNCTIONS

There are four main functions of the CSF. (1) The brain and spinal cord float in the CSF because the specific gravities of these central nervous system (CNS) structures are approximately the same. This buoyant effect of the CSF results in reduction of traction exerted upon the nerves and blood vessels connected with the CNS. (2) The CSF provides a cushioning effect on the CNS and dampens the effects of trauma. (3) The CSF also serves as a vehicle for removal of metabolites from the CNS. (4) Under normal conditions, the CSF provides a stable ionic environment for the CNS. However, the chemical composition of the CSF may change in certain situations such as administration of drugs that cross the blood-brain barrier.

COMPOSITION

Normally, very little protein is present in the CSF, and this is the primary difference between CSF and blood serum. The concentrations of glucose, as well as Ca^{2+} and K^+ ions, are slightly smaller in the CSF, and the concentrations of Na^+, Cl^-, and Mg^{2+} ions are slightly greater when compared with that of serum (Table 3-1).

Alteration of the Cerebrospinal Fluid in Pathological Conditions

Normally, the CSF is a clear and colorless fluid. However, it may be colored in pathological states. For example, xanthochromia (yellow color) of the CSF results several hours after subarachnoid hemorrhage when red blood cells undergo lysis and the liberated hemoglobin is broken down into bilirubin, which imparts a yellow color to the CSF. Because CSF is sterile, the results of microbiological studies on normal CSF should be negative, with a normal sample of CSF containing up to 5 lymphocytes/μL and no red blood cells (RBCs). Thus, an increased white blood cell (WBC) count in CSF is indicative of disease (e.g., **bacterial meningitis** or **viral encephalitis**). Gamma globulin levels are elevated in CSF of patients with multiple sclerosis (a disorder associated with localized areas of demyelination in the white matter of the CNS) or chronic infections of the CNS. CSF glucose level is low in acute bacterial and chronic fungal infections of the CNS. Increased glycolysis by polymorphonuclear leukocytes in these conditions may be responsible for decreased glucose levels. In contrast, CSF glucose levels are frequently normal in viral infections of the CNS. Alterations in the composition of CSF in some pathological states are listed in Table 3-2.

Table 3–1 Composition of Serum and CSF

Constituent	Serum	CSF
Protein (g/L)	60–78	0.15–0.45
Glucose (mmol/L)	3.9–5.8	2.2–3.9
Ca^{2+} (mmol/L)	2.1–2.5	1–1.35
K^+ (mmol/L)	4–5	2.8–3.2
Na^+ (mmol/L)	136–146	147–151
Cl^- (mmol/L)	98–106	118–132
Mg^{2+} (mmol/L)	0.65–1.05	0.78–1.26

CSF = cerebrospinal fluid.

Table 3–2 Alterations in CSF Composition in Some Pathological Conditions

Pathological Condition	Protein	Glucose	Cells
Subarachnoid hemorrhage	Increased (+)	Normal	Presence of RBC
Guillain-Barré syndrome	Increased (++)	Normal	Presence of a few WBC
Metastatic cancer in the meninges	Increased (+)	Normal or decreased	Presence of increased number of WBC (lymphocytes) Tumor cells
Viral meningitis	Increased (+)	Normal	Presence of excessive number of WBC (lymphocytes)
Tubercular meningitis	Increased (+)	Decreased	Presence of increased number of WBC (lymphocytes)
Bacterial meningitis	Increased (+)	Decreased	Presence of increased number of WBC (polymorphonuclear leukocytes)

CSF = cerebrospinal fluid; RBC = red blood cells; WBC = white blood cells.
Plus sign (+) indicates increase. Relatively greater increase is shown by two plus signs (++).

THE BLOOD-BRAIN BARRIER AND BLOOD-CSF BARRIER

Large molecules cannot pass from the blood into the interstitial fluid of the CNS. This is due to the existence of the **blood-brain barrier,** which is located at the interface between the capillary wall and brain tissue. The blood-brain barrier consists of: (1) endothelial cells lining the capillary wall with tight junctions between them, (2) processes of astrocytes abutting on the capillaries as perivascular end-feet (see Chapter 5), and (3) a capillary basement membrane. This arrangement of different cells or their processes prevents the passage of large molecules from the blood into the extracellular space between the neurons and neuroglia and forms the anatomical basis of the blood-brain barrier. One of the beneficial functions of the blood-brain barrier is to prevent entry of blood-borne foreign substances into the brain tissue. However, the existence of this blood-brain barrier also presents a problem when the goal is to deliver drugs into the CNS. In other organs, tight junctions do not exist between the neighboring endothelial cells lining the capillaries.

Large molecules cannot pass from the blood into the CSF. This is due to the presence of a **blood-CSF barrier**. In the choroid plexus, tight junctions do not exist between the neighboring endothelial cells lining the capillary wall. Unlike in other parts of the CNS, the capillary endothelium in the choroid plexuses is fenestrated. Therefore, large molecules can pass from blood through the capillary endothelium of the choroid plexus. However, the choroidal plexus has an outermost layer of epithelial cells. Tight junctions exist between choroidal epithelial cells that prevent large molecules in the blood from entering the CSF.

There are seven structures in the CNS that lack a blood-brain barrier. Called **circumventricular organs,** they are the **area postrema, pineal body, subcommissural organ, subfornical organ, organum vasculosum of lamina terminalis (OVLT), neurohypophysis** (the posterior pituitary gland), and the **median eminence** (Fig. 3-3B). They lack tight junctions in their capillaries. Instead, they have fenestrated capillaries, capillary loops, and large perivascular spaces that permit the passage of larger circulating molecules into the adjacent brain tissue. It is believed that some circulating hormones consisting of large molecules reach their target areas in the brain via the circumventricular organs. For example, the subfornical organ lies in the roof of the third ventricle. Blood-borne angiotensin II reaches the subfornical organ readily because of the lack of the blood-brain barrier in this organ and induces thirst for overall regulation of fluid balance and cardiovascular homeostasis.

DISORDERS OF THE CSF SYSTEM

Hydrocephalus

Dilation of the ventricles (or **hydrocephalus**) occurs when the circulation of CSF is blocked or its absorption is impeded, while the CSF formation continues to occur at a constant rate. This results in an increase in ventricular pressure that, in turn, causes ventricular dilation. The ventricular dilation exerts pressure on the adjacent tissue, causing impairment of such structures as the corticobulbar and corticospinal tracts. Therefore, a progressive loss of motor function ensues. Hydrocephalus may occur before birth and is usually noted during the first few months of life.

When movement of CSF out of the ventricular system is impeded (e.g., by blockage at the cerebral aqueduct or foramina of the fourth ventricle), the ensuing hydrocephalus is classified as a **noncommunicating hydrocephalus**. If the movement of the CSF into the dural venous sinuses is impeded or blocked by an obstruction at the arachnoid villi, hydrocephalus developed in this manner is called a **communicating hydrocephalus**. In communicating hydrocephalus, a tracer dye injected into the lateral ventricle appears in the lumbar CSF, indicating that there is no obstruction to the flow of CSF in the ventricular or extraventricular pathways. On the other hand, in noncommunicating hydrocephalus, a tracer dye injected into the lateral ventricle does not appear in the lumbar CSF, indicating that there is an obstruction to the flow of CSF in the ventricular pathways.

Increase in Intracranial Pressure

The craniovertebral cavity and its dural lining form a closed space. An increase in the size or volume of any constituent of the cranial cavity results in an increase in intracranial pressure (ICP). For example, the ICP may increase in the following situations: (1) when the total volume of brain tissue is increased by diffuse cerebral edema; (2) when regional increase in the volume of brain tissue results from an intracerebral hemorrhage or tumors; (3) when the CSF volume increases due to an obstruction in its flow; and (4) when a venous obstruction causes an increase in blood volume in the brain tissue.

The following symptoms may accompany increased ICP: headache (due to stretching of cranial pain-sensitive mechanisms), nausea and vomiting (due to the activation of a **chemoreceptor trigger zone** located near the **area postrema**), bradycardia (due to the increased pressure on the **nucleus ambiguus** and **dorsal motor nucleus of vagus in the medulla**), an increase in systemic blood pressure (due to the increased pressure on the ventrolateral medulla where vasomotor centers are located), and loss of consciousness. Nucleus ambiguus and the dorsal motor nucleus of vagus contain **preganglionic parasympathetic neurons** whose axons travel in the vagus nerve

and provide parasympathetic innervation to the heart. An elevation and blurring of the optic disk margin (**papilledema**) may occur due to increased pressure in the subarachnoid space along the optic nerve.

CLINICAL CASE

HISTORY

Charles is a 77-year-old man who has been having gait problems and urinary incontinence for the past 6 months. Although he was reluctant to see a physician, his daughter persevered and brought him to a neurologist. His daughter believed that his condition was worsening because, in the past month or so, she noticed that his short-term memory was deteriorating and that he was receiving notices from collection agencies for unpaid or incorrectly paid bills. The gait problem manifested itself as difficulty with climbing stairs and frequent, unexplained falls. During the Korean War, Charles had suffered a subarachnoid hemorrhage as a result of his close proximity to an exploding grenade. The neurologist was informed by the patient's daughter that, until the recent events, Charles had been an active, healthy, intelligent, and coherent person.

EXAMINATION

When the neurologist asked Charles to remember three random, unrelated objects, he was unable to recall any of them after 5 minutes. He did not know how many quarters are in $1.75, and he incorrectly spelled the word "world." A grasp reflex (squeezing the examiner's hand as a reflex reaction to stroking of the palm) was present. Although motor strength was normal in his arms and legs bilaterally, when asked to walk, Charles took many steps in the same place without moving forward and then started to fall. His cranial nerve, sensory, and cerebellar examinations were normal.

EXPLANATION

This case is an example of a condition called normal pressure hydrocephalus. Various meningeal and ependymal conditions, such as chronic meningitis and prior subarachnoid hemorrhages, may cause this condition by initially blocking CSF absorption. As a result, formation of CSF diminishes slightly, but so does its absorption. The ventricles compensate by enlarging due to the initial higher pressure, as well as the larger volume of CSF, and a new equilibrium is attained. If there is continued obstruction, this process will repeat itself. As a result, the force exerted by the larger ventricles causes hydrostatic impairment to the nerve fiber tracts in the central white matter surrounding the ventricles. The frontal lobe white matter absorbs maximal ventricular expansion with preservation of the cortical gray matter and subcortical structures. As a result, patients with normal pressure hydrocephalus have abnormal frontal lobe function, including gait apraxia (dysfunction of gait not explained by weakness, cerebellar problems, or sensory problems), urinary incontinence without bladder dysfunction, and dementia. Frontal lobe dysfunction may also cause the reappearance of primitive reflexes, which normally disappear shortly after birth, such as the grasp reflex, because this brain region normally suppresses them. Later, urinary incontinence may also manifest itself in a manner similar to that of a young child, where the patient may be indifferent to it. Headaches are rare in this particular type of hydrocephalus because ventricular expansion is slow, and increased ICP is transient. The symptoms of this disorder (e.g., incontinence, gait apraxia, and dementia) are commonly referred to as the 3Ws (wet, wobbly, and weird).

Normal pressure hydrocephalus is usually diagnosed through a neurologic examination, computed tomography (CT), or magnetic resonance imaging (MRI) of the brain and neuropsychological testing. The imaging studies of the brain show enlarged ventricles and occasionally interstitial fluid within the white matter adjacent to the lateral ventricles. Measurement of CSF pressures with a lumbar puncture (normal) and radionuclide cisternography (a procedure where a radionuclide is injected into the CSF and distribution is observed over a period of 24 hours) may be helpful but are not always necessary. Occasionally, shunting procedures allowing the CSF to drain into the peritoneal cavity or the bloodstream are helpful if performed early in the course of this condition.

CHAPTER TEST

QUESTIONS

Choose the best answer for each question.

1. A 50-year-old man was admitted to the emergency room after a head injury resulting from an automobile accident. The patient was diagnosed as having a subarachnoid hemorrhage. Which of the following changes are most likely in the composition of the cerebrospinal fluid of this patient?
   a. Decreased protein, normal glucose, and presence of a few WBCs
   b. Increased protein, normal glucose, and presence of RBCs
   c. Increased protein, decreased glucose, and presence of polymorphonuclear leukocytes
   d. Decreased protein, normal glucose, and presence of a small number of lymphocytes
   e. Decreased protein, decreased glucose, and presence of tumor cells

2. An adult male suffering from chills, fever, headache, nausea, vomiting, and pain in the back was admitted to the emergency room and diagnosed as having meningococcal meningitis. Which of the following changes are most likely in the composition of the cerebrospinal fluid of this patient?
   a. Increased protein, decreased glucose, and increased polymorphonuclear WBCs
   b. Increased protein, normal glucose, and excessive number of lymphocytes
   c. Increased protein, normal glucose, and a few WBCs

   d. Increased protein, normal glucose, and presence of tumor cells and WBCs
   e. Increased protein, increased glucose, and a few WBCs

3. A 75-year-old man was admitted to the emergency room complaining that he had trouble walking and that he could not move his arms as well. An MRI revealed the presence of a brain tumor. Tracer dye injected into the lateral ventricle did not appear in the lumbar CSF, suggesting that the patient had developed a noncommunicating hydrocephalus. Which one of the following is the most likely location of the tumor?
   a. Interventricular foramen
   b. Cerebellar cortex
   c. Cerebral cortex
   d. Lateral thalamus
   e. Lateral medullary reticular formation

4. A 22-year-old man was admitted to the emergency room after a motorcycle accident. A clinical examination showed that he had an elevated intracranial pressure due to head trauma. The patient suffered from severe bradycardia. In which of the following brain regions would elevated intracranial pressure most likely cause bradycardia?
   a. Cerebral cortex
   b. Basal ganglia
   c. Brainstem
   d. Thalamus
   e. Cerebellum

5. The membranes that line the cisterns in the cranial cavity are:
   a. Dura and arachnoid mater
   b. Dura mater and ependymal cell layer
   c. Neuronal cell membrane and the pia mater
   d. Pia and arachnoid mater
   e. Periosteal and meningeal layers of dura mater

ANSWERS AND EXPLANATIONS

1. Answer: b

Normal CSF may contain a few lymphocytes and polymorphonuclear leukocytes, but it contains no RBCs. The presence of RBCs in CSF is characteristic of subarachnoid hemorrhage. In viral and tubercular meningitis and metastatic cancer, the CSF will show an increased number of lymphocytes, while the number of polymorphonuclear leukocytes is increased in bacterial meningitis. Most pathologic conditions do not decrease protein levels in the CSF; glucose level may be decreased in metastatic cancer and tubercular or bacterial meningitis. The presence of WBCs in the CSF occurs in pathologies other than subarachnoid hemorrhage (see Table 3-2).

2. Answer: a

Increased protein, decreased glucose, and increased polymorphonuclear WBCs are observed in the CSF of patients with bacterial meningitis. The glucose levels in CSF decrease because the bacteria present in CSF (usually meningococcus, pneumococcus and *Haemophilus influenzae* organisms) use glucose. The CSF glucose levels are low in tubercular meningitis also; however, in this condition, the cells in CSF are predominantly lymphocytes. In viral meningitis, the glucose levels in CSF remain normal because, in this condition, the viruses do not use glucose. In addition, the number of lymphocytes present in the CSF is excessive (see Table 3-2).

3. Answer: a

In patients suffering from hydrocephalus, the circulation of CSF is blocked or its absorption is impeded, while the CSF formation continues to occur. The ventricles dilate, and pressure is exerted on the adjacent tissue, causing impairment of such structures as the corticobulbar and corticospinal tracts. Therefore, a progressive loss of motor function ensues. Hydrocephalus that develops when the movement of CSF out of the ventricular system is impeded is called a noncommunicating hydrocephalus. In noncommunicating hydrocephalus, a tracer dye injected into the lateral ventricle does not appear in the lumbar CSF, indicating that there is an obstruction to the flow of CSF in the ventricular pathways. Therefore, of the structures listed as choices, the interventricular foramen is the most likely site where the tumor is present. If the movement of the CSF into the dural venous sinuses is impeded or blocked by an obstruction at the arachnoid villi, this type of hydrocephalus is called a communicating hydrocephalus. A tracer dye injected into the lateral ventricle in this condition does appear in the lumbar CSF, indicating that there is no obstruction to the flow of CSF in the ventricular or extraventricular pathways.

4. Answer: c

The craniovertebral cavity and its dural lining form a closed space. An increase in the size or volume of any constituent of the cranial cavity results in an increase in intracranial pressure (ICP). The following symptoms may accompany increased ICP: loss of consciousness, headache, nausea and vomiting, increase in systemic blood pressure, and bradycardia. The bradycardia (decrease in heart rate) is usually due to the increased pressure on the nucleus ambiguus and dorsal motor nucleus of vagus located in the medulla. The other brain structures listed are not involved in the control of heart rate.

5. Answer: d

The cisterns are formed by enlargements of subarachnoid space located between the pia and arachnoid mater. Other choices listed are not appropriate. For example, there is no space between the dura and arachnoid mater. Ependymal cells line the ventricles. There is no space between the pia and brain tissue; the pia mater is tightly attached to the brain. The periosteal and meningeal layers of the dura mater are fused except at the places where venous sinuses are located.

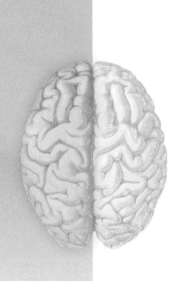

CHAPTER 4

BLOOD SUPPLY OF THE CENTRAL NERVOUS SYSTEM

OBJECTIVES

In this chapter, the student should be able to describe:

1. The major arteries (internal carotid and vertebral) and their prominent branches supplying the brain

2. The prominent neural structures supplied by these arteries

3. The cerebral arterial circle (circle of Willis)

4. The sinuses of the dura and the major veins draining the brain

5. The arterial blood supply and the venous drainage of the spinal cord

The central nervous system (CNS) represents one of the most metabolically active systems in the body. The metabolic demands of the brain must be met with the blood supply to this organ. Normal cerebral blood flow is about 50 mL/100 g of brain tissue/min. Thus, a brain of average weight (1400–1500 g) has a normal blood flow of 700–750 mL/min. Even a brief interruption of the blood supply to the CNS may result in serious neurological disturbances. A blood flow of 25 mL/100 g of brain tissue/min constitutes ischemic penumbra (a dangerously deficient blood supply leading to loss of brain cells). A blood flow of 8 mL/100 g of brain tissue/min leads to an almost complete loss of functional neurons. Consciousness is lost within 10 seconds of the cessation of blood supply to the brain. The effects of occlusion of different arteries supplying the CNS are described in Chapter 27. This chapter is focused on the arterial supply and venous drainage of the CNS.

ARTERIAL SUPPLY OF THE BRAIN

Blood supply to the brain is derived from two arteries: (1) the **internal carotid artery** and (2) the **vertebral artery**. These arteries and their branches arise in pairs that supply blood to both sides of the brain. The basilar artery (described later in the chapter) is a single artery located in the midline on the ventral side of the brain. The branches of the basilar artery also arise in pairs. The origin of the arteries supplying blood to the brain, their major branches, and the neural structures supplied by them are described in the following sections.

INTERNAL CAROTID ARTERY

This artery (Fig. 4-1) arises from the common carotid artery on each side at the level of the thyroid cartilage and enters the cranial cavity through the carotid canal. It penetrates the dura just ventral

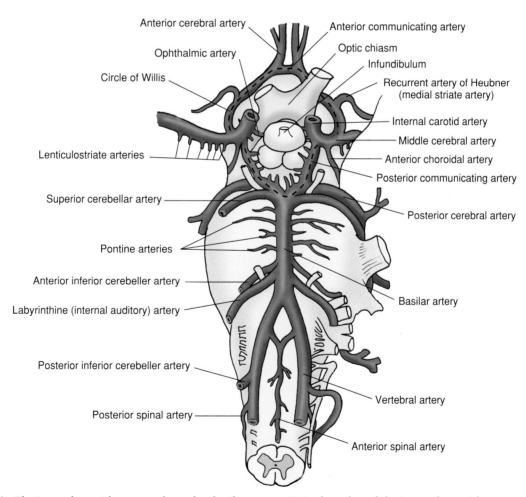

Figure 4–1 The internal carotid artery and vertebro-basilar system. Major branches of the **internal carotid** artery are the ophthalmic artery, the posterior communicating artery, the anterior choroidal artery, the anterior cerebral artery, and middle cerebral artery. The main branches of the **vertebral artery** are the anterior spinal artery and the posterior inferior cerebellar artery. The **basilar artery** is formed by the confluence of the two vertebral arteries; its major branches are the anterior inferior cerebellar artery, the pontine arteries, the superior cerebellar artery, and the posterior cerebral artery. Note the cerebral arterial circle (circle of Willis; marked by a thick dashed black line). The optic chiasm and infundibulum are shown for orientation purposes.

to the optic nerve. The main intracranial branches of each internal carotid artery are described in the next sections.

The Ophthalmic Artery

This artery (Fig. 4-1) enters the orbit through the optic foramen and gives rise to the **central artery of the retina,** which supplies the retina and cranial dura. Interruption of blood flow in the ophthalmic artery causes loss of vision in the **ipsilateral** eye.

The Posterior Communicating Artery

This artery (Fig. 4-1) arises at the level of the **optic chiasm** and travels posteriorly to join the posterior cerebral arteries. Small branches arising from this artery supply blood to the hypophysis, infundibulum, parts of the hypothalamus, thalamus, and hippocampus.

The Anterior Choroidal Artery

This artery (Fig. 4-1) arises near the optic chiasm and supplies the choroid plexus located in the **inferior horn of the lateral ventricle,** the **optic tract,** parts of the **internal capsule, hippocampal formation, globus pallidus,** and lateral portions of the thalamus.

The Anterior Cerebral Artery

At the level just lateral to the optic chiasm, the internal carotid artery divides into a smaller **anterior cerebral artery** and a larger middle cerebral artery (Fig. 4-1). The anterior cerebral artery travels rostrally through the interhemispheric fissure. It supplies blood to the medial aspect of the cerebral hemisphere, including parts of the frontal and parietal lobes. This artery also supplies blood to the postcentral gyrus (which is concerned with the processing of sensory information from the contralateral leg) and precentral gyrus (which is concerned with the motor control of the contralateral leg). Occlusion of one of the anterior cerebral arteries results in loss of motor control (paralysis) and loss of sensation in the contralateral leg. The symptoms associated with the occlusion of the anterior cerebral artery are consistent with the somatotopic representation of body parts in the cortex. The leg and foot are represented in the medial surface of the pre- and postcentral gyri. It should be noted that when the parts of the body are drawn in terms of the degree of their cortical representation (i.e., in the form of a somatotopic arrangement), the resulting disproportionate figure that is depicted is frequently called a **homunculus** (see Chapter 19 for more details). Other structures supplied by the anterior cerebral artery include the olfactory bulb and tract, anterior hypothalamus, parts of caudate nucleus, internal capsule, putamen, and septal nuclei.

The Anterior Communicating Artery

At the level of the optic chiasm, the **anterior communicating artery** connects the anterior cerebral arteries on the two sides (Fig. 4-1). A group of small arteries arising from the anterior communicating and anterior cerebral arteries penetrates the brain tissue almost perpendicularly and supplies blood to the anterior hypothalamus, including preoptic and suprachiasmatic areas. Intracranial aneurysms are often present (20–25% incidence) on the anterior communicating artery or the junction of this artery and the anterior cerebral artery. These aneurysms may cause visual deficits due to their proximity to the optic chiasm.

The Medial Striate Artery (Recurrent Artery of Heubner)

This artery (Fig. 4-1) arises from the anterior cerebral artery at the level of the optic chiasm and supplies blood to the anteromedial part of the head of the caudate nucleus and parts of the internal capsule, putamen, and septal nuclei. The medial striate and the lenticulostriate arteries penetrate the perforated substance.

The orbital branches: These branches (Fig. 4-2) arising from the anterior cerebral artery supply the orbital and medial surfaces of the frontal lobe.

The frontopolar branches: These branches (Fig. 4-2) of the anterior cerebral artery supply medial portions of the frontal lobe and lateral parts of the convexity of the hemisphere.

The callosomarginal artery: This artery (Fig. 4-2), arising from the anterior cerebral artery, supplies the paracentral lobule and portions of the cingulate gyrus.

The pericallosal artery: This artery (Fig. 4-2) continues caudally along the dorsal margin of the corpus callosum and supplies the precuneus (the portion of the parietal lobe caudal to the paracentral lobule).

The Middle Cerebral Artery

As mentioned earlier, the internal carotid artery divides into the smaller anterior cerebral artery and the larger **middle cerebral artery** (Figs. 4-1 and 4-3A) at the level just lateral to the optic chiasm. Branches of the middle cerebral artery supply blood to the lateral convexity of the cerebral hemisphere including parts of the temporal, frontal, parietal, and occipital lobes. The middle cerebral artery gives off the following major branches.

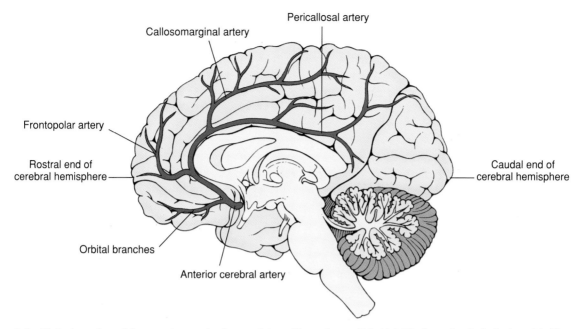

Figure 4–2 Major branches of the anterior cerebral artery (viewed from the medial side). The branches include the orbital branches, the frontopolar branches, the callosomarginal artery, and the pericallosal artery. The rostral and caudal ends of the cerebral hemisphere are shown for orientation purposes.

The lenticulostriate branches: This group of small arteries (Figs. 4-1 and 4-3A) are the first branches of the middle cerebral artery. They supply the putamen, caudate nucleus, and anterior limb of the internal capsule.

The orbitofrontal artery: It supplies parts of the frontal lobe (Fig. 4-3B).

The precentral (pre-Rolandic) and central (Rolandic) branches: These arteries (Fig. 4-3, A and B) supply different regions of the frontal lobe.

The anterior and posterior parietal arteries: These arteries (Fig. 4-3B) supply different regions of the parietal lobe.

The angular branch: This artery (Fig. 4-3B) supplies the **angular gyrus**.

The anterior, middle, and posterior temporal arteries: These arteries (Fig. 4-3, A and B) supply different regions of the temporal lobe. Branches of the posterior temporal artery also supply the lateral portions of the occipital lobe.

VERTEBRO-BASILAR CIRCULATION

This system includes the two **vertebral arteries**, the **basilar artery** (which is formed by the union of the two vertebral arteries), and their branches (Fig. 4-1). This arterial system supplies the medulla, pons, mesencephalon, and cerebellum. Different branches of the vertebral artery are described in the following sections.

THE VERTEBRAL ARTERY

The **vertebral artery** (Fig. 4-1) on each side is the first branch arising from the subclavian artery. It enters the transverse foramen of the sixth cervical vertebrae, ascends through these foramina in higher vertebra, and eventually enters the cranium through the foramen magnum. In the cranium, at the medullary level, each vertebral artery gives off the anterior spinal artery, the posterior inferior cerebellar artery, and the posterior spinal artery.

The Anterior Spinal Artery

At the confluence of the two vertebral arteries, two small branches arise and join to form a single anterior spinal artery (Fig. 4-1). This artery supplies the medial structures of the medulla, which include the pyramids, medial lemniscus, medial longitudinal fasciculus, hypoglossal nucleus, and the inferior olivary nucleus. It should be recalled that the axons contained within the pyramid originate in the cerebral cortex (see Chapter 1). At the caudal end of the medulla, near its juncture with the spinal cord, most of the fibers contained within the pyramid pass to the contralateral side through a commissure, the pyramidal decussation.

The Posterior Inferior Cerebellar Artery (PICA)

This artery (Fig. 4-1) arises from the vertebral artery and supplies the regions of the lateral medulla that include the spinothalamic tract, dorsal and ventral spinocerebellar tracts, descending sympathetic

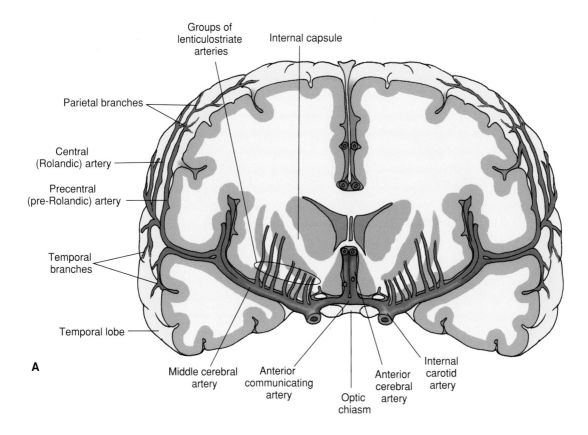

A

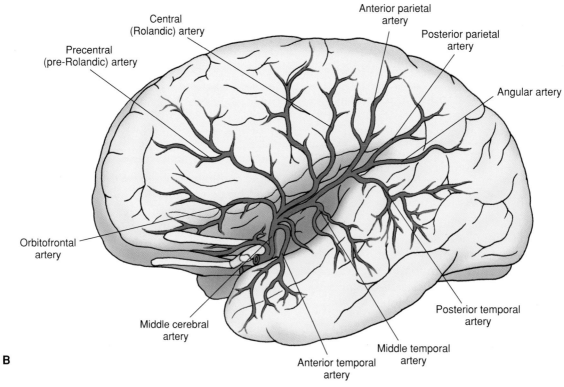

B

Figure 4–3 Major branches of the middle cerebral artery. (A) Coronal section showing some branches of the middle cerebral artery (the internal carotid, anterior cerebral, and anterior communicating arteries; optic chiasm, internal capsule, and temporal lobe of the brain are shown for orientation purposes). The main branches of the middle cerebral artery shown here are the group of lenticulostriate branches, and the precentral (pre-Rolandic), central (Rolandic), and temporal branches. (B) The branches of the middle cerebral artery. The major branches are the anterior, middle, and posterior temporal arteries; the angular artery; the posterior and anterior parietal arteries; the central (Rolandic) and precentral (pre-Rolandic) arteries; and the orbitofrontal arteries.

tract, descending tract of cranial nerve V, and nucleus ambiguus. Occlusion of this artery produces a Wallenberg's syndrome, which is characterized by damage to the lateral medulla where the nucleus ambiguus is located. Damage to the nucleus ambiguus, which provides innervation to laryngeal muscles, results in lack of coordination in speech (**dysphonia**), disturbance in articulation (**dysarthria**), and dysphagia (difficulty in swallowing). The PICA also supplies the vermal region and inferior-lateral surface of the cerebellar hemisphere.

The Posterior Spinal Artery (PSA)

It is the first branch of the vertebral artery in the cranium in about 25% of cases. However, in a majority of cases (75%), it arises from the posterior inferior cerebellar artery (Fig. 4-1). In the caudal medulla, this artery supplies the **fasciculus gracilis** and **cuneatus** as well as the gracile and cuneate nuclei, spinal trigeminal nucleus, dorsal and caudal portions of the inferior cerebellar peduncle, and portions of the solitary tract and dorsal motor nucleus of the vagus nerve.

THE BASILAR ARTERY

The two vertebral arteries join at the caudal border of the pons to form the single **basilar artery** (Fig. 4-1). The major branches of the basilar artery are described in the following sections.

The Anterior Inferior Cerebellar Artery (AICA)

The AICA is the most caudal branch arising from the basilar artery (Fig. 4-1). The **AICA** supplies the ventral and inferior surface of the cerebellum and lateral parts of the pons.

The Labyrinthine (Internal Auditory) Artery

The labyrinthine (internal auditory) artery (Fig. 4-1) is usually a branch of the AICA and supplies the cochlea and labyrinth.

The Pontine Arteries

Several pairs of pontine arteries (Fig. 4-1) arise from the basilar artery. Some pontine arteries (**the paramedian arteries**) enter the pons immediately and supply the medial portion of the lower and upper pons. The following structures are located in these regions: the pontine nuclei, corticopontine fibers, the corticospinal and corticobulbar tracts, and portions of the ventral pontine tegmentum, and medial lemniscus. Some pontine arteries (the **short circumferential arteries**) travel a short distance around the pons and supply substantia nigra and lateral portions of the midbrain tegmentum.

The Superior Cerebellar Artery

The superior cerebellar artery (Fig. 4-1) arises just caudal to the bifurcation of the basilar artery and supplies the rostral level of the pons, caudal part of the midbrain, and superior surface of the cerebellum. This artery supplies the following structures: portions of the superior and middle cerebellar peduncles, the medial and lateral lemniscus, part of the spinal trigeminal nucleus and tract, the spinothalamic tract, and superior cerebellar peduncle.

Posterior Cerebral Arteries

The posterior cerebral arteries arise at the terminal bifurcation of the basilar artery (Fig. 4-1). Branches of the **posterior cerebral arteries** (Fig. 4-4) supply most of the midbrain, thalamus, and subthalamic nucleus. The major branches arising from this artery after it passes around the midbrain (anterior and posterior temporal and parieto-occipital branches) supply the temporal lobes and medial and inferior occipital lobes of the cerebral cortex. The branch called the **calcarine artery** supplies the **primary visual cortex**.

CEREBRAL ARTERIAL CIRCLE (CIRCLE OF WILLIS)

The **cerebral arterial circle** (Fig. 4-1) surrounds the optic chiasm and the infundibulum of the pituitary. It is formed by the anastomosis of the branches of the internal carotid artery and the terminal branches of the basilar artery. The **anterior communicating artery** connects the two anterior cerebral arteries, thus forming a semicircle. The circle is completed as the **posterior communicating arteries** arising from the **internal carotid arteries** at the level of the optic chiasm travel posteriorly to join the **posterior cerebral arteries** that are formed by the bifurcation of the basilar artery. The circle of Willis is patent in only 20% of individuals. When it is patent, this arterial system supplies the hypothalamus, hypophysis, infundibulum, thalamus, caudate nucleus, putamen, internal capsule, globus pallidus, choroid plexus (lateral ventricles), and temporal lobe. When the blood flow in either the internal carotid arteries or vertebro-basilar system is reduced, collateral circulation in the circle of Willis provides blood to the deprived brain regions.

ARTERIES OF THE DURA

Meningeal arteries arise from the internal carotid artery as it passes through the cavernous sinus. The primary arterial supply to the dura is

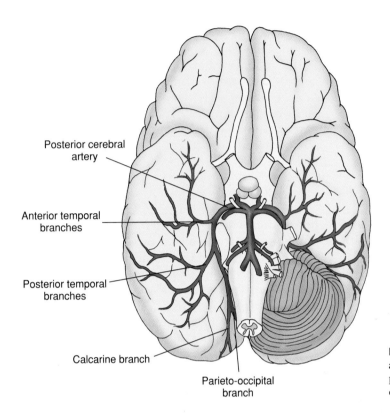

Posterior cerebral
artery

Anterior temporal
branches

Posterior temporal
branches

Calcarine branch

Parieto-occipital
branch

Figure 4–4 Major branches of the posterior cerebral artery. These include the anterior and posterior temporal branches, the parieto-occipital branch, and the calcarine branch.

provided by the **middle meningeal artery.** The anterior meningeal arteries supply the dura located in the anterior fossa, and the posterior meningeal arteries supply the dura located in the posterior fossa.

VENOUS DRAINAGE OF THE BRAIN

The brain is drained by a system of veins that empty into the **dural sinuses.** The sinuses empty into the right and left internal jugular veins.

THE SINUSES

The Superior Sagittal Sinus

The superior sagittal sinus (Fig. 4-5, A and B) lies along the superior border of falx cerebri and empties into the confluence of sinuses.

The Inferior Sagittal Sinus

The inferior sagittal sinus (Fig. 4-5B) lies in the inferior border of the falx cerebri. The **great cerebral vein of Galen** joins the **inferior sagittal sinus** to form the **straight sinus** (Fig. 4-5B) that runs caudally and empties into the caudal end of the superior sagittal sinus at the level of the confluence of sinuses.

The Transverse Sinuses

The transverse sinuses (Fig. 4-5, A and B) originate on each side of the **confluence of sinuses.** Each **transverse sinus** travels laterally and rostrally and curves downward to form the **sigmoid sinus** that empties into the **internal jugular vein** on the same side (Fig. 4-5A).

The Confluence of Sinuses

At this site, the superior sagittal, straight, transverse, and occipital sinuses join (Fig. 4-5, A and B). The occipital sinus ascends from the foramen magnum.

The Cavernous Sinuses

The cavernous sinuses are located on each side of the sphenoid bone. Ophthalmic and superficial middle cerebral veins drain into these sinuses.

The Sphenoparietal Sinuses

The sphenoparietal sinuses are located below the sphenoid bone and drain into the cavernous sinus.

THE CEREBRAL VEINS

The cerebral veins are usually divided into the superficial cerebral veins and the deep cerebral veins.

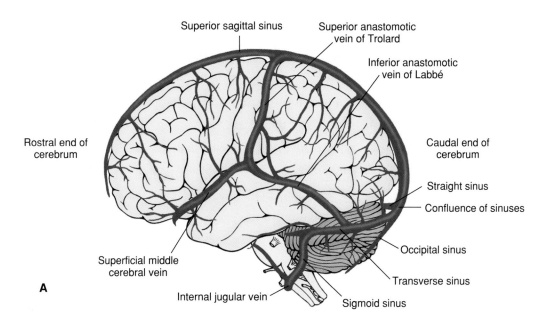

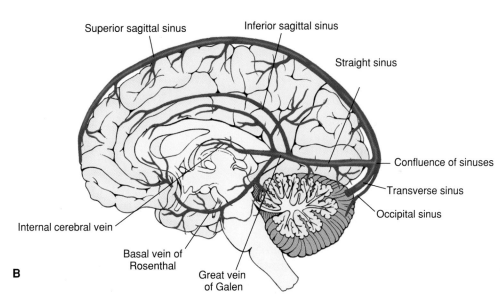

Figure 4–5 Major dural sinuses and veins. (A) Major dural sinuses shown here include the superior sagittal, straight, occipital, transverse, and sigmoid sinus. The superior sagittal, straight, transverse, and occipital sinuses join at the confluence of sinuses. Major veins include the superficial middle cerebral vein, the superior anastomotic vein of Trolard, and the inferior anastomotic vein of Labbé. (B) Major dural sinuses shown here include the superior sagittal, inferior sagittal, straight, occipital, and transverse sinuses, and their confluence. Major veins shown here include the great vein of Galen, the basal vein of Rosenthal, and the internal cerebral vein.

The Superficial Cerebral Veins

There are three major veins in the group of the superficial cerebral veins (Fig. 4-5A). (1) **The superficial middle cerebral vein,** which runs along the lateral sulcus, drains the temporal lobe and empties into the **cavernous sinus.** (2) **The superior anastomotic vein of Trolard** is the largest superficial vein; it travels across the parietal lobe, drains into the **superior sagittal sinus**, and connects the superficial middle cerebral vein with the superior

sagittal sinus. (3) **The inferior anastomotic vein of Labbé** connects the superficial middle cerebral vein with the transverse sinus. It is the largest vein draining into the transverse sinus. It travels across the temporal lobe.

The Deep Cerebral Veins

Three major veins are included in the group of the deep cerebral veins (Fig. 4-5B): (1) **the great cerebral vein of Galen,** (2) **the basal vein of Rosenthal,** and (3) **the internal cerebral vein.** The great cerebral vein of Galen is a short vein (about 2 cm long) and is formed by the union of two internal cerebral veins at the level of the splenium of corpus callosum. It courses caudally and joins the inferior sagittal sinus to form the straight sinus, which then empties into the confluence of sinuses. The basal vein of Rosenthal receives blood from the orbital surface of the frontal lobe, anterior part of corpus callosum, rostral parts of the cingulate gyrus, the insula, the opercular cortex (a portion of the motor area for speech), and the ventral parts of corpus striatum. The basal vein empties into the great cerebral vein of Galen. The internal cerebral veins receive venous blood from the thalamus, striatum, caudate nucleus, internal capsule, choroid plexus, and hippocampus. The cerebellum and medulla are drained by a network of veins that empty into the great cerebral vein of Galen, as well as the straight, transverse, and superior and inferior petrosal sinuses.

THE SPINAL CORD

ARTERIES

Posterior Spinal Arteries (PSAs)

As stated earlier, in a majority of cases (75%), the posterior spinal arteries arise from the PICA (Fig. 4-6A). They descend on the dorsolateral surface of the spinal cord slightly medial to the dorsal roots.

Anterior Spinal Arteries (ASAs)

Two small branches arise from the vertebral arteries as they ascend on the anterolateral surface of the medulla. These branches unite to form one single anterior spinal artery (Fig. 4-6A) that courses along the midline of the ventral surface of the spinal cord.

The Spinal Medullary and Radicular Arteries

The posterior and anterior spinal medullary and radicular arteries arise from the segmental arteries and communicate with the posterior and anterior spinal arteries (Fig. 4-6A). These arteries provide blood supply to the thoracic, lumbar, and sacral regions of the spinal cord.

VEINS

In the spinal cord, on the ventral side, **the anteromedian spinal vein** is located in the midline and two **anterolateral spinal veins** are located along the line of attachment of the ventral roots (Fig. 4-6B). On the dorsal side, the **posteromedian spinal vein** is located in the midline and two **posterolat-**

eral spinal veins are located along the line of attachment of the dorsal roots. The posteromedian and posterolateral veins are drained by posterior spinal medullary and radicular veins. The anterior median and anterolateral spinal veins are drained by anterior spinal medullary and radicular veins.

CLINICAL CASE

HISTORY

Stan is a 78-year-old man who was brought to the local emergency room (ER) because his family noted that he was suddenly not using his left arm and leg. In addition, he began to show some behavioral changes. When asked about his inability to move his right side, he said, "I am fine. What is wrong with you?" Although normally very cooperative, he appeared to be more withdrawn and irritable. The morning that he was brought to the ER, he only shaved the right half of his face, combed the right side of his hair, and wore a sock and shoe on the right foot.

EXAMINATION

A neurologist examined Stan and found a loud bruit (pronounced as "bru-ee"; a rumbling sound) over the right carotid artery in his neck. When asked to show his left hand, Stan ignored the question. When his hand was lifted and he was confronted with the question of whether, indeed, the hand was his; he denied it and insisted that the hand belonged to the doctor. He did not blink when a hand was waved over the left lateral aspect of his visual fields, and when asked to draw a clock, he put all of the numbers on the clock on the right side. He denied any problem with the clock that he drew. The left side of his face drooped, excluding his forehead, which was symmetrical, and although there was minimal movement on the left side of his body, he moved it very infrequently. When the lateral aspect of the plantar surface of his left foot was scratched, the great toe dorsiflexed and the other toes fanned upwards. When the same maneuver was performed on the other side, the toes deviated downward.

EXPLANATION

Stan has a classic example of a right parietal stroke, most often involving the superior parietal lobule. The artery infarcted is the right middle cerebral artery. Because the middle cerebral artery continues in nearly a straight line from the internal carotid artery, it is a common route for small emboli originating from the internal carotid artery. The bruit noted is most likely the result of a thrombus (clot) occluding the lumen of the carotid artery. When blood flows across the thrombus, a bruit is heard.

The parietal lobe is responsible for primary and secondary sensory information. One of the types of sensory information provided by this region is the ability to localize objects in space. People with lesions in the right parietal

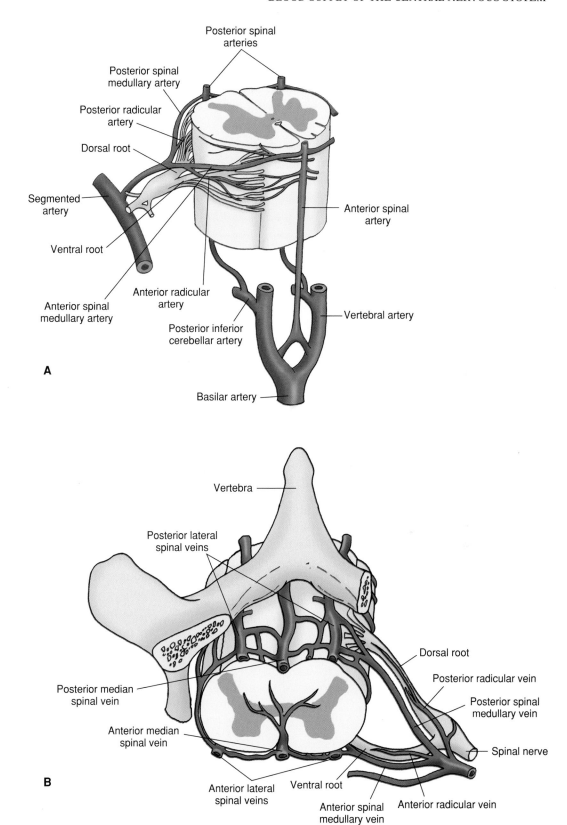

Figure 4–6 Vascular supply of the spinal cord. (A) Major **arteries supplying** the spinal cord. Note especially the two posterior and one anterior spinal arteries. The vertebral, posterior inferior cerebellar, and basilar arteries, and the dorsal and ventral roots of the spinal nerve are shown for orientation purposes. (B) Major **veins draining** the spinal cord. The vertebra and spinal nerve are shown for orientation purposes.

lobe live in "right-sided worlds" and ignore the left side of their bodies and all objects in space. Behavioral changes, including dulling of affect, accompany these deficits. These patients may become less cooperative, and it is not unknown for them to have several automobile accidents, colliding with objects on their left sides, before their deficits are recognized. Because the fibers from the lateral fields of

the optic tract run through the parietal lobe of the contralateral side, a visual defect often accompanies strokes in this region, and patients don't blink in response to hand-waving in this field. The motor strip may also be affected by an infarct of this artery, so genuine motor weakness with a Babinski sign (the up-going toe) would be present, signifying upper motor neuron weakness.

CHAPTER TEST

QUESTIONS

Choose the best answer for each question.

1. A 40-year-old man noticed that he had an almost complete loss of vision in his right eye. A funduscopic examination of his eye indicated a loss of blood supply to the right eye. The blood supply of which one of the following arteries may be occluded in this patient?

a. Posterior communicating artery
b. Ophthalmic artery
c. Posterior cerebral artery
d. Anterior choroidal artery
e. Middle cerebral artery

2. A neurologic examination of a 55-year-old woman indicated that she had weakness and loss of discriminative touch and vibratory sense on the left side of her body. When she attempted to protrude her tongue, it deviated to the right. The blood supply of which one of the following arteries may be occluded in this patient?

a. Basilar artery
b. Branches of the anterior spinal artery
c. Branches of the superior cerebellar artery
d. Posterior spinal artery
e. Anterior inferior cerebellar artery

3. A 65-year-old man suffering from lack of coordination in speech and disturbance of articulation was referred to a neurologist by his primary physician. The neurologist diagnosed the patient to be suffering from Wallenberg's syndrome and sent him for angiography. Which one of the following arteries is most likely to be occluded in this patient?

a. Anterior cerebral artery
b. Middle cerebral artery
c. Posterior cerebral artery

d. Anterior inferior cerebellar artery
e. Posterior inferior cerebellar artery

4. A 70-year-old woman suffering from loss of motor control and sensation in her left leg was examined by her neurologist. Subsequent angiographic procedures performed on the patient revealed that one of the arteries supplying the brain was 80% occluded. Which one of the following arteries most likely was occluded in this patient?

a. Right anterior cerebral artery
b. Left anterior cerebral artery
c. Posterior cerebral artery
d. Posterior communicating artery
e. The vertebral artery

5. Which one of the following statements regarding the circle of Willis is correct?

a. It is the primary source of blood supply to the pons and medulla.
b. It includes two vertebral arteries.
c. It is the site where most of the cerebrospinal fluid is formed.
d. The superior cerebellar artery arises from this circle of arteries.
e. It surrounds the optic chiasm, tuber cinereum, and the interpeduncular region.

ANSWERS AND EXPLANATIONS

1. Answer: b

The ophthalmic artery, which supplies the ipsilateral eye, arises from the internal carotid artery in the cranium. It enters the orbit through the optic foramen and gives rise to the central artery of the retina, which supplies the retina in the ipsilateral eye. Although the other arteries mentioned as alternative choices arise in the region of the optic chiasm, they do not supply the eye.

2. Answer: b

The anterior spinal artery supplies the medial structures of the medulla. These structures include the pyramids, medial lemniscus, and hypoglossal nucleus. It should be recalled that the axons contained within the pyramids originate in the cerebral cortex. At the caudal end of the medulla, near its juncture with the spinal cord, most of the fibers contained within the pyramid pass to the contralateral side. If the loss of senses occurs on the patient's left side, the corticospinal fibers on the right side must be impaired, implying that the branches of the anterior spinal artery supplying the right side of the caudal medulla must be occluded. The fibers that form the medial lemniscus arise from cells of nuclei gracilis and cuneatus. The cells of these nuclei are involved in mediating the sense of discriminative touch and vibration. These fibers cross in the lower medulla. Therefore, damage to these fibers on the right side will impair the sense of discriminative touch and vibration on the left side of the body. Normally, right hypoglossal nerve fibers innervate the left side of the tongue and vice versa. Activation of both hypoglossal nerves allows the tongue to remain straight when it is protruded. If the hypoglossal nerve fibers on the right side of the medulla are damaged, the tongue will deviate to the right when it is protruded (i.e., the tongue, when protruded, deviates to the side of the lesion). The other arteries listed do not supply blood to the medulla.

3. Answer: e

The posterior inferior cerebellar artery supplies the regions of lateral medulla that include the spinothalamic tract, dorsal and ventral spinocerebellar tracts, descending sympathetic tract, descending tract of cranial nerve V, and the nucleus ambiguus. Occlusion of this artery produces Wallenberg's syndrome. The symptoms (lack of coordination in speech and disturbance in articulation) are caused by damage to the nucleus ambiguus, which provides innervation to laryngeal muscles. The other arteries do not supply the lateral medulla.

4. Answer: a

The anterior cerebral artery supplies blood to the dorsal and medial parts of the cerebral hemisphere. This artery supplies the postcentral gyrus (which is concerned with the processing of sensory information from the contralateral leg) and the precentral gyrus (which is concerned with the motor control of the contralateral leg). Therefore, occlusion of the right anterior cerebral artery is likely to result in the loss of motor and sensory control in the patient's left leg. Other arteries listed do not supply blood to the pre- and postcentral gyri, and therefore, their occlusion would not elicit the symptoms observed in this patient. For example, the vertebral artery and its branches supply the medulla, the posterior cerebral arteries supply most of the midbrain, and the posterior communicating arteries supply blood to the hypophysis, infundibulum, and parts of the hypothalamus, thalamus, and hippocampus.

5. Answer: e

The cerebral arterial circle (circle of Willis) surrounds the optic chiasm and the infundibulum of the pituitary. It is formed by the anastomosis of the branches of the internal carotid artery and the terminal branches of the basilar artery. The arteries that form the circle of Willis include the anterior communicating artery, posterior communicating arteries, and the posterior cerebral arteries. Vertebral and superior cerebellar arteries are not included in the circle of Willis, which, under normal circumstances, does not supply blood to the pons and medulla. When the circle of Willis is patent (20% of individuals), it supplies the hypothalamus, hypophysis, infundibulum, thalamus, caudate nucleus, putamen, internal capsule, globus pallidus, choroid plexus (lateral ventricles), and temporal lobe. The choroid plexuses produce about 70% of the cerebrospinal fluid present in the brain and spinal cord.

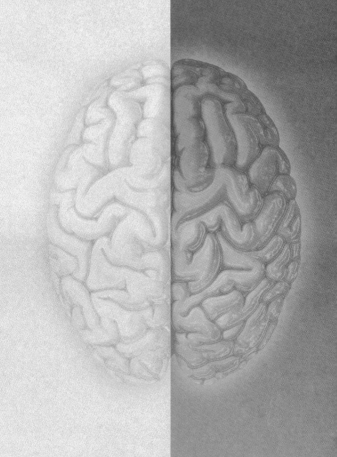

SECTION II

The Neuron

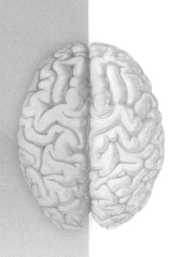

CHAPTER 5

HISTOLOGY OF THE NERVOUS SYSTEM

OBJECTIVES

In this chapter, the student is expected to know:

1. The composition and function of different components of the neuron (e.g., plasma membrane, cell body, nucleus, nucleolus, cytoplasm, dendrites, and axon)

2. The mechanism of axonal transport and its application to the study of neuroanatomy

3. Different types of neurons found within the nervous system

4. Different types of neuroglia and their functions

5. Nature of myelin formation

6. The composition of the peripheral nerves

7. The types of neuronal injury and the process of regeneration

THE NEURON

Signals from one nerve cell to another are transferred across special zones of contact between the neurons that are known as **synapses**. The mechanism by which neurons communicate with each other is called **synaptic transmission**. Chemical neurotransmission is the most prevalent mechanism of communication between neurons. It involves release of chemical substances (**neurotransmitters**) from the presynaptic terminals of neurons, which excite or inhibit one or more postsynaptic neurons. The details of synaptic neurotransmission are described in Chapter 7.

The human brain consists of about 10^{11} nerve cells. Each nerve cell (**neuron**) consists of a cell body (**perikaryon** or **soma**) from which numerous processes (**neurites**) arise. The neurites that receive information and transmit it to the cell body are called **dendrites** (Fig. 5-1, A and B). A long neurite conducts information from the cell body to different targets and is known as an **axon** (Fig. 5-1, A and B). The **cytoskeleton** of a neuron consists of fibrillar elements (e.g., neurofilaments and microfilaments) and their associated proteins (Fig. 5-1B). Descriptions of the different components of the neuron are provided in the following sections.

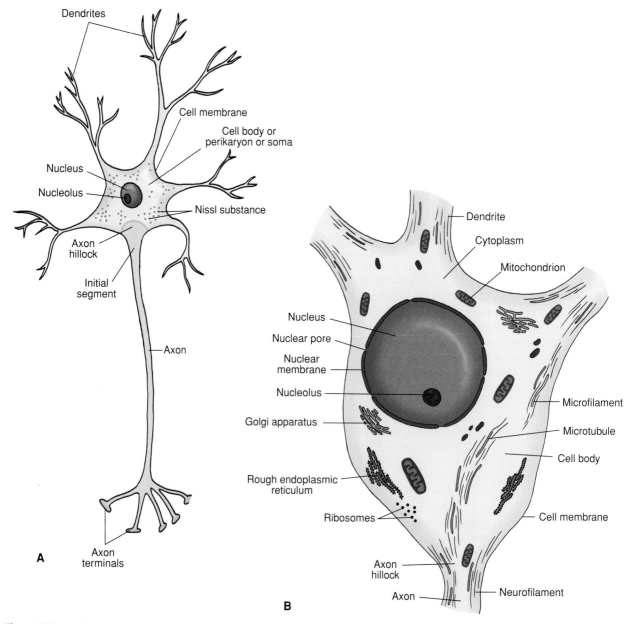

Figure 5–1 A schematic representation of a neuron. (A) Note the orientation of the dendrites, axon, and nucleus. The first few microns of the axon as it emerges from the axon hillock represent the initial segment of the axon. (B) Components of the neuron, including the cell membrane, nucleus, nuclear membrane, nucleolus, and the organelles are present in the cytoplasm of the neuron.

THE CELL MEMBRANE

The cell (plasma) membrane (Fig. 5-1, A and B) forms the external boundary of the neuronal cell body and its processes. It is about 6-8 nanometers (nm) thick and consists of a double layer of lipids in which proteins, including ion channels, are embedded. Inorganic ions enter and leave the neuron through the ion channels. Functions of the neuronal membrane are discussed in Chapter 6.

THE NERVE CELL BODY

The neuronal cell body, also called **perikaryon** or **soma** (Fig. 5-1, A and B), consists of a mass of cytoplasm bounded by an external membrane. The presence of neurites increases the surface area of the cell body for receiving signals from axons of other neurons. The total volume of cytoplasm present in the neurites is much greater than in the cell body proper. The cell body contains the nucleus and various **organelles** and is the metabolic and trophic (relating to nutrition) center of the neuron. Accordingly, the synthesis of most proteins, phospholipids, and other macromolecules occurs in the soma.

THE NUCLEUS

Histologically, the term **nucleus** refers to the round structure that is usually located in the center of the cell body (Fig. 5-1). It should be noted that, in neuroanatomy, the term nucleus also refers to a collection of neurons in the brain or spinal cord with similar morphological characteristics (e.g., nucleus ambiguus). The contents of the nucleus are enclosed within a **nuclear membrane**. The nuclear membrane is double-layered and contains fine pores through which substances can diffuse in and out of the nucleus (Fig. 5-1B). The genetic material of the nucleus, consisting of deoxyribonucleic acid (DNA), is called **chromatin**. When the nucleoplasm is homogenous and does not stain with basic dyes, the DNA is said to be widely dispersed and in **euchromatin** form. The nucleus contains a prominent (relatively large) **nucleolus** that is concerned with the synthesis of ribonucleic acid (RNA) and stains deeply. In the female, the **Barr body** represents one of the two X chromosomes and is located at the inner surface of the nuclear membrane.

THE CYTOPLASM

The following organelles and inclusions are present in the **cytoplasm**.

Nissl Substance or Bodies

This granular material is present in the entire cell body and proximal portions of the dendrites. However, it is not present in the **axon hillock** (portion of the soma from which the axon arises) and the axon (Fig. 5-1A). The **Nissl substance** consists of RNA granules called **ribosomes** (Fig. 5-1A). In all neurons, a net-like meshwork consisting of a highly convoluted single membrane, called the **endoplasmic reticulum**, extends throughout the cytoplasm. Many ribosomes are attached to the membrane of the endoplasmic reticulum and create regions known as rough endoplasmic reticulum (Fig. 5-1B). Many ribosomes lie free in the cytoplasm. The Nissl substance is basophilic and stains well with basic dyes (e.g., toluidine blue or basic aniline dyes). It is responsible for the synthesis of proteins that are carried into the dendrites and the axon.

Mitochondria

These spherical or rod-shaped structures consist of a double membrane (Fig. 5-1B). The inner membrane consists of folds projecting into the interior of the **mitochondria**, and many enzymes involved in the tricarboxylic cycle and cytochrome chains of respiration are located on this membrane. The mitochondria are present in the soma, dendrites, and the axon of the neuron and are involved in the generation of energy for the neuron.

Golgi Apparatus

The Golgi apparatus (Fig. 5-1B) consists of aggregations of flat vesicles of various sizes made up of smooth endoplasmic reticulum. Protein-containing vesicles that bud off from the **rough endoplasmic reticulum** are transported to the **Golgi apparatus** where the proteins are modified (with processes such as glycosylation or phosphorylation), packaged into vesicles, and transported to other intracellular locations (such as nerve terminals).

Lysosomes

Lysosomes are small (300–500 nm) membrane-bound vesicles formed from the Golgi apparatus that contain hydrolytic enzymes. They serve as scavengers in the neurons.

Cytoskeleton

This cytoplasmic component is the main determinant of the shape of a neuron. It consists of the following three filamentous elements: microtubules, neurofilaments, and microfilaments.

1. **Microtubules** (Fig. 5-1B) consist of helical cylinders made up of 13 protofilaments, which, in

turn, are linearly arranged pairs of alpha and beta subunits of tubulin. They are 25–28 nm in diameter and are required in the development and maintenance of the neuron's processes.

2. **Neurofilaments** (Fig. 5-1B) are composed of fibers that twist around each other to form coils. Two thin protofilaments form a protofibril. Three protofibrils form a neurofilament that is about 10 nm in diameter. Neurofilaments are most abundant in the axon. In Alzheimer's disease, neurofilaments become modified and form a neurofibrillary tangle (see Chapter 25 for more details regarding this disease).

3. **Microfilaments** (Fig. 5-1B) are usually 3–7 nm in diameter and consist of two strands of polymerized globular actin monomers arranged in a helix. They play an important role in motility of growth cones during development and in the formation of pre- and postsynaptic specializations.

DENDRITES

These short processes arise from the cell body; their diameter tapers distally, and they branch extensively (Fig. 5-1, A and B). Small projections, called dendritic spines, extend from dendritic branches of some neurons. The primary function of dendrites is to increase the surface area for receiving signals from axonal projections of other neurons. The presence of dendritic spines further enhances the synaptic surface area of the neuron. The cytoplasmic composition in the dendrites is similar to that of the neuronal cell body. Nissl granules, ribosomes, smooth endoplasmic reticulum, neurofilaments, microfilaments, microtubules, and mitochondria are found in the dendrites.

AXON

A single, long, cylindrical and slender process arising usually from the soma of a neuron is called an **axon.** The axon usually arises from a small conical elevation on the soma of a neuron that does not contain Nissl substance and is called an **axon hillock** (Fig. 5-1A). The plasma membrane of the axon is called the axolemma, and the cytoplasm contained in it is called axoplasm. The axoplasm does not contain the Nissl substance or Golgi apparatus, but it does contain mitochondria, microtubules, and neurofilaments. The first 50–100 μm of the axon, after it emerges from the axon hillock, is known as the initial segment (Fig. 5-1A). The action potential originates at the axon hillock. An action potential is a brief fluctuation in the membrane potential, which moves like a wave along the axon in order to transfer information from one neuron to another. Membrane potential is the voltage difference across the cell membrane brought about by differences in extracellular and intracellular ionic distributions (see Chapter 6). Axons are either myelinated or unmyelinated; the mechanism of myelination is described later in this chapter. Usually, the axons do not give off branches near the cell body. However, in some neurons, collateral branches arise from the axon near their cell body; these branches are called **recurrent collaterals.** At their distal ends, the axons branch extensively (Fig. 5-1A); their terminal ends, which are mostly enlarged, are called synaptic terminals (synaptic boutons).

AXONAL TRANSPORT

Various secretory products produced in the cell body are carried to the axon terminals by special transport mechanisms. Likewise, various constituents are carried from the axon terminals to the cell body. Three main types of axonal transport are fast anterograde transport, slow anterograde transport, and fast retrograde transport.

Fast Anterograde Transport

Fast anterograde transport (orthograde or forward flowing) is involved in the transport of materials that have a functional role at the nerve terminals (e.g., precursors of peptide neurotransmitters, enzymes needed for the synthesis of small molecule neurotransmitters, and glycoproteins needed for reconstitution of the plasma membrane) from the cell body to the terminals. Polypeptides much larger than final peptide neurotransmitters (prepropeptides) and enzymes needed for the synthesis of small molecule neurotransmitters are synthesized in the rough endoplasmic reticulum (Fig. 5-2A, a). Vesicles containing these propeptides and enzymes bud off from the rough endoplasmic reticulum and are transported to the Golgi apparatus (Fig. 5-2A, b) where they are modified and packaged into vesicles. The vesicles formed in the Golgi apparatus then become attached to the microtubules and are transported by fast axonal transport (at a rate of 100–400 mm/d) into the nerve terminal (Fig. 5-2A, c). The propeptides are then cleaved to smaller peptides (Fig. 5-2A, d). Small molecule neurotransmitters are synthesized in the neuronal terminal. The neurotransmitters (either small peptides or small molecule neurotransmitters) are packaged in vesicles (Fig. 5-2A, e). The neurotransmitters are then released into the synaptic cleft by **exocytosis.** During the process of

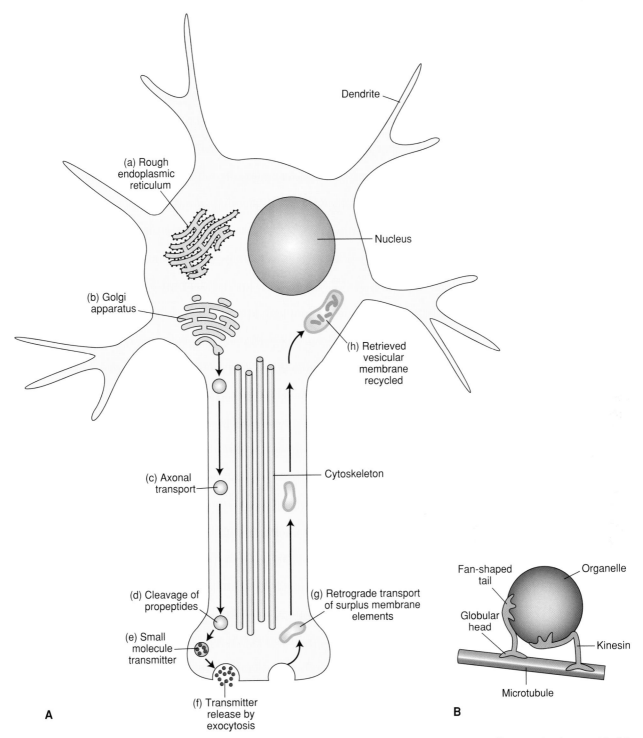

Figure 5–2   Axonal transport. (A) Large molecule peptides (pre-propeptides) are converted into smaller peptides (propeptides) in the rough endoplasmic reticulum (a). The propeptides and enzymes are packaged into vesicles that are transported to the Golgi apparatus, modified, and packaged into vesicles (b). The vesicles get attached to microtubules and are carried to the terminals by fast axonal transport (c). The propeptides are cleaved to produce smaller peptide transmitters in the terminal (d). Small molecule neurotransmitters are synthesized in the neuronal terminal and packaged into vesicles (e). The peptides and neurotransmitters are released into the synaptic cleft by exocytosis (f). Surplus membrane elements in the terminal are carried back to the cell body by retrograde transport (g). The retrieved vesicular membrane is degraded or recycled (h). (B) A model showing how kinesin (a microtubule-associated ATPase) can move an organelle along a microtubule.

exocytosis, the membranes of the vesicles and terminal membrane fuse together, an opening develops, and the contents of the vesicle are released in the synaptic cleft (Fig. 5-2A, f).

The rapid axonal transport depends on the microtubules. The microtubule provides a stationary track and a microtubule-associated ATPase (**kinesin**) forms a cross-bridge between the organelle to be moved and the microtubule. On one end, kinesin contains two globular heads that bind to the microtubule, and on the other end, it has a fan-shaped tail that binds to the surface of an organelle. The organelle then moves by sliding of the kinesin molecule along the microtubule (Fig. 5-2B).

Slow Anterograde Transport

Slow anterograde transport involves movement of neurofilaments and microtubules synthesized in the cell body to the terminals at a rate of 0.25–5 mm/d. Soluble proteins transported by this mechanism include actin, tubulin (which polymerizes to form microtubules), proteins that make up neurofilaments, myosin, and a calcium-binding protein (calmodulin).

Fast Retrograde Transport

Fast retrograde transport is slower than the fast anterograde transport (about 50–200 mm/d). Rapid retrograde transport carries materials from the nerve terminals to the cell body; the transported materials travel along microtubules. For example, when a transmitter is released from the synaptic terminal by exocytosis, the surplus membrane in the terminal is transported back to the cell body by retrograde fast axonal transport (Fig. 5-2A, g), where it is either degraded by lysosomes or recycled (Fig. 5-2A, h). Also transported by this mechanism is nerve growth factor (NGF), a peptide synthesized by a target cell and transported into certain neurons in order to stimulate their growth. Materials lying outside the axon terminals are taken up by **endocytosis** and transported to the cell body. Endocytosis is a mechanism by which materials lying outside the terminal that are no longer needed are taken up by the terminals, transported to the cell body, and degraded. Fast retrograde axonal transport is also involved in some pathological conditions. For example, the herpes simplex, polio, and rabies viruses and tetanus toxin are taken up by the axon terminals in peripheral nerves and carried to their cell bodies in the central nervous system (CNS) by rapid retrograde transport.

Axonal transport (anterograde as well as retrograde) has been used to trace target sites of neurons. A simplified procedure for **anterograde tracing techniques** involves the microinjection of a fluorescent dye at the desired site in the CNS. The dyes are taken up by the neuronal cell bodies and transported anterogradely to their axon terminals. The fluorescence of the axons and their terminals is then visualized under a microscope to ascertain the projections of the neuron.

Retrograde tracing techniques involve the microinjection of an enzyme (e.g., **horseradish peroxidase**; HRP), fluorescent dyes (e.g., Fluoro-Gold), cholera toxin, or viruses at the desired site. The injected substance (e.g., HRP) is taken up by axon terminals and transported retrogradely into the neuronal cell bodies. The neurons labeled with HRP are visualized by a chemical reaction in which a dense precipitate is formed and can be identified under dark- or bright-field illumination. Likewise, fluorescent substances such as Fluoro-Gold, microinjected at the desired site, are taken up by axon terminals and transported to the cell bodies where they are visualized under a fluorescent microscope.

TYPES OF NEURONS

Based on morphological characteristics, the neurons have been classified into the following groups: multipolar, bipolar, pseudo-unipolar, and unipolar.

MULTIPOLAR NEURONS

These neurons are most common in the brain and spinal cord. They possess three or more dendrites and one long axon issuing from the cell body (Fig. 5-3A). A large motor neuron of the anterior horn of the spinal cord is one example of such a neuron.

BIPOLAR NEURONS

In these neurons, two processes, one on each end, arise from an elongated cell body (Fig. 5-3B). One process ends in dendrites, and the other process, an axon, ends in terminals in the CNS. These neurons have sensory functions and transmit information received by the dendrites on one end to the CNS via the axon terminals on the other end. Retinal bipolar cells, sensory cells of the cochlear, and vestibular ganglia are included in this category.

PSEUDO-UNIPOLAR NEURONS

In this type of neuron, a single process arises from the cell body and divides into two branches. One of these branches projects to the periphery, and the other projects to the CNS (Fig. 5-3C). Each branch has the structural and functional characteristics of

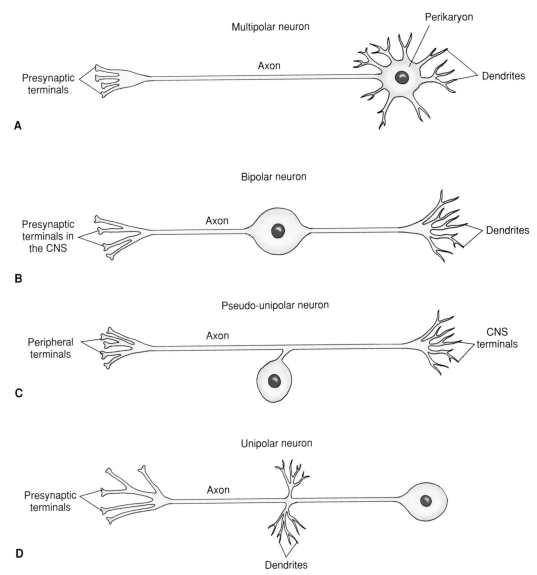

Figure 5–3 Different types of neurons. (A) Multipolar neuron. (B) Bipolar neuron. (C) Pseudo-unipolar neuron. (D) Unipolar neuron.

an axon. Information collected from the terminals of the peripheral branch is transmitted to the CNS via the terminals of the other branch. Examples of this type of cell are sensory cells in the dorsal root ganglion and baroreceptor-sensitive cells in the nodose ganglion, which sense changes in the systemic blood pressure and transmit this information to neurons in the dorsal medulla.

UNIPOLAR NEURONS

These types of neurons are relatively rare in vertebrates. In these neurons, dendrites arise from one end of the neuron, and an axon arises from the site where the dendrites are located (Fig. 5-3D).

OTHER TYPES OF NEURONS

Neurons can also be divided into two groups:

1. **Principal or projecting neurons** are also known as type I or **Golgi type I neurons**. Principal neurons (e.g., motor neurons in the ventral horn of the spinal cord) possess very long axons and form long fiber tracts in the brain and the spinal cord.

2. **Intrinsic neurons** are also known as type II or **Golgi type II neurons**. Intrinsic neurons have very short axons. These neurons are **interneurons** and are considered to have inhibitory function. They are abundant in the cerebral and cerebellar cortex.

NEUROGLIA

The supporting cells located in the CNS are called **neuroglia** or simply **glial cells**. They are nonexcitable and more numerous (5 to 10 times) than neurons. Neuroglia have been classified into the following groups: astrocytes, oligodendrocytes, microglia, and ependymal cells.

ASTROCYTES

Among the glial cells, astrocytes are the largest and have a stellate (star-shaped) appearance because their processes extend in all directions. Their nuclei are ovoid and centrally located. The astrocytes provide support for the neurons, a barrier against the spread of transmitters from synapses, and insulation to prevent electrical activity of one neuron from affecting the activity of a neighboring neuron. Some transmitters (for example, glutamate and γ-aminobutyric acid [GABA]), when released from nerve terminals in the CNS, are taken up by astrocytes, thus terminating their action. The neurotransmitters taken up by astrocytes are processed for recycling (see Chapter 8).

When extracellular K^+ increases in the brain due to local neural activity, astrocytes take up K^+ via membrane channels and help to dissipate K^+ over a large area because they have an extensive network of processes. They are further subdivided into the following subgroups: protoplasmic astrocytes, fibrous astrocytes, and Müller cells.

Protoplasmic Astrocytes

These cells are present in the gray matter in close association with neurons. Because of their close association with the neurons, they are considered satellite cells and serve as metabolic intermediaries for neurons. They give out thicker and shorter processes, which branch profusely. Several of their processes terminate in expansions called end-feet (Fig. 5-4A). The neuronal cell bodies, dendrites, and some axons are covered with end-feet of the astrocytes. The end-feet join together to form a limiting membrane on the inner surface of the pia mater (glial limiting membrane) and outer surface of blood vessels (called perivascular lining membrane) (Fig. 5-4A). The perivascular end-feet may serve as passageways for the transfer of nutrients from the blood vessels to the neurons. Abutting of processes of protoplasmic astrocytes on the capillaries as perivascular end-feet is one of the anatomical features of the blood-brain barrier.

Fibrous Astrocytes

These glial cells are found primarily in the white matter between nerve fibers (Fig. 5-4B). Several thin, long, and smooth processes arise from the cell body; these processes show little branching. Fibrous astrocytes function to repair damaged tissue, and this process may result in scar formation.

Müller Cells

These modified astrocytes are present in the retina (see Chapter 16).

OLIGODENDROCYTES

These cells are smaller than astrocytes and have fewer and shorter branches. Their cytoplasm contains the usual organelles (e.g., ribosomes, mitochondria, and microtubules), but they do not contain neurofilaments. In the white matter, oligodendrocytes are located in rows along myelinated fibers and are known as interfascicular oligodendrocytes (Fig. 5-4C). These oligodendrocytes are involved in the myelination process (described later). The oligodendrocytes present in the gray matter are called perineural oligodendrocytes (Fig. 5-4D).

MICROGLIA

These are the smallest of the glial cells (Fig. 5-4E). They usually have a few short branching processes with thorn-like endings. These processes arising from the cell body give off numerous spine-like projections. They are scattered throughout the nervous system. When the CNS is injured, the microglia become enlarged, mobile, and phagocytic.

EPENDYMAL CELLS

Ependymal cells consist of three types of cells: ependymocytes, tanycytes, and choroidal epithelial cells.

Ependymocytes are cuboidal or columnar cells that form a single layer of lining in the brain ventricles and the central canal of the spinal cord. They possess microvilli and cilia (Fig. 5-5A). The presence of microvilli indicates that these cells may have some absorptive function. The movement of their cilia facilitates the flow of the cerebrospinal fluid (CSF).

Tanycytes are specialized ependymal cells that are found in the floor of the third ventricle, and their processes extend into the brain tissue where they are juxtaposed to blood vessels and neurons (Fig. 5-5B). Tanycytes have been implicated in the

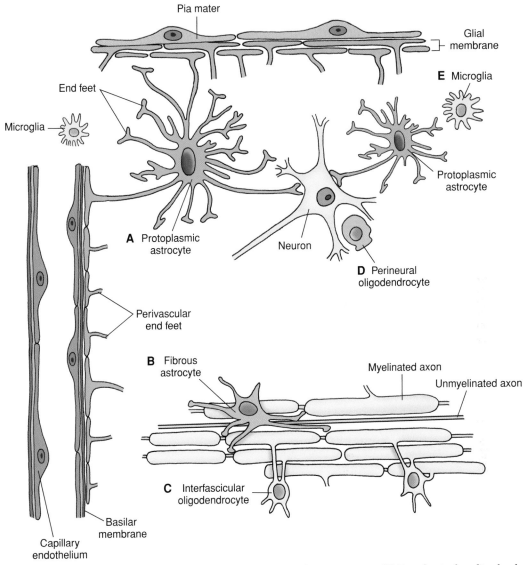

Figure 5–4 Different types of neuroglia. (A) Protoplasmic astrocyte. (B) Fibrous astrocyte. (C) Interfascicular oligodendrocyte. (D) Perineural oligodendrocyte. (E) Microglia.

transport of hormones from the CSF to capillaries of portal system and from hypothalamic neurons to the CSF.

Choroidal epithelial cells are modified ependymal cells. They are present in the choroid plexus and are involved in the production and secretion of CSF. They have tight junctions that prevent the CSF from spreading to the adjacent tissue.

MYELINATED AXONS

Myelinated axons are present in the peripheral nervous system and the CNS.

PERIPHERAL NERVOUS SYSTEM

In the peripheral nervous system (PNS), **Schwann cells** (Fig. 5-6A) provide myelin sheaths around axons. The myelin sheaths are interrupted along the length of the axons at regular intervals at the **nodes of Ranvier** (Fig. 5-6A). Thus, the nodes of Ranvier are uninsulated and have a lower resistance. These nodes of Ranvier are rich in Na^+ channels, and the action potential becomes regenerated at these regions. Therefore, the action potential traveling along the length of the axon jumps from one node of Ranvier to another. This type of propagation

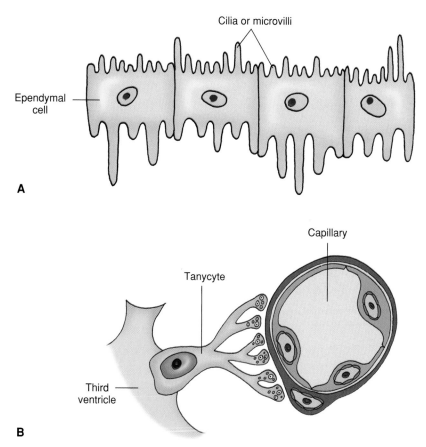

Figure 5–5 (A) Ependymocytes are cuboidal or columnar in shape and line the brain ventricles. (B) Tanycytes are specialized ependymal cells that are found in the floor of the third ventricle.

enables the action potential to conduct rapidly and is known as **saltatory conduction.** During the myelination, the axon comes in contact with the Schwann cell, which then rotates around the axon in clockwise or counterclockwise fashion. As the Schwann cell wraps around the axon, the cytoplasm becomes progressively reduced, and the inner layers of the plasma membrane come in contact and fuse together (Fig. 5-6, B–E).

CENTRAL NERVOUS SYSTEM

Within the brain and the spinal cord, **oligodendrocytes** form the myelin sheaths around axons of neurons. Several glial processes arise from one oligodendrocyte and wrap around a portion of the axon (Fig. 5-7). The intervals between adjacent oligodendrocytes are devoid of myelin sheaths and are called the nodes of Ranvier (Fig. 5-7). Unlike in peripheral axons, the process of an oligodendrocyte does not rotate spirally on the axon. Instead, it

may wrap around the length of the axon. The cytoplasm is reduced progressively, and the sheath consists of concentric layers of plasma membrane. Unlike in peripheral nerves, one oligodendrocyte forms myelin sheaths around numerous (as many as 60) axons of diverse origins.

DISORDERS ASSOCIATED WITH DEFECTIVE MYELINATION

Normal conduction of the nerve impulses is dependent on appropriate insulation provided by the myelin sheath surrounding the axons in the central and peripheral nervous systems. Demyelination of axons occurs in diseases such as **multiple sclerosis** and **Guillain-Barré syndrome.** In multiple sclerosis, axons are demyelinated in the CNS, whereas the Guillain-Barré syndrome involves axonal demyelination in the PNS. Because of the lack of myelination, conduction of action potentials along axons is slowed down or blocked in the brain and

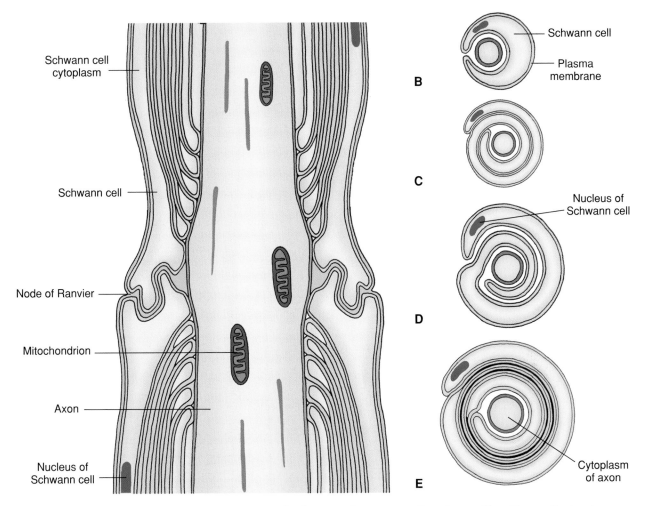

Figure 5–6 Myelination of peripheral nerves. (A) A longitudinal section showing a myelinated nerve fiber. The myelin sheaths are discontinuous along the length of the axons, and the intervals between these sheaths are called nodes of Ranvier. (B–E) Cross sections showing different stages of formation of a myelin sheath.

spinal cord, resulting in severe disturbances in motor and sensory functions.

COMPOSITION OF PERIPHERAL NERVES

Each peripheral nerve consists of the following components:

1. **Epineurium,** which consists of a dense connective tissue layer enclosing several bundles of nerve fibers (Fig. 5-8A)

2. **Perineurium,** which is a sheath of connective tissue enclosing each bundle of nerve fibers (Fig. 5-8A)

3. **Endoneurium,** which consists of a loose, delicate connective tissue layer in which nerve fibers are enclosed (Fig. 5-8A)

Nerve fibers have been classified into three major groups based on the diameters and conduction velocities (Table 5-1). Peripheral nerves include the following groups of nerves: cranial nerves, spinal nerves, and preganglionic and postganglionic nerves of the autonomic nervous system (Chapter 22). The axons in a peripheral nerve may be myelinated or unmyelinated. It should be noted that nerve bundles traversing the CNS (e.g., internal capsule) lack the connective tissue coverings (e.g., epineurium and perineurium) that enclose peripheral nerves.

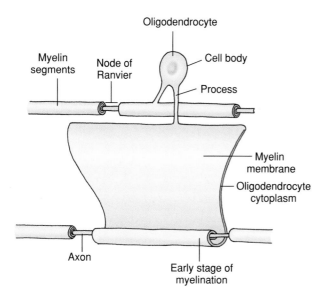

Figure 5–7   Myelination in the central nervous system (CNS). Within the CNS, oligodendrocytes form the myelin sheaths around neurons. Several glial processes arise from one oligodendrocyte and wrap around a portion of the axon. The intervals between adjacent oligodendrocytes are devoid of myelin sheaths and are called the nodes of Ranvier.

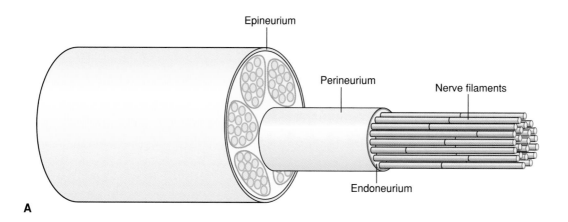

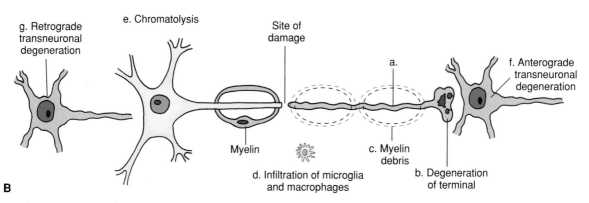

Figure 5–8   Composition of a peripheral nerve and neuronal injury. (A) The epineurium, perineurium, endoneurium, and nerve fibers in a peripheral nerve. (B) Effects of axonal injury. (a–d) Wallerian degeneration. (e) If the injury is close to the cell body, chromatolysis occurs in the cell body. (f) The neuron receiving input from a degenerated axon undergoes anterograde transneuronal degeneration. (g) The neuron, from which the inputs to the chromatolytic neuron arise, degenerates.

Table 5–1 General Classification of Nerve Fibers*

Type	Size (μm)	Conduction Velocity (m/sec)	Functions
Myelinated:			
A	1–20	5–120	Larger, faster conducting fibers (60–120 m/sec) transmit motor impulses to the skeletal muscle; smaller A fibers conduct afferent impulses from muscle spindles, Golgi tendon organs, and mechanoreceptors
B	1–3	3–15	Afferent and efferent innervation of the viscera
Unmyelinated:			
C	<2	0.6–2	Efferent: postganglionic fibers of the autonomic nervous system
			Afferent: impulses of poorly localized pain in the viscera or periphery

* Other nomenclature for the classification of nerve fibers is presented in Chapter 15 (Table 15-1).

NEURONAL INJURY

INJURY OF THE NEURONAL CELL BODY

The neuronal cell body may be damaged by disease, ischemia (lack of blood supply), or trauma. In the CNS (the brain and spinal cord), the debris produced by neuronal damage is phagocytosed (see below) by microglia. The adjacent fibrous astrocytes proliferate, and the neurons are replaced by scar tissue. In the PNS, macrophages are responsible for the removal of the debris produced by neuronal damage, and the scar tissue is produced by the proliferation of the fibroblasts.

Necrotic cell death is caused by acute traumatic injury that involves rapid lysis of cell membranes. Necrotic cell death is different from **apoptosis.** Apoptosis is defined as a genetically determined process of cell death and is characterized by shrinkage of the cell, cellular fragmentation, and condensation of the chromatin. During the process of formation of tissues from undifferentiated germinal cells in the embryo (**histogenesis**), more neurons (about 2 times more) are formed than the neurons present in the mature brain. The excess number of neurons is destroyed during the development by apoptosis. The mechanism of apoptosis involves activation of a latent biochemical pathway that is present in neurons and other cells of the body. The cellular debris after neuronal cell death is removed by **phagocytosis,** which involves transport of solid material into the cells (e.g., microglia) that remove the debris by indentation of the cell membrane of the phagocyte and formation of a vesicle. **Pinocytosis** is similar to phagocytosis, except that liquid material is removed. **Exocytosis** involves fusion of a vesicle inside the nerve terminal (e.g., a vesicle containing a neurotransmitter) with the plasma membrane and transportation of the contents of the vesicle outside the nerve terminal.

AXONAL DAMAGE

Wallerian Degeneration

This type of degeneration refers to the changes that occur *distally* to the site of damage on an axon. Because protein synthesis occurs primarily in the neuronal cell body, the segment distal to the damaged site on the axon is affected profoundly. Initially, the axon swells up and becomes irregular. Later, the axon and the terminal are broken down into fragments that are phagocytosed by adjacent macrophages and Schwann cells (Fig. 5-8B, a-d). **Myelin** is converted into fine drops of lipid material in the Schwann cells and is extruded from these cells; it is removed by macrophages in the PNS and microglial cells and invading macrophages in the CNS.

Alterations (similar to those mentioned earlier) may also be present in the *proximal* segment of the axon up to the first node of Ranvier.

Chromatolysis

Sectioning of an axon may produce changes in the cell body, and if the injury is close to the cell body, the neuron may degenerate. The cell body swells up due to edema and becomes round in appearance, and the Nissl substance gets distributed throughout the cytoplasm. This process is known as **chromatolysis** (Fig. 5-8B, e). The nucleus moves from its central position to the periphery due to edema. The degenerative changes start within hours and are complete within a relatively short time (about a week).

Anterograde Transneuronal Degeneration

This type of degeneration occurs in the CNS when damage to a neuron results in the degeneration of another postsynaptic neuron closely associated with the same function (Fig. 5-8B, f). For example, damage to an optic nerve results in the degeneration of the lateral geniculate neurons receiving inputs from this nerve.

Retrograde Transneuronal Degeneration

This type of degeneration occurs in neurons sending inputs to an injured neuron. In this situation, terminals of the neuron synapsing with a chromatolytic neuron withdraw and are replaced by processes of glial cells. The neuron, from which the inputs to the chromatolytic neuron arise, eventually degenerates.

RECOVERY OF NEURONAL INJURY (REGENERATION)

If the damage to the neurons is not severe and they survive the injury, regeneration is possible, but complete recovery may take as long as 3–6 months. Within about 3 weeks, the swelling of the cell subsides, the nucleus occupies a central position in the cell body again, and the Nissl bodies are normally distinguished. These events indicate that protein synthesis has been restored in the neuronal cell body. In severe damage, although sprouting occurs in axons in the CNS, this process ceases within a short time (about 2 weeks). In this situation, normal functions of the neurons in the CNS are not restored. However, in peripheral nerves, an axon can regenerate satisfactorily if the endoneurial sheaths are intact. In this situation, the regenerating axons reach the correct destination, and the chances of recovery of function are reasonable. The growth rate of an axon has been estimated to be 2–4 mm per day.

HISTORY

Roseanne is a 40-year-old woman who was brought to a local emergency room due to 7 days of progressive numbness and weakness, first appearing in her toes, then moving proximally to her feet, knees, and hands. She initially ignored the symptoms because she thought that the tingling in her feet was merely her feet "falling asleep." However, the symptoms progressed proximally, and she finally realized that something was wrong when she was unable to climb the stairs of her house and developed increasing shortness of breath.

EXAMINATION

Roseanne was short of breath continuously when she arrived at the emergency room. Her vital capacity (the greatest volume of air that can be exhaled from the lungs after maximal inspiration) was extremely low, which was consistent with severe weakness of the diaphragm and poor oxygenation. Her arms and legs were weak bilaterally, and she had no sensation in her legs or her arms below her elbows. She was able to feel a pin on her upper chest. No deep tendon reflexes could be elicited. Roseanne was transferred to the intensive care unit.

EXPLANATION

Roseanne has a condition called Guillain-Barré syndrome (GBS). GBS is an inflammatory demyelinating disease of peripheral nerves, which may be rapidly progressive. Conduction of action potentials in the affected nerves is either slowed down or blocked due to demyelination. Histologically, inflammatory cells are found within the nerves. Additionally, segmental demyelination and Wallerian degeneration progressing in a proximal direction may be found. Clinically, progressive motor and sensory loss is manifested, potentially affecting the limbs, face, trunk, and diaphragm. This damage also eliminates both reflex arcs of the deep tendon reflexes. GBS is thought to be an immunologic reaction resulting directly or indirectly from a prior infection or inflammatory process, although the precise cause is rarely found. Sometimes, the patient gives a history of a viral infection 2 or 3 weeks prior to the onset of the GBS symptoms. Most patients recover, however, and treatment is aimed at the immunological aspect, with gamma globulin administration and plasma exchange being the most common treatments.

CHAPTER TEST

QUESTIONS

Choose the best answer for each question.

1. Due to the neurologic findings of muscle weakness, spasticity, and impairment of vibratory/position, pain, temperature, and touch sensations, a 25-year-old woman was diagnosed with multiple sclerosis. Which one of the following options constitutes one of the mechanisms for the impairment of her motor and sensory functions?

   a. Schwann cells providing myelin sheaths on the axons in the central nervous system are degenerated.
   b. Oligodendrocytes providing myelin sheaths on the axons in the peripheral nervous system are degenerated.
   c. Oligodendrocytes providing myelin sheaths on the axons in the central nervous system are degenerated.
   d. Noradrenergic neurons in the central nervous system responsible for maintaining muscle tone are degenerated.
   e. A genetic defect resulting in proliferation of astrocytes impaired the insulation of neurons in the patient's central nervous system.

2. A 20-year-old young man was admitted to an emergency room with serious traumatic injury of the median nerve in his right forearm. The axons distal to the injured nerve were swollen and irregular, and the terminals were broken down into fragments. In addition, Schwann cells were filled with lipid material. Which of the following describes this type of neuronal injury?

   a. Chromatolysis
   b. Wallerian degeneration
   c. Transneuronal degeneration
   d. Necrosis
   e. Apoptosis

3. While out on a hike, a 23-year-old young man was bitten on his left leg by a raccoon. Being in the remote woods of a State Forest, he could not receive immediate medical attention. Several weeks later, he developed profound changes in his emotional state and suffered from bouts of terror and rage. A clinician who examined the young man suspected that the raccoon that bit him was rabid, and the rabies virus had affected his hippocampus. The rabies virus may have traveled to the young man's brain by which of the following mechanisms?

   a. Fast anterograde axonal transport
   b. Phagocytosis
   c. Transneuronal transport
   d. Fast retrograde transport
   e. Pinocytosis

4. Which one of the following statements regarding different types of neurons is correct?

   a. Multipolar neurons have many axons.
   b. Sensory cells of the cochlear ganglion are unipolar neurons.
   c. Pseudo-unipolar neurons in the nodose ganglion sense systemic blood pressure changes.
   d. Sensory cells in the dorsal root ganglion represent multipolar cells.
   e. Golgi type I neurons possess very short axons.

5. Which one of the following statements is correct regarding the components of a central nervous system neuron?

   a. The Nissl substance is not present in the axon hillock.
   b. The synthesis of proteins occurs in the mitochondria.
   c. The Barr body represents a Y chromosome.
   d. Nissl substance consists of DNA granules called ribosomes.
   e. The axoplasm contains Nissl substance and Golgi apparatus.

ANSWERS AND EXPLANATIONS

1. Answer: **c**

Multiple sclerosis (MS) is a chronic disease that begins in young adults. It is more common in women than in men. The symptoms and signs are diverse. Most common symptoms include muscle weakness, spasticity, and impairment of sensory pathways. The disease is characterized by demyelination in multiple areas in the central nervous system (CNS). In the CNS, oligodendrocytes are involved in the myelination process. Schwann cells provide myelin sheaths around axons in the peripheral nervous system. Noradrenergic neurons in the CNS are not involved in maintaining muscle tone (see Chapter 8).

2. Answer: b

Because the injury to the median nerve is in the forearm, the site of injury is distant from the cell body located in the ventral horn of the spinal cord. Wallerian degeneration occurs distal to the site of damage on an axon. The axon swells up and becomes irregular, and the axon and its terminals break down into fragments that are phagocytosed by adjacent macrophages and Schwann cells. Myelin is converted into fine drops of lipids in the Schwann cells and is extruded from these cells and removed by macrophages in the peripheral nervous system. The other choices are not relevant to the processes described in the question. In chromatolysis, sectioning of an axon may produce changes in the cell body, which swells up due to edema and becomes round in appearance, the Nissl substance gets distributed throughout the cytoplasm, and the nucleus moves from its central position to the periphery. Transneuronal degeneration occurs in the CNS when damage to one group of neurons results in the degeneration of another set of neurons closely associated with the same function. Necrotic cell death, or necrosis, is caused by acute traumatic injury that involves rapid lysis of cell membranes. Apoptosis is a genetically determined process of cell death.

3. Answer: c

Rabies virus infecting the leg muscles of the young man may have been taken up by nerve terminals and carried to the cell bodies of the neurons in the spinal cord by fast retrograde transport, thus infecting these neurons. The infection must have involved spread from neuron to neuron by transport across synapses (transneuronal transport) and, therefore, must have reached the hippocampus of the young man by this mechanism. This type of transport has been observed in tracing techniques in which viruses, such as the pseudorabies virus that does not infect humans, have been used to trace neuronal networks in experimental animals.

Anterograde transport involves transport of materials that have a functional role at the nerve terminals (e.g., neurotransmitters, lipids, and glycoproteins, which are necessary to reconstitute the plasma membrane) from the cell body to the terminals. Phagocytosis involves the transport of a solid into the cell by a process of indentation of the cell membrane and vesicle formation. Pinocytosis involves the transport of a liquid into the cell by a process of indentation of the cell membrane and vesicle formation.

4. Answer: c

In pseudo-unipolar neurons, a single axon arising from the cell body divides into two branches. One of the branches terminates as fine endings that serve as peripheral receptors, while the other branch terminates on neurons in the CNS. The peripheral nerve endings of the pseudo-unipolar neurons located in the nodose (vagus nerves) and petrosal (glossopharyngeal nerves) ganglia terminate in the vascular walls of the carotid sinus and aortic arch and sense blood pressure changes. Signals received from the vascular nerve endings are transmitted to the CNS for making appropriate adjustment in the systemic blood pressure. Other pseudo-unipolar neurons lie in the dorsal root ganglia. Golgi type I neurons have relatively long axons, while Golgi type II neurons have relatively short axons. Multipolar neurons (e.g., motor neurons in the anterior horn of the spinal cord) have several dendrites and one long axon arising from the cell body.

5. Answer: a

Nissl substance is present in the entire cell body and proximal portions of the dendrites. However, it is not present in the axon hillock (portion of the soma from which the axon arises) and the axon. Protein synthesis occurs in the cell body, the Barr body represents an X chromosome, Nissl substance consists of RNA, and the axoplasm does not contain Nissl substance or a Golgi apparatus.

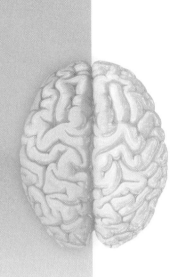

CHAPTER 6

ELECTROPHYSIOLOGY OF NEURONS

OBJECTIVES

In this chapter, the student is expected to:

1. Know the structure and permeability of the neuronal membrane

2. Know the mechanisms of different types of transport (simple diffusion, passive or facilitated diffusion, and active transport)

3. Understand the properties and functions of Na^+-K^+ ATPase

4. Know the general properties of ion channels and their major classes

5. Learn the ionic mechanisms contributing to the resting membrane potential

6. Learn the ionic mechanisms of the action potential

7. Learn the mechanism of propagation of an action potential along an axon

To understand the mechanisms by which the nervous system regulates complex functions and behaviors, it is important to have knowledge of the structure and function of its basic unit, the **neuron**. The most striking properties of neurons are their excitability and ability to conduct electrical signals. This chapter will first describe the organization of the neuronal membrane and its role in maintaining the internal ionic composition. Then, the mechanisms responsible for generating resting membrane potentials and action potentials will be discussed.

STRUCTURE AND PERMEABILITY OF THE NEURONAL MEMBRANE

The **neuronal membrane**, like other cell membranes, consists of a lipid bilayer in which proteins, including ion channels, are embedded. Although three major types of lipids (phospholipids, cholesterol, and glycolipids) are present in the neuronal membrane, **phospholipids** are the most abundant type. Phospholipids consist of long nonpolar chains of carbon atoms that are bonded to hydrogen atoms. A polar phosphate group (a phosphorus atom bonded to three oxygen atoms) is attached to one end of a phospholipid molecule. All lipids in the neuronal membrane are **amphiphilic;** that is, they have a **hydrophilic** (or "water-soluble") end, as well as a hydrophobic (or "water-insoluble") end. Phospholipids have a hydrophilic "polar" end (head) and a hydrophobic "nonpolar" end (tail). The lipids in the neuronal membrane form bilayers, with their hydrophobic tails facing each other and their hydrophilic heads oriented on opposite sides (Fig. 6-1).

The lipid bilayer isolates the cytosol (cytoplasm) of the neuron from the extracellular fluid, while the proteins embedded in it are responsible for most of the membrane functions, such as serving as specific receptors, enzymes, and transport proteins. The neuronal membrane is impermeable to (1) most polar molecules (e.g., sugars and amino acids), and (2) charged molecules (even if they are very small). Cations (positively charged ions) are attracted electrostatically to the oxygen atom of water (which bears a net negative charge). Anions (negatively charged ions) are attracted to the hydrogen atom of water (which bears a net positive charge). Therefore, cations and anions contain electrostatically bound water (water of hydration). The attractive forces between the ions and the water molecules make it difficult for the ions to move from a watery environment into the hydrophobic lipid bilayer of the neuronal membrane. Examples in this category include Na^+, K^+, Ca^{2+}, Mg^{2+}, Cl^-, and HCO_3^-.

STRUCTURE OF PROTEINS

Protein molecules are made up of different combinations of amino acids. Each amino acid has a carbon atom (called the alpha carbon) that is covalently bonded to a hydrogen (H) atom, an amino group (NH_3^+), a carboxyl group (COO^-), and an R group (this group varies in different amino acids). In a covalent bond, two atoms share electrons. Amino acids assemble to form proteins according to instructions provided by messenger RNA in cell organelles called **ribosomes**. The synthesis of proteins occurs in ribosomes in the neuronal cell body. The amino acids are connected by peptide bonds to form a chain. In a **peptide bond**, the amino group of one amino acid joins with the carboxyl group of another amino acid. When a protein is made of a single chain of amino acids, it is called a **polypeptide**. When different polypep-

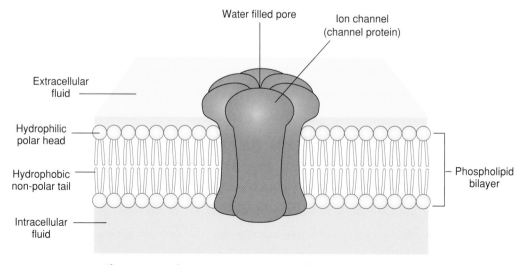

Figure 6–1 Schematic representation of the neuronal membrane.

tide chains assemble to form a large protein molecule, the protein is said to acquire a **quarternary** structure. In a protein with quarternary structure, each polypeptide is called a **subunit**.

MEMBRANE TRANSPORT-PROTEINS

Essential nutrients (e.g., sugars, amino acids, and nucleotides) need to enter the neuron, while metabolic waste products must be removed from the neuron. In addition, the concentration of various ions has to be maintained within the neuron. Therefore, this necessitates **influx** of some ions and **efflux** of others. These functions are carried out by different **membrane transport-proteins**. Two types of proteins are implicated in the transport of solutes across the neuronal membrane: (1) carrier proteins and (2) channel proteins.

CARRIER PROTEINS (CARRIERS OR TRANSPORTERS)

When a specific solute binds to a carrier protein, a reversible conformational change occurs in the protein which, in turn, results in the transfer of the solute across the lipid-bilayer of the membrane. A hypothetical scheme of how solutes are transported across neuronal membranes is as follows. When the carrier protein is in one conformational state, its binding sites may be exposed to the extracellularly located solute molecules. The binding of the solute to the carrier protein results in a change in the conformational state of the protein so that the solute is now exposed to the cytoplasmic side of the neuronal membrane. The solute then dissociates from its binding site on the carrier protein and enters the interior of the neuron.

CHANNEL PROTEINS

The channel proteins span the neuronal membrane and contain water-filled pores (Fig. 6-1). The inorganic ions of suitable size and charge (e.g., Na^+ and K^+) can pass through the pore when it is in the open state and, thus, pass through the membrane. Ion channels are discussed in the *Electrophysiology of the Neuron* section.

TRANSPORT OF SOLUTES ACROSS CELL MEMBRANE

SIMPLE DIFFUSION

The categories of substances that pass through the neuronal membrane by simple diffusion include: (1) all lipid-soluble (hydrophobic or nonpolar) substances (e.g., oxygen molecules), and (2) some polar (lipid-insoluble or water-soluble) molecules, provided they are small and uncharged (e.g., carbon dioxide, urea, ethanol, glycerol, and water molecules). The rate of transport of solutes during simple diffusion is proportional to the solute concentration; the solutes move from regions of high concentration to regions of low concentration (i.e., "downhill"). Such a difference in concentrations of the solute is called a **concentration gradient** (Fig. 6-2). No metabolic energy is needed when the molecules are transported across the cell membrane by simple diffusion.

PASSIVE TRANSPORT (FACILITATED DIFFUSION)

All channel proteins and some carrier proteins mediate passive transport (Fig. 6-2). The solutes are transported across the neuronal membrane passively, so no metabolic energy is needed for the transport of the molecules. If the molecule to be transported is uncharged, then the concentration gradient of the solute determines the direction in which it moves; it diffuses from the side where its concentration is higher to the side where its concentration is lower.

ACTIVE TRANSPORT

This type of transport is always mediated by specific carrier proteins and requires coupling of the carrier protein to a source of metabolic energy (e.g., hydrolysis of ATP) (Fig. 6-2). If the solute molecule has an electrical charge, the determinants of its movement are the concentration gradient and the **electrical potential** between the two sides. The combination of the concentration and electrical potential gradients is called the **electrochemical gradient.** There are many negatively charged organic molecules (e.g., proteins, nucleic acids, carboxylic groups, and metabolites carrying phosphate) within the cell that are unable to cross the neuronal membrane. *These are called fixed anions, and they change the charge inside the neuronal membranes to negative, as compared to the outside of the cell.* Therefore, entry of positively charged ions will be permitted, while negatively charged ions will not be able to enter. Under these conditions, some carrier proteins transport certain solutes by active transport (i.e., the solute is moved across the neuronal membrane against its electrochemical gradient, or "uphill"). Two examples of this type of carrier protein are the sodium-potassium (Na^+-K^+) and calcium pumps.

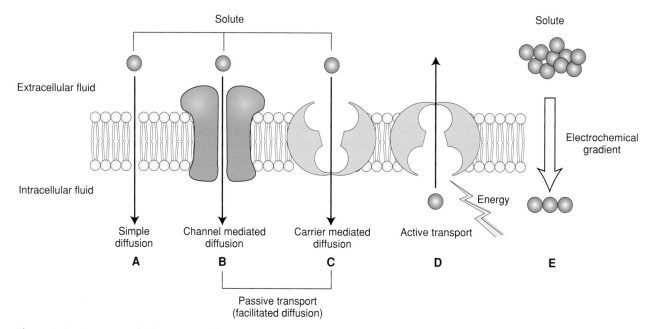

Figure 6–2 Transport of solutes across the neuronal membrane. (A) Simple diffusion. (B, C). Passive transport (facilitated diffusion) occurs either by channel-mediated (B) or carrier-mediated (C) diffusion. (D-E) Active transport occurs by specific carrier proteins, against the (E) electrochemical gradient. Active transport requires coupling of a carrier protein to a source of metabolic energy (e.g., hydrolysis of ATP).

Sodium-Potassium Ion Pump

The sodium-potassium ion pump (Na^+-K^+ pump), also known as **Na^+-K^+ ATPase**, is located in the membranes of neurons as well as other cells. The Na^+-K^+ ATPase consists of a small glycoprotein and a large multi-pass transmembrane catalytic subunit. Na^+ binds on the cytoplasmic side and K^+ binds on the external side of Na^+-K^+ ATPase. ATP binds on the cytoplasmic side of the ATPase and phosphorylates it, and a conformational change occurs, which results in the transfer of Na^+ to the outside and K^+ to the inside. Subsequently, a conformational change again occurs due to dephosphorylation, and the Na^+-K^+ ATPase reverts to its original conformation; then, the cycle is repeated. With each cycle, one molecule of ATP is hydrolyzed, and the energy generated is used to move Na^+ and K^+ ions across the neuronal membrane. There are three binding sites for Na^+ and two binding sites for K^+ on the Na^+-K^+ ATPase. Therefore, three Na^+ ions are transferred out of the neuron for every two K^+ ions that are taken in. A net outward ionic current is generated because of this unequal flow of Na^+ and K^+ ions across the neuronal membrane. Because a current is generated, the Na^+-K^+ pump is said to be **electrogenic**. Since the Na^+-K^+ pump drives more positive charges (Na^+) out of the neuron than it brings into the neuron (K^+), the inside of the neuron becomes more negative relative to the outside. It should be noted that the contribution of the Na^+-K^+ pump in making the inside of the neuron more negative relative to the outside is only about 10%; the major factor responsible for the negativity of the interior of the neuron is the presence of fixed anions.

Because the extracellular concentration of Na^+ ions is high, these ions leak into the neuron. The Na^+-K^+ ATPase pumps them out and, thus, maintains the high extracellular concentration of Na^+. It is necessary to keep the extracellular concentration of Na^+ ions high to prevent water from entering the neuron; a high intracellular concentration of solutes (fixed anions and accompanying cations) tends to pull water into the neuron. Thus, Na^+-K^+ ATPase plays an important role in maintaining (1) the ionic concentrations inside and outside the neuron and (2) the osmotic balance of the neuron.

Calcium Pump

The neuronal plasma membrane contains a calcium pump, which is an enzyme that actively transports Ca^{2+} out of the cell so that the concentration of this ion remains small inside the resting cell. One Ca^{2+} is transported for each ATP hydrolyzed.

INTRACELLULAR AND EXTRACELLULAR IONIC CONCENTRATIONS

As mentioned earlier, the concentration of various ions needs to be maintained within the neuron, necessitating flow of some ions into and out of the cell. Table 6-1 shows the differences in the intra-

Table 6–1 Approximate Neuronal Intracellular and Extracellular Concentrations of Some Important Ions

Ion	Extracellular concentration (mM)	Intracellular concentration (mM)
Cations		
Na^+	150	15
K^+	5	100
Ca^{2+}	2	0.0002
Anions		
Cl^-	150	13
A^- (fixed anions; organic acids and proteins)	—	385

mM = millimolar concentration.

cellular and extracellular concentrations of major ions. The concentration of Na^+ ions is much greater (approximately 10 times) outside the neuron compared with the concentration inside the neuron. On the other hand, the concentration of K^+ ions is greater (approximately 20 times) inside the cell than outside. The presence of many negatively charged fixed ions makes the interior of the cell more negative relative to outside. To balance these negative charges, positively charged K^+ ions are retained inside the neuron, and as such, the intracellular concentration of K^+ ions is much greater than the extracellular concentration. The intracellular concentration of Ca^{2+} is very small, and most of it is bound with proteins or stored in various organelles. Like Na^+ ions, the concentration of the Cl^- ions is greater outside relative to inside the neuron. The differences in intracellular and extracellular concentrations of different ions are maintained by Na^+-K^+ and Ca^{2+} pumps.

ELECTROPHYSIOLOGY OF THE NEURON

An understanding of the electrophysiology of neurons is likely to be facilitated if the student bears in mind the following terms.

TERMINOLOGY

Ions: Atoms or molecules that have an electrical charge.

Anions: Negatively charged ions (e.g., Cl^-).

Cations: Positively charged ions (e.g., Na^+, K^+, and Ca^{2+}).

Influx of ions: Flow of ions into the neuron.

Efflux of ions: Flow of ions out of the neuron.

Electrical Charge–Related Terms

Anode: Positive terminal of a battery; negatively charged ions (e.g., Cl^-) move towards an anode.

Cathode: Negative terminal of battery; positively charged ions (e.g., Na^+) move towards a cathode.

Electrical current: The movement of electrical charge. The flow of electrical current (I) depends on electrical potential and electrical conductance. It is measured in amperes (amps).

Electrical potential (voltage): The difference in charge between the anode and the cathode. More current flows when this difference is increased. Electrical potential is measured in volts (V).

Electrical conductance: The ability of an electrical charge to move from one point to another is determined by its electrical conductance (g). It is measured in siemans (S).

Electrical resistance: The inability of an electrical charge to move from one point to another is determined by electrical resistance (R). It is measured in ohms (Ω). Electrical resistance is the inverse of electrical conductance, and this relationship is expressed as R = 1/g.

Ohms law: This law describes the relationship between electrical current (I), electrical conductance (g), and electrical potential (V). According to this law, current is the product of the conductance and potential difference (I = gV).

Current Flow–Related Terms

Direction of current flow: In an ionic solution, cations as well as anions carry electrical current. Conventionally, current flow is defined as the direction of net movement of positive charge. Therefore, cations move in the same direction as the current. Anions move in the opposite direction as the current.

Inward current: When positively charged ions (e.g., Na^+) flow into the neuron.

Outward current: When positively charged ions (e.g., K^+) move out of the neuron or when negatively charged ions (e.g., Cl^-) move into the neuron.

Leakage current: The current due to the flow of ions through the nongated ion channels (discussed later).

Membrane Potential–Related Terms

Excitable membrane: Cells capable of generating and conducting action potentials have excitable membranes.

Membrane potential (V_m): The electrical potential difference across the neuronal membrane (i.e., between the interior and the exterior of the neuron) at any time is called the membrane potential.

Resting membrane potential: When a neuron is not generating action potentials, it is at rest. When the neuron is at rest, its cytosol along the inner surface of its membrane is negatively charged compared with the charge on the outside. Typically, the resting membrane potential (or resting potential) of a neuron is -65 millivolts (mV) (1 volt = 1000 mV).

Threshold potential: The level of membrane potential at which a sufficient number of voltage-gated sodium channels open and relative permeability of sodium ions is greater than that of potassium ions. Action potentials are generated when the membrane is depolarized beyond the threshold potential.

Depolarization: Occurs when there is a reduction in the negative charge inside the neuron (e.g., if the resting membrane potential is changed from -65 to -60 mV by flow of positively charged ions, like Na^+, into the neuron).

Hyperpolarization: Occurs when there is an increase in the negative charge inside the neuron (e.g., if the resting membrane potential changes from -65 to -70 mV by flow of positively charged ions, like K^+, out of the neuron or flow of negatively charged ions, like Cl^-, into the neuron).

ION CHANNELS

A brief description of ion channels is presented in this chapter. Further discussion of ion channels is provided in Chapters 7 and 8. Ion channels are made up of proteins that are embedded in the lipid bilayer of the neuronal membrane across which they span (Fig. 6-1). They are characterized by the following general properties.

1. The flow of ions through the channels does not require metabolic energy; the flow is passive.

2. The electrochemical driving force across the membrane, but not the channel itself, determines the direction and eventual equilibrium of this flow.

3. The ionic charge determines whether a channel allows an ion to flow through; some channels allow cations while others allow anions to flow through them.

4. Most cation-selective channels allow only one ion species (e.g., Na^+ or K^+ or Ca^{2+}) to flow through them. However, some channels allow more than one ion species to flow through them. For example, when L-glutamate (an excitatory amino acid neurotransmitter) activates an N-methyl-D-aspartic acid (NMDA) receptor (see Chapter 8), both Na^+ and Ca^{2+} ions flow through the NMDA receptor channel into the neuron.

5. Most anion-selective channels allow only Cl^- to flow through them.

6. Some blockers can prevent the flow of ions through the ion channels. For example, phencyclidine (PCP, or Angel Dust) blocks the NMDA receptor channel (see Chapter 8).

Classification of Ion Channels

The ion channels have been divided into the following two major classes: nongated and gated channels.

Nongated Channels

Although **nongated channels** are capable of opening as well as closing, most of the time they are in the open site. They control the flow of ions during the resting membrane potential. They are also known as "leak channels." Examples include nongated Na^+ and K^+ channels that contribute to the resting membrane potential.

Gated Channels

These channels are also capable of opening as well as closing. All gated channels are allosteric proteins (i.e., they exist in more than one conformation, and their function is altered when they shift from one conformation to another). Each **allosteric** channel exists in at least one open and one closed state. The transition of a channel between the open and closed states is called *gating*. At rest, these channels are mostly closed, and they open in response to different stimuli (e.g., change in membrane potential, ligand-binding, or mechanical forces). Individual channels are usually most sensitive to only one of these stimuli. Subtypes of the gated ion channels are described in the following paragraphs.

The channels that are opened or closed by a change in the membrane potential are called **voltage-gated channels**. The opening and closing of the channel is believed to be due to the movement of the charged region of the channel back and forth through the electrical field of the membrane. Voltage-gated channels exist in three states: (1) *resting state* (the channel is closed but can be activated), (2) *active state* (the channel is open), and (3) *refractory state* (the channel is inactivated). Changes in the electrical potential difference across the membrane provide the energy for gating in these channels. Genes encoding for voltage-gated Na^+, K^+, and Ca^{2+} channels belong to one family. These channels are described as follows.

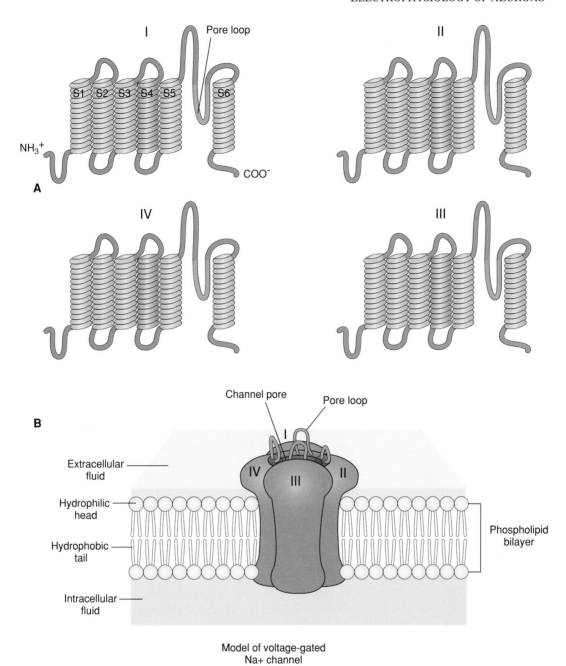

Figure 6-3 Voltage-gated Na$^+$ channel. (A) The channel is formed by a single long polypeptide that has four domains (I-IV). S1–S5 are hydrophobic alpha helices that span across the membrane. Note also the hydrophobic pore loop. The NH$_3^+$ and COO$^-$ terminals are exposed on the cytoplasmic side of the membrane. (B) The four domains clump together to form a channel with a pore. The wall of the channel pore is formed by the pore loops. The domains are shown in clockwise fashion in A and B to facilitate orientation.

The **voltage-gated Na$^+$ channel** is formed by a single long polypeptide (a string of amino acids containing peptide bonds) that has four domains (I-IV, Fig. 6-3A). Each domain has six hydrophobic alpha helices (S1–S6) that span back and forth within the cell membrane. The four domains join together and form an aqueous pore of the channel (Fig. 6-3B). An additional hydrophobic region connects the S5 and S6 alpha helical segments, forming a **pore loop** (Fig. 6-3B). The presence of this pore loop makes the channel more permeable to Na$^+$ than to K$^+$. The membrane-spanning S4 alpha helical segment is believed to be voltage sensitive. At the resting membrane potential, the channel pore is closed. The S4 segment undergoes a conformational change when the membrane potential changes (e.g., when the neuron is depolarized), the S4 segment is pushed away from the inner side of the membrane, and the channel gate opens, allowing an influx of Na$^+$ ions.

There are some cases where Na^+ permeability is blocked. Tetrodotoxin (TTX), a toxin isolated from the ovaries of Japanese puffer fish, binds to the sodium channel on the outside and blocks the sodium permeability pore. Consequently, neurons are not able to generate action potentials after the application of TTX. These channels are also blocked by local anesthetic drugs (e.g., lidocaine).

The basic structure of the **voltage-gated Ca^{2+}** channel is similar to that of the voltage-gated Na^+ channel. Ca^{2+} ions enter the postsynaptic neurons through these channels and activate enzymes. Depolarization of presynaptic nerve terminals results in entry of Ca^{2+} ions into the terminal via these channels. An increase in the levels of intracellular Ca^{2+} results in the release of transmitters from presynaptic nerve terminals.

Different varieties of **voltage-gated K^+** channels have been identified, and they serve different functions. The general scheme describing the components of this channel is similar to that of the voltage-gated Na^+ channel, except that the voltage-gated K^+ channel consists of four polypeptides. It should be recalled that each polypeptide contributing to the formation of a large protein molecule is called a subunit. Each subunit of a voltage-gated K^+ channel consists of six alpha-helical membrane-spanning segments (S1–S6). A pore loop makes the channel more permeable to K^+ than to Na^+. The S4 segment acts as an activation gate. The K^+ channels are generally blocked by chemicals such as tetraethylammonium (TEA) or 4-aminopyridine.

The **ligand-gated channels** are opened by noncovalent binding of chemical substances with their receptors on the neuronal membrane. These chemical substances include: (1) transmitters or hormones present in the extracellular fluid that bind to their receptors on the extracellular side of the channel and bring about a conformational change to open the channel (e.g., acetylcholine, γ-aminobutyric acid [GABA], or glycine); and (2) an intracellular second messenger (e.g., cyclic adenosine monophosphate, which is activated by a transmitter such as norepinephrine). The second messenger can open the channel (1) *directly* by binding to the channel and causing a conformational change or (2) *indirectly* by phosphorylating the channel protein in the presence of a protein kinase and causing a conformational change; this effect on the channel is reversed by dephosphorylation catalyzed by a protein phosphatase. Genes encoding for transmitter-gated channels (e.g., channels activated by acetylcholine, GABA, or glycine) and genes encoding for voltage-gated channels belong to different families.

Mechanically gated channels open by a mechanical stimulus and include the channels involved in producing generator potentials of stretch and touch receptors.

EQUILIBRIUM POTENTIALS

The **equilibrium potential** of an ion is the electrical potential difference at which the diffusional forces and electrical forces exerted on the ion are equal and opposite, and the net movement of the ion across the cell membrane ceases. The equilibrium potential of any ion that is present on the sides of the cell membrane, which is permeable to that ion, is calculated by the **Nernst equation** (Table 6-2). Using this equation, the value for the equilibrium potential of K^+ is -80 mV. If the membrane were permeable only to K^+, the resting membrane potential of a neuron would be equal to the equilibrium potential of K^+ (-80 mV). However, actual recordings show that the resting membrane potential of a neuron is usually -65 mV. The reason for this discrepancy is that the neuronal membrane is permeable to more than one ion species. The resting membrane potential of the neuron under these conditions is calculated by the **Goldman equation**, which takes into consideration the contribution of the permeability of each ion and its extracellular and intracellular concentrations (Table 6-2).

IONIC BASIS OF THE RESTING MEMBRANE POTENTIAL

When the neuron is at rest (i.e., when it is not generating action potentials), the cytosol along the inner surface of the cell membrane has a negative electrical charge compared with the outer surface of the cell membrane. Many negatively charged fixed ions (associated with proteins and amino acids) make the interior of the cell more negative relative to outside. The potential difference across the cell membrane during resting state is called the **resting membrane potential.** The lipid bilayer of the neuronal membrane maintains this separation of charges by acting as a barrier to the diffusion of ions across the membrane. The ion concentration gradients across the neuronal membrane are established by **ion pumps** that actively move ions into or out of neurons against their concentration gradients. The selective permeability of membranes is due to the presence of **ion channels** that allow some ions to cross the membrane in the direction of their concentration gradients.

The ion pumps and ion channels work against each other in this manner. If the neuronal mem-

Table 6–2 Nernst and Goldman Equations to Determine Equilibrium Potential of Ions and Membrane Potentials

Description	Components of the equation	Ionic equilibrium or membrane potentials
Nernst equation This equation is used to calculate equilibrium potential of an ion that is present on both sides of the cell membrane. Substitution of the values for R, T, F, and extra- and intracellular concentrations of the ion (see Table 6-1) in the equation yields the value of equilibrium potential of that ion.	$E_{ion} = 2.303 \dfrac{RT}{ZF} \log \dfrac{[ion]_o}{[ion]_i}$ Where: E_{ion} = ionic equilibrium potential R = gas constant (1.98 cal deg^{-1} mole^{-1}) T = temperature in Kelvin scale (273.15 + temperature in centigrade degrees) Z = valence of the ion F = Faraday constant (23,060 cal volt^{-1} equiv^{-1}) $[ion]_o$ = ionic concentration outside the cell $[ion]_i$ = ionic concentration inside the cell	$E_k = 61.5$ mV log 5/100 $= -80$ mV $E_{Na} = 61.5$ mV log 150/15 $= +62$ mV $E_{Ca} = 61.5$ mV log 2/0.0002 $= +123$ mV $E_{Cl} = 61.5$ mV log 150/13 $= -65$ mV If the membrane was permeable to only K$^+$, the neuronal membrane potential would be equal to E_k (-80 mV). Actual membrane potential of a neuron is usually -65 mV (see below)
Goldman equation Since the neuronal membrane is permeable to more than one ion, the Goldman equation is used to calculate membrane potential. This equation takes into consideration the contribution of the permeability of each ion and its extra- and intracellular concentrations.	$V_m = 61.5 \log$ $\dfrac{P_k [K^+]_o + P_{Na}[Na^+]_o + P_{Cl}[Cl^-]_i}{P_k [K^+]_i + P_{Na}[Na^+]_i + P_{Cl}[Cl^-]_o}$ where: V_m = membrane potential (mV) P = permeability of the specific ion Other abbreviations = same as in Nernst equation Note that the valence factor (Z) present in the Nernst equation is absent in this equation. Therefore, the concentration of negatively charged ion (Cl$^-$) has been inverted relative to the concentrations of positively charged ions; recall that $-\log(A/B) = \log(B/A)$.	If the membrane is permeable to Na$^+$ and K$^+$, but not Cl$^-$, the values related to Cl$^-$ = 0 and the derived value for $V_m = -65$ mV

brane is selectively permeable to only a K$^+$ ion, this ion will move out of the neuron down its concentration gradient. Therefore, more positive charges accumulate outside the neuron. The fixed negative charges inside the neuron impede the efflux of positively charged K$^+$ ions, and excess positive charges outside the neuron tend to promote influx of the K$^+$ ions into the neuron due to the electrostatic forces. It should be recalled that opposite charges attract, while similar charges repel each other. Thus, two forces are acting on the flow of K$^+$ ions out of the neuron; a higher concentration inside the neuron (concentration gradient) tends to expel them out of the neuron, while the electrostatic

forces tend to prevent their flow out of the neuron.

When the two opposing forces are equal, K$^+$ concentrations inside and outside the neuron are in equilibrium. The value of the membrane potential at this time is called the **K$^+$ equilibrium potential**. Thus, if the neuronal membrane contained only K$^+$ channels, the resting membrane potential would be determined by the K$^+$ concentration gradient and would be equal to the equilibrium potential for K$^+$ ions (approximately -80 mV). However, as stated earlier, the resting membrane potential of a neuron is usually -65 mV. This is because neurons at rest are permeable to the Na$^+$ ion also. The Na$^+$ ions tend to flow into the neuron due to two forces: (1) concentration gradient of Na^+ ions (extracellular Na^+ concentration is much higher than its intracellular concentration) and (2) electrostatic forces (there is an excess of positive charges outside and an excess of negative charges inside the neuron). Due to the influx of Na^+ ions, the resting membrane potential deviates from that of the K^+ equilibrium potential (i.e., it becomes -65 mV instead of -80 mV).

However, the membrane potential does not reach the equilibrium potential for Na^+. The reason for the neuron's inability to attain a resting membrane potential closer to the Na^+ equilibrium potential is that the number of open nongated Na^+ channels is much smaller than the number of open nongated K^+ channels in the resting state of a neuron. Therefore, the permeability of Na^+ is small despite large electrostatic and concentration gradient forces tending to drive it into the neuron. To maintain a steady resting membrane potential, the separation of charges across the neuronal membrane must be maintained at a constant. This is accomplished by the Na^+-K^+ pump described earlier.

IONIC BASIS OF THE ACTION POTENTIAL

As stated earlier, the resting membrane potential of a neuron is usually -65 mV. At rest, Na^+ influx into the neuron through open nongated Na^+ channels is balanced by the efflux of K^+ through open nongated K^+ channels. Thus, the membrane potential remains constant closer (but not equal) to the K^+ equilibrium. When a neuron receives an excitatory input, the neuronal membrane is depolarized, resulting in an opening of some voltage-gated Na^+ channels and influx of Na^+. It should be noted that voltage-gated Na^+ channels are normally closed. The accumulation of positive charges due to influx of Na^+ promotes depolarization of the neuronal membrane. When the membrane potential reaches **threshold potential**, the chances of generating an action potential are about 50%. However, when the membrane is depolarized beyond the threshold potential, a sufficient number of voltage-gated Na^+ channels open, relative permeability of Na^+ ions is greater than that of K^+ ions, and action potentials are generated with certainty. Generation of an action potential is an "all-or-nothing" phenomenon. Because the concentration of Na^+ channels is relatively high at the axon hillock, this is the site of generation of action potentials in a neuron.

The configuration of an action potential is shown in Figure 6-4A. During the rising phase of

the action potential, there is a rapid depolarization of the membrane due to increased permeability of Na^+ (Fig. 6-4B). The depolarization continues so that the membrane potential approaches the Na^+ equilibrium potential. The part of the action potential where the inside of the neuron is positive relative to the outside is called the **overshoot.** Towards the end of the rising phase of the action potential, voltage-gated Na^+ channels are inactivated, and the influx of Na^+ through these channels is stopped.

During the **falling phase** of the action potential, the neuron is repolarized by opening of voltage-gated K^+ channels, which allows increased efflux of K^+ from the neuron through these channels (Fig. 6-4B). The opening of voltage-gated K^+ channels is also caused by depolarization of the neuronal membrane. Because these voltage-gated K^+ channels open with a delay (about 1 msec) after the mem-

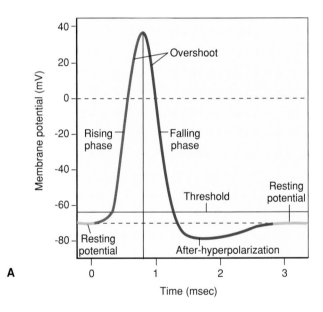

Configuration of action potential

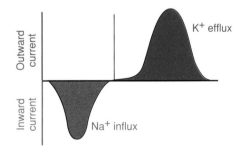

Figure 6–4 Configuration of an action potential. (A) Phases of an action potential. (B) Inward and outward current flows due to the influx of Na^+ and efflux of K^+, during the rising and falling phases of the action potential, respectively.

brane depolarization and their opening rectifies the membrane potential, they are called **delayed rectifier K$^+$ channels**. At the end of the falling phase, the membrane potential is more negative than the resting potential because of increased K$^+$ permeability caused by the opening of the delayed rectifier K$^+$ channels in addition to the already present resting K$^+$ permeability through nongated channels. The permeability is closer to the equilibrium potential of K$^+$ because there is little Na$^+$ permeability during this period. This portion of the action potential is called **after-hyperpolarization** or **undershoot** (Fig. 6-4A). Once after-hyperpolarization has occurred, the resting membrane potential is restored gradually as the voltage-gated K$^+$ channels close again.

The Na$^+$ channel has two hypothetical gates, the activation and inactivation gates. Depending on which gates are open or closed, the sodium channel exists in the following three states: resting, activated, or inactivated.

1. **Resting state**: During this state, the activation gate closes the channel pore while the inactivation gate is open (Fig. 6-5A). With the channel pore closed, Na$^+$ cannot flow into the neuron.

2. **Activated state**: During the rising phase of action potential, both activation and inactivation gates are open, and Na$^+$ ions flow into the neuron (Fig. 6-5B).

3. **Inactivated state**: During this state, the inactivation gate closes the channel pore while the activation gate is still open (Fig. 6-5C). Even though the activation gate is open, Na$^+$ cannot flow into the neuron. The neuron cannot be activated until the sodium channel reverts back to resting state (i.e., the inactivation gate opens the channel, and the activation gate closes the channel). This process is known as **de-inactivation**. Voltage-gated Na$^+$ channels get de-inactivated when the membrane potential becomes adequately negative.

The time required for the sodium channel to revert from inactivated to resting state (de-inactivation) determines the **refractory period** of the neuron. The period during which the voltage-gated Na$^+$ channels are in inactivated state and an action potential cannot be generated is called the **absolute refractory period**. Immediately after the absolute refractory period (the period at the end of the falling phase), when the neuron is hyperpolarized, until the time when voltage-gated K$^+$ channels are closed again, an action potential can be generated, but more depolarizing current is needed to shift the membrane potential to threshold level. This phase of action potential is called

the **relative refractory period.** The entire duration of an action potential in a neuron is about 2 msec. It should be noted that, during an action potential, there is a great surge of Na$^+$ influx into the cell via the voltage-gated Na$^+$ channels. However, the Na$^+$-K$^+$ pump is working all the time, including the duration of the action potential, and transports Na$^+$ out of the neuron via nongated channels to maintain the ionic concentration gradients across the cell membrane.

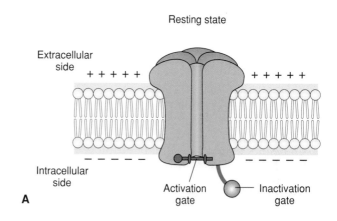

A

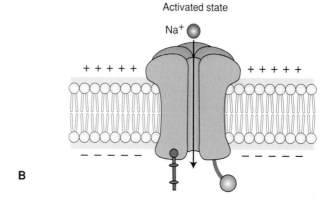

B

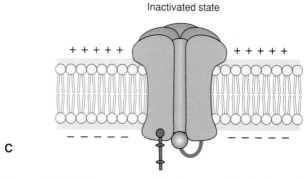

C

Figure 6–5 Different states of voltage-gated Na$^+$ channel. (A) Resting state. (B) Activated state. (C) Inactivated state. Note: the "bar" is the activation gate and the "circle" represents the inactivation gate. (See text for descriptions.).

PROPAGATION OF ACTION POTENTIALS

When a region (region 1 in Fig. 6-6A) of an unmyelinated axonal membrane is depolarized sufficiently by a depolarizing stimulus (e.g., a synaptic potential in a neuron) to reach a threshold potential, voltage-gated Na$^+$ channels open, Na$^+$ flows into the axoplasm, and an action potential is generated in that region of the axon (Fig. 6-6B). Some of the current generated by the action potential spreads by electrotonic conduction (passive spread) to an adjacent region (region 2 in Fig. 6-6A) of the axon. The passive spread of current occurs by movement of electrons, and movement of Na$^+$ ions is not required. At the adjacent region, the passive spread of current results in opening of voltage-gated Na$^+$ channels, influx of Na$^+$ into the axoplasm (Fig.6-6C, region 2), and generation of an action potential (Fig. 6-6D). In other words, the passive spread of voltage along the length of an axon results in an active regeneration process.

The propagation of an action potential along the axon depends on the cable properties of the axon. The larger the diameter of the axon, the lower the resistance there is to the flow of current along its length. Therefore, the conduction velocity (propagation of action potentials) along the length of the axon can be increased by increasing its diameter. For example, the axons of stellate ganglion neurons in the squid are about 1 mm in diameter (100–1000 times larger than the axons of mammalian neurons). The conduction of action potentials in these squid giant axons is faster than in mammalian axons. The squid needs these fast conducting axons for faster contraction of the mantle muscles that produce a jet propulsion effect needed for quick escape from predators.

In vertebrates, the conduction velocity is increased by myelination of axon. A myelin sheath consists of about 1-mm lengths of as many as 300 concentric layers of membrane around a single axon. In the peripheral nervous system, myelin is formed by Schwann cells. In the central nervous system, oligodendrocytes form the myelin (see Chapter 5). **Nodes of Ranvier** (bare segments of the axonal membrane with a very high density of voltage-gated Na$^+$ channels) are present in between the segments of the myelin sheath (Fig. 6-7, A and C). The myelinated segments of an axon are not excitable and have a high resistance to the leakage of current across them. On the other hand, passive spread of current can generate an intense current at the nodes of Ranvier due to the presence of a high density of voltage-gated Na$^+$ channels.

When a depolarizing stimulus (e.g., a synaptic potential in a neuron) arrives at a node of Ranvier (node 1 in Fig. 6-7A), Na$^+$ channels open, there is an influx of Na$^+$ ions, and an action potential is generated at that node (Fig. 6-7B). Some current generated by the action potential spreads passively to the next node of Ranvier (node 2 in Fig. 6-7A), and depolarization of the membrane at this node results in the generation of an action potential (Fig. 6-7D). By this time, Na$^+$ channels at the preceding node (node 1 in Fig. 6-7C) are inactivated, K$^+$ channels open, and repolarization occurs. Thus, the action potential propagates along a myelinated axon by **saltatory conduction** (i.e., the jumping of an action potential from one node to another). Myelination of an axon has two advantages: (1) conduction is very rapid along an axon, and (2) there is a conservation of metabolic energy because excitation is restricted to the nodal regions that are relatively small (0.5 μm).

CLINICAL CONSIDERATIONS

Many clinical syndromes have been attributed to malfunction of different ion channels and disturbances in the generation and conduction of action potentials. Some of these syndromes are briefly described here.

LAMBERT-EATON (EATON-LAMBERT) SYNDROME

This disorder is usually associated with small-cell carcinoma of the lung, which is derived from primitive neuroendocrine precursor cells expressing voltage-gated Ca^{2+} channels. An antibody is produced in the body against these Ca^{2+} channels, and its presence results in a loss of voltage-gated Ca^{2+} channels in the presynaptic terminals at the neuromuscular junction. Therefore, less Ca^{2+} enters the presynaptic terminal during depolarization and, consequently, there is a reduction in the release of the transmitter (acetylcholine) at the neuromuscular junction that results in muscle weakness. Loss of voltage-gated Ca^{2+} channels at the preganglionic nerve terminals of the sympathetic and parasympathetic autonomic nervous system results in a number of symptoms characteristic of autonomic dysfunction. These symptoms include dry mouth, constipation, reduced sweating, orthostatic hypotension (dizziness while standing or walking), and impotence.

GUILLAIN-BARRÉ SYNDROME

This syndrome has been described as a clinical case in Chapter 5.

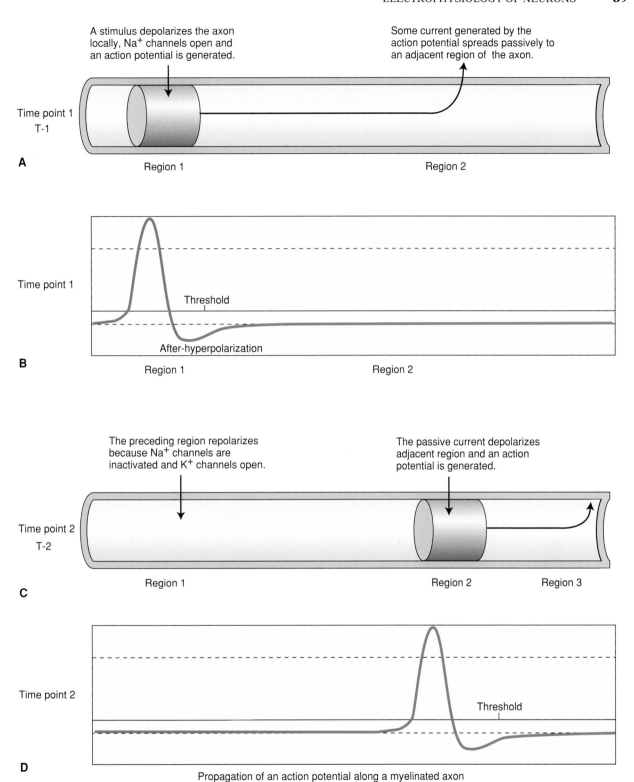

A stimulus depolarizes the axon locally, Na⁺ channels open and an action potential is generated.

Some current generated by the action potential spreads passively to an adjacent region of the axon.

Time point 1
T-1

Region 1   Region 2

A

Time point 1

Threshold

After-hyperpolarization

B

Region 1   Region 2

The preceding region repolarizes because Na⁺ channels are inactivated and K⁺ channels open.

The passive current depolarizes adjacent region and an action potential is generated.

Time point 2
T-2

Region 1   Region 2   Region 3

C

Time point 2

Threshold

D

Propagation of an action potential along a myelinated axon

Figure 6–6 Propagation of action potentials in unmyelinated axons, as described in the text. (A) Time point 1: region 1 of an unmyelinated axonal membrane is depolarized. (B) Depolarization in region 1 results in an action potential at time point 1. (C) Time point 2: passive spread of current by the action potential generated at time point 1 causes depolarization in region 2. (D) Depolarization in region 2 results in an action potential at time point 2.

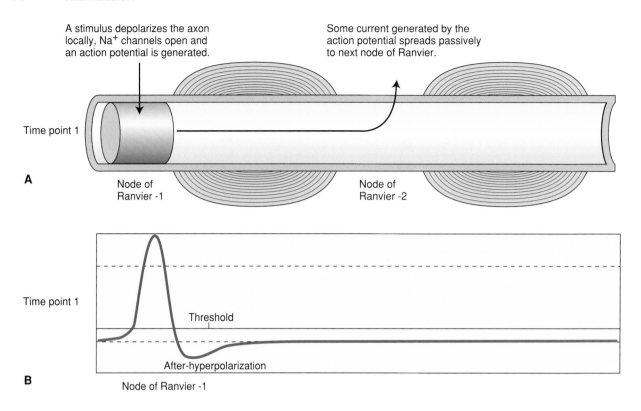

A stimulus depolarizes the axon locally, Na⁺ channels open and an action potential is generated.

Some current generated by the action potential spreads passively to next node of Ranvier.

Time point 1

A

Node of Ranvier -1

Node of Ranvier -2

Time point 1

Threshold

After-hyperpolarization

B

Node of Ranvier -1

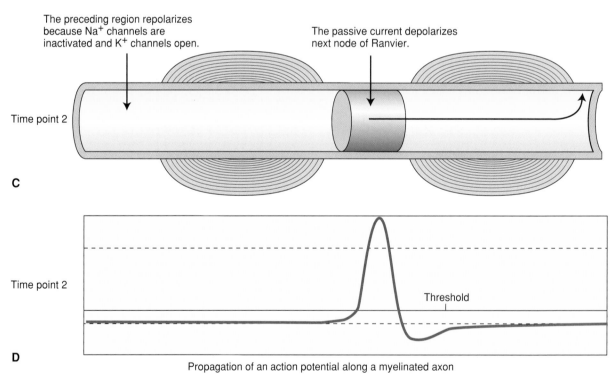

The preceding region repolarizes because Na⁺ channels are inactivated and K⁺ channels open.

The passive current depolarizes next node of Ranvier.

Time point 2

C

Time point 2

Threshold

D

Propagation of an action potential along a myelinated axon

Figure 6–7 Propagation of action potentials in myelinated axons. (A) Time point 1: a stimulus depolarizes node of Ranvier 1. (B) An action potential is generated at node 1 at time point 1. (C) Time point 2: passive spread of current due to action potential generated at time point 1 depolarizes node 2. (D) An action potential is generated at node 2 at time point 2.

MULTIPLE SCLEROSIS

Patients with this disease have muscle weakness, lack of coordination, and disturbances in speech and vision. The cause of this disease is unknown. It may be an autoimmune disease with inflammatory features. In these patients, myelination of axons in the optic nerves, brain, and spinal cord is disrupted. Assessment of the slowing of conduction in the optic nerve of these patients is used as one of the tests of this disease. Conduction in the optic nerve is tested by applying a visual stimulus consisting of a checkerboard pattern and monitoring visual evoked potentials from the scalp (for more on multiple sclerosis, see also Chapter 9).

CYSTIC FIBROSIS

Cystic fibrosis is an inherited disease that affects primarily the respiratory system (airways and the lungs). It is a recessive disorder (i.e., a person is afflicted with this disease when he/she inherits a copy of the mutated gene from each parent). The mutated gene is known as CFTR gene, which resides on chromosome 7. The genetic mutation stops production of a protein in the cells of the lungs (and other organs, e.g., pancreas). The lack of this protein impairs the function of Cl^- channels that are involved in the production of secretions in the lungs. Thus, the ability of these cells to transport Cl^- in and out of cells is impaired, and the chemical properties of secretions are changed, causing the mucus to be thicker than normal, which leads to obstructions in the respiratory tract and creates conditions that lead to repeated infections. Management of the respiratory symptoms of the disease include administration of antibiotics (for treating infections), decongestants and bronchodilators (to open airways), steroids (to reduce inflammation), chest or back clapping (to help loosen mucus from lungs), and postural drainage (to help drain mucus from lungs).

CLINICAL CASE

HISTORY

Martha is a 33-year-old woman who, until several months ago, was a normal, healthy individual who exercised regularly. She maintained an administrative position in the Department of Neurology at a northeastern medical school. On three separate occasions over the past 2 months, she began to experience weakness and numbness in her right arm and leg. In addition, she also began to have double vision and experienced a sensation as if insects were moving along the right side of her face and tongue. She consulted her physician, who then referred her to a neurologist.

EXAMINATION

The neurological examination revealed some nystagmus (see Chapters 14, 17, and 21) when she attempted to look to the right, some depressed vision in her right eye, weakness of the right eye when medial gaze was attempted, and some weakness of the right facial muscles. She also showed some tremor when attempting to point to her nose, a wide ataxic gait, and general difficulty in walking. The evoked potentials test revealed a longer than normal latency for the visual evoked response following stimulation of the right eye. A magnetic resonance imaging (MRI) scan of the head indicated the presence of what appeared to be small lesions over widespread regions of the brain. A lumbar puncture was done to collect a CSF sample that, on subsequent analysis, showed an increase in gamma globulin level above normal values.

EXPLANATION

Martha was diagnosed with multiple sclerosis, a syndrome described earlier in the text of this chapter. The MRI showed that there was no single locus of a lesion. Instead, a variety of lesions seemed to be present, affecting both sensory and motor systems, and visual evoked potential test revealed slower conduction velocity along visual neuronal pathways. These symptoms are consistent with a diagnosis of multiple sclerosis. Multiple sclerosis is a debilitating disease that frequently affects young people, especially women in their 30s. It typically affects such systems as the white matter of the cerebellum, spinal cord, and projections of the corticospinal tract and basal ganglia, causing an upper motor neuron weakness, as well as sensory systems such as the visual and somatosensory pathways, resulting in numbness and some loss of vision.

The course of this disease can vary. There may be no re-occurrence after the first event. In other cases, there may be a series of episodes followed by periods of remission. In the worst cases, the disease is progressive in which few or no periods of remission are present. Treatment strategies include the administration of steroids. Another treatment includes administration of interferon β-1b, which has been shown to reduce the frequency and severity of relapses. In the case of Martha, she was treated with oral prednisone in the hospital for 5 days. She showed an excellent recovery and soon resumed her professional life.

CHAPTER TEST

QUESTIONS

Choose the best answer for each question.

1. Which of the following statements is correct regarding the Na$^+$-K$^+$ pump?
   a. Binding sites for ATP are located on the extracellular side of the pump.
   b. It drives more positive charges into the neuron.
   c. Binding sites for K$^+$ ions are located on the cytoplasmic side of the pump.
   d. It pumps out two Na$^+$ ions and pumps three K$^+$ ions into the neuron.
   e. It pumps out of the neuron three Na$^+$ ions and pumps in two K$^+$ ions.

2. Which of the following statements is correct regarding the voltage-gated Na$^+$ channel?
   a. It is in an open state at the resting membrane potential.
   b. It is blocked by local anesthetic drugs.
   c. It is formed by several long polypeptide chains.
   d. It is equally permeable to Na$^+$ as well as K$^+$ ions.
   e. It can be activated during the falling phase of the action potential.

3. Which of the following statements is correct regarding the rising phase of an action potential in a neuron?
   a. The membrane potential becomes more negative during this phase.
   b. There is an influx of Na$^+$ through the nongated ion channels.
   c. Na$^+$ flows into the neuron through voltage-gated Na$^+$ channels.
   d. K$^+$ flows into the neuron through the voltage-gated K$^+$ channels.
   e. Energy for influx of Na$^+$ is provided by the Na$^+$-K$^+$ pump.

4. A 25-year-old woman complained to her neurologist of a sudden onset of blurred vision, loss of visual acuity, and loss of color vision in her right eye. The patient also experienced pain behind her right eye. The neurologist suspected that this was a case of optic neuritis and ordered a magnetic resonance imaging (MRI) scan. The MRI showed changes consistent with demyelinating disease. The optic neuritis with this history was associated with which one of the following disorders?
   a. Myasthenia gravis
   b. Lambert-Eaton syndrome
   c. Guillain-Barré Syndrome
   d. Multiple sclerosis
   e. Cystic fibrosis

5. A patient visiting a neurologist complained of spells of dizziness while standing, dry mouth, constipation, and muscle weakness. A routine chest x-ray revealed a tumor in the lung. Biopsy of the tissue suggested the presence of small-cell carcinoma of the lung. Which one of the following is likely to account for muscle weakness in this patient?
   a. Loss of voltage-gated Ca^{2+} channels in the presynaptic terminals
   b. Loss of voltage-gated K$^+$ channels in the neuronal cell body
   c. Excessive release of acetylcholine from nerve terminals
   d. Blockade of voltage-gated Na$^+$ channels in the neurons
   e. Excessive increase in the conductance of Cl$^-$ channels in the spinal motor neurons

ANSWERS AND EXPLANATIONS

1. Answer: **e**

The Na$^+$-K$^+$ pump is located in the neuronal membrane. Binding sites for ATP and Na$^+$ ions are located on the cytoplasmic side. It pumps out three Na$^+$ ions for the two K$^+$ ions it pumps in. Thus, it drives more positive charges out of the cell than it brings into the cell. Binding site for K$^+$ is located on the extracellular side of the pump.

2. Answer: **b**

This channel is formed by a single long polypeptide that has four domains (I-IV). Each domain has six hydrophobic alpha helices (S1–S6) that span back and forth within the cell membrane. The four domains join together and form an aqueous pore of the channel. These channels open during the rising phase of the action potential. At the resting membrane potential, the channel pore is closed. When the neuron is depolarized, the channel gate opens, allowing an influx of Na$^+$ ions. They are blocked by a poison, called tetrodotoxin (TTX), obtained from the puffer fish, and local anesthetic drugs (e.g., lidocaine). At the end of the rising phase of the action potential, the voltage-gated Na^+ channels are inactivated. They cannot be activated to generate an action potential until the membrane potential becomes adequately negative and the Na^+ channels get de-inactivated. The period during which the Na^+ channels are in an inactivated state and an action potential cannot be generated is called the absolute refractory period.

3. Answer: c

When the membrane depolarizes beyond the threshold potential, a sufficient number of voltage-gated Na^+ channels open, and there is an influx of Na^+ during the rising phase of the action potential. The membrane potential becomes less negative during depolarization. The flow of ions through the voltage-gated channels during the rising phase of the action potential does not require energy. At the end of the depolarization, there is an efflux of K^+, and the neuron repolarizes.

4. Answer: d

In patients with multiple sclerosis, demyelination of axons in the optic nerves, brain, and spinal cord occurs. Therefore, neural conduction in the CNS is disrupted. On the other hand, in Guillain-Barré syndrome, demyelination occurs in peripheral nerves, innervating the muscles and skin. In the other syndromes listed, there is not demyelination of axons.

5. Answer: a

The patient is suffering from Lambert-Eaton syndrome. In patients with this syndrome, a specific antibody causes loss of voltage-gated Ca^{2+} channels in the presynaptic terminal at the neuromuscular junction. Therefore, depolarization of the terminal does not result in opening of a sufficient number of Ca^{2+} channels, and the release of the transmitter (acetylcholine) is reduced. This results in muscle weakness. The patient's other symptoms are caused by the loss of voltage-gated Ca^{2+} channels in the presynaptic terminals of the sympathetic and parasympathetic divisions of the autonomic nervous system.

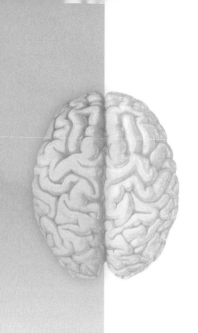

CHAPTER 7

SYNAPTIC TRANSMISSION

OBJECTIVES

In this chapter, the student is expected to:

1. Know the salient features of chemical transmission

2. Know the characteristics of electrical transmission

3. Know the components of receptors

4. Define indirectly gated ion channels

5. Know the mechanism of directly gated synaptic transmission at the peripheral synapse (nerve-muscle synapse)

6. Know the mechanism of directly gated synaptic transmission at the central synapses

7. Know the diseases affecting chemical transmission at the nerve-muscle synapse

One of the unique features of nerve cells is their capability to communicate with each other with great precision even when they are separated by long distances. The mechanism by which neurons communicate with each other is called **synaptic transmission,** which is defined as the transfer of signals from one cell to another. A **synapse** is described as a special zone of contact at which one neuron communicates with another. In this chapter, the different types of synapses and various aspects of synaptic transmission are described.

TYPES OF SYNAPTIC TRANSMISSION

Two types of synaptic transmission—electrical and chemical—are recognized in the nervous system. It should be noted that the electrical synapses are relatively less common than the chemical synapses in the mammalian nervous system.

ELECTRICAL TRANSMISSION

In electrical transmission between the nerve cells, the current generated by an impulse in one neuron spreads to another neuron through a pathway of low electrical resistance. Electrical synapses occur at gap junctions (described later in this section). In an electrical synapse, ion channels connect the cytoplasm of the presynaptic and postsynaptic cells. In the adult mammalian central nervous system, electrical synapses are present where the activity of neighboring neurons needs to be highly synchronized. For example, hormone-secreting neurons in mammalian hypothalamus are connected with electrical synapses so that they fire almost simultaneously and secrete a burst of hormone into the circulation.

At an electrical synapse, the current generated by voltage-gated channels at the presynaptic neuron flows directly into the postsynaptic neuron. Therefore, transmission at such a synapse is very rapid (<0.1 msec). At some synapses (e.g., in the giant motor synapse of crayfish), the current can pass in one direction (from presynaptic to postsynaptic neuron) but not in the reverse direction. Such synapses are called **rectifying** or **unidirectional synapses.** At other synapses, the current can pass equally well in both directions. Such synapses are called **nonrectifying** or **bidirectional synapses.** Most electrical synapses in mammalian nervous system are believed to be the nonrectifying type.

At this point, it is important to understand the morphology of a gap junction. The area where the two neurons are apposed to each other, at an electrical synapse, is called a **gap junction** (Fig. 7-1A). The channels that connect the neurons at the gap junction are called **gap junction channels** (Fig. 7-1B). The extracellular space between pre- and postsynaptic neurons at an electrical synapse is 3–3.5 nm, which is much smaller than the usual extracellular space (about 20–50 nm) between neurons. The narrow space between these neurons is bridged by gap junction channels. These channels are formed by two hemichannels, one in the presynaptic neuron and the other in the postsynaptic neuron. Each hemichannel is called a **connexon** (Fig. 7-1C), which is composed of six subunits of identical proteins called **connexins** (Fig. 7-1D). In the connexon, the connexins are arranged in a hexagonal pattern (Fig. 7-1C). Each connexin consists of four membrane-spanning regions (Fig. 7-1E). The hemichannels located in pre- and postsynaptic neurons meet each other at the gap between the membranes of the two neurons and form a conducting channel. Rotation of the connexins, in a manner similar to the opening of a shutter in a camera, results in the opening of the pore of the gap junction channel.

It should be noted that gap junctions are relatively rare in adult mammalian nervous system. However, they are more common in nonneural cells, such as the epithelial cells, smooth and cardiac muscle cells, liver cells, some glandular cells, and glia. In Schwann cells of the myelin sheath, successive layers of myelin are connected with gap junctions, which allow flow of ions and small metabolites between these myelin layers. A form of **Charcot-Marie-Tooth disease** is characterized by demyelination, which is caused by a mutation in one of the connexin genes expressed in the Schwann cells. As a result of this mutation, connexin fails to form functional gap junction channels, which are essential for the normal flow of metabolites in the Schwann cells. One of the consequences of this defect is the impairment in the myelination process.

CHEMICAL TRANSMISSION

At chemical synapses (Fig. 7-2A), there is no continuity between the cytoplasm of the presynaptic terminal and postsynaptic neuron. Instead, the cells are separated by **synaptic clefts,** which are fluid-filled gaps (about 20–50 nm). The presynaptic and postsynaptic membranes adhere to each other due to the presence of a matrix of extracellular fibrous protein in the synaptic cleft. The presynaptic terminal contains synaptic vesicles that are filled with several thousand molecules of a specific chemical substance, the **neurotransmitter**.

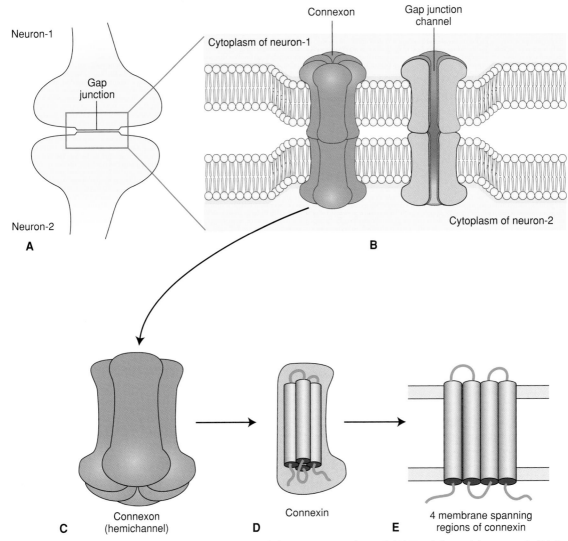

Figure 7–1 Morphology of a gap junction. (A) Gap junction. (B) Gap junction channel. (C) Hemichannel (connexon). (D) Connexin. (E) Membrane-spanning regions of connexin.

Pyramid-like structures consisting of proteins arise from the intracellular side of the presynaptic terminal membrane and project into the cytoplasm of the presynaptic terminal. These pyramids and the membranes associated with them are called **active zones** and are the specialized release sites in the presynaptic terminal. The vesicles containing the neurotransmitter are aggregated near the active zones.

TYPES OF CENTRAL NERVOUS SYSTEM SYNAPSES

Axodendritic synapse: when the postsynaptic membrane is on a dendrite of another neuron (Fig. 7-2B).

Axosomatic synapse: when the postsynaptic membrane is on the cell body (soma) of another neuron (Fig. 7-2C).

Axoaxonic synapse: when the postsynaptic membrane is on the axon of another neuron (Fig. 7-2D).

Dendrodentritic synapse: when some dendrites of some specialized neurons form synapses with each other.

Symmetric synapse: when postsynaptic and presynaptic membranes are similar in thickness. This type of synapse is usually inhibitory (Fig. 7-2E).

Asymmetrical synapse: when the postsynaptic membrane of a synapse is thicker than the presynaptic membrane. This type of synapse is usually excitatory (Fig. 7-2F).

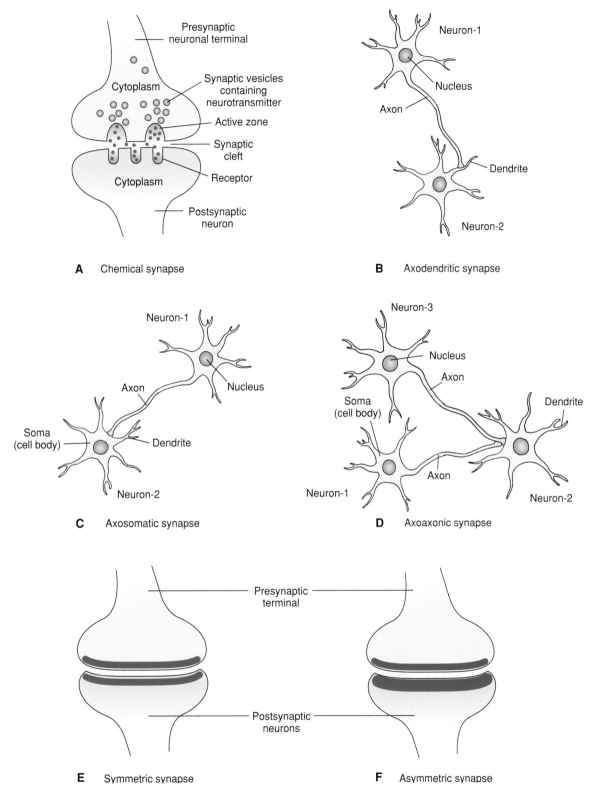

Figure 7–2 Morphology of a chemical synapse. (A) The presynaptic terminal and postsynaptic neuron are separated by a fluid-filled synaptic cleft. Note that the presynaptic terminal contains synaptic vesicles, which contain neurotransmitter and active zones. Receptors for the transmitter are located on the postsynaptic membrane. Different types of CNS synapses are (B) axodendritic synapse, (C) axosomatic synapse, and (D) axoaxonic synapse. (E) In a symmetrical synapse, the presynaptic and postsynaptic membranes are similar in thickness. (F) In an asymmetrical synapse, the postsynaptic membrane of a synapse is thicker than the presynaptic membrane.

MECHANISMS OF TRANSMITTER RELEASE

An action potential depolarizes the presynaptic nerve terminal, voltage-gated Ca^{2+} channels located in the presynaptic terminal membrane open, Ca^{2+} permeability increases, and Ca^{2+} enters the terminal (Fig. 7-3A) (see Chapter 6 for a description of voltage-gated channels). These events cause the membrane of the vesicles to fuse with the presynaptic membrane at the active zone and release the neurotransmitter into the synaptic cleft (Fig. 7-3B). This process of transmitter release is called **exocytosis**. Details of the mechanism of fusion of the vesicular and presynaptic membranes are described in Chapter 8. The neurotransmitter then diffuses across the synaptic cleft to the membrane of the postsynaptic neuron, interacts with its specific receptors, and opens or closes several thousand channels in the postsynaptic membrane, through which specific ions enter or leave the neuron (i.e., the permeability of different ion species is changed) (Fig. 7-3C).

The nature of the response (i.e., excitatory or inhibitory) elicited at the postsynaptic neuron does not depend on the chemical nature of the transmitter. Instead, it depends on the type of receptor being activated and the ion species that becomes more permeable. For example, acetylcholine produces synaptic excitation at the neuromuscular junction (skeletal muscle contraction) by binding with the **nicotinic cholinergic receptor**, while the same transmitter produces an inhibitory response (decrease in heart rate) by interacting with a **muscarinic cholinergic receptor** located in the cardiac tissue. As stated earlier, chemical synapses are much more common than electrical synapses in the nervous system. They are involved in mediating complex functions. One of the important characteristics of chemical synapses is that they can amplify signals (i.e., a small presynaptic nerve terminal can change the potential of a large postsynaptic cell).

RECEPTORS

Receptors consist of membrane-spanning proteins. The recognition sites for the binding of the chemical transmitter are located on the extracellular components of the receptor. As indicated earlier, when a neurotransmitter binds to its receptor, the result is opening or closing of ion channels on the postsynaptic membrane. The ion channels are gated either directly or indirectly (by activating a second-messenger system within the postsynaptic cell). Details regarding different receptors and their subtypes are described in Chapter 8.

DIRECTLY GATED ION CHANNELS

The classification of different types of gated channels has been described in Chapter 6. In a directly gated ion channel, several protein subunits (four or

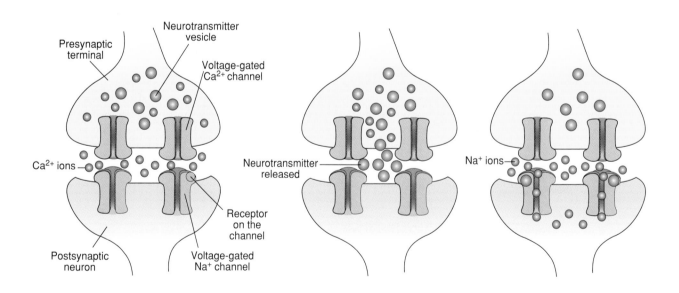

A Action potential depolarizes the presynaptic terminal membrane, Ca^{2+} channels open and Ca^{2+} ions enter the terminal.

B Ca^{2+} ions in the terminal promote fusion of vesicular and terminal membranes and the neurotransmitter is released in the synaptic cleft.

C Neurotransmitter binds with the receptor on the channel which opens, Na^+ ions enter the postsynaptic neuron, depolarize it, and excite it.

Figure 7–3 Mechanism of transmitter release.

five) are arranged in such a way that the recognition site for the neurotransmitter is part of the ion channel. This type of receptor is called an **ionotropic receptor**. A transmitter binds to its receptor and brings about a conformational change that results in the opening of the ion channel. Receptors of this type usually bring about fast synaptic responses that last for only a few milliseconds. In the central nervous system (CNS), examples of such ionotropic receptors include those associated with specific neurotransmitters (e.g., acetylcholine, glutamate, gamma aminobutyric acid [GABA], and glycine) (see Chapter 8).

DIRECTLY GATED SYNAPTIC TRANSMISSION AT A PERIPHERAL SYNAPSE (NEUROMUSCULAR JUNCTION)

The cell bodies of motor neurons are located in the ventral horn of the spinal cord (Fig. 7-4A). At the **neuromuscular junction**, the axons of motor neurons innervate skeletal muscle fibers (Fig. 7-4B). As the motor axon reaches a specialized region on the muscle membrane, called the **motor end-plate**, it loses its myelin sheath and gives off several fine branches. Many varicosities (swellings), called synaptic boutons, are present at the terminals of these branches (Fig. 7-4C). These boutons lie over depressions in the surface of the muscle fiber membrane. At these depressions, the muscle fiber membrane forms several folds called postsynaptic junctional folds (Fig. 7-4D) that are lined by a basement membrane (connective tissue consisting of collagen and glycoproteins).

The presynaptic boutons enclose the synaptic vesicles that contain acetylcholine. When the motor axon is stimulated, an action potential reaches the axon terminal and depolarizes the membrane of the presynaptic bouton; the result is that the **voltage-gated Ca^{2+} channels** open. Influx of Ca^{2+} into the terminal promotes fusion of the vesicle with the terminal membrane and subsequent release of acetylcholine by exocytosis. Acetylcholine acts on the nicotinic cholinergic receptors (see Chapter 8) located at the crest of the junctional folds to produce an excitatory postsynaptic potential in the muscle fiber, which is generally referred to as an **end-plate potential (EPP).**

During the EPP, Na$^+$ flows into the postsynaptic cell while K$^+$ flows out of the cell because the transmitter-gated ionic channel at the motor end-plate is permeable to both Na$^+$ and K$^+$. The current for the EPP is determined by: (1) the total number of end-plate channels, (2) the probability of the opening of the channel, (3) the conductance of each open channel, and (4) the driving forces acting on the ions. In the junctional folds, the muscle cell membrane has a high density of voltage-gated channels that are selective for Na$^+$. The amplitude of the EPP is large enough (about 70 mV) to activate the voltage-gated Na$^+$ channels in the junctional folds and generate an action potential that then propagates along the muscle fiber and brings about muscle contraction. Released acetylcholine is then inactivated by the enzyme **acetylcholinesterase** that is present in the basement membrane at the end-plate. Acetylcholinesterase is synthesized in the endoplasmic reticulum of the presynaptic neuronal cell body. The enzyme is transported to its active site (e.g., presynaptic axonal terminal) by the axonal microtubules.

The following features of the transmission at the nerve-muscle synapse (peripheral synapse) contribute to its relative simplicity compared to the transmission at a central synapse: (1) only one motor neuron innervates a muscle fiber, (2) only excitatory input (no inhibitory input) is received by each muscle fiber, (3) only one neurotransmitter (acetylcholine) activates the muscle fibers, and (4) only one kind of receptor channel (nicotinic acetylcholine receptor channel) mediates the actions of acetylcholine.

DIRECTLY GATED TRANSMISSION AT A CENTRAL SYNAPSE

The directly gated synaptic transmission at a **central synapse** is more complex than that at the nerve-muscle synapse. The transmission at a synapse in the CNS involves many inhibitory as well as excitatory inputs to a central neuron. These inputs release different transmitters that are targeted for different receptor channels in the neuronal membrane.

When a neuron is stimulated (e.g., by a neurotransmitter), **graded potentials** are produced, which are brief local changes in membrane potential that occur in neuronal dendrites and cell bodies but not in axons. They are called graded potentials because their amplitude is directly proportional to the intensity of the stimulus; the larger the stimulus, the greater the change in membrane potential. Graded potentials travel through the neuron until they reach the **trigger zone**. In the efferent neurons, the trigger zone is at the axon hillock. The purpose of the graded potentials is to drive the axon hillock to threshold membrane potential so that an **action potential** is generated. **Threshold** is a membrane potential at the trigger zone at which action potentials become self-propagating (self-generating), which means that an ac-

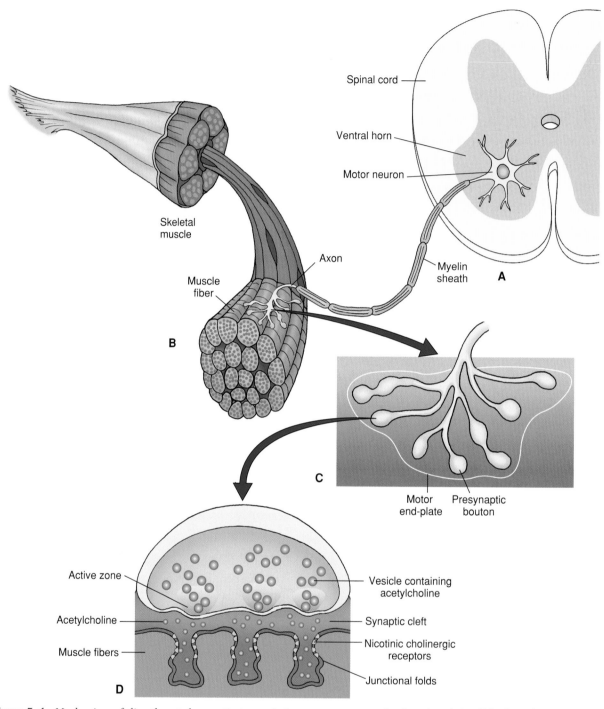

Figure 7–4 Mechanism of directly gated synaptic transmission at a neuromuscular junction. (A) Cell bodies of motor neurons. (B and C) Myelinated axons of motor neurons innervate skeletal muscle fibers. As the motor axon reaches a specialized region on the muscle membrane (motor end-plate), it loses its myelin sheath and gives off several fine branches. Presynaptic boutons (swellings) are present at the terminals of these branches. (D) The presynaptic boutons have synaptic vesicles containing acetylcholine.

tion potential automatically triggers the adjacent membrane regions into producing an action potential (see Chapter 6). An action potential is a brief all-or-nothing reversal in membrane potential that is brought about by rapid changes in membrane permeability of Na^+ and K^+. When multiple signals arrive at the trigger zone, they are superimposed (summed). In **spatial summation**, the multiple signals arrive simultaneously, whereas in **temporal summation**, the signals arrive at different times. Comparison of the graded and action potentials is shown in Table 7-1.

Table 7–1 Comparison of Graded and Action Potentials

Graded Potentials	Action Potentials
Amplitude varies with the intensity of stimulus, i.e., the response is graded	Once the threshold is reached, the amplitude of an action potential is not dependent on the initial stimulus, i.e., it is an all-or-none phenomenon
There is no threshold	There is a threshold
There is no refractory period	There is a refractory period
Duration is dependent on the initial stimulus	Duration is constant
Conduction decreases with distance (decremental conduction)	Conduction is not decremental
Can be depolarizing or hyperpolarizing	Are always initiated by depolarization
Summation can occur	No summation occurs
Are mediated by a receptor	Are mediated by voltage-gated ion channels

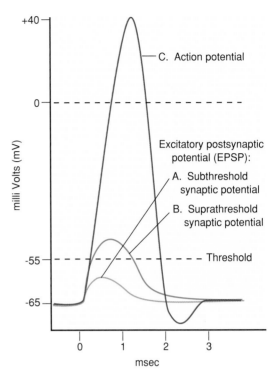

Figure 7–5 Generation of an action potential by an excitatory postsynaptic potential (EPSP). (A) Subthreshold EPSPs do not elicit an action potential. (B) When the EPSP is large enough, the membrane potential of the axon-hillock of the spinal motor neuron is raised beyond the threshold (suprathreshold synaptic potential), and (C) an action potential is generated.

Neurotransmitters produce depolarizing graded potentials when Na^+ channels open. A depolarizing graded potential that drives the membrane potential towards the threshold and excites the neuron is called an **excitatory postsynaptic potential (EPSP)**. For example, an EPSP is elicited in a spinal motor neuron following the stimulation of afferent fibers arising from one of the thigh muscles (e.g., quadriceps). This EPSP is generated by the opening of directly gated ion channels, which permit influx of Na^+ and efflux of K^+. Subthreshold depolarizations (synaptic potentials) do not elicit an action potential (Fig. 7-5). When the depolarization produced by the EPSP is large enough, the membrane potential of the axon-hillock of the spinal motor neuron is raised beyond threshold (suprathreshold synaptic potential), and an action potential is generated. In the CNS, glutamate is one of the major excitatory neurotransmitters (see Chapter 8).

Neurotransmitters can also produce graded potentials that may be hyperpolarizing (i.e., K^+ or Cl^- channels open). A hyperpolarizing graded potential that drives the membrane potential away from the threshold and inhibits the neuron is called an **inhibitory postsynaptic potential (IPSP)**. In the CNS, gamma aminobutyric acid (GABA) and glycine are major inhibitory neurotransmitters (see Chapter 8).

INDIRECTLY GATED ION CHANNELS

In this type of channel, the ion channel and the recognition site for the transmitter (receptor) are separate. These receptors are called **metabotropic receptors**. When a transmitter binds to the metabotropic receptor, a guanosine-5′-triphosphate (GTP)-binding protein (G-protein) is activated, which, in turn, activates a second-messenger system. The second messenger can either act directly on the ion channel to open it or it can activate an enzyme that, in turn, opens the channel by phosphorylating the channel protein. Dephosphorylation of the channel results in the closure of the channel. Activation of this type of channel elicits slow and long-lasting synaptic actions (see Chapter 8 for further details).

DISEASES AFFECTING THE CHEMICAL TRANSMISSION AT THE NERVE-MUSCLE SYNAPSE

MYASTHENIA GRAVIS

Myasthenia gravis means "severe muscle weakness." It is an autoimmune disease in which the number of functional nicotinic acetylcholine receptors in the postsynaptic membrane at the motor end-plate is reduced (for a description of different subtypes of acetylcholine receptors, see Chapter 8). In this disorder, antibodies against the nicotinic acetylcholine receptors (probably produced by T and B lymphocytes) are present in the serum of patients who have the disease. The antibodies bind with nicotinic acetylcholine receptors at the motor end-plate and reduce the number of these receptors. Thus, muscular weakness is elicited due to a decrease in the response of the muscle fiber to acetylcholine. The symptoms of myasthenia gravis include weakness of the eyelids, eye muscles, oropharyngeal muscles, and limb muscles. The muscle weakness is increased during exercise and reduced by rest. Standard therapy for patients with myasthenia gravis includes administration of anticholinesterase drugs (e.g., neostigmine). These drugs can reverse the muscle weakness. Inhibition of acetylcholinesterase allows the released acetylcholine to remain unhydrolyzed for a longer time and increases the chances of its interaction with the nicotinic acetylcholine receptors.

In some patients, removal of the thymus improves the symptoms. It should be recalled that T lymphocytes, which are responsible for cell-mediated immunity, develop in the thymus; and B lymphocytes, which produce antibodies, develop in bone marrow. In myasthenia gravis, T cells become reactive against the nicotinic acetylcholine receptor. Infection with a virus containing an amino acid sequence similar to that in the nicotinic acetylcholine receptor may activate the T cells.

LAMBERT-EATON SYNDROME

This disorder has been described in Chapter 6. See also the clinical case that follows.

CLINICAL CASE

HISTORY

Sonia is a 49-year-old woman with a history of heavy smoking for many years. For the past couple of months, she noticed a generalized progressive weakness in her neck, arms, and leg muscles. She also suffered from constipation, and her mouth remained dry. When she stood up or walked, she often experienced a short period of dizziness. She consulted her internist, who gave her a battery of tests in the local hospital. She was then admitted to the hospital for further examination and treatment.

EXAMINATION

An initial evaluation resulted in a diagnosis of lung cancer, as a result of having smoked for many years. This diagnosis was confirmed by a histological examination revealing the presence of a small-cell carcinoma of the lung. The physical examination also showed weakness of the neck flexors, arms, and legs. Electromyograms (EMGs) and nerve conduction tests were given. These tests involved electrical stimulation of the ulnar nerve, by placing an electrode on her wrist, and recording of compound motor action potentials in the muscles controlling her little finger. The amplitude of the compound motor action potential in this muscle was reduced. She was asked to exercise her hand muscles vigorously, and nerve conduction and EMG tests were repeated. Following the exercise, a marked improvement was observed in the amplitude of the compound motor action potential in the muscle being recorded. In addition, Sonia's muscle function improved briefly after the intravenous administration of edrophonium (Tensilon).

EXPLANATION

This is an example of an autoimmune disorder, called the Lambert-Eaton (Eaton-Lambert) syndrome. The disorder occurs frequently in patients who have lung or breast cancer. Antibodies to Ca^{2+} channels have been demonstrated to be present in these patients. A reduction of presynaptic Ca^{2+} channels results in reduced release of acetylcholine from these terminals at the neuromuscular junction. It should be noted that, in another autoimmune disorder, myasthenia gravis, antibodies to nicotinic acetylcholine receptors are present, which also cause muscle weakness. In both the Lambert-Eaton syndrome and myasthenia gravis, administration of a short-acting acetylcholinesterase inhibitor (edrophonium [Tensilon]) improves muscle function. The enzyme, acetylcholinesterase, present at the neuromuscular junction, normally hydrolyzes acetylcholine released from the nerve terminals innervating the skeletal muscle (see Chapter 8). Inhibition of this enzyme by edrophonium increases the availability of acetylcholine at the neuromuscular junction, causing an improvement in the muscle function. The two disorders can be distinguished by EMG and nerve conduction tests. Repetitive nerve stimulation or vigorous muscle exercise improves muscle function in patients with the Lambert-Eaton syndrome, while the muscle function deteriorates following vigorous exercise in patients with myasthenia gravis. Sonia was administered the corticosteroid prednisone intravenously for several days, which was then followed by further administration of this drug orally. Other approaches used to treat patients suffering from Lambert-Eaton syndrome include direct treatment of the tumor by standard radiation and chemotherapy and attempts at suppression of the immune system.

CHAPTER TEST

QUESTIONS

Choose the best answer for each question.

1. A 50-year-old man complained to his neurologist that he was suffering from a generalized muscle weakness that was exacerbated when he exercised. The patient's history revealed that he had suffered from a viral infection 4 to 5 weeks prior to the onset of muscle weakness. The neurologist suspected that the patient was suffering from myasthenia gravis and prescribed drug treatment with neostigmine. Following this treatment, the patient reported a significant improvement in his symptoms. Which one of the following could have accounted for muscle weakness in this patient?

   a. Reduction of voltage-gated Ca^{2+} channels on the presynaptic terminals
   b. Reduction in the number of functional nicotinic acetylcholine receptors on the muscle end-plates
   c. Reduction in the release of acetylcholine at the muscle end-plates
   d. Demyelination of nerves innervating the muscle end-plates
   e. Demyelination of axons in the central nervous system

2. Which of the following statements is correct concerning chemical transmission at a synapse?

   a. Continuity of the cytoplasm between the pre- and postsynaptic neurons is necessary.
   b. Ca^{2+} entry into the presynaptic terminal is an important step in this type of transmission.
   c. The nature of the response elicited depends upon the chemical nature of the transmitter.
   d. It involves transmitter release by endocytosis.
   e. This type of transmission is uncommon in the central nervous system.

3. Which of the following statements is correct concerning indirectly gated ion channels?

   a. A G-protein is activated by the binding of the transmitter to its receptor.
   b. The ion channel and the transmitter recognition site are identical.
   c. Activation of these channels usually elicits fast synaptic actions.

   d. The channel can open when the channel proteins are dephosphorylated.
   e. Activation of these channels usually elicits brief synaptic actions.

4. Which of the following statements is correct concerning directly gated transmission at the nerve-muscle synapse?

   a. The presynaptic boutons include synaptic vesicles containing norepinephrine.
   b. Norepinephrine released from the presynaptic terminal acts on α-adrenergic receptors located at the end-plate.
   c. The transmitter-gated ion channel at the end-plate is permeable only to Ca^{2+}.
   d. Voltage-gated channels selective for Na^+ are present in the junctional folds of the muscle-cell membrane.
   e. Each muscle fiber receives both excitatory and inhibitory inputs.

5. Which of the following statements is correct concerning a gap junction?

   a. The neurons at a gap junction are separated by a large (20–50 nm) space.
   b. Gap junction channels are formed by two hemichannels connecting pre- and postsynaptic neurons.
   c. These channels are transmitter gated.
   d. At the gap junction, the current generated by an impulse in one neuron spreads to another neuron through a pathway of high resistance.
   e. Usually gap junctions allow flow of current in only one direction.

ANSWERS AND EXPLANATIONS

1. Answer: **b**

The patient is suffering from myasthenia gravis. The virus that had infected the patient 4 to 5 weeks prior to the onset of muscle weakness may have contained an amino acid sequence similar to that present in the nicotinic acetylcholine receptor. The patient's T cells may have become reactive and produced an antibody against the nicotinic acetylcholine receptor. The circulating antibody may have bound to the nicotinic acetylcholine receptors on the muscle end-plates, thus reducing the number of functional nicotinic acetylcholine receptors. Consequently, acetylcholine released from the presynaptic terminals did not activate a sufficient number of nicotinic acetylcholine receptors at the neuromuscular junction, thus producing muscle weakness. Neostigmine, an acetylcholinesterase inhibitor, may have increased the probability of interaction of the neurotransmitter with the remaining functional nicotinic acetylcholine receptors by reducing the destruction of released acetylcholine. Therefore, the patient's muscle weakness was reversed. In myasthenia gravis, there is no defect in myelination of axons either in the CNS or peripheral nervous system. Reduction in the number of functional voltage-gated Ca^{2+} channels does not occur in myasthenia gravis; it is a characteristic of Lambert-Eaton syndrome.

2. Answer: b

At the chemical synapses, there is no continuity between the cytoplasm of the pre- and postsynaptic cell. Instead, the cells are separated by fluid-filled gaps that are relatively large (about 20–50 nm). Ca^{2+} entry into the presynaptic nerve terminal is necessary for the release of the transmitter. The neurotransmitter then interacts with its specific receptors and opens or closes several thousand channels in the postsynaptic membrane. The nature of the response (i.e., excitatory or inhibitory) elicited at the postsynaptic neuron does not depend on the chemical nature of the transmitter. Instead, it depends on the type of receptor being activated and the ion species that becomes more permeable. Transmitter release involves a process called exocytosis, in which the vesicles containing the transmitter fuse with the presynaptic membrane and release their contents into the synaptic cleft. Neurotransmission in the nervous system involves predominantly chemical synapses.

3. Answer: a

In the indirectly gated ion channels, a GTP-binding protein (G-protein) is activated when a transmitter binds with the recognition site on the receptor and a second-messenger system (e.g., cAMP) is activated. The second messenger can either act directly on the ion channel to open it or it can activate an enzyme that, in turn, opens the channel by phosphorylating the channel protein. In this type of channel, the ion channel and the recognition site for the transmitter (receptor) are separate. Activation of these channels elicits slow and long-lasting synaptic actions. Dephosphorylation of the channel results in its closure.

4. Answer: d

At the neuromuscular junction, many varicosities (swellings), called synaptic boutons, are present at the terminals of the presynaptic neuron. The presynaptic boutons include the synaptic vesicles that contain acetylcholine. When the motor axon is stimulated, acetylcholine is released, which acts on the nicotinic cholinergic receptors located at the crest of the junctional folds to produce an endplate potential (EPP). During the end-plate potential, Na^+ flows into the postsynaptic cell, while K^+ flows out of the cell (the transmitter-gated ionic channel at the end-plate is permeable to both Na^+ and K^+). In the junctional folds, the muscle cell membrane has a high density of voltage-gated channels that are selective for Na^+; these channels convert the end-plate potential into an action potential in the muscle fiber that eventually results in muscle contraction. The muscle fibers receive only excitatory inputs.

5. Answer: b

In electrical transmission between the nerve cells, the current generated by an impulse in one neuron spreads to another neuron through a pathway of low resistance (these channels are not transmitter gated). Such a pathway has been identified at gap junctions. The area where the two neurons are apposed to each other, at an electrical synapse, is called a gap junction. The extracellular space between pre- and postsynaptic neurons at an electrical synapse is 3–3.5 nm, which is much smaller than the usual extracellular space (about 20–50 nm) between neurons. These channels are formed by two hemichannels, one in the presynaptic and the other in the postsynaptic neuron. Most gap junctions allow ion flow in both directions.

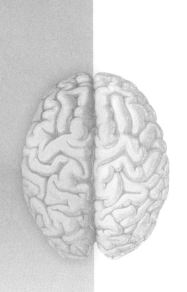

CHAPTER 8

NEUROTRANSMITTERS

OBJECTIVES

In this chapter, the student is expected to know:

1. The definition of a neurotransmitter, criteria for accepting a substance as a neurotransmitter, and the major classes of neurotransmitters and the differences between them

2. Individual neurotransmitters: synthesis, release, removal, the receptors on which they act, and their role in physiological functions

3. Clinical conditions related to transmitter dysfunction

Chemical transmission is the major mechanism of synaptic communication in the brain. To understand how neurotransmitters function, several issues must be addressed. These issues include how neurotransmitters are synthesized, released, removed from the synaptic cleft, and metabolized. In addition, it is important to identify the characteristics, anatomical loci, and functional properties of the receptors that mediate the actions of these transmitters. Moreover, wherever possible, the role of these transmitters in the central nervous system (CNS) functions and their linkage to clinical disorders need to be considered.

DEFINITION

A **neurotransmitter** is defined as a chemical substance that is synthesized in a neuron, released at a synapse following depolarization of the nerve terminal (usually dependent on influx of calcium ions), which binds to receptors on the postsynaptic cell and/or presynaptic terminal to elicit a specific response.

CRITERIA USED FOR IDENTIFYING NEUROTRANSMITTERS

The criteria for accepting a substance as a transmitter include: (1) the substance must be synthesized in the neuron, and the enzymes needed for its synthesis must be present in the neuron; (2) it must be released in sufficient quantity to elicit a response from the postsynaptic neuron or cell located in the effector organ; (3) mechanisms for removal or inactivation of the neurotransmitter from the synaptic cleft must exist; and (4) it should mimic the action of the endogenously released neurotransmitter when administered exogenously at or near a synapse.

MAJOR CLASSES OF NEUROTRANSMITTERS

Neurotransmitters in the nervous system can be classified into the following major categories: small molecule transmitters, neuroactive peptides, and gaseous neurotransmitters (Table 8-1).

STEPS INVOLVED IN NEUROTRANSMITTER RELEASE

SMALL MOLECULE NEUROTRANSMITTERS

The following steps are involved in the synthesis, transport, and release of small molecule neurotransmitters (Fig. 8-1A).

1. The enzymes required for synthesis of small molecule transmitters are synthesized in the

Table 8–1   Major Classes of Neurotransmitters

Small Molecule Neurotransmitters	Neuropeptides	Gaseous Neurotransmitters
Acetylcholine	Opioid peptides	Nitric oxide
Excitatory amino acids	β-endorphin,	
Glutamate	Methionine-enkephalin	
Aspartate	Leucine-enkephalin	
Inhibitory amino acids	Endomorphins	
GABA	Nociceptin	
Glycine		
Biogenic amines	Substance P	
Catecholamines		
Dopamine		
Norepinephrine		
Epinephrine		
Indoleamine		
Serotonin (5-hydroxytryptamine,		
[5-HT])		
Imidazole amine		
Histamine		
Purines		
ATP		
Adenosine		

ATP = adenosine triphosphate; GABA = gamma aminobutyric acid.

neuronal cell body in the **rough endoplasmic reticulum.**

2. They are transported to the Golgi apparatus.

3. In the Golgi apparatus, they are modified (e.g., sulfation, glycosylation).

4. Soluble enzymes (e.g., **acetylcholinesterase, tyrosine hydroxylase**) are transported along the axon to the nerve terminal by slow axonal transport (0.5–5 mm/day) via microtubules. The remaining enzymes are transported by **fast axonal transport.**

5. The precursor needed for the synthesis of small molecule neurotransmitters is taken up via transporter proteins located in the plasma membrane of the nerve terminal, and the neurotransmitter is synthesized in the presynaptic nerve terminal from the precursor. The enzyme needed for the synthesis of the neurotransmitter is synthesized in the neuronal cell body and transported to the terminal.

6. The synthesized pool of the neurotransmitter in the cytoplasm is taken up into small vesicles by vesicular membrane transport proteins. Small molecule transmitters are usually contained in **clear-core vesicles.** Serotonin and norepinephrine are exceptions because they are contained in **dense-core vesicles.**

7. The appropriate stimulus results in the release of the neurotransmitter by **exocytosis.** In this process, depolarization of the presynaptic terminal membrane by an action potential results in the influx of Ca^{2+} ions into the terminal through voltage-gated Ca^{2+} channels (see Chapter 6). Increase in Ca^{2+} concentration within the presynaptic terminal promotes fusion of the vesicle membrane with the presynaptic terminal membrane. The mechanism of the fusion of the vesicular and terminal membranes is believed to be as follows. Proteins in the vesicular (e.g., synaptobrevin) and presynaptic terminal membranes (e.g., syntaxin) form complexes that bring the two membranes together. Ca^{2+} binds to another protein (synaptotagmin) on the vesicular membrane causing it to insert into the presynaptic terminal membrane, and fusion of two membranes occurs. An opening develops in the fused membranes, and the contents of the synaptic vesicle are discharged into the synaptic cleft. The synaptic vesicle membrane is retrieved after the contents are released by exocytosis and recycled within the presynaptic terminal to make new synaptic vesicles, which are then filled with the transmitter for subsequent release. The neurotransmitter released into the synaptic cleft binds with specific receptors, and a response is elicited. The released transmitter en-

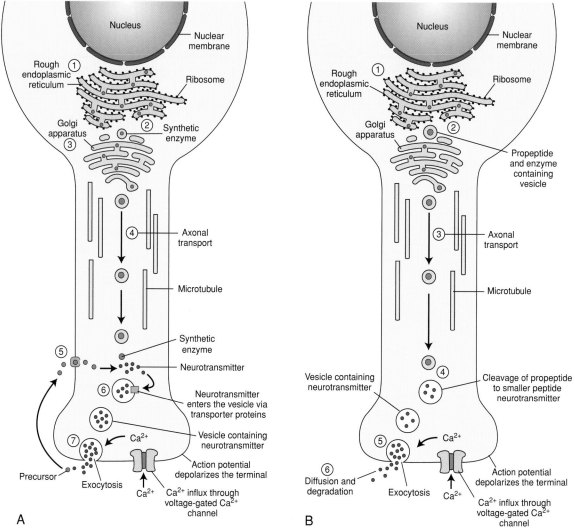

Figure 8–1 Steps involved in the synthesis, transport, and release of neurotransmitters. (A) Small molecule neurotransmitters. (B) Neuropeptides.

ters back into the terminal by an uptake mechanism and is recycled for subsequent release. Some neurotransmitters (e.g., acetylcholine) are degraded in the synaptic cleft, and one or more of their degradation products are taken back into the terminal and reused to synthesize the neurotransmitter in the terminal.

The vesicles that contain the neurotransmitter are produced in the rough endoplasmic reticulum and Golgi apparatus and transported to the nerve terminal. The surplus vesicular membrane remaining in the nerve terminal after the neurotransmitter is released by exocytosis is transported back into the cell body where it is either degraded or recycled (see Chapter 5). Briefly, fused vesicular membrane is retrieved and transported back into the cytoplasm of

the nerve terminal by endocytosis. The retrieved vesicular membrane goes through several intracellular compartments (e.g., coated vesicles and endosomes). During continuous neuronal activity, the retrieved vesicular membrane is recycled in the terminal to form new synaptic vesicles and filled with the neurotransmitter that is then released. In this manner, rapid replacement of synaptic vesicles during continuous neuronal activity becomes possible because synaptic vesicles form in the terminal. The synaptic vesicles produced in the neuronal cell body would not be rapidly available due to the long distance between the neuronal cell body and the terminal. Some of the vesicular membrane retrieved into the cytoplasm of the nerve terminal is transported back into the cell body and is either degraded or recycled.

NEUROPEPTIDE NEUROTRANSMITTERS

These neurotransmitters usually mediate slow on-going brain functions. Only a few important peptides (e.g., substance P and enkephalins) will be discussed in this chapter. The following steps are involved in the synthesis, transport, and release of neuropeptide neurotransmitters (Fig. 8-1B).

1. Polypeptides much larger than the final peptide transmitter (called pre-propeptides) are synthesized in rough endoplasmic reticulum where they are converted into a propeptide (pre-propetide from which the signal sequence of amino acids is removed). The enzymes needed for the cleavage of polypeptides are also synthesized in the rough endoplasmic reticulum.

2. The propeptide and the enzymes are transported to the Golgi apparatus where they are packaged into vesicles.

3. The propeptide and enzyme-filled vesicles are carried along the axon to the nerve terminal by fast axonal transport (400 mm/day) via microtubules. Adenosine triphosphate (ATP)-requiring "motor" proteins, such as **kinesins**, are needed for this transport.

4. Enzymes cleave the propeptide to produce a smaller peptide transmitter that remains in the large dense-core vesicles.

5. The peptide neurotransmitter is then released into the synaptic cleft by exocytosis.

6. After the release, the peptide transmitter then diffuses away and is degraded by proteolytic enzymes; it is not taken back into the nerve terminal as is the case with small molecule neurotransmitters.

More than one transmitter (usually a small molecule transmitter and a neuroactive peptide) coexist in many mature neurons (e.g., most spinal motor neurons contain acetylcholine and calcitonin gene-related peptide).

INDIVIDUAL SMALL MOLECULE NEUROTRANSMITTERS

ACETYLCHOLINE

Synthesis

The following steps are involved in the synthesis and release of acetylcholine (Fig. 8-2).

1. Glucose enters the nerve terminal by passive transport (facilitated diffusion).

2. **Glycolysis** occurs in the neuronal cytoplasm, and pyruvate (pyruvic acid) molecules are generated.

3. Pyruvate is transported into the mitochondria, and an acetyl group derived from pyruvic acid combines with coenzyme-A present in the mitochondria to form acetylcoenzyme-A, which is transported back into the cytoplasm.

4. Choline, the precursor for acetylcholine, is actively transported into the neuronal terminal from the synaptic cleft via Na^+ and choline transporters.

5. Acetylcholine is synthesized in the cytoplasm of the nerve terminal from choline and acetylcoenzyme-A in the presence of an enzyme, choline acetyltransferase.

6. Acetylcholine is then transported into vesicles and stored there.

7. It is then released into the synaptic cleft by exocytosis and hydrolyzed by acetylcholinesterase (see *Removal* below).

Removal

High concentrations of an enzyme, acetylcholinesterase, are present on the outer surfaces of the nerve terminal (prejunctional site) and the effector cell (postjunctional site). Acetylcholinesterase is synthesized in the endoplasmic reticulum of neuronal cell bodies and major dendrites and is transported to the presynaptic terminal membrane by microtubules. This enzyme hydrolyses acetylcholine in the junctional extracellular space; choline liberated in this reaction re-enters the nerve terminal and is again used for the synthesis of acetylcholine.

Distribution

There are two constellations of cholinergic neurons (Fig. 8-3).

1. **The basal forebrain constellation** is located in the telencephalon, medial and ventral to the basal ganglia. It includes the basal nucleus of Meynert, which provides cholinergic innervation to the entire neocortex, amygdala, hippocampus, and thalamus. The medial septal nuclei provide cholinergic innervation to the cerebral cortex, hippocampus, and amygdala.

2. The second constellation includes cholinergic neurons located in the **dorsolateral tegmentum of the pons** that project to the basal ganglia, thalamus, hypothalamus, medullary reticular formation, and deep cerebellar nuclei.

Physiological and Clinical Considerations

Cholinergic neurons in the dorsolateral tegmentum of pons have been implicated in the regulation of forebrain activity during cycles of sleep and wakefulness. Cholinergic neurons of the basal

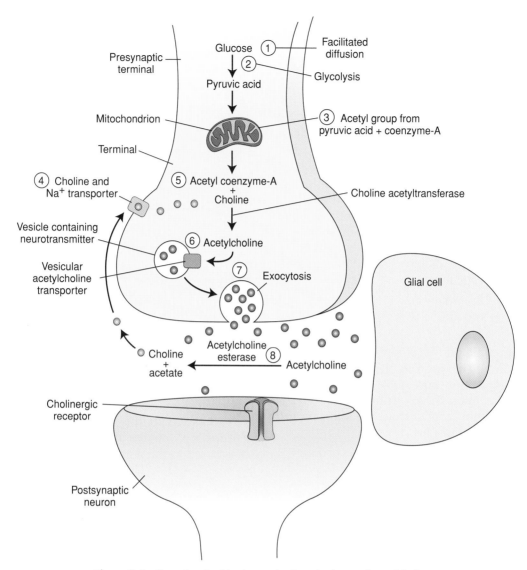

Figure 8–2 Steps involved in the synthesis and release of acetylcholine.

forebrain constellation are involved in learning and memory and have been implicated in **Alzheimer's disease**. In this disease, there is extensive neural atrophy, especially in the cortex and hippocampal formation. Patients with this disease suffer from memory loss, personality change, and dementia. There is a dramatic loss of cholinergic neurons in the basal nucleus of Meynert and acetylcholine in the cortex of these patients. These observations prompted attempts to treat Alzheimer's disease by acetylcholine replacement therapy. For example, treatment with donepezil (Aricept), an acetylcholinesterase inhibitor, is indicated for mild to moderate dementia in patients with Alzheimer's disease. However, these attempts have not shown dramatic results in relieving the symptoms of the disease, indicating that the mechanisms of neuronal degeneration in Alzheimer's disease must involve multiple transmitter systems.

EXCITATORY AMINO ACIDS: GLUTAMATE

Glutamate is discussed as an example of the excitatory class of neurotransmitters. It occurs in high concentrations in the brain. Although it plays a role in other functions, such as synthesis of proteins and peptides, glutamate is considered to be an important excitatory neurotransmitter because it fulfills the criteria for a substance to be accepted as a neurotransmitter.

Synthesis

Glutamate is synthesized in the brain by two processes. In one process, glucose enters the neuron by facilitated diffusion and is metabolized via the Krebs (tricarboxylic acid) cycle. α-oxoglutarate generated during the Krebs cycle is transaminated by α-oxoglutarate transaminase

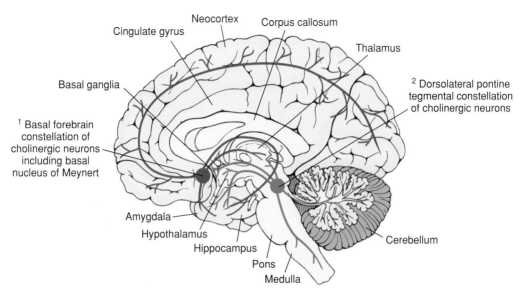

Figure 8-3 Major cholinergic cell groups. Note two major constellations of cholinergic neurons: cholinergic neurons located in the basal forebrain constellation, including the basal nucleus of Meynert, and cholinergic neurons located in the dorsolateral tegmentum of the pons.

(GABA transaminase or GABA-T) to form glutamate. The following steps are involved in the second process of the synthesis of glutamate (Fig. 8-4).

1 and 2. Glial cells and nerve terminals reuptake the glutamate released from the nerve terminals via glutamate transporters located in their cell membranes.

3. In the glia, glutamate is converted into glutamine by an enzyme, glutamine synthetase.

4. Glutamine is transported out of the glia into the neuronal terminal via glutamine transporters located in the glial and neuronal terminal membranes.

5. In the neuronal terminal, glutamine is converted into glutamate by an enzyme, glutaminase. Glutamate is taken up into the vesicles by active transport, stored, and subsequently released by exocytosis. Released glutamate is then actively taken up by the glia and neuronal terminals via glutamate transporters. In the neuronal terminal, it is repackaged into the vesicles for subsequent reuse. In the glia, it is converted into glutamine as described earlier.

Removal

As described earlier, glutamate transporters are located on the plasma membrane of the presynaptic nerve terminal and on glial cells. Glutamate is taken up by a high-affinity, sodium-dependent, re-uptake mechanism into the nerve terminals and glial cells via these transporters.

Physiological and Clinical Considerations

Some of the important physiological and clinical considerations relevant to glutamate are as follows.

1. Glutamate has been implicated as a transmitter in a variety of circuits in the brain. For example, excitatory amino acids may be involved in learning and memory processes, as well as motor functions.

2. Glutamate has also been implicated in some chronic neuropathological conditions such as **amyotrophic lateral sclerosis** (ALS, also known as Lou Gehrig's disease), which is characterized by degeneration of the motor neurons in the anterior horn of the spinal cord, brainstem, and cerebral cortex. Patients suffering from this disease exhibit widespread muscle fasciculations, flaccid weakness, and atrophy of the muscles. The mechanism of the involvement of glutamate in the symptoms of ALS is not clearly known (see also Chapter 9).

3. Prolonged stimulation of neurons by excitatory amino acids results in neuronal death or injury. This effect is known as **excitotoxicity**. There is predominantly a loss of postsynaptic neurons. Neuronal loss due to excitotoxicity has been implicated in cerebrovascular stroke. Occlusion of arteries supplying the brain results in brain ischemia. Concentrations of excitatory amino acids (glutamate and aspartate) increase in the extracellular spaces in the brain perhaps due to slowing of their uptake by neurons and glia. The

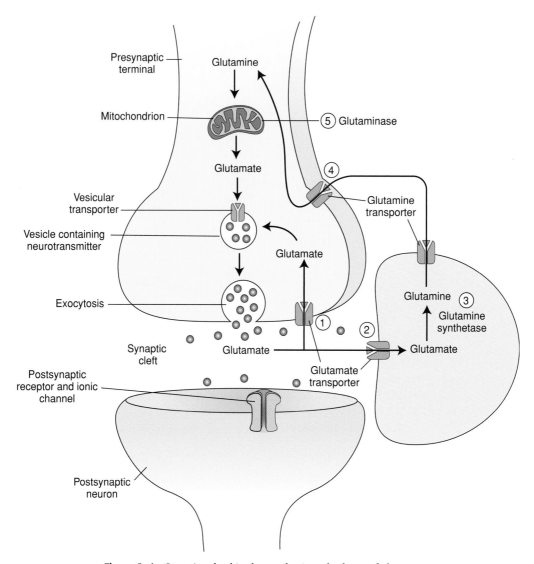

Figure 8–4 Steps involved in the synthesis and release of glutamate.

neurons are excited excessively, and a chain of events, not fully identified yet, causes neuronal death. Excessive intracellular Ca^{2+} concentrations have been implicated in the neuronal death due to excitotoxicity.

4. Excitotoxic action of glutamate has been implicated in Alzheimer's disease. One of the mechanisms of the loss of neurons concerned with memory in this disease is believed to be overexcitation and, finally, loss of these neurons by glutamate-induced activation of N-methyl-D-aspartic acid (NMDA) receptors (described later in this chapter in the *Ionotropic Receptors* section). Memantine (Namenda), an NMDA receptor antagonist, is reported to mitigate this effect and slow down the symptoms of the disease.

INHIBITORY AMINO ACIDS

Gamma Aminobutyric Acid (GABA)

Synthesis and Removal

The following steps are involved in the synthesis of GABA and its removal from the synaptic cleft (Fig. 8-5).

1. Glutamine is converted into glutamate by an enzyme, glutaminase.

2. GABA is formed by α-decarboxylation of glutamate. This reaction is catalyzed by a cytosolic enzyme, **L-glutamic acid-1-decarboxylase (GAD)**, which is present almost exclusively in GABAergic neurons. GAD is not present in neurons using glutamate as transmitter or in glia. It requires

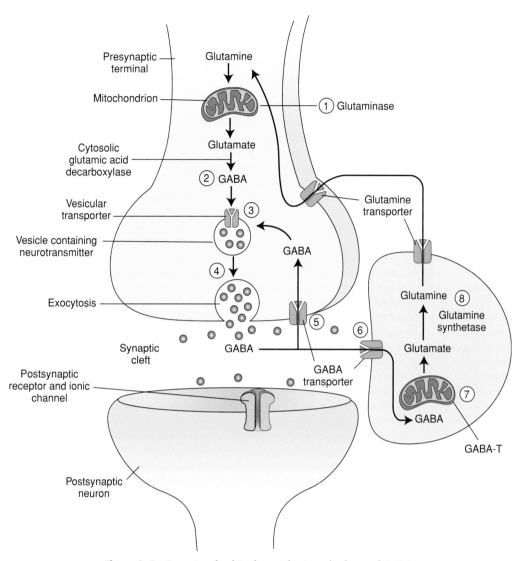

Figure 8–5 Steps involved in the synthesis and release of GABA.

pyridoxyl phosphate (a form of vitamin B_6) as a coenzyme.

3. Synthesized GABA is taken up into vesicles where it is stored.

4. It is released into the synaptic cleft by exocytosis.

5. After its release, GABA is taken up into presynaptic terminal via GABA transporters and repackaged into vesicles for subsequent use.

6. GABA is also taken up into the glia via GABA transporters.

7. In glia, GABA is converted to glutamate by a mitochondrial enzyme, GABA transaminase (GABA-T).

8. Another enzyme, glutamine synthetase, converts glutamate into glutamine, which is then transported into the neighboring nerve terminals where it is processed to synthesize glutamate.

Distribution

GABA is found in high concentrations in the brain and spinal cord but is absent in peripheral nerves or peripheral tissues. Unlike glutamate, GABA is not an essential metabolite, and it is not incorporated into a protein.

Physiological and Clinical Considerations

Some of the important physiological and clinical considerations regarding this neurotransmitter are as follows.

1. GABA is an inhibitory transmitter in many brain circuits. For example, GABA is used as an inhibitory neurotransmitter by the Purkinje cells in the cerebellum. Alteration of GABAergic circuits has been implicated in neurological and psychiatric disorders like Huntington's chorea, **Parkinson's disease**, senile dementia, Alzheimer's disease, and schizophrenia.

2. As mentioned earlier, GAD requires vitamin B_6 as a coenzyme. Therefore, dietary deficiency of vitamin B_6 can lead to diminished GABA synthesis. In a disastrous series of infant deaths, it was noted that vitamin B_6 was omitted in an infant feeding formula. GABA content in the brain of these infants was reduced. Subsequently, there was a loss of synaptic inhibition that caused seizures and death.

3. Since epileptic seizures can be facilitated by lack of neuronal inhibition, increase in the inhibitory transmitter, GABA, is helpful in terminating them. Thus, valproic acid (dipropylacetic acid) is useful as an anticonvulsant because it inhibits **GABA transaminase**, which is an enzyme that metabolizes GABA, and increases GABA levels in the brain.

4. Barbiturates act as agonists or modulators on postsynaptic GABA receptors and are used to treat epilepsy.

Glycine

Synthesis and Removal

In the nerve terminal, serine is formed from glucose. Glycine is formed from serine by an enzyme, serine transhydroxymethylase. This reaction is folate-dependent. After its release, glycine is taken up by neurons by an active sodium-dependent mechanism involving specific membrane transporters.

Distribution

Glycine is found in all body fluids and tissue proteins in substantial amounts. It is not an essential amino acid, but it is an intermediate in the metabolism of proteins, peptides, and bile salts. It is also a neurotransmitter in the CNS.

Physiological and Clinical Considerations

Glycine has been implicated as an inhibitory neurotransmitter in the spinal cord, lower brainstem, and retina. Glycine hyperpolarizes neurons by opening chloride channels. Mutations of genes coding for some of the membrane transporters needed for removal of glycine result in **hyperglycinemia**, which is a devastating neonatal disease characterized by lethargy and mental retardation.

CATECHOLAMINES

The chemical structure of these neurotransmitters includes a catechol (a benzene ring containing two adjacent hydroxyl groups). The steps involved in the synthesis of catecholamine neurotransmitters are shown in Figure 8-6. Individual members of this group of neurotransmitters are discussed in the following sections.

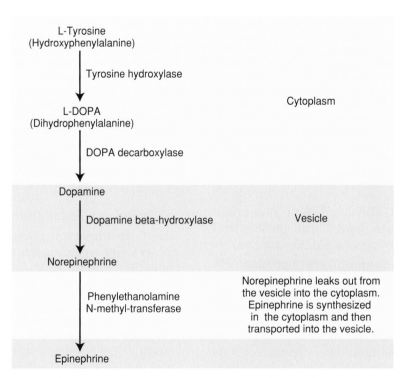

Figure 8–6 Steps involved in the synthesis of catecholamines.

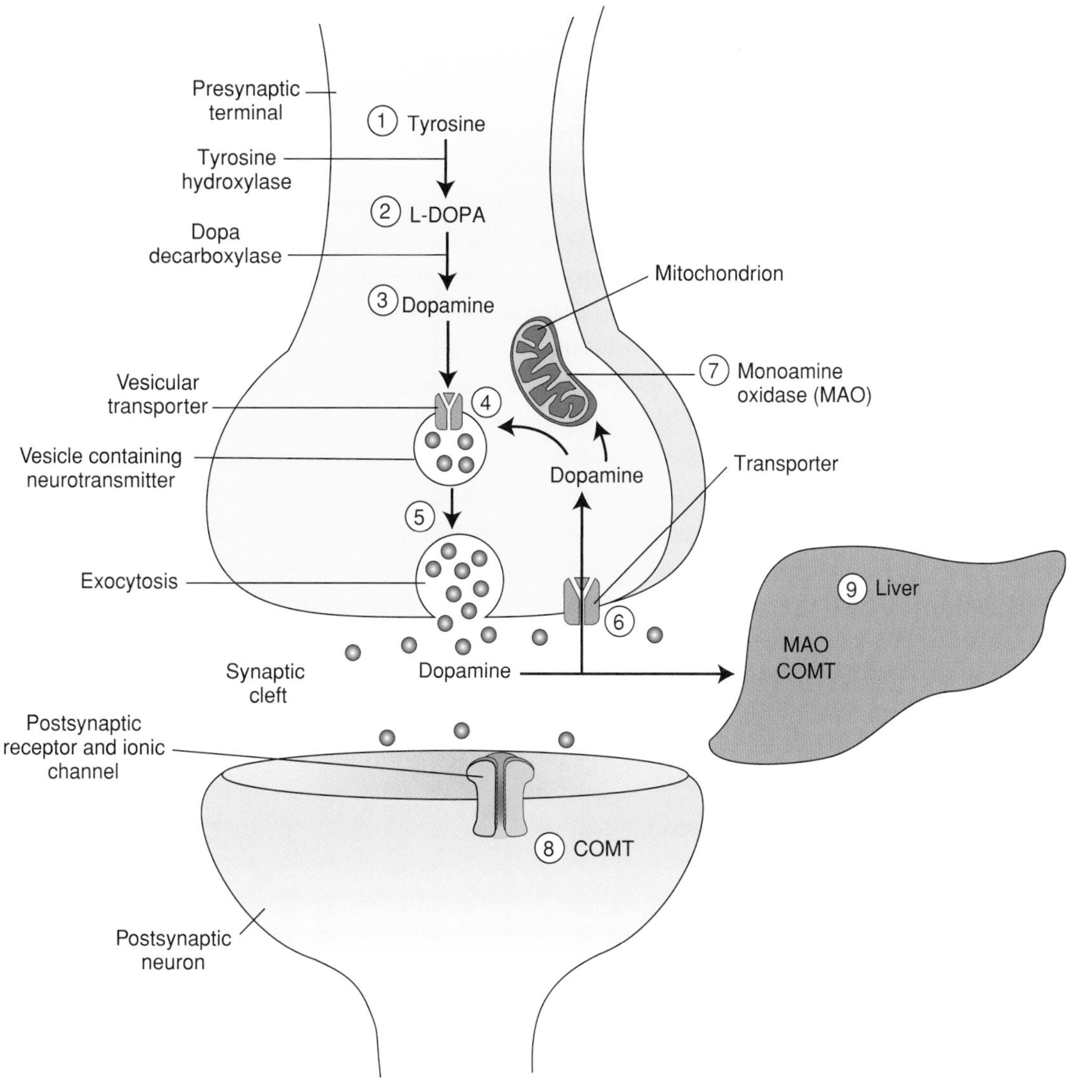

Figure 8–7 Steps involved in the synthesis and release of dopamine.

Dopamine

Synthesis and Removal

The steps involved in the synthesis, removal, and metabolism of dopamine are as follows (Fig. 8-7).

1. The amino acid tyrosine (hydroxy-phenylalanine) is present in all food products and can be synthesized from phenylalanine. It enters the neuron by active transport.

2. In the cytoplasm of the dopaminergic neuron, tyrosine is converted into dihydroxyphenylalanine (DOPA) by **tyrosine hydroxylase** enzyme. This enzyme is rate-limiting for the synthesis of all three catecholamines.

3. DOPA is converted to dopamine in the cytoplasm by the enzyme aromatic L-amino acid decarboxylase (DOPA-decarboxylase).

4. Dopamine is then actively transported into the storage vesicles by vesicular transport mechanism.

5. In the dopaminergic neuron, dopamine remains unchanged in the storage vesicles and is ready for release by exocytosis.

6. Dopamine released into the synaptic cleft is actively transported back into the neuronal terminal. This process is called **reuptake-1** and is the most important mechanism by which dopamine and other catecholamines are removed from the synaptic cleft. Some of the dopamine entering the neuronal terminal (about 50%) is transported into the vesicles for storage and release.

7. Remaining dopamine that enters the neuronal terminal is destroyed by a mitochondrial enzyme, **monoamine oxidase (MAO)**.

8. Some of the dopamine that is released into the synaptic cleft (about 10%) is actively transported into the effector cells. This process is known as **reuptake-2.** Dopamine entering the effector cells is inactivated primarily by an enzyme, **catechol-O-methyltransferase (COMT).** Although MAO is also present in the effector cells, its role in the inactivation of dopamine is unclear.

9. Remaining dopamine in the synaptic cleft diffuses into the circulation and is destroyed in the liver by COMT and MAO. The end products of metabolism of catecholamine are organic acids and alcohols, which are excreted in urine.

Distribution

Dopaminergic neurons are located in the following nuclei (Fig. 8-8).

1. **Substantia nigra,** which is located bilaterally in the midbrain. Axons of the dopaminergic neurons located in the **substantia nigra (pars compacta)** ascend rostrally as **nigrostriatal projection**, providing dopaminergic innervation to neurons located in the **corpus striatum (caudate nucleus and putamen).** Dopaminergic neurons in the substantia nigra are selectively degenerated in Parkinson's disease.

2. **Ventral tegmental area,** which is located just medial to the substantia nigra pars compacta. Dopaminergic neurons, located in this area, project as either the mesolimbic or the mesocortical pathway. In the **mesolimbic pathway,** axons of the dopaminergic neurons ascend in the brainstem and forebrain in the median forebrain bundle to supply limbic structures (amygdala, septal area, and hippocampal formation) and the **nucleus accumbens** (which is embedded in the ventral striatum). In the **mesocortical pathway,** axons of the dopaminergic neurons ascend in the median forebrain bundle to provide dopaminergic innervation to the frontal and cingulate cortices.

3. **The arcuate nucleus,** which is located in the ventrolateral aspect of hypothalamus (not shown in Fig. 8-8). Dopaminergic neurons located in the arcuate nucleus project to the median eminence and release dopamine directly into the **hypophyseal portal circulation,** which is then carried to the anterior lobe of the pituitary to inhibit the release of prolactin (the hormone primarily responsible for lactation).

Physiological and Clinical Considerations

Parkinson's Disease. This disease is characterized by an expressionless face (clinicians sometimes refer to it as "mask-like face"), slowness of movement (bradykinesia or hypokinetic syndrome), rigidity of extremities and neck, and

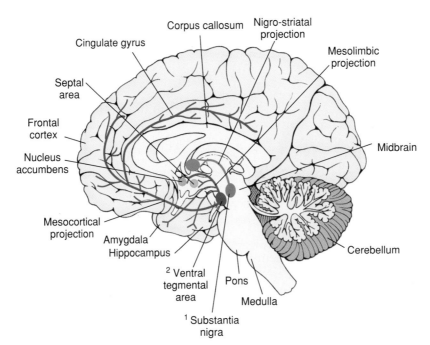

Figure 8–8 Dopaminergic neurons and their projections. Axons of dopaminergic neurons located in the substantia nigra pars compacta ascend rostrally as the nigrostriatal pathway and provide dopaminergic innervation to neurons located in the caudate nucleus and putamen (striatum). Axons of another group of dopaminergic neurons that are located in the ventral tegmental area ascend in the median forebrain bundle to provide dopaminergic innervation to the frontal and cingulate cortices.

tremors in the hands. Patients with Parkinson's disease have a gait that is characterized by short wide-based steps (sometimes referred to as fenestrating gait), stooped posture, and scarcity of normal limb movements. These symptoms are often accompanied by dementia. Dopaminergic neurons located in the substantia nigra are degenerated in this disease, and the release of dopamine in the caudate/putamen is decreased. The mechanism of bradykinesia in Parkinson's disease is discussed in Chapter 20.

The main aim of drug **therapy** for this disease is to replace the deficiency of the transmitter (dopamine) in the basal ganglia (target of nigrostriatal projection). Because dopamine does not cross blood-brain barrier, its immediate metabolic precursor (**L-DOPA**, or **levodopa**), which does cross this barrier, is administered orally. L-DOPA is transported into the brain via a large neutral amino acid transporter, and it permeates the striatal tissue, where it is decarboxylated to dopamine. In recent years, a combination of L-DOPA and **carbidopa** (Sinemet) has been prescribed for this disease. Carbidopa is an inhibitor of dopa-decarboxylase and reduces the decarboxylation of L-DOPA in the peripheral tissues, enabling a greater concentration of this precursor to reach the brain. Carbidopa does not cross the blood-brain barrier. Therefore, conversion of L-DOPA to dopamine does not diminish in the brain.

Another potentially useful but controversial approach is to implant fetal midbrain or adrenal medullary tissue into the deteriorating caudate nucleus and putamen. An attractive possibility in the future is transplantation of genetically engineered cells capable of expressing tyrosine hydroxylase that is involved in the synthesis of dopamine.

Psychotic Disorders. Many adult psychotic disorders, including schizophrenia, are believed to involve increased activity at dopaminergic synapses. Many drugs that are effective in the treatment of these disorders (e.g., phenothiazines, thioxanthines, and butyrophenones) are believed to reduce the dopamine synaptic activity in the limbic forebrain. Further discussion of dopamine and other neurotransmitters in psychiatric disorders is considered in Chapter 28.

Cocaine Drug Abuse. Cocaine (a local anesthetic drug) blocks the reuptake of dopamine (and norepinephrine) into the nerve terminals. Elevated levels of dopamine in certain brain circuits may be responsible for the euphoric effects of cocaine. This mechanism is not responsible for the local anesthetic effect of cocaine that is mediated via the blockade of neuronal voltage-gated Na^+ channels.

Dopaminergic projections from the ventral tegmental area to the limbic structures, especially the projections to nucleus accumbens, may be involved in emotional reinforcement and motivation associated with cocaine drug addiction. Levels of dopamine in these projections are increased in individuals addicted to cocaine.

Norepinephrine

Synthesis and Removal

Initial steps in the synthesis of norepinephrine (up to the step of transport and storage of dopamine into the storage vesicles) are described in the section about dopamine. The noradrenergic neurons contain an enzyme, **dopamine β-hydroxylase** (DBH), which converts dopamine into norepinephrine. It should be noted that the synthesis of norepinephrine takes place in the storage vesicles (Fig. 8-9). The norepinephrine thus formed is ready to be released by exocytosis. Norepinephrine released into the synaptic cleft is removed by the mechanisms described in the dopamine section.

Autoinhibition and Negative Feedback Mechanisms

Activation of presynaptic adrenergic receptors results in inhibition of the release of norepinephrine. This process is known as **autoinhibition** and is distinct from negative feedback in which synthesis of the transmitter (norepinephrine in this case) is blocked at its rate-limiting step (i.e., conversion of tyrosine to DOPA by tyrosine hydroxylase).

Distribution

The major concentration of noradrenergic neurons is in the **locus ceruleus** (also known as A_6 group of neurons) that is located in the pons. These neurons send projections through the central tegmental tract and the medial forebrain bundle to the thalamus, hypothalamus, limbic forebrain structures (cingulate and parahippocampal gyri, hippocampal formation, and amygdaloid complex), and the cerebral cortex. This group of neurons modulates a variety of physiological functions (e.g., sleep and wakefulness, attention, and feeding behaviors).

Physiological and Clinical Considerations

Norepinephrine is released as a transmitter from postganglionic sympathetic nerve terminals. Its role in the CNS as a transmitter is not clearly understood. Norepinephrine is believed to play a role in psychiatric disorders such as depression. Drugs used in the treatment of depression (e.g., tricyclic antidepressants like desimipramine) are known to inhibit the reuptake of norepinephrine at the nerve terminals and increase the synaptic levels of

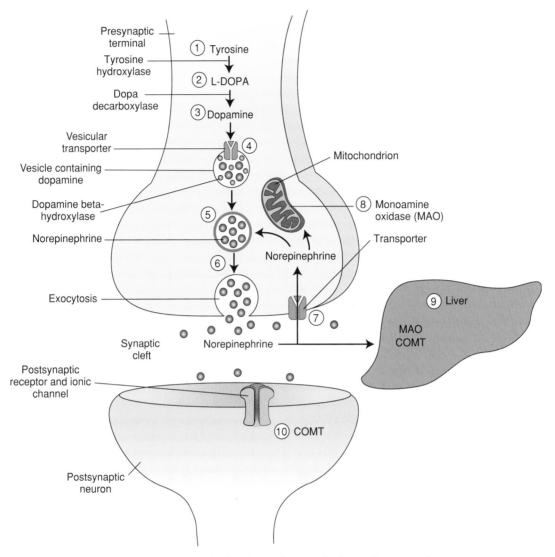

Figure 8–9 Steps involved in the synthesis and release of norepinephrine.

norepinephrine. The exact mechanism by which increased levels of norepinephrine in the CNS mediate the antidepressant action of these drugs is not clearly known.

Epinephrine

Synthesis and Removal

The initial steps (up to synthesis and storage of norepinephrine in the storage vesicles) in the synthesis of epinephrine are identical to those of norepinephrine. In the adrenergic neuron (Fig. 8-10), norepinephrine stored in the vesicles leaks out into the cytoplasm and is converted into epinephrine by the enzyme **phenylethanolamine-N-methyl-transferase (PNMT)**. Epinephrine thus formed in the cytoplasm is actively transported back into storage vesicles in the nerve terminal (or chromaffin granules in the adrenal medulla) and stored for subsequent release. The mechanisms for removal

of epinephrine are the same as those for norepinephrine and dopamine.

Distribution

Two major groups of adrenergic cells have been identified in the medulla: **C_1 neurons** located in the rostral ventrolateral medulla, and **C_2 neurons** located in the nucleus tractus solitarius (or solitary nucleus).

Physiological and Clinical Considerations

The function of adrenergic neurons in the CNS has not been clearly established.

Immunohistochemical Identification of Catecholaminergic Neurons

Antibodies, developed for enzymes involved in the synthesis of different catecholamine neurotransmitters, have been used for immunohistochemical iden-

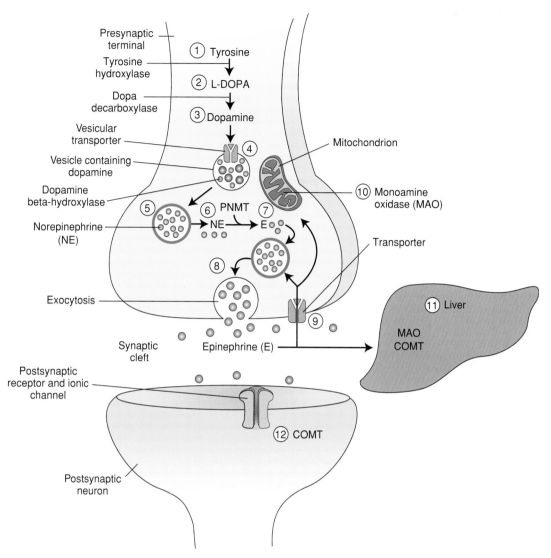

Figure 8–10 Steps involved in the synthesis and release of epinephrine.

tification of these neurons. For example, positive staining for tyrosine hydroxylase indicates that the neuron contains a catecholamine. Positive staining for tyrosine hydroxylase, but not DBH, indicates that the neuron contains dopamine. Positive staining for DBH, but not PNMT, indicates that the neuron contains norepinephrine. Positive staining for PNMT indicates that the neuron contains epinephrine.

INDOLEAMINES: SEROTONIN (5-HYDROXYTRYPTAMINE; 5-HT)

Synthesis and Removal

Because serotonin does not cross the blood-brain barrier, brain cells must synthesize their own serotonin. Dietary tryptophan serves as a substrate for serotonin synthesis. Plasma tryptophan enters the brain by an active uptake process and is hydroxylated by tryptophan hydroxylase to form 5-hydroxytryptophan, which is immediately decar-

boxylated by aromatic L-amino acid decarboxylase to form serotonin. Serotonin is then actively taken up and stored in vesicles where it is ready for release. After its release, serotonin is removed from the synaptic cleft by the mechanisms of reuptake and metabolism. Reuptake involves entry of serotonin into the neuronal terminals by active transport via serotonin transporter proteins. Metabolism involves deamination of serotonin by monoamine oxidase to form 5-hydroxyindoleacetaldehyde, which is then oxidized by aldehyde dehydrogenase to form 5-hydroxyindoleacetic acid. The latter is excreted through the urine.

Distribution

Serotonin-containing neurons have been identified in the midline **raphe nuclei** of the medulla, pons, and upper brainstem. The serotonin-containing cell groups of the rostral raphe nuclei (e.g., dorsal and median raphe nuclei) send their projections to the diencephalon and telencephalon. The caudal raphe nuclei (e.g., raphe magnus) send their projections to the spinal cord.

Physiological and Clinical Considerations

Serotonin-containing cells in the raphe regions of the brainstem are believed to play a role in descending pain-control systems. Other serotonin-containing neurons may play a role in mediating affective processes such as aggressive behavior and arousal. Serotonin synthesized in the **pineal gland** serves as a precursor for the synthesis of **melatonin**, which is a neurohormone involved in regulating sleep patterns. Serotonin is also believed to play an important role in depression. Serotonin uptake inhibitors, belonging to different chemical families, have been found to be beneficial in the treatment of depression; this effect may be due to an increase in serotonin levels in the brain. For example, **fluoxetine (Prozac)** selectively blocks reuptake of serotonin and enhances serotonin levels in the brain. It may produce beneficial effects in mental depression via enhancement of transmission through 5-HT$_{1A}$ receptors. **Sumatriptan (Imitrex)** is a 5-HT$_{1D}$ receptor agonist. It is a vasoconstrictor and has proved useful in treating migraine headaches.

Designer Drugs of Abuse and Their Relationship With Serotonin

Some drugs of abuse mediate their effects through serotonin-containing neurons. For example, **Ecstasy** has been used as a recreational drug by young adults, especially in large dance parties know as "raves." Ecstasy includes two drugs, MDMA (3,4, methylene-dioxy-methamphetamine) and MDEA (3,4, methylene-dioxy-ethamphetamine). These drugs, generally called "Adam" and "Eve," respectively, by drug abusers, have been reported to induce sensory enhancement (a feeling that all is right with this world) and empathogenesis (a feeling of closeness with others and removal of barriers in communication, especially in intimate relationships). These effects are believed to be due to initial release of serotonin by these drugs. Toxic effects of these drugs are dehydration, hyperthermia, tachycardia (increase in heart rate), and sweating. Undesirable side effects following prolonged use of Ecstasy are believed to be caused by the degeneration of the projections of serotonin-containing neurons.

IMIDAZOLEAMINES: HISTAMINE

Synthesis and Removal

In the periphery, histamine is synthesized in mast cells. Histamine circulating in the blood does not cross the blood-brain barrier. Brain cells synthesize their own histamine from histidine, which enters the brain by active transport. Histidine is then decarboxylated by histidine decarboxylase to form histamine. Histamine is metabolized by two enzymes—histamine methyltransferase and diamine oxidase (histaminase)—to organic aldehydes and acids.

Distribution

The highest density of histamine-containing neurons has been found in the median eminence and premammillary regions of the hypothalamus. These neurons send projections to almost all areas of the brain and spinal cord.

Physiological and Clinical Considerations

Histamine has been implicated as a transmitter in the regulation of food and water intake, as well as in thermoregulation and autonomic functions.

PURINES

Recently, ATP has been implicated as a neurotransmitter. Since it contains a purine ring, it has been included in a new class of neurotransmitters called **purines**. Purinergic transmission has been demonstrated in autonomic neurons innervating the bladder, intestinal smooth muscles, and vas deferens. ATP has also been implicated in pain mechanisms. For example, when ATP is released by tissue damage, it excites the peripheral nerve endings of the dorsal root ganglion cells via a subtype of ionotropic purine receptor. Subsequently, ATP is released at the terminal of the central axon of the dorsal root ganglion cell, and neurons in the dorsal horn of the spinal cord are activated via another subtype of ionotropic purine receptor. Adenosine is also considered to be a purinergic neurotransmitter. However, it is not a classical neurotransmitter in the sense that it is not stored in presynaptic vesicles and is not released in a Ca^{2+}-dependent manner. It is generated by degradation of ATP by extracellular enzymes.

NEUROACTIVE PEPTIDES

More than 100 pharmacologically active peptides have been identified in neurons and implicated as neurotransmitters. However, representatives of only two groups will be discussed in this chapter because some of their functions have been delineated.

OPIOID PEPTIDES

There are three endogenous opioid peptide families: β-endorphins, enkephalins, and dynorphins.

1. **β-endorphin:** The pre-propeptide, pre–proopiomelanocortin, is synthesized in rough endoplasmic reticulum of neurons in the anterior pituitary, in the intermediate lobe of pituitary, and in the arcuate nucleus of hypothalamus. Removal of a signal peptide from the pre-propeptide within the rough endoplasmic reticulum results in the generation of the propeptide pro-opiomelanocortin (POMC), which is then transported to the Golgi apparatus where it is packaged into vesicles. These vesicles are transported to the axon terminal by fast axonal transport. Further proteolytic processing in the terminal results in the generation of the active peptides, adrenocorticotropic hormone (ACTH) and β-lipotropin. β-lipotropin is further cleaved into γ-lipotropin and β-endorphin (31-amino acid C-terminal fragment). The term "endorphin" refers to a substance that has morphine-like properties. β–endorphin–containing neurons are located in the hypothalamus and send projections to periaqueductal gray (PAG) and noradrenergic cells in the brainstem.

2. **Enkephalins:** The pre-propeptide, pre-proenkephalin A, is synthesized in the rough endoplasmic reticulum of neurons in the hindbrain. Removal of the signal peptide from the pre-propeptide within the rough endoplasmic reticulum results in the generation of the propeptide, proenkephalin A, which is then transported to the Golgi apparatus where it is packaged into vesicles. The vesicles are transported to the axon terminal by fast axonal transport. Further proteolytic processing in the terminal results in the generation of the active peptides, methionine and leucine enkephalin. Both of these peptides are pentapeptides. Met-enkephalin contains methionine, and leu-enkephalin contains leucine at position 5. Enkephalins are then packaged into dense-core vesicles and are released by exocytosis as transmitters.

3. **Dynorphin (1-13):** This peptide can be isolated from the pituitary and consists of C-terminally extended form of Leu^5-enkephalin.

In the CNS, the action of most of the peptides is terminated by their degradation due to the presence of peptidases.

Physiological and Clinical Considerations

Blood-borne peptides do not cross the blood-brain barrier. Intracerebroventricular injection of opioid peptides (e.g., β-endorphin) produces only transient analgesia. However, β-endorphin is much more potent than morphine in these tests. A search for better analgesics, devoid of side effects like addiction, is going on in many laboratories. Enkephalinergic interneurons in the spinal cord have been shown to play a role in the modulation of pain sensation (see Chapter 15). Opioid peptides have been implicated in regulating blood pressure, temperature, feeding, aggression, and sexual behavior.

TACHYKININS: SUBSTANCE P

Substance P will be discussed as a representative of this group. This substance is an undecapeptide (it is composed of 11 amino acids). The dorsal root ganglia projecting to the substantia gelatinosa of the spinal cord are rich in substance P-containing neurons. These neurons have been called nociceptors because they transmit information regarding tissue damage to the pain-processing areas located in the CNS. The sensation of pain is initiated at the peripheral terminals of these sensory neurons. These terminals are stimulated by noxious chemical, thermal, and mechanical stimuli. The central terminals of these sensory neurons release substance P in the substantia gelatinosa. Substance P has been implicated as one of the neurotransmitters in mediating pain sensation (see Chapter 15).

In recent years, a topical cream containing capsaicin has been used as an analgesic in the treatment of painful disorders such as viral neuropathies (e.g., shingles) and arthritic conditions (e.g., osteoarthritis and rheumatoid arthritis). Capsaicin, the pungent substance present in hot chili peppers, mediates its actions via vanilloid receptors, which are present exclusively on the membranes of primary afferent neurons. The mechanism by which capsaicin acts as an analgesic is not fully understood. Initially, it causes a burning sensation, which is consistent with activation of peripheral terminals of primary afferent neurons. With repeated applications, the vanilloid receptors may become desensitized, thus reducing pain sensations. With prolonged use, capsaicin causes death of primary afferent neurons as a consequence of increased intracellular Ca^{2+} concentrations. Reduction in the population of primary afferent neurons results in a reduction in the release of one of the primary neurotransmitters (substance P) mediating pain sensation. This mechanism may provide a novel approach for designing topical analgesics with fewer side effects.

GASEOUS NEUROTRANSMITTERS: NITRIC OXIDE

This is a new class of neurotransmitters. **Nitric oxide** (NO) and **carbon monoxide** (CO) are two important members of this class. In this chapter, NO is discussed as a representative of this group because relatively more information is available for this neurotransmitter.

In isolated vascular smooth muscle preparations, acetylcholine and other vasodilators release a short-acting substance from the endothelial cells that relaxes blood vessels. This relaxing factor was named endothelium-derived relaxing factor (EDRF). Subsequent studies have shown that EDRF and nitric oxide (NO) are the same molecule. It is now well recognized that NO plays an important role in mediating vasodilation. Nitric oxide is also produced in many other cells including neurons where it has been implicated as a neurotransmitter.

Differences From Other Transmitters

Nitric oxide does not satisfy some of the criteria formulated for classical transmitters (small molecule and peptide transmitters), and it differs from conventional neurotransmitters in the following respects:

1. It is not stored in vesicles and is generated when it is needed.

2. It is not released by calcium-dependent exocytosis from a presynaptic terminal. NO is an uncharged molecule; it diffuses freely across cell membranes and modifies the activity of other cells.

3. Inactivation of NO is passive (there is no active process that terminates its action). It decays spontaneously and is converted to nitrites, nitrates, oxygen, and water.

4. It does not interact with receptors on target cells. Its sphere of action depends on the extent to which it diffuses, which may include several target cells. Therefore, the action of NO is not confined to the conventional presynaptic-postsynaptic direction.

5. NO acts as a retrograde messenger and regulates the function of axon terminals presynaptic to the neuron in which it is synthesized.

Synthesis and Removal

In the CNS, the enzyme needed for the synthesis of nitric oxide, **nitric oxide synthase (NOS)**, is present in discrete populations of neurons, but it is not present in glia. Three isoforms of NOS have been cloned; isoform I (nNOS or cNOS) is found in neurons and epithelial cells, isoform II (iNOS) is induced by cytokines and is found in macrophages and smooth muscle cells, and isoform III (eNOS) is found in endothelial cells lining blood vessels (Table 8-2). All three isoforms require tetrahydrobiopterin as a cofactor and nicotinamide adenine dinucleotide phosphate (NADPH) as a coenzyme. Isoforms I and III of NOS are activated by the influx of extracellular calcium into the cell. Isoform II (iNOS), the inducible form of NOS, is activated by cytokines. The steps involved in the activation of constitutive forms of NOS (cNOS and eNOS) are as follows (Fig. 8-11).

1. Glutamate is released from a presynaptic neuron.

2. Glutamate acts on NMDA receptors located on the postsynaptic neuron, and Ca^{2+} enters the postsynaptic neuron and binds with calmodulin (calcium-binding protein).

3. Ca^{2+}-calmodulin complex activates NOS.

4. Activation of NOS results in the formation of NO and citrulline from L-arginine.

5. Once generated, NO interacts with the heme moiety of soluble guanylate cyclase; this results in an allosteric transformation and activation of this enzyme.

6. The stimulation of soluble guanylate cyclase results in the formation of cyclic guanosine monophosphate (cGMP) from guanosine

Table 8–2 Isoforms of Nitric Oxide Synthase

Property	Isoform I	Isoform II	Isoform III
Name	cNOS or nNOS	iNOS	eNOS
Expression	Constitutive	Inducible by cytokines	Constitutive
Calcium dependence	Yes	No	Yes
Tissue	Neurons, epithelial cells	Macrophages, smooth muscle cells	Endothelial cells

NOS = nitric oxide synthase.

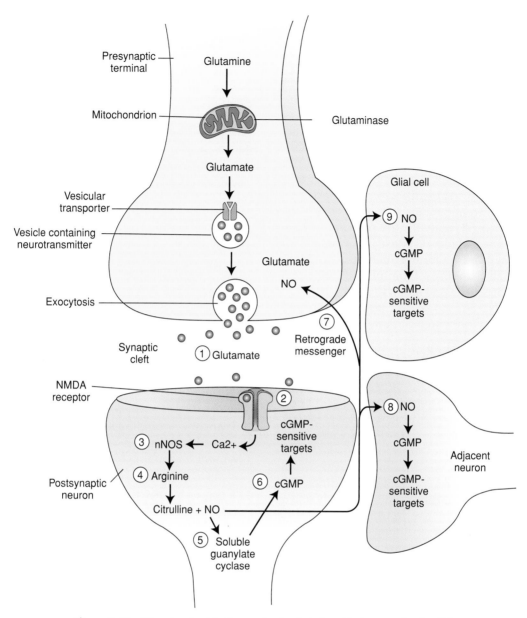

Figure 8–11 Steps involved in the synthesis of nitric oxide (see text for details).

triphosphate (GTP) in the postsynaptic neuron. Increased levels of cGMP in the postsynaptic neuron result in a physiological response.

7. NO generated in the postsynaptic neuron can diffuse out to the presynaptic terminal. Diffusion of NO to the presynaptic terminal suggests that it serves as a **retrograde messenger.** This action is believed to result in enhanced and prolonged transmitter release from the presynaptic neuron.

8. NO can also diffuse out to the adjacent neuron and (9) adjacent glial cells. In each of these sites, NO stimulates soluble guanylate cyclase and increases cGMP levels, which then brings about a response.

As mentioned earlier, NO decays spontaneously and is converted to nitrites, nitrates, oxygen, and water.

Physiological and Clinical Considerations

In the CNS, the role of NO as a transmitter is still under investigation.

RECEPTORS

Receptors are proteins located on neuronal membranes with which neurotransmitters bind; the result is the opening or closing of specific ion channels. There are two families of receptors: (1) ionotropic or ligand-gated receptors, and

(2) metabotropic or G-protein–coupled receptors (for classification of different ion channels, see Chapter 7).

IONOTROPIC RECEPTORS

Ionotropic receptors usually consist of multimeric proteins (different proteins, usually five). Each subunit spans the plasma membrane and contributes to the formation of the pore of the ion channel. They are called ligand-gated receptors because they combine transmitter-binding and channel functions into one molecular entity. When the neurotransmitter binds with the receptor site, an ion channel opens and a response is elicited. These types of receptors generally mediate rapid and short-duration responses. Examples of ionotropic receptors for different neurotransmitters are shown in Table 8-3. Some of these receptors are discussed in the following sections.

Nicotinic Acetylcholine Receptor (nAChR)

These receptors are located at the neuromuscular junction (NMJ) as well as at central neurons. Nicotinic acetylcholine receptor at the NMJ consists of 5 protein subunits (2 alpha, 1 beta, 1 gamma, and 1 delta subunit) (Fig. 8-12A). Each subunit spans the membrane four times (Fig. 8-12B). Twenty transmembrane domains from 5 subunits surround a central pore of the channel (Fig. 8-12C); the transmembrane domains of only one α-subunit are shown in the figure. Acetylcholine binds to the α-subunits and opens the channel to allow influx of Na^+ and efflux of K^+ (agonists: acetylcholine and nicotine; antagonist: d-tubocurarine, which is one of the muscle relaxants used in surgical procedures).

Clinical Disorders Associated With the Neuromuscular Junction

There are two major autoimmune disorders associated with the NMJ. In the **Lambert-Eaton syndrome**, an antibody develops against the Ca^{2+} channels on the presynaptic terminal at the NMJ. Details of this syndrome are described in Chapter 6 (see also the clinical case in this chapter). In **myasthenia gravis**, antibodies develop against the nicotinic acetylcholine receptor at the NMJ. Details of this disorder are described in Chapter 6.

N-Methyl-D-Aspartic Acid (NMDA) Receptor

This ionotropic glutamate receptor is distributed widely in the CNS. Current evidence suggests that the NMDA receptor consists of 5 subunits (NMDAR1, NMDAR2A, NMDAR2B, NMDAR2C, and NMDAR2D). Each NMDA receptor subunit consists of 4 transmembrane domains (TM1-TM4). The TM2 domain forms a kink and does not fully traverse the membrane (Fig. 8-13). The TM2 domain of each subunit lines the pore of the NMDA receptor channel. The activity of this receptor can be altered through the following binding sites (Fig. 8-13):

1. Transmitter binding site where L-glutamate and related agonists act and promote opening of the channel through which Na^+ and Ca^{2+} ions enter and K^+ ions leave the cell.

2. A region of the transmitter binding site where NMDA receptor antagonists bind.

3. The strychnine-insensitive glycine modulatory site, which must be occupied by glycine in order for L-glutamate to be effective at this receptor. Glycine increases the frequency of the opening of this receptor channel. At the glycine binding

Table 8–3 Ionotropic and Metabotropic Receptors for Different Neurotransmitters

Neurotransmitter	Ionotropic Receptor	Metabotropic Receptor
Acetylcholine (ACh)	Cholinergic nicotinic	Cholinergic muscarinic
Glutamate	NMDA, AMPA, kainate	$mGlu_1$–$mGlu_8$
GABA	$GABA_A$	$GABA_B$
Glycine	Strychnine-sensitive glycine receptor	—
Dopamine	—	D_1-D_5
Norepinephrine	—	α- and β-adrenergic receptors
Epinephrine	—	α- and β-adrenergic receptors
Serotonin	$5-HT_3$	$5HT_1$, $5HT_2$, $5HT_4$–$5HT_7$
Histamine	—	H_1, H_2, H_3
Adenosine	—	A_1–A_3
Opioid peptides	—	Mu, delta, kappa, ORL_1

AMPA = alpha-amino-3-hydroxy-5-methyl-4-isoxazole-propionate; GABA = gamma aminobutyric acid; NMDA = N-methyl-D-aspartic acid.

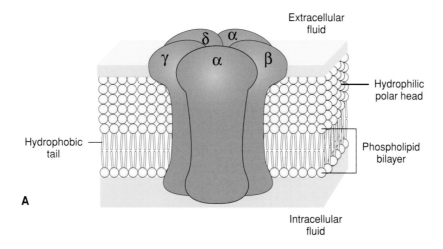

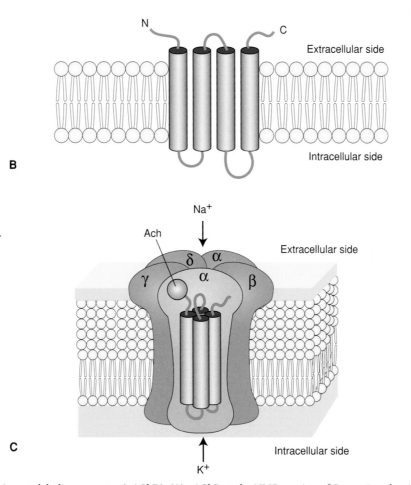

Figure 8–12 Nicotinic acetylcholine receptor (nAChR). (A) nAChR at the NMJ consists of 5 protein subunits (alpha, beta, gamma, and delta). (B) Each subunit spans the membrane 4 times. N and C represent NH_2 and COOH terminals, respectively. (C) The transmembrane domains from 5 subunits surround a central pore of the channel. Acetylcholine (Ach) binds to the α-subunit and opens the channel to allow influx of Na^+ and efflux of K^+.

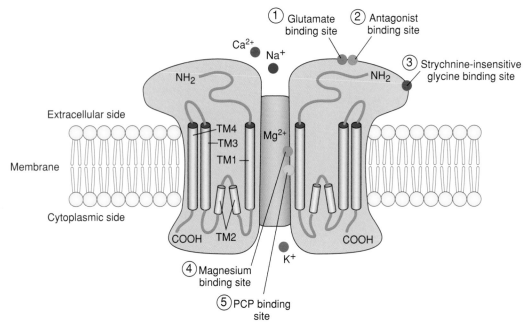

Figure 8–13 Components of an NMDA receptor.

site of the NMDA receptor, strychnine does not act as an antagonist; therefore, it is called the strychnine-insensitive glycine site. It should be noted that, in the synapses where glycine acts as a neurotransmitter, strychnine acts as an antagonist, and these sites are called strychnine-sensitive glycine sites (see the section on glycine receptor).

4. Voltage-dependent magnesium binding site where Mg^{2+} binds at normal resting potentials or when the cell is hyperpolarized and blocks the NMDA receptor channel. Therefore, NMDA receptor cannot be activated at normal resting potentials or when the cell is hyperpolarized. When the cell is depolarized, Mg^{2+} is dislodged from its binding site in the channel, and Na^+ and Ca^{2+} enter, while K^+ leaves the cell through the same channel.

5. The phencyclidine binding site is located within the channel where phencyclidine (PCP; Angel dust) binds and elicits the side-effects associated with its use.

Kainate Receptor

The binding of kainic acid to this ionotropic glutamate receptor results in the opening of an ion channel, permitting influx of Na^+ (but not Ca^{2+}) and efflux of K^+ through the same channel; and the neuron is depolarized.

AMPA/Quisqualate Receptor

AMPA (alpha-amino-3-hydroxy-5-methyl-4-isoxazole-propionate) and quisqualic acid are agonists for this ionotropic glutamate receptor. Binding of these agonists to this receptor results in the opening of an ion channel, permitting influx of Na^+ (but not Ca^{2+}) and efflux of K^+; and the neuron is depolarized.

GABA$_A$ Receptors

These ionotropic receptors are distributed throughout the CNS. They consist of a combination of 5 subunits (2 alpha, 2 beta, and 1 gamma) (Fig. 8-14). Each subunit has four transmembrane domains (TM1-TM4). Present on these receptors are major binding sites: (1) for agonists (e.g., GABA), (2) for antagonists (e.g., bicuculline), (3) for barbiturates (e.g., phenobarbital), and (4) for benzodiazepines (e.g., diazepam [Valium]). Activation of the GABA receptor site by GABA agonists results in the opening of the chloride channel; negatively charged chloride ions (Cl^-) enter the neuron and hyperpolarize and inhibit it. GABA receptor antagonists bind to their receptor site, and the conformation of the receptor changes so that subsequent application of the GABA receptor fails to elicit a response. Barbiturates bind to another site and prolong the opening of chloride channel. Antianxiety (anxiolytic) drugs (e.g., diazepam) that bind to the benzodiazepine site enhance the electrophysiological effects of GABA on these neurons.

Glycine Receptor

Glycine has been implicated as a neurotransmitter in the spinal cord, lower brainstem, and retina. Activation of glycine receptors results in an influx

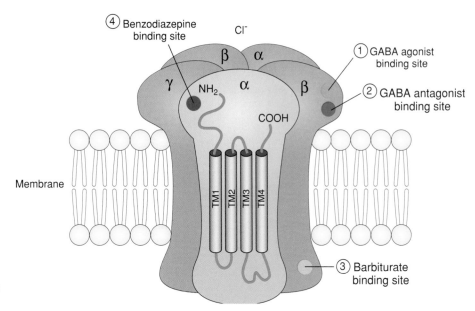

Figure 8–14 Components of a GABA$_A$ receptor.

of chloride ions into the neuron, which is then hyperpolarized and inhibited. Strychnine blocks the glycine receptors at the synapses where glycine acts as a neurotransmitter. As stated earlier, the glycine sites on the NMDA receptors are strychnine-resistant.

Serotonin Receptors

At least seven subtypes of serotonin receptors have been identified. Only 5-HT$_3$ receptors are ionotropic receptors. All other subtypes are metabotropic receptors (see Table 8-3). 5-HT$_3$ receptors are located in central and peripheral neurons. Their function remains to be established.

METABOTROPIC RECEPTORS

These receptors do not have the ion channel as part of the receptor. The flow of ions through the channels associated with these receptors depends on one or more metabolic steps. Therefore, these receptors are called metabotropic receptors. The opening or closing of the ion channels associated with these receptors involves activation of intermediate molecules called **G-proteins**. For this reason, metabotropic receptors are also called G-protein–coupled receptors.

Metabotropic receptors consist of a single protein (monomeric) molecule that has membrane-spanning domains (I-VII) (Fig. 8-15A) (see also Chapter 7). Portions of domains II, III, VI, and VII make up the extracellular domain where a neurotransmitter binding site is located. G-proteins bind to the intracellular loop between domain V and VI and to portions of the C terminus. Heterotrimeric G-proteins consist of three subunits (alpha, beta,

and gamma) (Fig. 8-15B). The α-subunit binds guanine nucleotides, such as guanosine-5′-triphosphate (GTP) and guanosine-5′-diphosphate (GDP). When GDP is bound to the α-subunit, the three subunits are bound together and form an inactive trimer.

The steps involved in the binding of the neurotransmitter to the metabotropic receptor and the events that follow are shown in Figure 8-15C. The neurotransmitter binding to the metabotropic receptor results in the replacement of GDP by GTP on the α-subunit. The activated GTP–α-subunit dissociates from the β-γ–subunit complex. Either one of these complexes can bind to effector molecules (e.g., enzymes) and stimulate them (e.g., adenylate cyclase) and generate second messengers (e.g., cyclic adenosine monophosphate, cAMP). The second messengers (e.g., cAMP) stimulate enzymes (e.g., protein kinase-A), which then phosphorylate appropriate ion channels.

Usually phosphorylation of ion channels by protein kinases results in opening of the channel; ions flow across the neuronal membrane, the neurons are depolarized, and the amplitude of neurotransmitter-induced excitatory postsynaptic potentials (EPSPs) is increased. Hence, the neuron is made more excitable. The onset and duration of responses mediated by the metabotropic receptors is longer than those mediated by ionotropic receptors. Dephosphorylation of ion channels by protein phosphatases results in the closing of the channel.

Examples of metabotropic receptors for different neurotransmitters are shown in Table 8-3.

Some of them are discussed in the following sections.

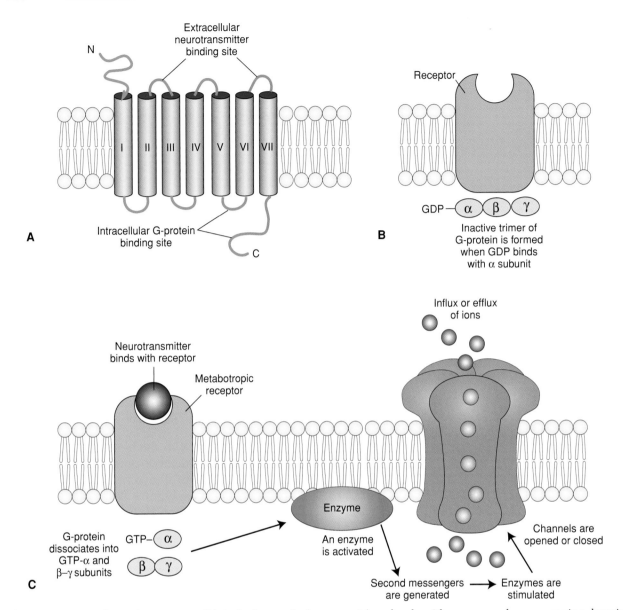

Figure 8–15 Metabotropic receptors. (A) A single protein (monomeric) molecule with seven membrane-spanning domains (I-VII). A neurotransmitter-binding site is located in the extracellular domain (made up of portions of domains II, III, VI, and VII). G-proteins bind to the intracellular loop between domains V and VI and to portions of the C terminus. N and C denote NH_2 and COOH terminals, respectively. (B) Heterotrimeric G-proteins consist of three subunits (alpha, beta, and gamma). When GDP is bound to the α-subunit, the α-subunit binds to β- and γ-subunits, and an inactive trimer is formed. (C) The steps of a neurotransmitter binding to the metabotropic receptor and the events that follow.

Cholinergic Muscarinic Receptors

The steps involved in the binding of acetylcholine (ACh) to the muscarinic receptor and the events that follow are shown in Fig. 8-16A. ACh binds with muscarinic receptor; a G-protein (G_o) is activated; the enzyme phospholipase-C is stimulated; and two second messengers (inositol triphosphate [IP_3] and diacylglycerol [DAG]) are produced. IP_3 releases Ca^{2+} from intracellular stores, which leads to opening of Ca^{2+}-activated K^+ and Cl^- channels. DAG activates protein kinase-C, which can directly open Ca^{2+}-activated K^+ channels.

Opening of Ca^{2+}-activated K^+ and Cl^- channels results in the hyperpolarization and inhibition of the neuron.

Metabotropic Glutamate Receptors (mGLURs)

Eight subtypes of mGLURs have been identified so far. Based on their amino acid sequence and their transduction mechanisms, mGLURs have been assigned to three groups.

- Group I: includes mGLUR1 and mGLUR5. They stimulate phospholipase C and phosphoinositide hydrolysis.

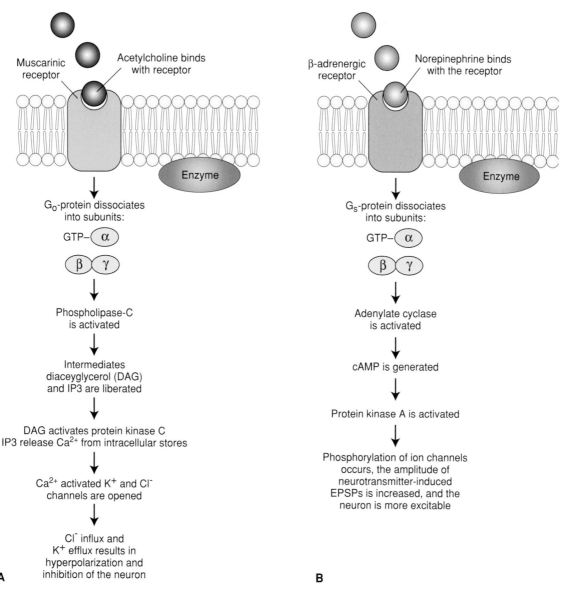

Figure 8–16 Mechanisms by which metabotropic receptors mediate responses to different transmitters. (A) Events that follow binding of ACh to a muscarinic receptor. (B) Events that follow binding of norepinephrine to a β-adrenergic receptor.

- Group II: includes mGLUR2 and mGLUR3.
- Group III: includes mGLUR4, mGLUR6, mGLUR7, and mGLUR8. These two groups inhibit adenylyl cyclase and cAMP formation.

Dopamine Receptors

At least five subtypes of dopamine receptors (D_1-D_5) have been identified. All of them are metabotropic receptors.

Adrenergic Receptors

Norepinephrine and epinephrine mediate their actions via adrenergic receptors. These receptors are divided into two major classes: α- and β-adrenergic receptors. These classes have been further subdivided into many subtypes of adrenergic receptors.

The action of norepinephrine mediated via β-adrenergic receptors is used as an example to illustrate how catecholamines act via metabotropic receptors (Fig. 8-16B). The binding of norepinephrine with β-adrenergic receptor results in the activation of a G-protein (G_s). Adenylyl cyclase enzyme is activated, which generates the second messenger, cAMP. The latter activates protein kinase-A, which phosphorylates appropriate channels and opens them. The neurons are depolarized, the amplitude of neurotransmitter-induced excitatory postsynaptic potentials (EPSPs) is increased, and the neurons become more excitable.

GABA$_B$ Receptors

These metabotropic GABA receptors are not linked to a chloride channel. They are coupled to calcium or potassium channels via second-messenger systems. Activation of presynaptic GABA$_B$ receptors by baclofen decreases calcium conductance and reduces transmitter release.

Opioid Receptors

Three major classes of opioid receptors have been identified in the CNS: μ-, δ-, and κ-receptors. Morphine and endogenous opioid peptides produce their supraspinal analgesic (pain-relieving) effect via μ-opioid receptors that are present in the periaqueductal gray matter (PAG), thalamus, and raphe magnus (structures implicated in processing of pain sensation). Leu- and met-enkephalins act mainly on δ-receptors. Dynorphin acts mainly on κ-receptors. β-endorphin acts on all three (mu, delta, and kappa) opioid receptors. Recently, two tetrapeptides, **endomorphin-1** and **endomorphin-2**, have been identified as endogenous μ-opioid receptor ligands. Naloxone blocks them. A new opiate receptor, called ORL1 receptor, has been identified. Its endogenous ligand is **nociceptin**. Naloxone does not block ORL1 receptor. The physiological functions of these peptides are not clearly established yet.

Serotonin Receptors

At least five subtypes of serotonin receptors have been identified. Identification of the function of 5-HT receptors in the CNS remains an active area of research.

Histamine Receptors

At least three subtypes of histamine receptors (H$_1$, H$_2$, and H$_3$) have been identified. All of the subtypes are metabotropic. Their function in the CNS remains to be elucidated.

Adenosine Receptors

At least three adenosine receptors (A$_1$-A$_3$) have been identified, all of which are metabotropic receptors. Identification of their function in the CNS is an active area of research at present.

MECHANISMS OF REGULATION OF RECEPTORS

Desensitization

Prolonged exposure of a receptor (e.g., β-adrenergic receptor) to endogenous or exogenous agonists often reduces the responsiveness of the receptor. This phenomenon is called **desensitization**. Interaction of norepinephrine with a β-adrenergic receptor will be used as an example to demonstrate the mechanisms by which desensitization occurs. Norepinephrine binds with the β-adrenergic receptor; a G-protein (G$_s$) is stimulated; and cAMP is formed, which stimulates protein kinase-A. This kinase phosphorylates the β-adrenergic receptor and uncouples it from the G-protein. Therefore, the receptor no longer responds to the agonist, causing desensitization.

Down-Regulation

When the number of receptors decreases, it is called **down-regulation** of receptors. One of the mechanisms by which down-regulation of receptors occurs is that the receptors are internalized and sequestered inside the cell.

CLINICAL CASE

HISTORY

Helena is a 22-year-old woman who had no prior medical problems. Insidiously, one day, she felt very fatigued and thought that she might be pregnant. She went to her internist and had a positive pregnancy test, so she attributed all of her fatigue to the pregnancy. However, throughout several months after her pregnancy, she continued to feel fatigued and worse in the evening than in the morning. Her eyes frequently drooped, and she was often told that her eyes did not move synchronously. Many times, she thought that she had trouble swallowing liquids. She felt that her face changed, in that it appeared more lax than previously. She felt generally weak and noticed that the more she exercised, such as walking around, the worse she felt. Noticing the persistence of Helena's symptoms, her internist referred her to a neurologist.

EXAMINATION

The neurologist observed that Helena was unable to abduct both eyes and that there was a ptosis (drooping) of both eyelids. When he asked her to flex her finger extensors repetitively, she was only able to keep it up for 5 repetitions, while most normal subjects were able to keep it up for more than 20. An edrophonium test (Tensilon test) was administered where edrophonium was given before and after testing of finger extensors, respiratory function, and eye movement function, all of which improved with the drug.

EXPLANATION

Helena has myasthenia gravis, an autoimmune disease directed against the nicotinic acetylcholine (nACh) receptor. There is a marked reduction in the number of nACh receptors as well as folds on the postsynaptic membrane of the neuromuscular junction. Neurophysiologically, there is a decrease in miniature end-plate potentials (MEPPs) upon repetitive stimulation. This demonstrates a progressive fatigue of the muscle. Treatment with anticholinesterase drugs, which increase the amount of acetylcholine in the neuromuscular junction, reverses the pathological process. Thymomas may be found in 10% to 15% of the cases and appear to play a role in the autoimmune process. Clinical features of this disease vary, depending on the type and age of the patient, but it is almost always characterized by fatigue, often involving the eyelids and ocular muscles,

muscles of facial expression and mastication, swallowing, and speech. In advanced cases, all of the muscles may become weak, including the diaphragm and abdominal and intercostal muscles, causing respiratory dysfunction. Weakness is usually least severe earlier in the day and progresses during the course of the day. Treatment includes administration of anticholinesterase drugs, thymectomy, corticosteroids, and immunosuppressant therapy.

CHAPTER TEST

QUESTIONS

Choose the one answer that is best for each question.

1. The neurologic examination of a 60-year-old man revealed that he is suffering from Parkinson's disease. Which one of the following statements is true concerning this disease?

   a. It involves a degeneration of cholinergic neurons in the basal nucleus of Meynert.
   b. It involves a degeneration of noradrenergic neurons of the locus ceruleus.
   c. It involves a degeneration of dopaminergic neurons of the substantia nigra.
   d. Oral administration of dopamine is likely to relieve the symptoms of Parkinson's disease.
   e. It is usually associated with hyperkinetic syndrome.

2. A 35-year-old woman suffering from severe migraine headache was prescribed sumatriptan (Imitrex) by her neurologist. The patient's headache was relieved after she took the drug. Which one of the following mechanisms is responsible for the beneficial effects of sumatriptan in treating migraine headache?

   a. It dilates meningeal arteries via β-adrenergic receptors.
   b. It constricts meningeal arteries via α-adrenergic receptors.
   c. It constricts meningeal arteries via 5-HT$_{1D}$ receptors.
   d. It dilates systemic arterioles via cholinergic muscarinic receptors.
   e. It dilates meningeal arteries via histamine receptors.

3. A neuropathologist received a brain specimen from a deceased Alzheimer's patient for postmortem histological examination. Which one of the following neuronal groups is likely to be degenerated in this specimen?

   a. Basal nucleus of Meynert
   b. Raphe magnus
   c. Locus ceruleus
   d. Nucleus ambiguus
   e. Substantia nigra

4. Which of the following statements is correct regarding norepinephrine?

   a. The main mechanism of its removal from the synaptic cleft involves its reuptake.
   b. Tyrosine is the immediate precursor for its synthesis.
   c. Neurons containing this transmitter are present only in the peripheral nervous system.
   d. Deficiency of this transmitter in substantia nigra causes Parkinson's disease.
   e. It is synthesized in the cytoplasm of the neuronal terminal.

5. Which one of the following statements is correct regarding nitric oxide?

   a. It stimulates soluble guanylate cyclase.
   b. Its precursor is alanine.
   c. Tyrosine hydroxylase is involved in its biosynthesis.
   d. It mediates its actions through NMDA receptors.
   e. Its actions are mediated by cAMP.

ANSWERS AND EXPLANATIONS

1. Answer: **c**

Parkinson's disease is characterized by tremor at rest, slowness of movement (bradykinesia or hypokinetic syndrome), rigidity of extremities and neck, and an expressionless face. Dopaminergic neurons located in the substantia nigra are degenerated in this disease, and the release of dopamine in the caudate/putamen is decreased. Drug treatment of this disease is aimed at replacement of the deficiency of the transmitter (dopamine) in the basal ganglia (target of nigrostriatal projection). Since dopamine does not cross the blood-brain barrier, its immediate metabolic precursor (levodopa or L-DOPA), which does cross this barrier, is administered orally. L-DOPA is transported into the brain via a large neutral amino acid transporter, and it permeates the striatal tissue where it is decarboxylated to dopamine. The levels of DOPA in the plasma are increased by simultaneous administration of carbidopa and L-DOPA. Carbidopa inhibits dopa-decarboxylase, which converts DOPA into dopamine. Carbidopa does not cross the blood-brain barrier.

2. Answer: c

One of the causes of migraine headaches is believed to be dilatation of meningeal arteries. Sumatriptan (Imitrex) is a vasoconstrictor and mediates this effect via 5-HT_{1D} receptors. Adrenergic, histaminergic, and cholinergic receptors are not involved in mediating migraine headaches.

3. Answer: a

In Alzheimer's patients, there is a dramatic loss of cholinergic neurons in the basal nucleus of Meynert. The other nuclei mentioned are not implicated in this disease. The raphe magnus, locus ceruleus, and nucleus ambiguus are concerned with descending control of pain sensation, forebrain activity during sleep and wakefulness cycles, and heart rate regulation, respectively. Dopaminergic neurons in the substantia nigra are degenerated in Parkinson's disease.

4. Answer: a

Re-uptake is the main mechanism by which norepinephrine is removed from the synaptic cleft. Norepinephrine is synthesized from dopamine by dopamine β-hydroxylase within the vesicle. Thus, its immediate precursor is dopamine. Noradrenergic neurons are present in the peripheral as well as the central nervous system. Alteration of adrenergic transmission has been implicated in some forms of depression but not in Parkinson's disease. In Parkinson's disease, there is degeneration of dopaminergic neurons in the substantia nigra.

5. Answer: a

Nitric oxide is a gas at normal atmospheric conditions and represents a new class of transmitters. It interacts with the heme moiety of soluble guanylate cyclase, which results in allosteric transformation and activation of this enzyme. Stimulation of soluble guanylate cyclase results in the formation of cGMP from GTP in the postsynaptic neuron, and the appropriate response is elicited. Alanine and tyrosine hydroxylase are not involved in its synthesis. Nitric oxide is synthesized from arginine by nitric oxide synthase. NMDA receptors do not mediate the responses of nitric oxide.

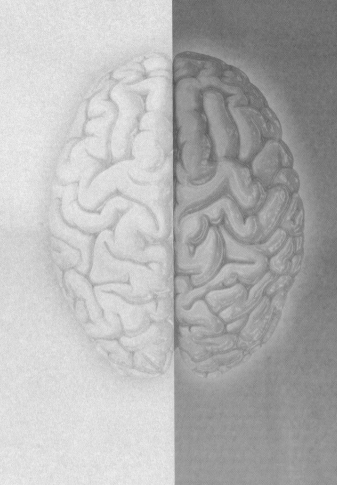

SECTION III

Organization of the Central Nervous System

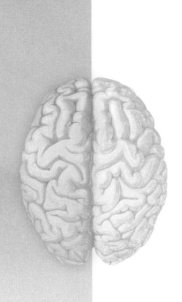

CHAPTER 9

THE SPINAL CORD

OBJECTIVES *In this chapter, the student is expected to know:*

1. The gross anatomy of the spinal cord
2. Internal structure of the spinal cord
3. Spinal segmentation: morphological differences among the different levels of spinal cord
4. Cytoarchitectural organization of the spinal cord: cellular laminae
5. The major spinal cell groups or nuclei
6. The course of the afferent fibers to the spinal cord
7. The locations and functions of the ascending and descending tracts in the spinal cord
8. The difference between the lower and upper motor neurons
9. The effects of lesions of the spinal cord and dorsal and ventral roots
10. The spinal reflexes

The spinal cord is a critical component for the transmission of sensory information to the brain as well as for the regulation of motor and autonomic functions. It receives sensory information from somatic and visceral receptors through dorsal roots, transmits this information to higher centers in the brain through ascending tracts, receives signals from higher centers through descending tracts, and transmits the signals to somatic and visceral target sites via the ventral roots. A number of reflexes are also mediated at the level of the spinal cord. These functions of the spinal cord and the anatomical, physiological, and clinical considerations associated with them are presented in this chapter.

GROSS ANATOMY

The spinal cord is located within the vertebral canal and extends from the **foramen magnum** to the rostral edge of the second lumbar vertebra (Figs. 9-1 and 9-2). The coverings (meninges) of the spinal cord (the dura, arachnoid, and pia mater) are described in Chapter 3. The caudal end of the spinal cord and the structures associated with it are shown in Figure 9-2. The conical-shaped caudal end of the spinal cord, known as the **conus medullaris**, is located at the rostral edge of the second lumbar vertebra. A thin filament enclosed in pia and consisting of glial cells, ependymal cells, and astrocytes emerges from the conus medullaris. This filament is called the **filum terminale internum**. It extends from the conus medullaris and passes through the caudal end of the dural sac. At this level, a caudal thin extension of the spinal dura, called the **coccygeal ligament (filum terminale externum)** surrounds the filum terminale. The coccygeal ligament, with filum terminale in it,

attaches to the coccyx and thus anchors the spinal cord and the fluid-filled dural sac to the caudal end of the vertebral canal.

The spinal cord occupies the whole length of the vertebral canal up to the third month of fetal life. Then it lengthens at a slower rate than the vertebral column. As a result, in an adult, the spinal cord occupies only the upper two thirds of the vertebral column. For this reason, the caudal end of the spinal cord in the normal adult is located at the rostral edge of the second lumbar vertebra (or caudal edge of the first lumbar vertebra). Therefore, the lumbar and sacral nerve roots have to descend some distance within the vertebral canal before they exit from their respective intervertebral foramina. The lumbosacral nerve roots surround the filum terminale and form a cluster that resembles the tail of a horse and that is called the **cauda equina** (Fig. 9-2). The subarachnoid space is widest from the caudal end of the spinal cord (i.e., caudal edge of the *first lumbar* vertebra) to the *second sacral* vertebra and contains no central nervous system (CNS) structures except the filum terminale and the nerve roots of cauda equina. This space is known as the lumbar cistern (see Chapter 3). Because of this anatomic feature, this space is most suitable for the withdrawal of cerebrospinal fluid (CSF) by lumbar puncture. The site for performing a lumbar puncture changes with age in childhood. For example, in children, the caudal end of the spinal cord is usually located at the third lumbar vertebra (L3); therefore, the needle for lumbar puncture is inserted at the L4–L5 level (see Chapter 3).

Spinal segmentation is based on the sites where spinal nerves emerge from the spinal cord. Thirty-one pairs of spinal nerves emerge from the spinal cord. At each level, the spinal nerves exit through

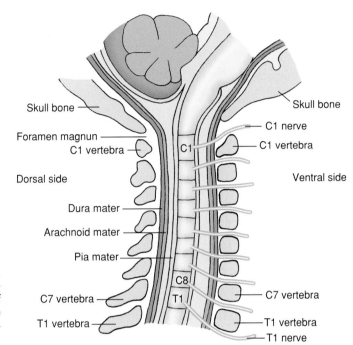

Figure 9–1 Cervical spinal cord. Note that the spinal nerves from spinal segments C1–C7 exit through the intervertebral foramen located rostral to the cervical vertebra of the same name. The spinal nerve from C8 segment of the spinal cord exits through the intervertebral foramen located caudal to T1 vertebra.

the intervertebral foramina. In the thoracic, lumbar, and sacral regions of the cord, spinal nerves exit through the intervertebral foramina *just caudal* to the vertebra of the same name. In the cervical region, these nerves exit through the intervertebral foramina *just rostral* to the vertebra of the same name. The eighth cervical spinal nerve (C8) exits through the intervertebral foramen just rostral to the first thoracic vertebra (Fig. 9-1).

Each **spinal nerve** consists of a dorsal root (containing afferent fibers) and a ventral root (containing efferent fibers). The dorsal root is absent in the first cervical and coccygeal nerves. The dorsal and ventral roots travel a short distance within the dural sac surrounding the spinal cord, penetrate the dura, and enter the intervertebral foramen. The spinal ganglion (dorsal root ganglion) is located within the intervertebral foramen and contains the neurons that give rise to afferent fibers entering the spinal cord. The dorsal and ventral roots are joined distal to the spinal ganglion and form the common spinal nerve trunk (Fig. 9-3). The common spinal nerve trunk is connected with the sympathetic chain of paravertebral ganglia that are located on either side of the vertebral column through the white and gray rami (rami communicantes; see Chapter 22).

The spinal cord is cylindrical in shape and is enlarged at the cervical and lumbar regions. The cervical enlargement includes four lower cervical segments and the first thoracic segment. The nerve roots emerging from this enlargement form the brachial plexus and innervate the upper extremities. The lumbar plexus (comprising the nerve roots from L1–L4) and sacral plexus (consisting of nerve roots from L4–S2) emerge from the lumbar enlargement. The lumbar plexus innervates the lower extremities. The sacral spinal nerves emerging from the conus medullaris contain parasympathetic fibers and motor fibers innervating the bladder and its sphincters, respectively.

INTERNAL STRUCTURE

Examination of a transverse section of the spinal cord reveals the presence of a central gray matter, shaped like a butterfly, which contains cell columns oriented along the rostro-caudal axis of the spinal cord. This butterfly-shaped gray area is surrounded by white matter consisting of ascending and descending bundles of myelinated and unmyelinated axons that are called **tracts** or **fasciculi**. The neurons comprising these tracts have similar origins and sites of termination. A bundle containing one or more tracts or fasciculi is called a **funiculus**. In each half of the spinal cord, there are three funiculi: (1) the **dorsal (posterior) funiculus**, which is located between the dorsal horn and a midline structure called the dorsal (posterior) median

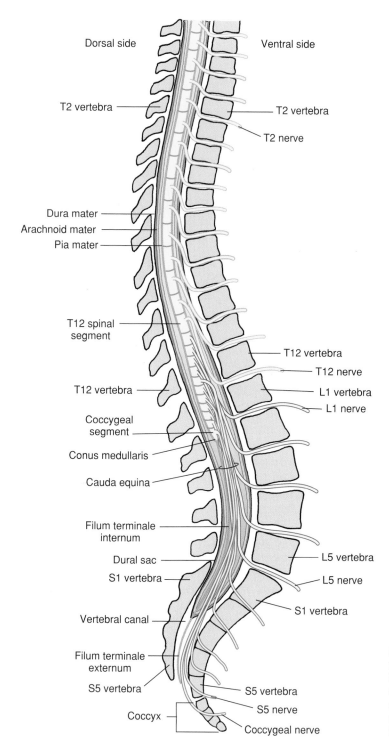

Figure 9–2 Spinal segments caudal to the cervical region. Note that the spinal nerves from thoracic (T), lumbar (L), and sacral (S) segments of the spinal cord exit through the intervertebral foramen located caudal to the vertebra of the same name. Note also the conus medullaris (caudal end of the spinal cord) and the cauda equina.

septum; (2) the **lateral funiculus**, which is located between the sites where the dorsal roots enter and ventral roots exit from the spinal cord; and (3) the **anterior (ventral) funiculus**, which is located between the **anterior (ventral) median fissure** and the site where the ventral roots exit (Fig. 9-4A).

In each half of the spinal cord, the dorsal horn of the butterfly-shaped **gray matter** reaches the surface where the dorsal rootlets of the spinal nerves

enter. The ventral horn of this butterfly-shaped gray matter does not reach the ventral surface of the spinal cord. The two sides of the gray matter are connected by a band of gray matter called the **gray commissure**. The **anterior white commissure**, consisting of decussating axons of nerve cells, is located ventral to the gray commissure. The **central canal** is located in the gray commissure (Fig. 9-4A). The lumen of the central canal in the

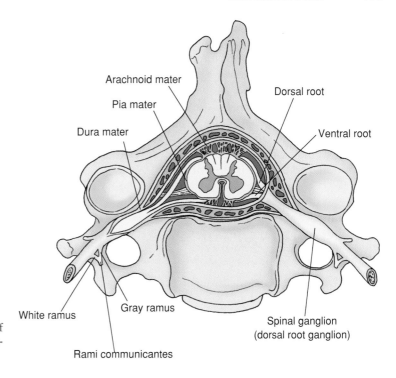

Figure 9–3 Spinal nerves. Note the location of dorsal and ventral roots and the dorsal root ganglion (as described in the text).

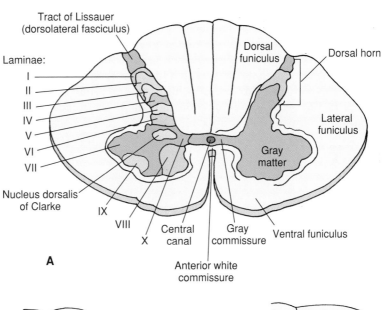

A

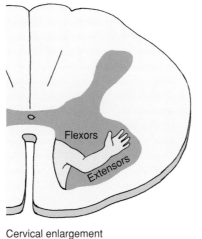

B Cervical enlargement

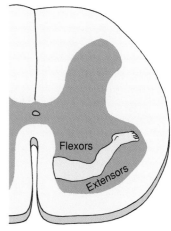

C Lumbar enlargement

Figure 9–4 Gross anatomy of the spinal cord in transverse section. (A) The central gray matter is shaped like a butterfly. Note the three funiculi in each half of the spinal cord: the dorsal (posterior) funiculus, the lateral funiculus, and the ventral (anterior) funiculus. The two sides of the gray matter are connected by the gray commissure. Note the location of laminae I through X. Lamina VII contains the nucleus dorsalis of Clarke. (B and C) Note the somatotopic arrangement of neurons in laminae VIII and IX and the location of the neurons innervating the flexors and extensors. See text for other details.

adult spinal cord may be filled with debris consisting of macrophages and neuroglial processes.

The gray matter of the spinal cord contains primarily neuronal cell bodies, dendrites, and myelinated and unmyelinated axons, which are either projecting from the white matter to innervate neurons located in the gray matter or exiting from the gray matter to the white matter. The white matter consists of ascending and descending tracts of myelinated and unmyelinated fibers.

CYTOARCHITECTURAL ORGANIZATION OF THE SPINAL GRAY MATTER

The architectural organization of the spinal gray matter was described by Rexed in 1952. He reported that clusters of cells are arranged in the spinal cord in 10 zones. A description of these zones, referred to as Rexed laminae I-X, is provided in the following paragraphs, and their location is shown in Fig. 9-4A. For important structures located in these laminae, see Table 9-1.

The **zone of Lissauer** (dorsolateral fasciculus) consists of fine myelinated and unmyelinated dorsal root fibers that enter the medial portion of this zone. A large number of propriospinal fibers, which interconnect different levels of the **substantia gelatinosa** (described later in this section), are also present in this zone. Laminae I through IV are located in the dorsal horn of the spinal cord. The cells situated in these laminae receive primarily exteroceptive (i.e., pain, temperature, and tactile) inputs from the periphery.

Lamina I contains terminals of dorsal root fibers mediating pain and temperature sensations that synapse, in part, on the group of cells called the **posteromarginal nucleus**. The axons of the cells in the posteromarginal nucleus cross to the opposite side and ascend as the lateral spinothalamic tract. *Lamina II* is located immediately below lamina I and contains the substantia gelatinosa. The neurons in the substantia gelatinosa modulate the activity of pain and temperature afferent fibers. Activation of peripheral pain receptors results in the release of substance P and glutamate in the substantia gelatinosa. *Laminae III and IV*, both of which contain the **proper sensory nucleus**, are located in the lower aspect of the dorsal horn. The proper sensory nucleus receives inputs from the substantia gelatinosa and contributes to the spinothalamic tracts mediating pain, temperature, and crude touch. *Lamina V* is located at the neck of the dorsal horn; neurons located in this lamina receive descending fibers from the corticospinal and rubrospinal tracts and give rise to axons that contribute to the spinothalamic tracts. *Lamina VI* is present only in cervical and lumbar segments. It contains a medial segment that receives muscle spindle and joint afferents, and also contains a lateral segment that receives fibers from descending corticospinal and rubrospinal pathways. Neurons in this region are involved in the integration of so-

Table 9–1   Key Structures in the Spinal Rexed Laminae

Laminae	Key Structures
I	Dorsal root fibers mediating pain, temperature, and touch sensations; posteromarginal nucleus
II	Substantia gelatinosa neurons mediating pain transmission
III & IV	Proper sensory nucleus that receives inputs from substantia gelatinosa and contributes to spinothalamic tracts mediating pain, temperature, and touch sensations
V	Neurons receiving descending fibers from corticospinal and rubrospinal tracts; neurons that contribute to ascending spinothalamic tracts
VI	Present only in cervical and lumbar segments; lateral segment receives descending corticospinal and rubrospinal fibers; medial segment receives afferents from muscle spindles and joint afferents
VII	Nucleus dorsalis of Clarke extending from C8–L2 receives muscle and tendon afferents; axons from this nucleus form spinocerebellar tract; intermediolateral cell column containing sympathetic preganglionic neurons from T1–L3; parasympathetic neurons located in S2–S4 segments; Renshaw cells
VIII & IX	Located in the ventral horn; alpha and gamma motor neurons innervating skeletal muscles; neurons in medial aspect receive inputs from vestibulospinal and reticulospinal tracts and innervate axial musculature for posture and balance; neurons in lateral aspect receive inputs from corticospinal and rubrospinal tracts and innervate distal musculature
X	Gray matter surrounding central canal

matic motor processes. *Lamina VII*, which is located in an intermediate region of the spinal gray matter, contains the **nucleus dorsalis of Clarke**, which extends from C8 through L2. This nucleus receives muscle and tendon afferents. Axons of this nucleus form the **dorsal spinocerebellar tract**, which relays this information to the ipsilateral cerebellum.

Other important neurons located in lamina VII include the sympathetic preganglionic neurons, which constitute the **intermediolateral cell column (IML) in the thoracolumbar cord (T1–L2)**, parasympathetic neurons located in the lateral aspect of sacral cord (S2–S4), and numerous interneurons such as **Renshaw cells**. The output of alpha motor neurons, which are located in the ventral horn of the gray matter, is regulated by Renshaw cells through a mechanism called "**recurrent inhibition**." Renshaw cells are interneurons that make inhibitory (glycinergic) synapses on the alpha motor neurons and receive excitatory (cholinergic) collaterals from the same neurons. When an alpha motor neuron is excited, it activates Renshaw cells via the excitatory (cholinergic) collaterals. Renshaw cells, in turn, inhibit, via glycinergic synapses, the activity of the same alpha motor neuron.

Laminae VIII and *IX* are located in the ventral horn of the gray matter of the spinal cord. Neurons in this region, which receive inputs from the descending motor tracts from the cerebral cortex and brainstem, give rise to both alpha and gamma motor neurons that innervate skeletal muscles. Neurons in these laminae are somatotopically arranged; neurons providing innervation to the extensor muscles are located ventral to those innervating the flexors, and neurons providing innervation to the axial musculature are medial to those innervating muscles in the distal parts of the extremity (Fig. 9-4, B and C). Neurons situated in the medial aspect of the ventral horn receive afferents from the vestibulospinal and reticulospinal systems and, in turn, innervate the axial musculature. This anatomical arrangement allows descending pathways to regulate the axial musculature (i.e., posture and balance). In contrast, neurons situated in the lateral aspect of the ventral horn receive afferents from the corticospinal and rubrospinal pathways. Axons of these neurons mainly innervate the distal musculature. This arrangement provides a basis by which these descending pathways can have a preferential influence upon the activity of the distal musculature. Thus, in the ventral horn, motor neurons are located according to the muscle that they innervate. Neurons providing innervation to the extensor muscles are located ventral to those inner-

vating the flexors. Neurons providing innervation to the axial and limb girdle musculature are medial to those innervating muscles in the distal parts of the extremity. In the cervical part of the spinal cord (segments C3, C4, and C5), lamina IX contains phrenic motor neurons that provide innervation to the diaphragm. Thoracic respiratory motor neurons, which innervate intercostal and other rib cage and back muscles, are located in lamina IX of the thoracic segments. The gray matter surrounding the central canal constitutes *lamina X*.

SPINAL SEGMENTS

The spinal cord consists of 31 segments (8 cervical, 12 thoracic, 5 lumbar, 5 sacral, and 1 coccygeal) based on the existence of 31 pairs of spinal nerves. Each segment (except the first cervical and coccygeal segments) receives dorsal and ventral root filaments on each side. A schematic representation of different spinal segments is shown in Figure 9-5. The functions of various tracts and neuronal groups located in these segments are described later in this chapter in the section *Spinal Cord Tracts*.

Cervical segments are the largest spinal cord segments. In each half of the spinal cord, the **dorsal funiculus** is divided into two major ascending pathways called the **fasciculus gracilis** and **fasciculus cuneatus.**

Thoracic segments are smaller than the cervical segments because they contain a smaller amount of gray and white matter. A lateral horn, which contains the **IML** (described earlier), is present in all thoracic segments (Fig. 9-5). The IML of the thoracic and lumbar spinal cord contains preganglionic sympathetic neurons. In all thoracic segments, a prominent structure called the **dorsal nucleus of Clarke** contains large cells and is located medially at the base of the dorsal horn. At rostral levels of the thoracic cord (T1–T6), both the fasciculi gracilis and cuneatus are present, whereas at caudal levels (e.g., T10), only the fasciculus gracilis is present. The spinal nerves emerging from the rostral levels of the thoracic cord (except T1) provide motor innervation to the back and intercostal muscles (axial muscles). The spinal nerves emerging from the caudal thoracic levels innervate abdominal muscles in addition to axial muscles.

The lumbar segments appear circular in transverse sections (Fig 9-5). The segments at L1 and L2 are similar to those located at lower thoracic levels. These segments contain the IML. The lumbar segments located at L3 to L5 do not contain IML. These segments provide motor innervation to the large muscles in the lower extremities.

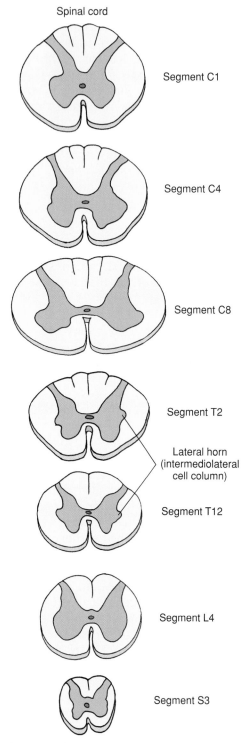

Spinal cord

Segment C1

Segment C4

Segment C8

Segment T2

Lateral horn
(intermediolateral
cell column)

Segment T12

Segment L4

Segment S3

Figure 9–5 Spinal cord segments. Cervical segments are the largest segments. The thoracic and sacral segments are relatively small. Note the presence of intermediolateral cell column (IML) in the thoracic and sacral segments.

The sacral segments are relatively small. They contain relatively small amounts of white matter and more abundant quantities of gray matter. The IML of sacral segments S2–S4 contains the parasympathetic preganglionic neurons (see

Chapter 22). The coccygeal segments resemble the sacral segments.

A **dermatome** is defined as the area of skin supplied by the right and left dorsal roots of a single spinal segment. Dermatomal maps of the peripheral distribution of spinal nerves reveal a set of bands on the surface of the body (Fig. 9-6). If one dorsal root is sectioned, the sensation in the corresponding dermatome is not lost because several adjacent dorsal roots innervate overlapping areas on the skin. Usually three adjacent dorsal roots have to be sectioned in order to lose sensation in one dermatome.

SPINAL CORD TRACTS

As noted earlier, tracts or fasciculi are defined as bundles of fibers that have the same origin, course, and termination. Different tracts are clustered together in the white matter of the spinal cord and are referred to as **dorsal**, **ventral**, and **lateral funiculi**. The dorsal funiculus (dorsal column) contains two ascending tracts, the fasciculus gracilis and fasciculus cuneatus, which are described in the following sections. The lateral aspect of the funiculi contains long ascending and descending tracts, whereas the region adjacent to the gray matter contains the short tracts that connect different spinal segments.

LONG ASCENDING TRACTS

Fasciculus Gracilis

A schematic representation of the course of this tract is shown in Figure 9-7. This tract exists at all levels of the spinal cord and contains long ascending fibers from the lower and upper limbs. Myelinated afferents from the *dorsal root ganglion* enter the dorsal (posterior) funiculus, medial to the dorsal horn, and the ascending fibers occupy a medial position in this funiculus. Myelinated afferent fibers from the *lumbosacral regions*, which mediate sensations from the lower limbs (i.e., sacral, lumbar, and caudal six thoracic segments), ascend medially; and those fibers from upper limbs (i.e., upper thoracic and lower cervical segments) ascend laterally in this tract.

The neurons located in the dorsal root ganglion represent the **first-order neurons** (i.e., neuron I). The peripheral processes of the first-order neuron innervate the Pacinian corpuscle (sensing tactile and vibratory stimuli) and Meissner's corpuscle (sensing touch) in the skin, as well as proprioceptors in joints that are involved in kinesthesia (sense of position and movement). The central processes of the first-order neuron ascend ipsilaterally in the spinal cord (i.e., the ascending fibers of first-order

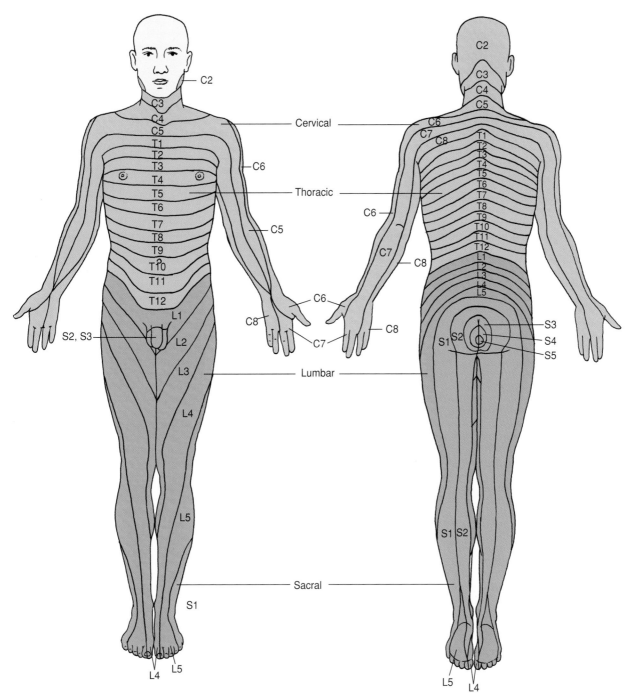

Figure 9–6 Dermatomal maps of the peripheral distribution of spinal nerves. (A) Front view. (B) Back view. Labels indicate the innervation of each dermatome. (Used with permission from Bear MF, et al.: Neuroscience: Exploring the Brain, 2nd ed. Philadelphia: Lippincott, Williams & Wilkins, 2001, p. 406.)

neurons are uncrossed) and terminate somatotopically on **second-order neurons** (i.e., neuron II) in the ipsilateral **nucleus gracilis** in the medulla. Axons of the second-order neuron in the nucleus gracilis travel ventromedially as **internal arcuate fibers** and cross in the midline to form the **medial lemniscus (decussation of medial lemniscus).**

This crossed tract ascends through the medulla, pons, and midbrain and finally terminates on the **third-order neurons** (i.e., neuron III) located in the contralateral **ventral posterolateral nucleus of the thalamus.** Axons of the third-order neurons terminate in the **sensorimotor cortex.** The fasciculus gracilis is involved in mediating conscious propri-

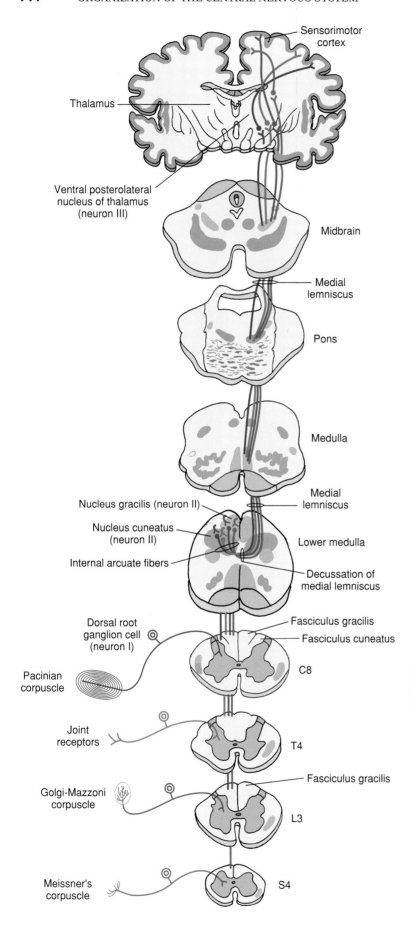

Figure 9–7 Diagram showing the course of fibers in the dorsal columns. Fasciculus gracilis exists at all levels of the spinal cord and contains long ascending fibers from the upper and lower limbs. The fasciculus cuneatus exists in thoracic segments above T6 and cervical segments and contains long ascending fibers from the upper limbs. Spinal ganglia and afferent fibers entering the spinal cord at different levels are color coded (red, sacral; purple, lumbar; green, thoracic; blue, cervical). The axons of second-order neurons in the nucleus gracilis travel as internal arcuate fibers and cross in the midline to form the medial lemniscus, which ascends through the medulla, pons, and midbrain and terminates in the contralateral ventral posterolateral nucleus of the thalamus. Axons of third-order neurons in the thalamus travel in the internal capsule and terminate in the sensorimotor cerebral cortex. For other details, see text.

oception that includes kinesthesia and discriminative touch.

Fasciculus Cuneatus

A schematic representation of the course of this tract is shown in Figure 9-7. It exists in thoracic segments above T6 and cervical segments and contains long ascending fibers from the upper limbs. Myelinated afferents from the dorsal root ganglion enter the dorsal funiculus, medial to the dorsal horn, and the ascending fibers occupy a lateral position in the dorsal funiculus. The peripheral processes of the first-order neuron innervate Pacinian and Meissner's corpuscles in the skin and proprioceptors in joints, and central processes of the first-order neuron ascend ipsilaterally to terminate on second-order neurons located in the ipsilateral **nucleus cuneatus** of the medulla. As noted earlier, axons of these second-order neurons travel as internal arcuate fibers, crossing the midline to form the medial lemniscus, and terminate on third-order neurons located in the contralateral ventral posterolateral nucleus of thalamus. The axons of these third-order neurons then terminate in the sensorimotor cortex. The fasciculus cuneatus is also involved in mediating conscious proprioception.

The fasciculi gracilis and cuneatus are also referred to as the **dorsal (posterior) columns**. *Damage to these tracts* results in symptoms that appear *ipsilateral* to the affected dorsal columns in the dermatomes *at and below* the level of the spinal cord lesion. The symptoms include loss of tactile sense (vibration, deep touch, and two-point discrimination) and kinesthetic sense (position and movement). The patient with a lesion affecting the cervical cord cannot identify an object placed in his/her hand ipsilateral to the lesion. If the lesion is located at the level of the lumbar cord, then the loss of these forms of sensation will be restricted to an ipsilateral lower limb. The patient perceives passive movements, such as touch or pressure, and his or her movements are poorly coordinated and clumsy because of the loss of conscious proprioception of his or her position in space.

Dorsal (Posterior) Spinocerebellar Tract

The course of this tract is shown in Figure 9-8A. The peripheral processes of the first-order neurons (located in the dorsal root ganglion) innervate mainly muscle spindles and, to a lesser extent, Golgi tendon organs (located at the junction of the muscle and tendon). The central processes of these sensory neurons project to the nucleus dorsalis of Clarke that extends from C8 to L2. Axons of neurons located in the dorsal nucleus of Clarke ascend ipsilaterally (i.e., the tract is uncrossed), reach the **inferior cerebellar pe-**duncle (**restiform body**) in the medulla, and terminate ipsilaterally in the cerebellar vermis of the anterior lobe. Although the nucleus dorsalis of Clarke receives afferents from all parts of the body except the head and neck, functionally it transmits information about muscle spindle and tendon afferents from the ipsilateral caudal aspect of the body and legs. In so doing, this tract provides the cerebellum with information about the status of individual muscles as well as groups of muscles, thus enabling this region to coordinate and integrate neural signals controlling movement of individual lower limb muscles and posture.

Cuneocerebellar Tract

The course of this tract is shown in Figure 9-8B. It should be recalled that the nucleus dorsalis of Clarke is not present in the spinal segments rostral to C8. Therefore, afferent fibers entering the spinal cord rostral to this level ascend ipsilaterally in the fasciculus cuneatus and project to neurons located in the **accessory cuneate nucleus of the lower medulla**. Neurons located in this nucleus then give rise to the cuneocerebellar tract, which is functionally related to the *upper limb*, conveying unconscious proprioception. (Recall that the dorsal spinocerebellar tract is functionally related to the lower limb). The fibers in this tract then terminate in the cerebellar cortex.

Ventral (Anterior) Spinocerebellar Tract

The course of this tract is shown in Figure 9-9. The first-order neurons in this system are located in the dorsal root ganglion; their peripheral processes innervate the Golgi tendon organs that are located at the junction of the muscle and tendon of the *ipsilateral lower limbs*. The central processes of the first-order neurons project to the second-order neurons located in the lateral part of the base and neck of the dorsal horn. The axons of the second-order neurons *cross in the spinal cord* and ascend through the medulla to the pons. The fibers then join the **superior cerebellar peduncle (brachium conjunctivum)** in the pons, cross again to the other side, and terminate in the vermal region of the anterior lobe of the cerebellum. Thus, the ventral (anterior) spinocerebellar tract crosses first in the spinal cord and then crosses again when it joins the superior cerebellar peduncle and crosses to terminate in the cerebellum. This tract conveys information about whole limb movements and postural adjustments to the cerebellum.

Anterolateral System of Ascending Tracts

Conventionally, it was believed that the *lateral* **spinothalamic tract** transmits pain and tempera-

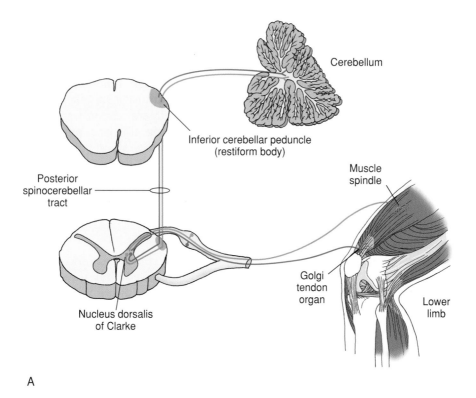

A

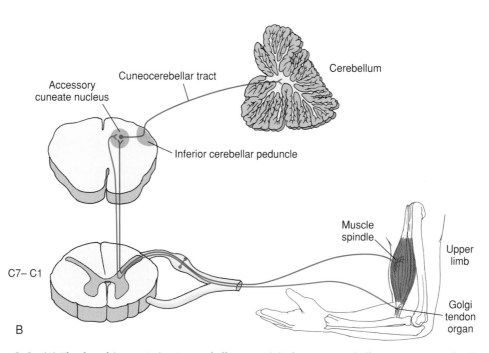

B

Figure 9–8 (A) The dorsal (posterior) spinocerebellar tract. (B) The cuneocerebellar tract. See text for details.

ture sensations, whereas the *anterior* spinothalamic tract transmits the sensation of nondiscriminative touch to the primary sensory cortex. This concept has recently been revised. Currently, it is believed that all components of the anterolateral ascending spinal system carry all somatosensory modali-

ties (i.e., pain, temperature, and simple tactile sensations) but that the routes carrying them are different. The *direct pathway*, consisting of the *neospinothalamic tract*, mediates pain, temperature, and simple tactile sensations; whereas several *indirect pathways* mediate the affective and arousal

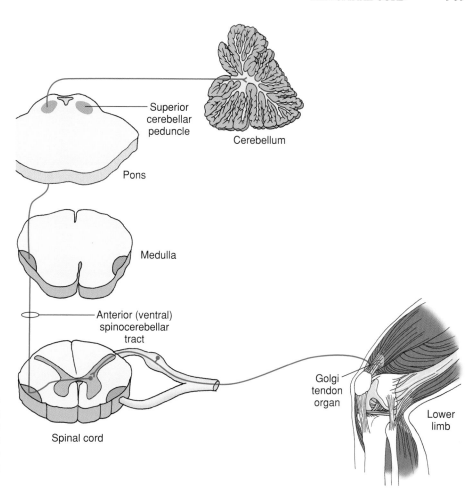

Figure 9–9 The ventral (anterior) spinocerebellar tract. Note that the tract first crosses in the spinal cord, and then it crosses a second time in the superior cerebellar peduncle and terminates in the cerebellum.

components of these sensations. These revised concepts and new terminology for various tracts transmitting these sensations are presented in the following sections.

Direct Pathway

Neospinothalamic Tract The course of this tract is shown in Figure 9-10. The neurons that give rise to this tract arise mainly from the **nucleus proprius (proper sensory nucleus)** that is located in lamina II of the dorsal horn. The axons of these neurons cross obliquely via the **ventral (anterior) white commissure** to enter the contralateral white matter where they ascend in the lateral funiculus. This tract has a somatotopic organization throughout its course, including in the spinal cord. Fibers arising from the lowest part of the body (the sacral and lumbar levels of spinal cord) ascend dorsolaterally, whereas those arising from the upper extremities and neck (the cervical cord) ascend ventromedially. The ascending axons synapse on third-order neurons located primarily in the ventral posterolateral nucleus of thalamus that, in

turn, project to the primary sensory cortex in the postcentral gyrus.

Deficits After Damage to the Direct Neospinothalamic Pathway Sectioning of the direct neospinothalamic pathway at the cervical level on one side results in complete loss of pain (anesthesia), temperature (thermoanesthesia), and simple tactile sensations on the *contralateral* side of the body (upper and lower limbs and trunk). The loss of pain sensation is experienced about 1 to 2 levels below the lesion because the first-order afferent fibers contained in the zone of Lissauer ascend or descend 1 to 2 levels before making synaptic contact with second-order neospinothalamic neurons. If a lesion is present at the lumbar level, then there would be a loss of pain, temperature, and simple tactile sensations in the contralateral lower limb and trunk.

Loss of pain, temperature, and tactile sensations can also occur at a specific segment after damage to the area around the central spinal canal. This occurs in a condition called **syringomyelia,** in which there is an expansion of the central canal of the

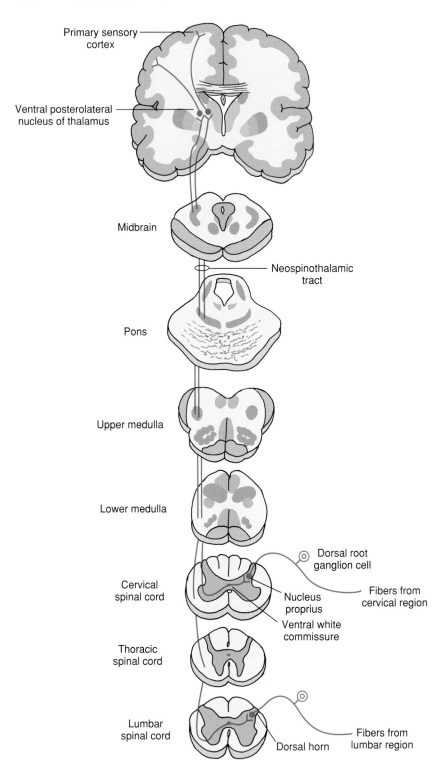

Figure 9–10 Neospinothalamic tract. The peripheral processes of these dorsal root ganglion cells end as receptors sensing pain, temperature, and simple tactile sensations. The central processes of these dorsal root ganglion cells synapse with the neurons of the nucleus proprius. The axons of these second-order neurons cross via the anterior white commissure, enter the contralateral white matter, ascend in the lateral funiculus, and synapse on third-order neurons located in the ventral posterolateral nucleus of the thalamus. The axons of third-order neurons project to the primary sensory cortex.

spinal cord. In addition, the glial cells proliferate around the central canal. In this case, the crossing fibers from the neospinothalamic tract on each side are affected but only in or about the segment in which the lesion is present. Accordingly, such a disorder results in *bilateral* loss of pain, temperature, and simple tactile sensations *at the affected segment.*

As noted earlier, the neospinothalamic tract is somatotopically organized in such a manner that sacral and lumbar fibers lie dorsolateral to the thoracic and cervical fibers. Accordingly, an expanding lesion or tumor located in the gray matter within the spinal cord is likely to affect the thoracic and cervical fibers first, while the sacral and lumbar fibers would be affected later, if at all. This clinical phenomenon in which damage to the spinothalamic tracts leaves intact the pain, temperature, and simple tactile sensations in sacral dermatomes is referred to as **"sacral sparing."**

Damage to the dorsal columns as well as to the neospinothalamic tracts on one side elicits the following symptoms. On the ipsilateral side below the level of the lesion, there is a loss of conscious proprioception, but the sensations of pain, temperature, and simple touch are preserved. On the contralateral side below the level of the lesion, just the reverse is true; that is, there is a loss of pain, temperature, and simple tactile sensations, while conscious proprioception is preserved.

Indirect Pathways

These pathways are involved in the autonomic, endocrine, motor, and arousal components of pain, temperature, and simple tactile sensations. Indirect pathways are also involved in activation of pain-inhibiting mechanisms (see Chapter 15). The axons of these neurons ascend in the spinal cord bilaterally, show poor somatotopic organization, and make multiple synapses in the reticular formation, hypothalamus, and limbic system. The pathways described in the following sections are included in this system.

Paleospinothalamic Tract In the spinal cord, the course of this tract is similar to that of the neospinothalamic tract. The neurons of this pathway are located in the deep dorsal horn and intermediate gray matter. The axons of these neurons ascend contralaterally as well as ipsilaterally (not shown in Fig. 9-11) in the ventrolateral quadrant of the spinal cord. The course of this tract rostral to the spinal cord is shown in Figure 9-11A. The axons ascending in the spinal cord make several synapses in the reticular formation of the brainstem (medulla, pons, and midbrain) and finally project to the midline and intralaminar thalamic nuclei (see Chapter 13). These nuclei, in turn, project in a diffuse manner to the cerebral cortex, especially to limbic regions such as the cingulate gyrus.

Spinoreticular Tract The course of this tract in the spinal cord is similar to the neo- and paleospinothalamic tracts. The neurons of this pathway are also located in the deep dorsal horn and intermediate gray matter. One group of these axons terminates in the medullary reticular formation and another ascends to the pontine reticular formation (Fig. 9-11B) (see also Chapters 10 and 11). The projections from the spinal cord to the brainstem are both crossed and uncrossed (not shown in Fig. 9-11B). A key feature about these pathways is that ascending spinoreticular fibers

are believed to transmit sensory information to the reticular formation, which, in turn, activates the cerebral cortex through secondary and tertiary projections via the midline and intralaminar thalamic nuclei (see Chapter 26). The thalamocortical projections, in turn, are highly diffuse and influence wide areas of the cerebral cortex.

Spinomesencephalic Tract The neurons of this pathway are also located in the deep dorsal horn and intermediate gray matter. The axons of these neurons ascend to the midbrain where they terminate in **periaqueductal gray**, a region surrounding the cerebral aqueduct (Fig. 9-11C). Similar to spinoreticular fibers, details regarding the distribution of these fibers have not been clearly established. It is believed that sensory information associated with this tract is transmitted to the amygdala via parabrachial nuclei.

LONG DESCENDING TRACTS

These tracts mediate motor functions including voluntary and involuntary movement, regulation of muscle tone, modulation of spinal segmental reflexes, and regulation of visceral functions. The corticospinal tract arises from the cerebral cortex, and the tectospinal and rubrospinal tracts arise from the midbrain. The remaining tracts arise from different nuclear groups within the lower brainstem. These tracts include the lateral and medial vestibulospinal and reticulospinal tracts that arise from the pons and medulla. In addition, other descending pathways that arise from medullary nuclei modulate autonomic functions. It should be noted that the corticospinal and rubrospinal pathways are mainly concerned with control over the flexor motor system and fine movements of the limbs, whereas the vestibulospinal and reticulospinal systems principally regulate antigravity muscles, posture, and balance.

Corticospinal Tract

This tract is involved in the control of fine movements. It is the largest and perhaps the most important descending tract in the human CNS. A schematic representation of the course of this tract is shown in Figure 9-12. It arises from the cerebral cortex, passes through the medullary pyramids, and terminates in the spinal cord. The corticospinal tract is somatotopically organized throughout its entire projection, and its structure and function are described in detail in Chapter 19. In brief, the cells of origin functionally associated with the arm are located in the lateral convexity of the cortex, whereas the cells of origin functionally

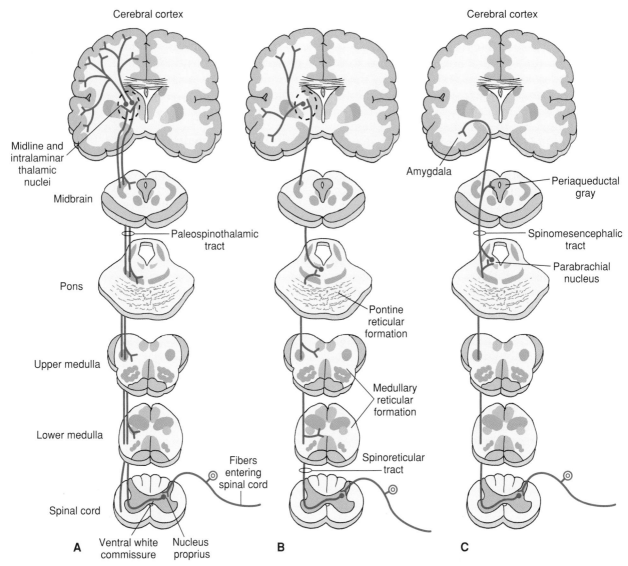

Figure 9–11 Indirect spinothalamic pathways. These pathways mediate the affective and arousal components of pain, temperature, and simple tactile sensations. (A) The ascending axons in the paleothalamic tract synapse in the brainstem reticular formation and neurons in midline and intralaminar thalamic nuclei, which then project diffusely to the cerebral cortex including the cingulate gyrus. (B) In the spinoreticular tract, one group of ascending axons projects to the medullary reticular formation, and the other group projects to the pontine reticular formation. The neurons in the reticular formation then project to neurons located in the midline and intralaminar thalamic nuclei. These thalamic neurons then project to the cerebral cortex. (C) In the spinomesencephalic tract, ascending axons terminate on the periaqueductal gray neurons that, in turn, project to neurons in the amygdala via the parabrachial nuclei.

associated with the leg are located along the medial wall of the hemisphere. This somatotopic organization is called a **cortical homunculus**. Many of these axons control the *fine movements of the distal parts of the extremities*. The axons arising from the cortex converge in the corona radiata and then descend through the internal capsule, crus cerebri in the midbrain, pons, and medulla. A majority (about 90%) of the fibers cross to the contralateral side at the juncture of the medulla and spinal cord, forming the **lateral corticospinal tract**, which descends to all levels of the spinal cord and terminates in the spinal gray matter of both the dorsal

and ventral horns. The remaining fibers do not cross at the juncture of the medulla and spinal cord; these uncrossed fibers constitute the **anterior corticospinal tract**. The fibers in this tract descend through the spinal cord and ultimately cross over at different segmental levels to synapse with anterior horn cells on the contralateral side.

There is a continuation of the anterior median fissure of the spinal cord on the ventral (anterior) surface of the medulla. The medullary pyramids are located on either side of this fissure. The pyramids carry descending corticospinal and corticobulbar fibers. As mentioned earlier, the cor-

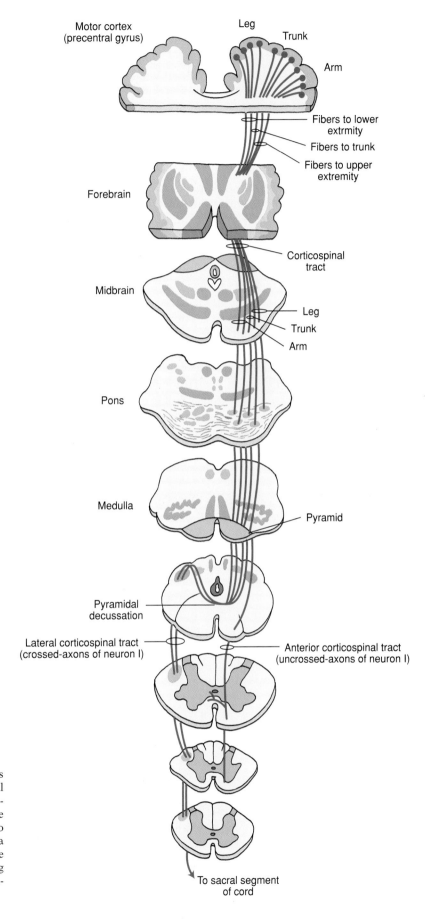

Figure 9–12 The corticospinal tract. This tract arises from the motor cortex (precentral gyrus), passes through the medullary pyramids, and terminates in the spinal cord. Note that a majority of corticospinal fibers cross to the contralateral side in the caudal medulla (pyramidal decussation) and descend as the lateral corticospinal tract and the remaining fibers descend ipsilaterally as anterior corticospinal tract.

ticospinal fibers in the pyramids cross to the contralateral side at the juncture of the medulla and spinal cord. This decussation, known as the **pyramidal decussation,** forms the anatomical basis for the voluntary motor control of one half of the body by the contralateral cerebral hemisphere. The corticobulbar fibers leave the pyramids as they descend in the medulla and project to the cranial nerve and other brainstem nuclei.

The corticospinal tract controls voluntary movements of both the contralateral upper and lower limbs. Depending on the extent of the lesion, these functions are lost when the corticospinal tract is *damaged*. After a stroke, first the affected *muscles lose their tone*. After several days or weeks, the *muscles become spastic*, (i.e., they resist passive movement in one direction) and *hyperreflexia occurs* (i.e., the force and amplitude of the myotatic reflexes is increased, particularly in the legs). The *superficial reflexes* (abdominal, cremasteric, and normal plantar) are *either lost or diminished*. A **Babinski sign**, which usually indicates damage of the corticospinal tract, is also present. This sign is characterized by an *abnormal plantar response* (extension of great toe while the other toes fan out) when the sole of the foot is stroked by a blunt instrument (see Chapter 19, Fig. 19-12) The *normal plantar response* consists of a brisk flexion of all toes when the sole of the foot is stroked by a blunt instrument.

At this time, it is useful to define the terms upper and lower motor neurons and their corresponding forms of paralyses. A **lower motor neuron** is a neuron whose cell body lies in the CNS but whose axon innervates muscles. An **upper motor neuron** is a neuron that descends from the cerebral cortex to the brainstem or spinal cord or a neuron that descends from the brainstem to spinal cord and synapses with a lower motor neuron. In general, a lower motor neuron is usually thought of as spinal cord motor neuron or cranial nerve motor neuron, while upper motor neurons are thought of as corticospinal or corticobulbar (neurons projecting from cerebral cortex to the brainstem nuclei) neurons.

The symptoms of damage to the corticospinal tract (i.e., loss of voluntary movement, spasticity, increased deep tendon reflexes, loss of superficial reflexes, and **Babinski sign**) comprise an *"upper motor neuron paralysis."* The symptoms of *"lower motor neuron paralysis"* include: loss of muscle tone, atrophy of muscles, and loss of all reflex and voluntary movement. When both the arm and leg on one side of the body are paralyzed, the disorder is referred to as *hemiplegia*. When one limb on a given side is paralyzed, it is called *monoplegia*. A paralysis involving both arms is called *diplegia*.

Paralysis of both legs is called *paraplegia*. *Quadriplegia* refers to paralysis of all limbs.

Rubrospinal Tract

The course of this tract is shown in Figure 9-13. The rubrospinal tract arises from neurons in the red nucleus (see Chapter 12). This nucleus is located in the rostral half of the midbrain tegmentum. The axons of these neurons cross the midline in the ventral midbrain (called the **ventral tegmental decussation**) and descend to the contralateral spinal cord. Fibers in the rubrospinal tract are somatotopically arranged. The cervical spinal segments receive fibers from the dorsal part of the red nucleus, which, in turn, receive inputs from the upper limb region of the sensorimotor cortex; the lumbosacral spinal segments receive fibers from the ventral half of the red nucleus, which in turn, receive inputs from the lower limb region of the sensorimotor cortex. The fibers of the rubrospinal tract end on interneurons that, in turn, project to the dorsal aspect of ventral (motor) horn cells. The neurons in the red nucleus are activated monosynaptically by projections from the cortex. The function of this tract is to facilitate flexor motor neurons.

Tectospinal Tract

The neurons from which this tract arises are located in the superior colliculus (Fig. 9-13). The axons of these neurons terminate in upper cervical segments. This tract is believed to aid in directing head movements in response to visual and auditory stimuli.

Lateral Vestibulospinal Tract

A schematic representation of the course of this tract is shown in Figure 9-14. This tract arises from neurons of the lateral vestibular nucleus, which is located at the border of the pons and medulla. The fibers in this tract are *uncrossed* and descend the entire length of the spinal cord. The descending fibers terminate predominantly on interneurons that activate motor neurons innervating extensor muscles of the trunk and ipsilateral limb. The lateral vestibular nucleus receives inhibitory inputs from the *cerebellum* and excitatory inputs from the vestibular apparatus. Impulses transmitted to the spinal cord by the lateral vestibular nucleus powerfully facilitate ipsilateral extensor motor neurons and their associated gamma motor neurons, thereby increasing extensor motor tone. Thus, the main functions of this tract are to control the muscles that maintain upright posture and balance.

Medial Vestibulospinal Tract

This tract arises from ipsilateral and contralateral medial vestibular nuclei, descends in the ventral funiculus of the cervical spinal cord, and terminates

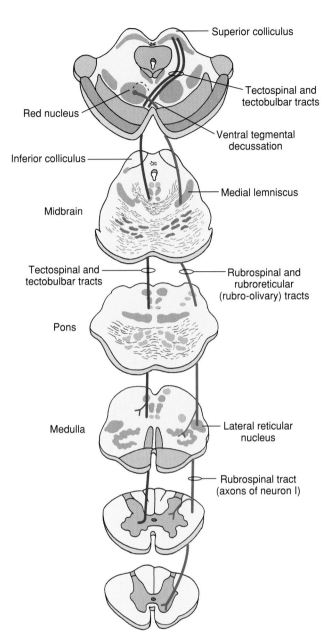

Figure 9–13 Rubrospinal and tectospinal tracts. The **rubro-spinal** tract (shown in red) arises from neurons in the red nucleus (located in the midbrain). The axons of these neurons cross the midline in the ventral midbrain (called the ventral tegmental decussation) and descend to the contralateral spinal cord. Fibers of the rubrospinal tract end on interneurons that, in turn, project to the dorsal aspect of ventral (motor) horn cells. The neurons giving rise to the **tectospinal** tract (shown in blue) are located in the superior colliculus. The axons of these neurons descend around the periaqueductal gray, cross the midline (called the dorsal tegmental decussation), join the medial longitudinal fasciculus in the medulla, and descend in the anterior funiculus of the spinal cord. They terminate in upper cervical segments.

in the ipsilateral ventral horn (Fig. 9-14). The main function of this tract is to adjust the position of the head in response to changes in posture, such as keeping the head stable while walking.

Reticulospinal Tracts

The reticular formation gives rise to three functionally different fiber systems. One component of this system mediates motor functions, a second component mediates autonomic functions, and a third component modulates pain impulses.

Fibers arising from the medulla emerge from a group of large cells located medially called the **nucleus gigantocellularis**. These cells project bilaterally to all levels of the spinal cord, and this pathway is referred to as the **medullary (lateral) reticulospinal tract** (Fig. 9-15). A key function of this pathway is that it powerfully suppresses extensor spinal reflex activity. In contrast, a separate reticulospinal pathway arises from two distinct nuclear groups in the medial aspect of the pontine reticular formation; these two nuclear groups are called the nucleus reticularis pontis caudalis and nucleus reticularis pontis oralis. These neurons project ipsilaterally to the entire extent of the spinal cord, and their principal - function is to facilitate extensor spinal reflexes. This fiber bundle is called the **pontine (medial) reticulospinal tract** (Fig. 9-15).

A second group of descending reticulospinal fibers mediates autonomic functions. These fibers arise largely from the ventrolateral medulla and project to the intermediolateral cell column of the thoracolumbar cord. This fiber system excites sympathetic preganglionic neurons in the intermediolateral cell column, and these neurons provide sympathetic innervation to visceral organs (see Chapter 22).

A third group of descending fibers is involved in pain modulation. The first limb of this pathway consists of enkephalinergic neurons located in the **midbrain periaqueductal gray** that project to serotonergic neurons located in the **nucleus raphe magnus** of the medulla. The second limb of this pathway consists of projections of these serotonergic neurons to the dorsal horn of the spinal cord, making synaptic contacts with a second group of enkephalinergic interneurons, which, in turn, synapse upon primary afferent pain fibers. Therefore, a key function of this descending fiber system is to modulate the activity of pain impulses that ascend in the spinothalamic system (see Chapter 15).

Medial Longitudinal Fasciculus

Medial longitudinal fasciculus (MLF) is a bundle of fibers that consists of mainly ascending fibers.

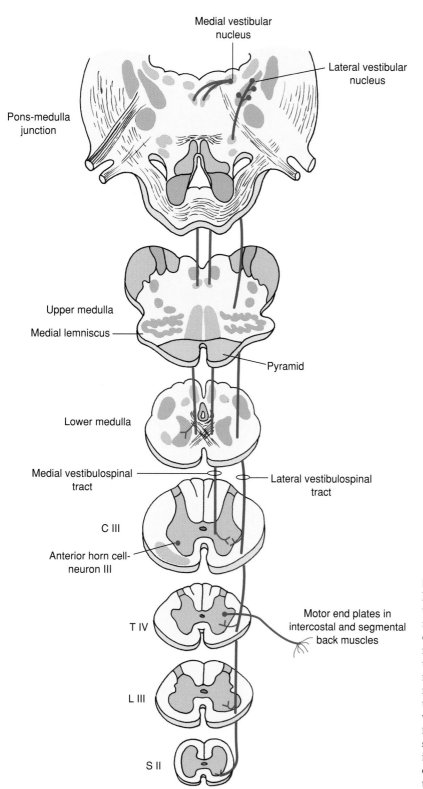

Medial vestibular
nucleus

Lateral vestibular
nucleus

Pons-medulla
junction

Upper medulla

Medial lemniscus

Pyramid

Lower medulla

Medial vestibulospinal
tract

Lateral vestibulospinal
tract

C III

Anterior horn cell-
neuron III

T IV

Motor end plates in
intercostal and segmental
back muscles

L III

S II

Figure 9–14 Lateral and medial vestibulospinal tracts. The **lateral** vestibulospinal tract (shown in blue) is uncrossed and arises from neurons of the lateral vestibular nucleus (located at the border of the pons and medulla) and descends the entire length of the spinal cord. The descending fibers terminate on interneurons that activate motor neurons innervating extensor muscles in the trunk and ipsilateral limb. The **medial** vestibulospinal tract (shown in red) arises from ipsilateral and contralateral (not shown) medial vestibular nuclei, descends in the ventral funiculus of the cervical spinal cord, and terminates in the ipsilateral ventral horn.

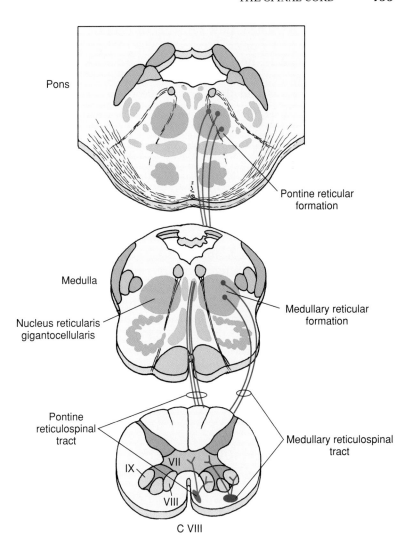

Figure 9–15 Reticulospinal tracts. The **medullary** (lateral) reticulospinal tract (shown in blue) arises from the nucleus gigantocellularis and projects bilaterally to all levels of the spinal cord (only ipsilateral projections are shown). The **pontine** (medial) reticulospinal tract (shown in red) arises from the pons and projects ipsilaterally to the entire extent of the spinal cord. (Used with permission from Parent A: Carpenter's Human Neuroanatomy, 9th ed. Baltimore: Williams & Wilkins, 1996, p. 395).

However, it also contains a descending component. Most of the ascending and descending fibers arise from different vestibular nuclei (lateral, superior, medial and vestibular nuclei) located in the pons. Descending fibers of the MLF are situated in the dorsal part of the ventral funiculus and project principally to upper cervical segments of the spinal cord. These fibers monosynaptically inhibit motor neurons located in the upper cervical cord. By virtue of its connections with motor neurons in the cervical cord, this pathway controls the position of the head in response to excitation by the labyrinth of the vestibular apparatus.

Fasciculi Proprii

The fasciculi proprii include fibers (ascending and descending, crossed or uncrossed) that arise and end in the spinal cord. They connect different segments of the spinal cord. These fibers mediate intrinsic reflex mechanisms of the spinal cord, such as the coordination of upper and lower limb move-ments. Signals entering the spinal cord at any segment are thus conveyed to upper or lower segments and finally transmitted to ventral horn cells either directly or through interneurons.

LESIONS OF THE SPINAL CORD

SPINAL CORD TRANSECTION

A complete transection of the spinal cord results in loss of muscle tone, motor function, reflex activity, visceral sensation, and somatic sensation *below* the level of the transection. Immediately after the spinal cord damage, there is a period during which all spinal reflexes below the level of transection are attenuated or absent. This condition is called *spinal shock* and results from a sudden interruption of descending excitatory influences on the spinal cord. Bladder and bowel function are also impaired because of the disruption of autonomic reflexes of these organs. In humans, spinal shock lasts for about 1 to 6 weeks. Then, slow recovery of neural function occurs: first, minimal reflex activity with a Babinski sign appears; next, flexor spasms are observed, which are then followed by alternate flexor and extensor spasms and the appearance of predominant extensor spasms.

BROWN-SÉQUARD SYNDROME

This syndrome involves a *hemisection of the spinal cord. The primary characteristic is the dissociation of function between conscious proprioception and pain and temperature sensations*. Loss of conscious proprioception and two-point discrimination occurs below the level of the lesion on the ipsilateral side, and loss of pain and temperature sensation occurs one or two segments below the level of the lesion on the contralateral side as well as bilaterally. There is also an upper motor neuron paralysis below the level of the lesion on the ipsilateral side and a lower motor neuron paralysis at the level of the lesion on the ipsilateral side. This kind of incomplete transection may occur by fracture dislocation of vertebrae, tumor, or missile wounds.

AMYOTROPHIC LATERAL SCLEROSIS (LOU GEHRIG'S DISEASE)

Amyotrophic lateral sclerosis (ALS) is a progressive degenerative disease in which the corticospinal tracts (upper motor neuron) and ventral horn cells (lower motor neuron) degenerate, often beginning with the lower limbs and later involving the upper limbs. Degeneration of the ventral horn cells in the cervical spinal cord results in weakness and ultimately in loss of control in muscles of the hand, trunk, and lower limbs. Involuntary twitching of muscle fascicles (fasciculations) occurs in these muscles. Bladder and bowel functions are also impaired due to the loss of descending autonomic pathways. The cause of this disease is not known.

SYRINGOMYELIA

This disease is due to a developmental or acquired abnormality and is characterized by an expansion of the central canal of the spinal cord (see Chapter 2). Such expansion produces proliferation of glial cells in this region, especially at the levels of the lower cervical and upper thoracic cord. In this condition, there is a segmental loss of pain and thermal sensation because there is an interruption of crossing fibers of the spinothalamic tracts in the same and adjoining segments at the level of the lesion. Because tactile sensation is

largely preserved, while pain and thermal sensation is lost, it is another example of *"dissociated sensory loss."*

TABES DORSALIS

This syndrome represents late consequences of syphilitic infection of the nervous system and is also referred to as **tertiary syphilis** or **neurosyphilis**. In this syndrome, the large diameter central processes of the dorsal root ganglion neurons (primary afferent sensors) degenerate, especially in the lower thoracic and lumbosacral segments. Therefore, the fibers in the fasciculus gracilis degenerate, and there is a loss of vibration sensation, two-point discrimination, and conscious proprioception. The loss of conscious proprioception results in ataxia (uncoordinated muscular movements) because the patient is now deprived of the "conscious" sensory feedback of signals that detect the position of the lower limbs at any given point in time.

MULTIPLE SCLEROSIS

As described in Chapter 6, multiple sclerosis is a demyelinating disease of the CNS. Impairment of mobility, paralysis, and disturbances in vision and bowel and bladder function occur in about one third of patients with multiple sclerosis. No single known cause of the disease has been identified. It has been proposed that, in genetically susceptible individuals, an infectious agent (as yet unidentified) may trigger an immune response against the nervous tissue. Although antibody titers to numerous viruses have been reported to be increased in serum and CSF in these patients, viral RNA or antigen have not been detected in the brain or spinal cord tissue. Since multiple sclerosis is currently believed to be an autoimmune disease, a number of immunosuppressants and immunomodulating agents have been used to treat the disease. However, no treatment has been reported to alter the progression of the disease significantly.

COMBINED SYSTEMS DISEASE

This disease results from a deficiency of enzymes necessary for vitamin B_{12} absorption. Deficiency of vitamin B_{12} results in pernicious anemia as well as degenerative changes in the dorsal and lateral funiculi of the spinal cord. These patients have defects in both sensory and motor function. The symptoms of sensory loss include tingling and the loss of senses of vibration and position. Disturbance in motor function includes upper motor neuron dysfunction. This may include a weakness of the lower limbs and an ataxic gait.

LESIONS OF THE DORSAL ROOT

Section of three consecutive dorsal roots causes abolition of all sensory function in a particular dermatome (anesthesia of the dermatome); section of one dorsal root does not cause much sensory loss because of overlap between dermatomes that are associated with intact dorsal roots and those that are damaged. With muscle tone also dependent on segmental reflexes, interruption of the afferent limb of these reflexes caused by the section of a dorsal root results in loss of muscle tone innervated by the affected segment.

LESIONS OF THE VENTRAL ROOT

These lesions abolish motor functions of the muscles innervated by the affected segment. For example, section of the ventral root of C8 will result in paralysis of the muscles of the hand. Similarly, section of thoracic ventral roots will result in disturbances in the function of visceral organs innervated by them.

SPINAL REFLEXES

A **spinal reflex** involves *discharge of an efferent motor neuron* in response to *afferent stimulation* of sufficient intensity. Spinal reflexes are modulated by supraspinal mechanisms. However, when continuity of supraspinal pathways is interrupted (e.g., by damage to the spinal cord), the spinal reflexes remain intact below the level of the lesion and are often exaggerated. Clinically, symptoms of motor dysfunctions can be readily identified by testing the integrity of spinal reflexes. The neural mechanisms involved in different important spinal reflexes are summarized in the following sections.

MYOTATIC REFLEX (ALSO CALLED STRETCH OR DEEP TENDON REFLEX)

Receptors

The myotatic reflex is the basis of the knee jerk response routinely tested in neurologic examinations. The primary receptor involved in the initiation of the myotatic reflex is the **muscle spindle.** Muscle spindles are present in all skeletal muscles with a few exceptions (e.g., the muscles in the middle ear). Each spindle consists of a connective tissue capsule in which there are 8 to 10 specialized

muscle fibers called **intrafusal fibers** (see Chapter 15). The intrafusal fibers and the connective tissue capsule in which they are located are *oriented parallel* to the surrounding larger skeletal muscle fibers called **extrafusal fibers,** which are involved in the movement of the limb. In larger intrafusal muscle fibers, the nuclei are located in the center of the fiber. These fibers are called the **nuclear bag fibers**. In other intrafusal fibers, the nuclei are arranged in a single file. These fibers are called **nuclear chain fibers**. Fast-conducting, large myelinated axons (called Group Ia afferents) encircle the middle of both types of intrafusal fibers, and these axon terminals constitute the *primary sensory ending* of the spindle. Group II afferent axons provide the secondary sensory innervation to the intrafusal fibers. The intrafusal fibers contract when gamma motor neurons are activated because these fibers are innervated by the spinal gamma motor neurons.

Circuitry and Mechanisms

A schematic representation of the circuitry involved in the myotatic reflex is shown in Figure 9-16. The mechanism of muscle contraction in response to its stretching is summarized as follows using the quadriceps muscle (extensor) as an example. When a quick tap is delivered to the patellar tendon, the quadriceps muscle is stretched briefly, the intrafusal fibers in the muscle spindle are deformed briefly, and action potentials are initiated by activating mechanically gated ion channels in the afferent axons coiled around the intrafusal fibers, resulting in a volley of discharge in group Ia afferent fibers emerging from the spindle (see Chapter 15 for structure of muscle spindle). These fast-conducting afferent fibers synapse directly on alpha motor neurons in the spinal cord, which innervate extrafusal muscle fibers of the same muscle in which the muscle spindle is located (*homonymous muscle*). The impulses conducted through the Ia afferent fibers result in excitation of alpha motor neurons, which, in turn, elicit contraction of the homonymous muscle (quadriceps in this case) causing extension of the leg. Thus, the myotatic reflex is *monosynaptic* and *involves a two-neuronal arc* consisting of the Ia fiber from the stimulated muscle spindle and the alpha motor neuron that innervates the *homonymous* muscle. Note that this reflex is of short duration because of the inhibitory action of the Renshaw cell on the alpha motor neuron (see page 141).

Reciprocal Inhibition in the Myotatic Reflex

Group Ia fibers from a muscle spindle also make an *excitatory synapse with an inhibitory interneuron* in

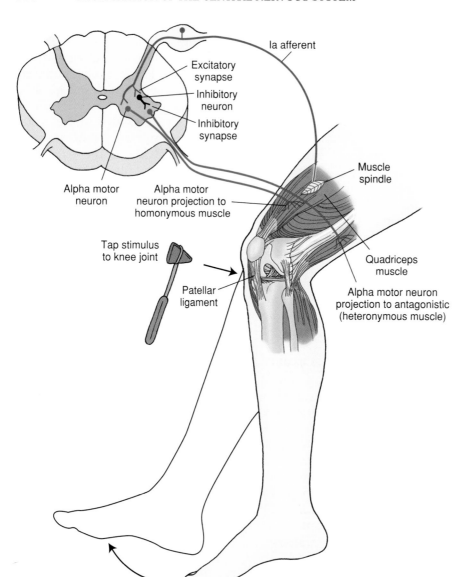

Figure 9–16 Myotatic reflex. When a quick tap is delivered to the patellar tendon, the quadriceps muscle is stretched, and the reflex response is a contraction of the homonymous muscle (quadriceps in this case). In the myotatic reflex, there is reciprocal inhibition of the antagonist muscle (heteronymous muscle). (Reproduced with permission from Bear MF, et al.: Neuroscience: Exploring the Brain, 2nd ed. Philadelphia: Williams & Wilkins, 2001, p. 454.)

the spinal cord, which, in turn, makes *an inhibitory synapse with an alpha motor neuron innervating the antagonist (heteronymous) muscle* (Fig. 9-16). An antagonist muscle is one that controls the same joint but has an antagonistic mechanical function. For example, an extensor has an antagonistic action to that of a flexor. Thus, activation of group Ia muscle spindle afferents causes contraction of homonymous muscles while producing *reciprocal inhibition* of antagonist muscles. The end result of this process is to resist the changes in muscle length through a negative feedback loop.

Inverse Myotatic Reflex

A schematic representation of the circuitry involved in the inverse myotatic reflex is shown in Figure 9-17. The Golgi tendon organ is another sensory receptor that plays an important role in regulating the motor unit activity. It is located in the tendon of the muscle (see also Chapter 15). The Golgi tendon organ is a high-threshold receptor that senses tension of the muscle; the muscle spindle, which has a much lower threshold, senses length of the muscle. Contraction of the muscle or stretching of the muscle (e.g., in whole-limb movement) constitutes the sufficient stimulus required for activation of the Golgi tendon organ. Activation of the Golgi tendon organ produces a volley in the associated afferent fiber (called a Ib fiber). This afferent fiber makes an excitatory synapse with an interneuron that inhibits the alpha motor neuron that innervates the homonymous muscle group. The net effect is that the period of contraction of the muscle in response to a stretch is reduced. This type of response (i.e., reduction of contraction of homonymous muscle) elicited by stimulation of Golgi tendon organs is referred to as the **"inverse myotatic reflex."**

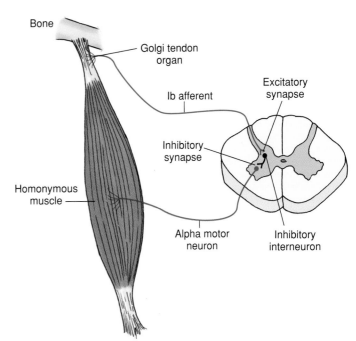

Figure 9–17 Inverse myotatic reflex. Contraction of the muscle or stretching of the muscle (e.g., in whole-limb movement) activates the Golgi tendon organs, and a volley of discharge is produced in the Ib fibers. Inhibitory interneurons are excited and alpha motor neurons innervating the homonymous muscle group are inhibited; the result is a reduction in the period of muscle contraction. (Used with permission from Bear MF, et al.: Neuroscience: Exploring the Brain, 2nd ed. Philadelphia: Williams & Wilkins, 2001, p. 457.)

Resetting of the Muscle Spindle Through the Gamma Loop

Gamma motor neurons, located in the ventral horn of the spinal cord and intermingled among alpha motor neurons, constitute lower motor neurons because they innervate skeletal muscle. As stated earlier, gamma motor neurons innervate the *polar ends of intrafusal muscle fibers.* Their activation produces contraction of the intrafusal muscle fibers at their polar ends, which results in stretching of the muscle spindle in the middle, causing the spindle to discharge. Thus, the primary function of the gamma motor neuron is not to cause the direct contraction of the extrafusal muscle but to *reset the spindle mechanism and increase the likelihood of discharge of Ia afferent fibers.* In this manner, the gamma motor neurons indirectly lead to contraction of the extrafusal muscle fibers because of their actions upon the spindle mechanism, which results in reflex activation of alpha motor neurons.

Modulation of Muscle Tone by Gamma Motor Neurons

It is also important to point out that the gamma motor neurons are under supraspinal control. Descending motor fibers principally from the reticular formation (i.e., the lateral and medial reticulospinal tracts) but also from other regions, such as the cerebral cortex and lateral vestibular nucleus, can modulate muscle tone by exciting or inhibiting gamma motor neurons. For example, excitation of gamma motor neurons by the medial reticulospinal tract causes an increase in muscle tone and a general facilitation of the stretch reflex. Conversely, activation of the lateral reticulospinal tract causes inhibition of gamma motor neurons and subsequent inhibition of the stretch reflex. In general, the descending motor fibers function in concert in order to constantly regulate muscle tone by providing converging inputs onto gamma motor neurons.

FLEXION (WITHDRAWAL) REFLEX

Receptors

The flexion reflex is primarily mediated by pain receptors (nociceptors) consisting of free nerve endings. Noxious stimuli activate these receptors.

Circuitry and Mechanism

A schematic representation of the circuitry involved in the flexion reflex is shown in Figure 9-18. When a noxious stimulus is applied to the skin or deeper structures, free nerve endings are stimulated, and the resulting impulses are conducted through myelinated afferent fibers of small diameter (group III fibers) and unmyelinated afferent fibers (group IV fibers) (see Chapter 15; Table 15-1). These fibers synapse with a number of alpha motor neurons located in the spinal cord. These connections are polysynaptic, and at least three to four interneurons are involved. Activation of these polysynaptic pathways in the spinal cord results in contraction of ipsilateral flexor muscles, producing flexion and relaxation of ipsilateral antagonist extensor muscles. The net effect of this reflex is to withdraw the limb in response to a noxious stimulus.

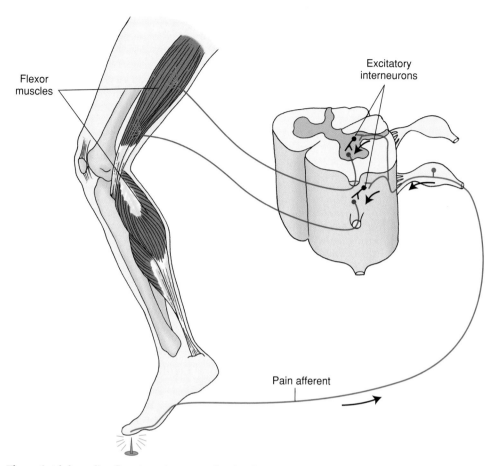

Figure 9–18 Flexor (withdrawal) reflex. A noxious stimulus (in this case stepping on a thumbtack) applied to the skin or deeper structures stimulates free nerve endings, and the resulting impulses are conducted through small-diameter myelinated afferent fibers and unmyelinated afferent fibers. These fibers make polysynaptic connections with at least three to four excitatory interneurons. The result is that ipsilateral flexor muscles contract, ipsilateral antagonist extensor muscles relax, and the person withdraws the limb in response to the noxious stimulus. (Used with permission from Bear MF, et al.: Neuroscience: Exploring the Brain, 2nd ed. Philadelphia: Williams & Wilkins, 2001, p. 459.)

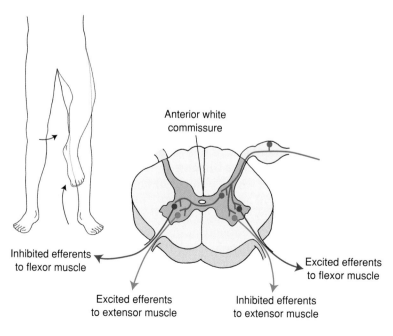

Figure 9–19 Crossed extension reflex. Noxious stimulation (in this case stepping on a thumbtack) activates pain fibers, and the impulses generated are conducted to the spinal cord via afferents that send collaterals through the anterior commissure to alpha motor neurons innervating contralateral flexor and extensor muscles. Activation of these polysynaptic pathways results in relaxation of contralateral flexor muscles, while contralateral extensor muscles are contracted. This neuronal circuitry of the flexion and crossed extension reflexes permits extension of the limb contralateral to the site of noxious stimulation and withdrawal (flexion) of the limb ipsilateral to it. (Used with permission from Bear MF, et al.: Neuroscience: Exploring the Brain, 2nd ed. Philadelphia: Williams & Wilkins, 2001. p. 460).

CROSSED EXTENSION REFLEX

Receptors

Nociceptors are also involved in the crossed extension reflex.

Circuitry and Mechanism

A schematic representation of the circuitry involved in the crossed extension reflex is shown in Figure 9-19. As noted with reference to the flexion reflex, a noxious stimulation activates pain fibers, and the impulses generated are conducted to the spinal cord via afferents, which send collaterals through the anterior commissure of the spinal cord that make multisynaptic connections with alpha motor neurons that innervate contralateral flexor and extensor muscles. Activation of these pathways produce effects opposite to those described for ipsilateral flexor and extensor muscles following activation of the flexor reflex. For example, contralateral flexor muscles are relaxed (note that in the flexion reflex, ipsilateral flexor muscles are contracted), while contralateral extensor muscles are contracted (note that in the flexion reflex, ipsilateral extensor muscles are relaxed). This neuronal circuitry of the flexion and crossed extension reflexes permits extension of the limb contralateral to the site of noxious stimulation and withdrawal (flexion) of the limb ipsilateral to it.

SYNCHRONIZATION OF REFLEXES OF UPPER AND LOWER LIMBS

Dorsal root fibers branch after they enter the spinal cord. Some of these collaterals synapse directly on alpha motor neurons. Other collaterals synapse on interneurons; the axons of these interneurons synapse on motor neurons in the same segment, rostral segments, or caudal segments. These ascending and descending axons, crossed or uncrossed, begin and end in the spinal cord and connect many segments. This intersegmental collection of fibers is referred to as *"fasciculus proprius"* or *"spinospinal columns." The reflexes of upper and lower limbs are thus synchronized by the "fasciculus proprius" system.* Therefore, as indicated, the function of this system is to synchronize movements and functions of the upper and lower limbs on each side of the body.

LOCOMOTION

Rhythmic stepping involves coordination of contraction of several muscle groups. The neural circuits that coordinate this rhythmic stepping are located in the spinal cord. However, supraspinal systems are also necessary for normal goal-directed locomotion. Humans with complete spinal cord transections cannot exhibit rhythmic stepping. Thus, corticospinal, rubrospinal, and reticulospinal descending systems are phasically active during locomotion.

HISTORY

Steve is a 37-year-old man who was well until he developed a weakness of his left leg for a few weeks. During this period of time, he gradually began to drag the leg when he walked, and he also noticed that his left leg was numb over the entire leg. He was no longer able to participate in his weekly golf game.

EXAMINATION

Steve went to a neurologist. The neurologist examined him and found no problems with his using language, his cranial nerves, or the sensory or motor function of his arms. His left leg was extremely weak, and the knee and ankle jerk reflexes were very brisk. While vibration and position sense were absent on the left leg, pain and temperature sense were absent on the right leg. Pain sensation, when tested with a pin prick was absent on the right aspect of the trunk below the level of the umbilicus, and, at this level, there was also some segmental bilateral loss of pain sensation. When the lateral plantar surface of Steve's left foot was scratched, the great toe dorsiflexed, and the other toes fanned. When this maneuver was repeated on the opposite side, the toes curled under.

EXPLANATION

The spinal cord syndrome described in Steve's case is called the Brown-Séquard syndrome, or hemisection of the spinal cord. In this case, the left side of the spinal cord was injured, causing damage to the corticospinal tract and resulting in upper motor neuron weakness on the ipsilateral side. The weakness is ipsilateral because the damage is caudal to the level at which the corticospinal tracts cross in the medullary pyramid. Position and vibratory sense are also lost on the ipsilateral side because the tracts in which these fibers travel (fasciculus gracilis) also cross above the lesion in the medulla. The loss of pain and temperature are on the contralateral side because first-order pain and temperature fibers enter the dorsal root and make synaptic contact with neospinothalamic tract neurons, whose axons cross over to the opposite side. Although the sensory level of diminished function was perceived to be at the umbilicus (approximately T10), the actual lesion was localized to T8 or T9. This is due to the fact that the first-order fibers carrying pain sensation in the zone of Lissauer ascend and descend 1 to 2 segments before making synaptic contact with second-order neospinothalamic neurons. The reason for the bilateral segmental loss of pain sensation at the approximate level of the lesion is that hemisection of the cord destroys the crossing neospinothalamic fibers from both sides in the anterior white commissure.

The Brown-Séquard syndrome results from a variety of causes, including tumors and infections of the spinal cord. In Steve's case, his neurologist ordered a magnetic resonance imaging (MRI) study of his thoracic spine, which revealed a meningioma, a type of usually benign tumor that was compressing the spinal cord at the level of T8. Several therapies were presented to Steve for relief of his symptoms, including the possible removal of the tumor.

CHAPTER TEST

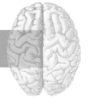

QUESTIONS

Choose the best answer for each question.

1. A 27-year-old male was involved in a street brawl, and during the fight, he was stabbed in the back. He lost consciousness and was rushed to the emergency room of a local hospital. After regaining consciousness, the patient received a neurologic examination. The patient indicated to the neurologist that he could not feel any pricks of a safety pin when tested along a band of an approximately 4-cm ring, which included both sides of his back. The patient was able to recognize tactile stimulation when tested on his arms and legs of both sides of the body as well as on the back or chest. Motor functions appeared to be intact. The neurologist concluded that the patient suffered damage of the:
   a. Substantia gelatinosa
   b. Dorsal root ganglion of the left side
   c. Lateral funiculus of both the lumbar and thoracic cords of the left side
   d. Region surrounding the central canal of thoracic cord
   e. Dorsal columns at the level of thoracic cord, bilaterally

2. A security guard at a bank was shot in the back during an attempted bank robbery. He was admitted to the emergency room, and when he regained consciousness, he was given a neurologic examination. The patient indicated that he could not detect tactile stimulation of the left leg, although sensation in the left arm after similar stimulation was intact. When a pin prick was applied to all four limbs, the patient said that he could not feel the sensation in his right leg, whereas this sensation was present in his left leg and both arms. In addition, further neurologic examination indicated that the patient could not move his left leg. The neurologist concluded that there was damage to the:
   a. Dorsal horn of the right side of the thoracic cord
   b. Region surrounding the central canal of the lumbar cord
   c. Region of the dorsal columns, bilaterally
   d. Ventral horn of the left side of the thoracic cord
   e. Left half of lower thoracic cord

3. A 69-year-old woman was admitted to a local hospital after she reported that she couldn't move her legs. Neurologic examination indicated that, not only did she lose motor functions in both of her legs, but that she could not detect any sensation in either leg when probed with a safety pin. However, she was aware of sensation in both legs when the neurologist applied tactile stimulation to them. It was concluded that the patient suffered damage to the:
   a. Anterior half of both sides of the spinal cord at the lumbar level
   b. Posterior half of both sides of the spinal cord at the lumbar level
   c. Region surrounding the central canal of the lumbar cord
   d. Left half of the cervical cord
   e. Dorsal roots of the lower thoracic cord, bilaterally

4. A 61-year-old man complained to his local physician that his legs had begun to feel weak over the past few months and that the weakness was progressive over time. Some time following the initial examination, the patient was unable to move his legs and then, several months later, his arms began to show weakness as well. Eventually, he couldn't move his limbs

at all, and in addition, he also began to lose bladder control. Sensation seemed to be relatively intact. A comprehensive neurologic examination led the neurologist to conclude that the patient was suffering from:

a. Syringomyelia
b. Amyotrophic lateral sclerosis
c. Multiple sclerosis
d. Combined systems disease
e. Tabes dorsalis

5. As a result of a vascular lesion of the brainstem, an afflicted individual displays a rather extensive marked rigidity in his limbs. The pathway most likely responsible for this rigidity is the:

a. Medial longitudinal fasciculus
b. Rubrospinal tract
c. Tectospinal tract
d. Lateral reticulospinal tract
e. Lateral vestibulospinal tract

ANSWERS AND EXPLANATIONS

1. Answer: d

Bilateral segmental loss of pain is the result of damage to the region surrounding the central canal of the spinal cord. This is due to damage to the crossing fibers of the lateral spinothalamic tracts (on each side) at a specific level of the cord. Damage to the substantia gelatinosa or dorsal root ganglia could only account for unilateral loss of pain. Damage to the lateral funiculus at both lumbar and thoracic levels on one side would likewise not account for bilateral loss of pain and, additionally, such a lesion would not be segmental. Dorsal column lesions would not affect the pathways mediating pain but, instead, would affect conscious proprioception.

2. Answer: e

This disorder is a classic example of a Brown-Séquard syndrome, in which there is damage to one side of the spinal cord. Such a lesion would cause loss of conscious proprioception below the lesion on the same side (i.e., left leg in this case) and loss of pain in the contralateral limb below the lesion (i.e., right leg). Sensation from other regions would remain intact. Because of the damage to the ventral horn and lateral funiculus, there would be loss of ability to move the limb at the level of the lesion or below it (i.e., left leg). A dorsal horn lesion of the right side could not account for the loss of sensation on the left side. Damage to the region of the cen-

tral canal would only produce loss of pain bilaterally and segmentally (see answer to Question 1). Damage to the dorsal columns would only affect conscious proprioception but not pain. A ventral horn lesion would not affect sensory functions such as pain and conscious proprioception.

3. Answer: a

This is an example of an individual who suffered an occlusion of the anterior spinal artery, affecting the ventral half of the spinal cord. Such an occlusion would affect the ventral horns on both sides, causing paralysis of both legs. Damage to the ventral half of the spinal cord would also affect the spinothalamic tracts, resulting in the loss of pain impulses below the lesion bilaterally. Damage to the posterior half of the spinal cord would affect conscious proprioception but would not affect transmission of pain and temperature. Damage to the region of the central canal would only produce segmental loss of pain and temperature but would have no motor effects. Damage to the left half of the cervical cord would produce a Brown-Séquard syndrome (see answer to Question 2). Dorsal root ganglion damage would only produce sensory loss but would not cause limb paralysis.

4. Answer: b

Progressive loss of motor functions, starting with the lower limbs and extending to the upper limbs, is characteristic of amyotrophic lateral sclerosis (ALS), which results in the destruction of ventral horn cells and, eventually, descending motor pathways. There is little or no sensory loss. In contrast, the other choices produce disorders that include components of sensory loss.

5. Answer: e

Impulses transmitted to the spinal cord by the lateral vestibular nucleus powerfully *facilitate* ipsilateral extensor motor neurons and increase extensor motor tone. The main function of this tract is to control the muscles that maintain upright posture and balance. The descending fibers of the medial longitudinal fasciculus do not descend beyond the cervical level and have no effect on functions of the lower limbs. The rubrospinal tract is known to facilitate the flexor musculature, and the lateral reticulospinal tract inhibits spinal reflex activity. Damage to the tectospinal tract does not produce rigidity. The tectospinal tract is believed to aid in directing head movements in response to visual and auditory stimuli.

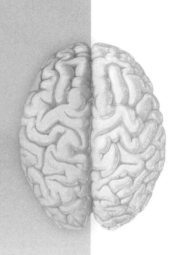

CHAPTER 10

BRAINSTEM I: THE MEDULLA

OBJECTIVES

In this chapter, the student is expected to:

1. Develop a general understanding of the gross anatomical arrangement of the medulla

2. Know the internal organization of the major fiber pathways that ascend and descend through the medulla

3. Be able to identify the major cell groups at different levels of the medulla

4. Develop the basis for an understanding of why syndromes associated with damage to the lateral aspect of the lower brainstem differ from those associated with the medial aspect of the lower brainstem

GROSS ANATOMICAL VIEW AND INTERNAL ORGANIZATION

GROSS ANATOMICAL VIEW

The purpose of this chapter is to begin to develop an understanding of the organization of the brainstem by considering the neuroanatomy of the medulla. Knowledge of the anatomy of the principal neural cell groups and pathways of the medulla is essential in acquiring an appreciation of their functions and insight into the clinical disorders resulting from damage to particular areas of this region of the brainstem. One may view the medulla as an extension of the spinal cord in that it contains a number of the fiber tracts present in the spinal cord and, like the spinal cord, also includes sensory, motor, and autonomic neurons. Thus, the principal pathways include long ascending and descending fiber systems that begin or terminate in the spinal cord and that pass through the medulla. Several other pathways mediating sensory, motor, and autonomic functions arise from the medulla and, to a considerable extent, are linked to cranial nerves. In addition, one of the three cerebellar peduncles, which connect the cerebellum to the brainstem, includes the **inferior cerebellar peduncle**. This massive fiber bundle represents an important conduit for transmission of information from the spinal cord and medulla to the cerebellum and is attached to the cerebellum from the dorsolateral aspect of the rostral medulla.

The **medulla,** or myelencephalon, is located between the pons and spinal cord. At its caudal end, it is continuous with the spinal cord. At its rostral end, the medulla is continuous with the pons (Fig. 10-1). Within the caudal half of the medulla, one can observe the positions of the **fasciculus gracilis** and **fasciculus cuneatus**, which ascend from the spinal cord (Fig. 10-1B). These tracts mediate conscious proprioception, vibratory sensation, and some tactile sensation from the body to the brain. As these structures pass in a rostral direction, they form two swellings (seen on the dorsal surface) referred to as the gracile and cuneate tubercles (Figs. 10-1 to 10-3). They reflect the underlying **nucleus gracilis** and **nucleus cuneatus** (the latter lies immediately lateral to the nucleus gracilis); these nuclei receive inputs from the fasciculus gracilis and cuneatus, respectively, and thus constitute a relay system for the transmission of conscious proprioception, vibratory sensation, and tactile impulses to higher regions of the brain. The gracile and cuneate tubercles extend rostrally to a level where the fourth ventricle begins. The rostral third of the medulla, which contains a portion of the fourth ventricle, is known as the "open" part of the medulla (described later in *Levels of the Medulla* section). The part of the medulla where the central canal is present is referred to as the "closed" part of the medulla (described later). At the rostral end of the medulla, the dorsolateral surface is expanded to form the inferior cerebellar peduncle, which conveys proprioceptive and vestibular fibers to the cerebellum (see Chapter 1, Fig. 1-8 for orientation).

Along the medial aspect of the ventral surface of the medulla, there is a swelling referred to as the pyramid, which is also present throughout the rostro-caudal extent of the medulla. The **pyramid** is composed of numerous nerve fibers that arise from the precentral, postcentral, and premotor regions of the cerebral cortex. These nerve fibers pass to the spinal cord as the **corticospinal tracts** or terminate within the medulla as **corticobulbar fibers**. As described in Chapter 19, the corticospinal tract mediates voluntary control over movements of the body. Similarly, the corticobulbar tract mediates voluntary control over movements of the head region.

At the *caudal* end of the medulla immediately above the rostral end of the spinal cord, the pyramid is considerably smaller because, at this level, 90% of the fibers are crossed in a dorsolateral direction to the opposite side in a series of bundles called the **decussation** of the pyramids. The decussated axons then descend into the spinal cord as the lateral corticospinal tract (Fig. 10-3). The remaining (uncrossed) component of the corticospinal tract passes ipsilaterally into the ventral white matter of the spinal cord as the ventral corticospinal tract (see Chapter 9).

At the level of the *rostral* half of the medulla, another swelling located just lateral to the pyramids is referred to as the inferior olivary nucleus.

INTERNAL ORGANIZATION

Major Fiber Tracts and Associated Nuclei (Figs. 10-2 and 10-3)

Pyramidal (Corticospinal) Tract

The pyramidal tract is situated in a ventromedial position throughout most of the medulla but changes position at its caudal end. Here, approximately 90% of the fibers, en route to the spinal cord, pass in a dorsolateral direction while crossing the midline to reach the dorsolateral aspect of the caudal medulla. The fibers, which cross to the contralateral side of the brainstem, form the decussation of the pyramid and descend into the dorsolateral aspect of the lateral funiculus of the spinal cord as the lateral corticospinal tract. As described in Chapter 9, the corticospinal tract mediates voluntary control over motor responses, and

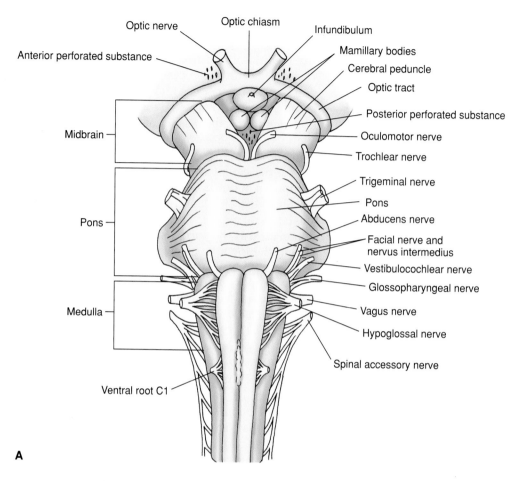

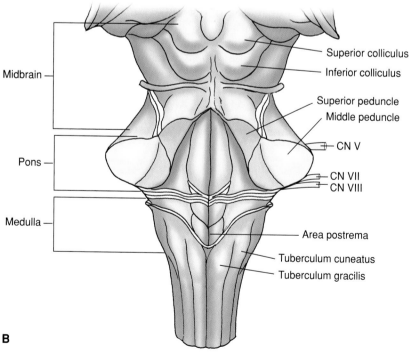

Figure 10–1 Different views of brainstem. (A) Anterior view of the medulla. (B) Posterior view of the medulla. Note the position at which the fourth ventricle begins (the "open" part of the medulla) at the level of the area postrema. In this illustration, the cerebellum has been removed in order to see the structures situated on the dorsal surface of the medulla. The midbrain and pons are included for purposes of orientation. CN VII-X and XII are presented to illustrate their medial or lateral positions along the neuraxis of the medulla.

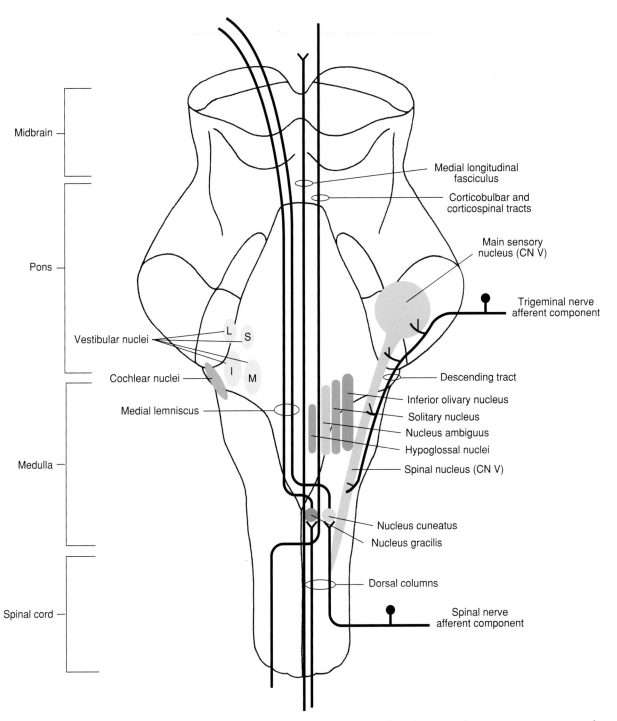

Figure 10–2 Ascending and descending pathways of fiber tracts and associated nuclei. Note the most prominent *ascending* pathways (the dorsal column-medial lemniscus) and *descending* pathways (the MLF, corticospinal and corticobulbar tracts, and descending tract of CN V) that traverse the medulla. In the lower half of the medulla, the nucleus gracilis and nucleus cuneatus are shown. At more rostral levels, the relative positions of the nucleus ambiguus (CN IX and X), spinal nucleus of CN V and its rostral extension in the pons, the main sensory nucleus of CN V, hypoglossal nucleus (CN XII), inferior olivary nucleus, inferior (I), medial (M), lateral (L), and superior (S) vestibular nuclei, and cochlear nuclei (CN VIII) are depicted.

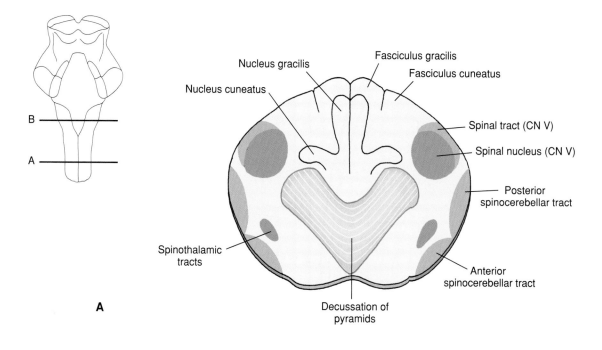

A

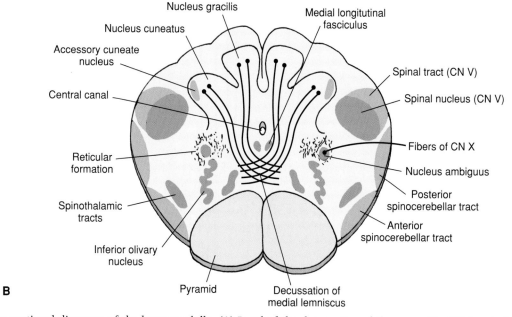

B

Figure 10–3 Cross-sectional diagrams of the lower medulla. (A) Level of the decussation of the pyramids. (B) Level of the decussation of the medial lemniscus.

damage to this pathway results in an upper motor neuron paralysis.

Medial Lemniscus

The medial lemniscus originates from the dorsal column nuclei (described on pages 170–171). These fibers collectively pass ventrally for a short distance in an arc-like trajectory and are referred to as **internal arcuate fibers**. These second-order so-

matosensory fibers then cross to the opposite side of the medulla as the decussation of the medial lemniscus. The medial lemniscal fibers then pass rostrally in a medial position throughout the remainder of their trajectory through the medulla and continue into the pons. The function of the medial lemniscus is to transmit information associated mainly with conscious proprioception and vibratory stimuli to the thalamus (Fig. 10-2).

The Medial Longitudinal Fasciculus (MLF)

The medial longitudinal fasciculus tract is located in a dorsomedial position within the medulla and consists of both ascending and descending axons (Fig. 10-2 and Fig. 10-3B). *Ascending* axons arising from the **lateral, medial, and superior vestibular nuclei** project to the pons and midbrain; they provide information about the position of the head in space to cranial nerve nuclei that mediate control over the position and movements of the eyes. The *descending* fibers, which arise from the medial vestibular nucleus and pass caudally to cervical levels of the cord, are often called the **medial vestibulospinal tract**. This tract serves to adjust changes in the position of the head in response to changes in vestibular inputs.

Descending Tract of Nerve V

The descending fibers of the **trigeminal nerve** extend caudally as far as the second cervical segment and occupy a far lateral position within the medulla immediately lateral to the **spinal nucleus of the trigeminal nerve** (cranial nerve [CN] V) (Figs. 10-2 and 10-3). The spinal nucleus of CN V is present throughout the entire length of the medulla, extending from the level of the lower pons caudally to the spinal cord–medulla border, where it becomes continuous with the **substantia gelatinosa**. In the middle of the pons, the spinal nucleus is replaced by the main sensory nucleus of CN V.

The descending fibers of CN V constitute first-order axons that mediate somatosensory inputs from the head region to the brain; they synapse at different levels along the rostro-caudal axis of the spinal nucleus. Therefore, the spinal nucleus constitutes the second-order neuron, which transmits **somatosensory** information from the head region to the thalamus (for subsequent transmission to the cerebral cortex). Further details concerning functions of the trigeminal nuclei are presented in Chapter 14.

Other Fiber Tracts

Several other tracts, shown in part in Figure 10-3, reflect pathways that mediate sensory and motor functions. Sensory tracts include the **spinothalamic** and **spinocerebellar** fibers. The spinothalamic and spinocerebellar fibers are situated laterally within the medulla and thus retain the same general positions that they occupied within the **lateral funiculus** of the spinal cord. The lateral spinothalamic tract mediates pain and temperature sensation from the contralateral side of the body to the thalamus, and the spinocerebellar tracts mediate unconscious proprioception (i.e., from muscle spindles and Golgi tendon organs) to the cerebellum. Tracts mediating

motor functions in addition to the corticospinal tract include the **tectospinal tract**, which follows the MLF to cervical levels and mediates postural movements from the superior colliculus; the **rubrospinal tract**, which passes in a ventrolateral position in the medulla from the red nucleus to all levels of the spinal cord and facilitates spinal cord flexor motor neuron activity; and the lateral and medial **reticulospinal tracts**, which arise from the medulla and pons, respectively, pass to different levels of the spinal cord, and modulate muscle tone. The functions of these tracts are considered in greater detail in Chapters 9, 19, 23, and 26.

Internal Nuclei of the Brainstem

Reticular Formation

The internal core of the entire brainstem contains mainly a complex set of neuronal groups (coupled with related fiber bundles) that are collectively referred to as the **reticular formation**. The nature of the structural and functional organization of this complex region of the brainstem is considered in detail in Chapter 23. In brief, it appears to be involved in such processes as modulation of sensory transmission to the cortex, regulation of motor activity, autonomic regulation, sleep and wakefulness cycles, and modulation of emotional behavior.

Major Nuclei of the Medulla

In the lower levels of the medulla, the principal nuclei of the **caudal** (or lower) **medulla** include the nucleus gracilis and nucleus cuneatus, which receive first-order somatosensory fibers from the fasciculus gracilis and fasciculus cuneatus, respectively, and the spinal nucleus of CN V, which receives first-order pain and temperature signals from the region of the head (Fig. 10-2).

In the upper levels of the medulla, numerous important nuclei are present. The **spinal nucleus** is present at this level, as it is at lower levels of the medulla. Other sensory neurons include the cochlear nuclei, which receive first-order auditory fibers (CN VIII), and vestibular nuclei, which also receive first-order vestibular inputs (CN VIII). In addition, a number of different cranial nerve nuclei appear. These include somatomotor nuclei (hypoglossal nucleus [CN XII] and nucleus ambiguus of CN X and CN IX) and sensory and motor autonomic nuclei (dorsal motor nucleus of CN X and the solitary nucleus [CN IX and X]).

Levels of the Medulla

In describing the anatomy of the medulla, we can distinguish at least two levels. The caudal half, which includes the **"closed"** medulla, contains two decussations: (1) the pyramidal decussation and (2) a second level that contains the decussation of the medial lemniscus. The upper half of the medulla, which includes the **"open" medulla**, contains the **inferior olivary nucleus**. The following sections consider the neuroanatomical organization of the medulla on the basis of the structures contained at each of these levels.

Level of the Pyramidal Decussation

At the level of the pyramidal decussation, the general organization of the medulla is very similar to that of the cervical spinal cord. For example, the dorsal aspect of this level of the medulla contains the fasciculus gracilis and fasciculus cuneatus (Figs. 10-3 and 10-4). The spinocerebellar and spinothalamic tracts also lie in the same general lateral position they occupy within the spinal cord. Some anterior horn cells can generally be seen at this level as well.

There are major new features found at this level of medulla that are not present in the spinal cord. The most obvious change is the presence of the **pyramidal decussation**. As indicated earlier, about 90% of the fibers of each pyramid cross over to the contralateral side of the brain in their descent into the spinal cord as the lateral corticospinal tract.

Approximately 8% of the fibers continue to descend uncrossed into the spinal cord as the anterior corticospinal tract and are situated in a ventromedial position; ultimately, these fibers cross over to the opposite side of the spinal cord. The remaining 2% of the corticospinal tract supplies the ipsilateral spinal cord grey matter. A second change is the presence of the **spinal nucleus of the trigeminal nerve**. It replaces the substantia gelatinosa in that it is situated in the dorsolateral aspect of the medulla, which is the approximate position occupied by the substantia gelatinosa in the dorsal horn of the spinal cord. The anatomical similarities between the substantia gelatinosa and the spinal nucleus of CN V are matched by their functional similarities as well. Both structures mediate pain and temperature modalities of sensation. The difference between the two relates to the fact that the substantia gelatinosa mediates these sensations from the body, whereas the spinal nucleus mediates sensations associated with the region of the anterior two thirds of the head, oral and nasal cavities, and the cutaneous surfaces of the ear and external auditory meatus.

Level of the Decussation of the Medial Lemniscus

At a level slightly rostral to that of the pyramidal decussation, a second major decussation called the

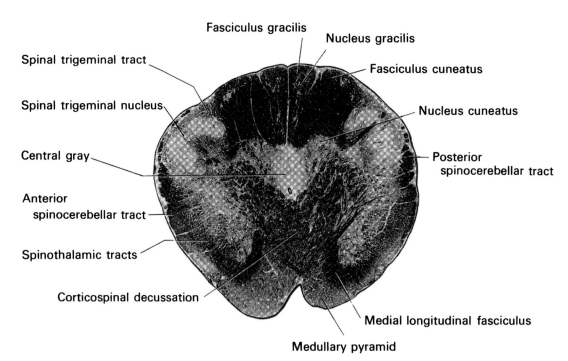

Figure 10–4 Photograph of a cross section of the human medulla at the level of the decussation of the pyramids (Weigert myelin stain). Note that the fasciculus gracilis and fasciculus cuneatus are still clearly present at this level, and note the positions occupied by the ascending sensory axons. (Reproduced with permission from Parent A: Carpenter's Human Neuroanatomy, 9th ed. Baltimore: Williams & Wilkins, 1996, P. 424.)

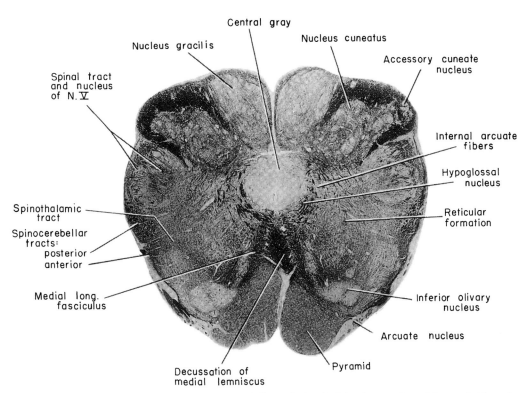

Central gray

Nucleus gracilis

Nucleus cuneatus

Accessory cuneate nucleus

Spinal tract and nucleus of N. Ⅴ

Internal arcuate fibers

Hypoglossal nucleus

Spinothalamic tract

Reticular formation

Spinocerebellar tracts: posterior anterior

Medial long. fasciculus

Inferior olivary nucleus

Arcuate nucleus

Decussation of medial lemniscus

Pyramid

Figure 10–5 Photograph of a cross section of the human medulla at the level of the decussation of the medial lemniscus (Weigert stain). Note that the nucleus gracilis and nucleus cuneatus are quite prominent at this level and that the accessory cuneate nucleus can be seen situated just lateral to the cuneate nucleus. In this section, one can see that internal arcuate fibers, which arise from the dorsal column nuclei, pass in a ventromedial direction to the opposite side to form the medial lemniscus. (Reproduced with permission from Parent A: Carpenter's Human Neuroanatomy, 9th ed. Baltimore: Williams & Wilkins, 1996, p. 426.)

decussation of the medial lemniscus is present (Figs. 10-3 and 10-5). While the pyramidal decussation involves fibers from sensorimotor cortex that are specifically involved in motor functions, the decussation of the medial lemniscus is part of an overall sensory pathway that contains fibers that arise from the nucleus gracilis and nucleus cuneatus (located immediately lateral to the nucleus gracilis) and mediates somesthetic impulses from the body to the thalamus and, ultimately, to the postcentral gyrus. Axons of the medial lemniscus initially pass ventrally in an arc (where fibers arising from the nucleus gracilis emerge prior to those of the nucleus cuneatus and collectively are called internal arcuate fibers) and then cross over to the contralateral side via the decussation of the medial lemniscus. These fibers then turn rostrally as they ascend toward the forebrain where they terminate in the ventral posterolateral (VPL) nucleus of the thalamus.

At this level of the medulla, another nucleus, called the **accessory cuneate nucleus**, is attached to the lateral edge of the nucleus cuneatus (Fig. 10-5). This structure receives inputs from muscle spindles and **Golgi tendon organs** associated with the skeletal muscles of the upper limbs that are conveyed by first-order fibers passing in the fasciculus cuneatus. Axons of the accessory cuneate nucleus, called **external arcuate fibers**, form the **cuneocerebellar tract** as they pass ipsilaterally into the **inferior cerebellar peduncle**. Thus, they mediate unconscious proprioception from the upper limbs to the cerebellum and represent the upper limb equivalent of the dorsal spinocerebellar tract.

Other structures that are prominent at the level of the decussation of the medial lemniscus are also present more caudally within the medulla. These include the pyramidal, spinocerebellar, and spinothalamic tracts, as well as the spinal nucleus and tract of the trigeminal nerve.

Rostral Half of the Medulla

At this level of the medulla, a number of new structures make their appearance, including important cranial nerve nuclei. It is useful to recall the section of Chapter 2 (pages 22–26) that described the development of the brainstem. On developmental

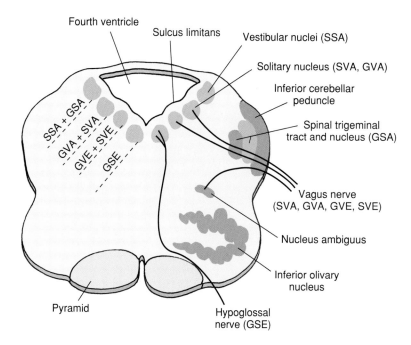

Fourth ventricle

Sulcus limitans

Vestibular nuclei (SSA)

Solitary nucleus (SVA, GVA)

Inferior cerebellar peduncle

Spinal trigeminal tract and nucleus (GSA)

SSA + GSA
GVA + SVA
GVE + SVE
GSE

Vagus nerve (SVA, GVA, GVE, SVE)

Nucleus ambiguus

Inferior olivary nucleus

Pyramid

Hypoglossal nerve (GSE)

Figure 10–6 The arrangement of sensory and motor nuclei of cranial nerves. The key point is that the region derived from the basal plate is located medially and contains motor nuclei, while the region derived from the alar plate is located more laterally and contains sensory nuclei. The region in between these two regions, which is formed from the sulcus limitans, contains neurons that relate to autonomic functions. Abbreviations: SSA, special sensory afferent neurons; GSA, general somatic afferent neurons; SVA, special visceral afferent neurons; GVA, general visceral afferent neurons; GSE, general somatic efferent fibers.

principles, the arrangement of sensory and motor nuclei, especially those of cranial nerves, is reviewed in the following paragraphs and is depicted in Fig. 10-6.

In brief, the locations of neuronal cell groups associated with cranial nerve function can be determined by knowing the following medial-to-lateral arrangement. Cell groups located in the most medial position, derived from the basal plate, are classified as general somatic efferent (GSE) neurons; they innervate skeletal muscle of somite origin. The clearest example of such a cell group that is

situated at this level of the brainstem is the **hypoglossal nucleus**, which can be easily seen in Figures 10-7 and 10-8 and lies just above the MLF in a dorsomedial position within the medulla. Axons of the hypoglossal nucleus innervate the intrinsic and extrinsic muscles of the tongue and thus control its movements.

The next column includes those cell groups that are derived from mesenchyme of the **branchial arches** and are classified as **special visceral efferent** (SVE) neurons, which also innervate skeletal muscle (Fig. 10-6). An example of this type of cell group is

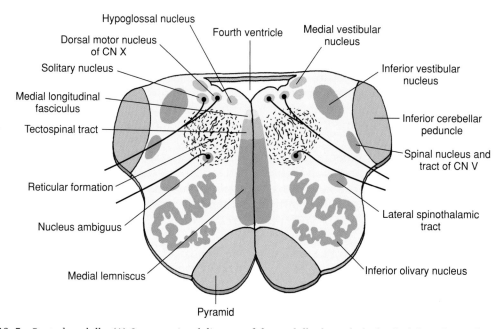

Hypoglossal nucleus

Dorsal motor nucleus of CN X

Solitary nucleus

Medial longitudinal fasciculus

Tectospinal tract

Reticular formation

Nucleus ambiguus

Medial lemniscus

Fourth ventricle

Medial vestibular nucleus

Inferior vestibular nucleus

Inferior cerebellar peduncle

Spinal nucleus and tract of CN V

Lateral spinothalamic tract

Inferior olivary nucleus

Pyramid

Figure 10–7 Central medulla. (A) Cross-sectional diagram of the medulla through the level of the inferior olivary nucleus.

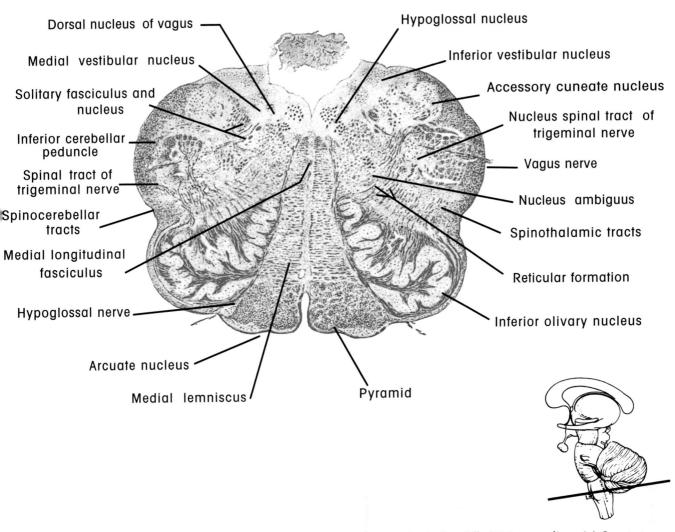

Dorsal nucleus of vagus

Medial vestibular nucleus

Solitary fasciculus and nucleus

Inferior cerebellar peduncle

Spinal tract of trigeminal nerve

Spinocerebellar tracts

Medial longitudinal fasciculus

Hypoglossal nerve

Arcuate nucleus

Medial lemniscus

Hypoglossal nucleus

Inferior vestibular nucleus

Accessory cuneate nucleus

Nucleus spinal tract of trigeminal nerve

Vagus nerve

Nucleus ambiguus

Spinothalamic tracts

Reticular formation

Inferior olivary nucleus

Pyramid

Figure 10–7 (*continued*) (B) Photograph of a cross section through the same level of medulla (Weigert myelin stain). Insert at bottom right indicates the level at which the section was taken. (Panel B: Reproduced with permission from Parent A: Carpenter's Human Neuroanatomy, 9th ed. Baltimore: Williams & Wilkins, 1996, p. 942.)

the **nucleus ambiguus**, which gives rise to axons of CN IX and X. Axons of the nucleus ambiguus travel, in part, in the **vagus nerve** and innervate the muscles of the larynx and pharynx, thus controlling phonation, gagging, and swallowing. Drawing a line from the dorsolateral tip of the **inferior olivary nucleus** to the hypoglossal nucleus can identify the position of the nucleus ambiguus. The nucleus ambiguus is located at the mid-point of this line.

Continuing in a lateral direction, the third column includes those cell groups that comprise the general visceral efferent (GVE) neuronal groups (Fig 10-6). These represent preganglionic parasympathetic fibers whose axons innervate autonomic ganglia. Postganglionic parasympathetic neurons are present either in these ganglia or within the wall of the target organs, and their axons innervate smooth muscles and glands.

Two groups of such neurons can be detected within the medulla. The first group of neurons includes the dorsal motor nucleus of the vagus nerve (CN X), whose axons contribute to the vagus nerve. The dorsal motor nucleus lies dorsolateral to the hypoglossal nucleus just medial to the **sulcus limitans** at the rostral end of the closed medulla (see Chapter 2). The second group of neurons constitutes the **inferior salivatory nucleus**, whose axons form part of CN IX and which contribute to the process of salivation. Axons of these neurons form **preganglionic parasympathetic fibers** that innervate the **otic ganglion**, from which **postganglionic parasympathetic fibers** innervating the **parotid gland** arise.

Immediately lateral to the sulcus limitans lies the general visceral afferent (GVA) column (Fig. 10-6). Cells in this region, which are derived from the alar plate, receive afferent signals from visceral organs, such as blood vessels, that are mediated via branches of the glossopharyngeal (CN IX) and vagus (CN X) nerves. The principal nucleus that receives and processes such information is the caudal por-

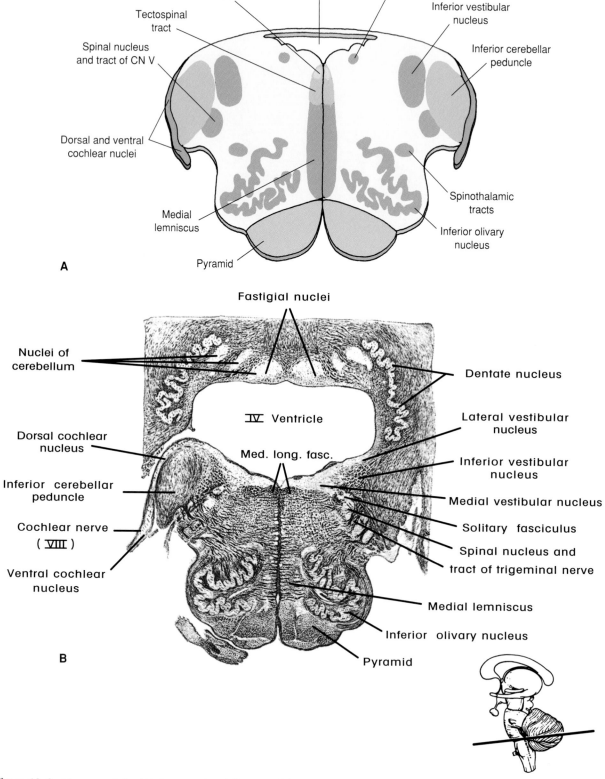

Figure 10–8 Upper medulla. (A) Cross-sectional diagram of the upper medulla just caudal to the pons. (B) Photograph of a cross section through the same level of medulla (Weigert myelin stain). Insert at bottom right indicates the level at which the section was taken. (Panel B: Reproduced with permission from Parent A: Carpenter's Human Neuroanatomy, 9th ed. Baltimore: Williams & Wilkins, 1996, p. 944.)

tion of the nucleus solitarius, which lies in a position slightly ventrolateral to the dorsal motor nucleus of the vagus nerve. Superimposed on this column is the **special visceral afferent** (SVA) column (Fig. 10-6), which includes the rostral half of the solitary nucleus (gustatory portion). The reason for the proximity of these two groups of separately classified cell types of neurons is that the primary neuron for both functions at this level of the brain is the solitary nucleus. Thus, different groups of cells within the solitary nucleus mediate two distinctly separate processes, one associated with GVA functions (i.e., cardiovascular and respiratory reflexes) and the other associated with SVA functions (i.e., taste).

The final categories of cell groups include **general sensory afferent** (GSA) neurons and **special sensory afferent** (SSA) neurons. They both lie in a most lateral position within the medulla. The primary GSA neuronal cell group found at this level of the brainstem is the spinal nucleus of the trigeminal nerve. Within the medulla, separate groups of SSA neurons can be detected. One such group is the vestibular nuclei. There are four **vestibular nuclei** that receive direct inputs from the vestibular apparatus: the inferior, medial, lateral, and superior nuclei. The inferior and medial vestibular nuclei are located in the rostral medulla at the approximate level of the rostral portions of the inferior olivary nucleus. The superior and lateral vestibular nuclei lie in a more rostral position at the transition region between the medulla and pons. The medial and inferior vestibular nuclei are best seen in the rostral open medulla, while the superior and lateral vestibular nuclei are best seen in the junction between the pons and medulla just lateral to the fourth ventricle and medial to the inferior cerebellar peduncle.

The other group of SSA neurons is the **cochlear nuclei**, which lie on the dorsolateral shoulder of the inferior cerebellar peduncle at the rostral aspect of the medulla. These neurons receive inputs from primary auditory fibers and thus constitute part of a complex auditory pathway that eventually transmits auditory signals to the cerebral cortex.

This discussion has indicated how nuclei related to cranial nerve function are organized within the lower brainstem. Thus, when taken together with the analysis of the structures of the lower medulla considered earlier in this chapter, it is now possible to reconstruct the organization of the rostral half of the medulla. As is shown in Figure 10-6, the structures seen in more caudal levels of the medulla that are present at more rostral levels are again represented in the same general locations as noted in sections of the lower medulla.

Structures Situated in the Medial Medulla The arrangement of structures when going from a ventral to a dorsal level is as follows. On the ventromedial aspect of the rostral half of the medulla are the pyramids (Figs. 10-7 and 10-8). Dorsal to them, lies the medial lemniscus, and dorsal to the medial leminiscus lies two descending pathways: (1) the tectospinal tract, which contains descending fibers from the **superior colliculus** to the cervical cord that are presumed to mediate postural adjustments to visual stimuli; and (2) the **MLF**, whose descending component mediates head movements in response to postural changes in concert with the position of the eyes. Just dorsal to the position of these two pathways is the **hypoglossal nucleus** whose action is to protrude the tongue. Further discussion concerning functions and dysfunctions of the hypoglossal nerve is found in Chapter 14.

Structures Situated in the Lateral Medulla On the lateral side, the **inferior olivary nucleus** is most conspicuous because it is situated in a ventrolateral position just lateral to the pyramids (Figs. 10-7 and 10-8). The inferior olivary nucleus consists of many groups of cells, which project to the contralateral cerebellar cortex. The inferior olivary nucleus receives inputs from the spinal cord and red nucleus. The fibers from the spinal cord reach the inferior olivary nucleus via **spino-olivary fibers** (see Chapter 21), whereas fibers from the red nucleus reach the inferior olivary nucleus via rubro-olivary fibers contained in a larger bundle called the central tegmental tract (see Chapter 11). The primary function of the inferior olivary nucleus appears to be that of an important relay for the transmission of afferent signals to the cerebellum that are required for smooth, coordinated movements to be made.

Situated dorsally to the inferior olivary nucleus is the **reticular formation**, which contains many different groups of nerve cells as well as ascending and descending fibers. Within the core of the brainstem that forms the reticular formation lie several of the structures previously mentioned that are associated with cranial nerves. Two of these structures include the nucleus ambiguus and the solitary nucleus. Located just under the dorsolateral surface of the brainstem are two vestibular nuclei, the medial and inferior vestibular nuclei. The inferior vestibular nucleus can be easily recognized by its stippled appearance, which is due to the presence of descending fibers from the lateral vestibular nucleus that form the lateral vestibulospinal tract (Fig. 10-7B). The vestibular nuclei receive sensory information from the vestibular apparatus and transmit this information to the cerebellum, CN III, IV, and VI, and the spinal cord.

In its ventral half, the far lateral aspect of the medulla contains the ascending dorsal and ventral spinocerebellar and spinothalamic pathways as well as the descending rubrospinal tract. In a more dorsal position, the spinal nucleus and tract of CN V can be easily seen, and dorsolateral to these structures is the inferior cerebellar peduncle, which is quite prominent at this level. At the most rostral aspect of the medulla, the primary afferent fibers of CN VIII terminate upon two additional nuclear groups, the ventral and dorsal cochlear nuclei, which lie off the dorsolateral shoulder of the inferior cerebellar peduncle and constitute part of the relay system for the transmission of auditory impulses from the periphery to the cerebral cortex (Fig. 10-8). In the human brain, the dorsal cochlear nucleus is small, whereas the ventral cochlear nucleus is large, extending into the junction between the medulla and pons.

CLINICAL CONSIDERATIONS

Typically, damage to a part of the brainstem results from a vascular lesion. Although the neurologic effects of vascular lesions are described in detail in Chapter 27, it is useful to briefly summarize several of the classical disorders of the medulla, not only because of its basic importance, but because it also serves as a helpful review and guide to understanding the organization of the lower brainstem.

As a general rule, there are certain deficits that are common to lesions of the lateral aspect of the brainstem. Likewise, there are several deficits that are common to lesions of the medial aspect.

LATERAL MEDULLARY SYNDROME

The lateral medullary syndrome (Wallenberg's syndrome) results from a vascular lesion of the vertebral and posterior inferior cerebellar arteries (PICA). This syndrome most often involves loss of pain and temperature on the opposite side of the body and the ipsilateral face, loss of coordination, loss of the gag reflex, hoarseness, and difficulty with speech and swallowing. In addition, damage to descending autonomic fibers from regions such as the hypothalamus will cause a loss of some sympathetic functions, an example of which is Horner's syndrome (see Chapter 22). The structures affected include the spinothalamic tracts, spinal nucleus and tract of the trigeminal nerve, nucleus ambiguus and its associated axons, descending autonomic fibers from higher regions of the brainstem and forebrain, and vestibular nuclei.

MEDIAL MEDULLARY SYNDROME

The medial medullary syndrome (Dejerine's syndrome) results from a vascular lesion of the anterior spinal or paramedian branches of the vertebral arteries. The syndrome involves the pyramid, medial lemniscus, and root fibers of the hypoglossal nerve. Three typical neurologic signs include: (1) loss of conscious proprioception, touch, and pressure from the contralateral side of the body, (2) contralateral upper motor neuron paralysis, (3) paralysis of the ipsilateral aspect of the tongue and deviation of the tongue upon protrusion to the side contralateral to the lesion.

DORSAL MEDULLARY SYNDROME

This syndrome, which overlaps somewhat with the lateral medullary syndrome, results from a vascular lesion of a medial branch of the PICA artery. The affected structures typically include the inferior cerebellar peduncle and the adjacent vestibular nuclei. The major symptoms are nystagmus (see Chapters 14 and 17), vomiting, and vertigo caused by involvement of the vestibular nuclei and ataxia due to damage to cerebellar afferent fibers that arise in the spinal cord and parts of the brainstem.

CLINICAL CASE

HISTORY

Eleanor is an 84-year-old woman who had heart bypass surgery 10 years ago. While baking bread in her apartment, she suddenly became very dizzy, feeling as if the room was spinning. She became very nauseated, and as she ran to the bathroom to vomit, she fell to the right side. As she pulled herself back to her feet, she felt that her legs were unsteady, but her left leg felt numb, as if she had received an injection of novocaine. While attempting to brush her teeth, she felt that the right side of her face was numb, and she felt as if the toothpaste was going into her windpipe. She continued to experience nausea and feel as if the world was not only spinning, but also bouncing up and down. Eleanor pressed her emergency call button, and when she spoke, she noted that her voice sounded hoarse, and she was hiccupping. An ambulance arrived, and she was taken to the local emergency room.

EXAMINATION

When the doctors examined Eleanor at the hospital, she was unable to stand unassisted, and she tended to fall to the right. Her right arm and leg had jerking movements, and her sensation to pinprick was diminished on the left side of her body and the right side of her face. She was hoarse and hiccupped continuously. Her eyes jerked rhythmically when she looked to the right side, and the gag reflex was diminished on the right side. Her right eyelid drooped slightly, the right pupil was smaller than the left, and the right side of her face produced no sweat. Eleanor had a magnetic resonance imaging (MRI) scan of her head and was admitted to the hospital.

EXPLANATION

Eleanor's multifaceted problem is an example of lateral medullary syndrome or Wallenberg syndrome, occurring as a result of infarction of the lateral portion of the medulla. This often results from infarction of an intrinsic branch of the posterior inferior cerebellar artery (PICA), although it may also occur from occlusion of the vertebral as well. Because of the large number of tracts running through the lateral portion of the medulla, classic cases may exhibit many symptoms. A review of the anatomy of the medulla predicts the possible symptoms patients with this syndrome may have.

Tracts running through the lateral medulla include the descending tract and nucleus of the fifth nerve (CN V), causing ipsilateral facial numbness, and the vestibular nuclei and their connections, causing the sensation of spinning (vertigo), jerking movements of the eyes (nystagmus), vomiting, and a bouncing sensation (oscillopsia). The jerking, ataxic movements of the limbs most likely result from involvement of the inferior cerebellar peduncle and possibly a portion of the cerebellar hemispheres, if involved. Infarction of descending sympathetic fibers cause a Horner syndrome, or partial drooping of the eyelid (pseudoptosis), pupillary constriction (miosis), and diminished sweating ipsilateral to the lesion. Although the origin of the hiccupping is uncertain, hoarseness, diminished gag reflex, difficulty with swallowing, and vocal cord paralysis occur as a result of involvement of fibers of CN IX and CN X. Contralateral numbness over the body results from infarction of the spinothalamic tract.

CHAPTER TEST

QUESTIONS

Choose the best answer for each question.

1. A 56-year-old man was admitted to the emergency room after fainting in a hallway of his apartment building. Two days later, he was able to open his eyes and began to regain some basic functions. However, a neurologic examination revealed that he was not able to move his left arm or leg. In addition, he also lost some sensation in his left leg and arm, and when he tried to extend his tongue, it deviated to the right side. Where was the location of the lesion?

   a. At the border of spinal cord and medulla
   b. In the dorsomedial medulla
   c. In the ventromedial medulla
   d. In the dorsolateral medulla
   e. At the border between medulla and pons

2. A 43-year-old woman had herself admitted to the hospital after complaining of headaches. Two days later, she was unable to move either her hands or feet and was, in effect, a quadriplegic. A neurologic examination revealed no loss of either cranial nerve reflexes or sensation from the body or head. Subsequent MRIs and other neurologic diagnoses indicated that the damage to the central nervous system was quite limited. The most likely focus of the lesion was in the:

   a. Dorsomedial aspect of the rostral medulla
   b. Dorsolateral aspect of the rostral medulla
   c. Ventromedial aspect of the rostral medulla
   d. Midline at the border of medulla and spinal cord
   e. Dorsomedial aspect of the border of medulla and pons

3. An elderly female patient was diagnosed as having had a stroke, which caused loss of pain to the left side of her face and head and to the right side of her body and flushing of the left side of her face. Where was the locus of the lesion?

   a. Ventromedial aspect of the right caudal medulla
   b. Dorsolateral aspect of the left rostral medulla
   c. Dorsomedial aspect of the right caudal medulla
   d. Midline region of the medulla-spinal cord border
   e. Dorsomedial aspect of the medulla-pons border

4. An 80-year-old man was brought to the emergency room after complaining of an inability to swallow food. The structure most closely linked to this dysfunction is:

a. Inferior olivary nucleus
b. Pyramids
c. Spinal trigeminal nucleus
d. Nucleus ambiguus
e. Hypoglossal nucleus

5. Conscious proprioception from the upper limbs to the thalamus is mediated through the:

a. Nucleus gracilis
b. Nucleus cuneatus
c. Spinal trigeminal nucleus
d. Inferior olivary nucleus
e. Nuclei of reticular formation of rostral medulla

ANSWERS AND EXPLANATIONS

1. Answer: c

The fiber bundle mediating upper motor neuron control over movements of the contralateral arm and leg is the pyramids, which are situated in the ventromedial aspect of the medulla. Sensory impulses from the left limbs are mediated through the right brainstem medial lemniscus as a result of a decussation of this pathway at its site of origin. Lesions of the hypoglossal nerve result in deviation of the tongue to the side of the lesion due to the unopposed action of the contralateral hypoglossal nerve upon the tongue muscles when the tongue is protruded (see Chapter 14 for further discussion). All of these structures lie in the ventromedial aspect of the medulla. Thus, the other choices are incorrect because they do not contain all of these structures.

2. Answer: d

The decussation of the pyramids occurs at the most caudal aspect of the medulla near its border with the spinal cord. Therefore, damage to the midline region would most likely affect corticospinal fibers that arise from both sides of the cerebral cortex and that normally pass to both the cervical and lumbar levels on both sides of the spinal cord. The net result here would result in an upper motor neuron paralysis of all four limbs. The position of the decussation of the pyramids is the only locus where a single lesion (among the choices presented) could affect pyramidal fibers bilaterally. Therefore, the other choices are incorrect because lesions at any of these other sites could not affect pyramidal fibers bilaterally (i.e., ventromedial medulla) or at all with respect to several choices (i.e., dorsolateral and dorsomedial aspects of the caudal or rostral medulla).

3. Answer: b

A lesion of the dorsolateral aspect of the left medulla would affect first-order pain fibers (and second-order neuronal cell bodies of the trigeminal complex) associated with the left side of the face. Pain fibers associated with the body have already crossed in the spinal cord. Thus, this lesion would affect pain sensation from the right side of the body. The flushing of the face would result from the loss of descending autonomic fibers from the hypothalamus, which controls the sympathetic nervous system, thus producing a flushing of the face known as Horner's syndrome. The medial aspect of the medulla does not contain pain fibers from either the head or body.

4. Answer: d

Swallowing is controlled by neurons of the 9th and 10th cranial nerves, which innervate the pharyngeal and laryngeal muscles. These neurons arise from the nucleus ambiguus, which contributes to the motor outputs of both cranial nerves. The inferior olivary nucleus serves as a relay for information from the spinal cord and red nucleus that is transmitted to the cerebellum and, thus, plays no role in swallowing. The pyramids at the level of the medulla contain mostly corticospinal fibers that control movements of the limbs. The spinal trigeminal nucleus receives inputs from the face associated mainly with pain and temperature. The hypoglossal nucleus regulates movements of the tongue.

5. Answer: b

First-order neurons mediating conscious proprioception from the body pass from the periphery through the dorsal columns of the spinal cord to the dorsal column nuclei of the lower medulla, where they terminate. Fibers associated with this type of sensation from the upper limbs terminate upon the nucleus cuneatus, while fibers associated with the lower limb terminate upon the nucleus gracilis. These nuclei then project their axons to the contralateral thalamus.

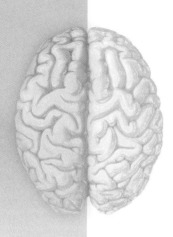

CHAPTER 11

BRAINSTEM II: PONS AND CEREBELLUM

OBJECTIVES

In this chapter, the student is expected to:

1. Learn the gross anatomy of the pons

2. Learn the gross anatomy of the cerebellum (details concerning cerebellar anatomy and function will be discussed in Chapter 21)

3. Know the organization and relationships of the major fiber pathways that traverse the pons

4. Identify the major cell groups that lie within the pons and cerebellum

5. Understand the bases for syndromes associated with different regions of the pons and cerebellum

In the previous chapter, we examined the organization of the medulla. In this chapter, a parallel analysis will be made with respect to the pons and cerebellum. Similar to the medulla, the pons consists of different kinds of nuclear groups belonging to cranial nerves as well as other groups that are unrelated to cranial nerves. There are also long ascending and descending fiber pathways that pass through the pons, the majority of which are also present in the medulla. In addition, two of the cerebellar peduncles linking the cerebellum with the brainstem (the middle and superior cerebellar peduncles) pass directly from or through the pons, respectively.

GROSS ANATOMICAL VIEW OF THE PONS

In its gross appearance, the **pons** serves as a connection between the medulla, which is attached to its caudal end, and the **midbrain**, which is attached at its rostral end (Fig. 11-1). From an anatomical perspective, the pons is typically divided into two regions, a ventral part, called the **basilar pons**, and a dorsal part, called the **tegmentum** (Fig. 11-2). The basilar pons consists of two different groups of fibers and neurons distributed throughout much of this region. One group of fibers, present throughout both the dorsoventral and rostro-caudal aspects of the basilar pons, runs in a transverse direction across the pons. This massive group of fibers is thus referred to as **transverse pontine fibers (ponto-cerebellar)** and arises from the neurons scattered throughout the basilar pons called **deep pontine nuclei**. The second group of fibers consists of corticospinal and corticobulbar fibers, which descend from the cerebral cortex and pass in a longitudinal manner with respect to the neuraxis of the brainstem to the spinal cord and lower brainstem, respectively, and are thus positioned perpendicular to the orientation of the transverse pontine fibers.

Along the midline of the basilar pons is a groove called the **basilar sulcus**, which is formed by the basilar artery. Laterally, another massive fiber bundle, called the **middle cerebellar peduncle**, is a continuation of the transverse pontine fibers. This peduncle passes laterally and dorsally into the cerebellum from the lateral aspect of the pons, thus forming a "bridge" between these two structures. The dorsal aspect of the pons (tegmentum) forms the floor of the fourth ventricle and the roof of the pons. Along the floor of the fourth ventricle, a bulge can be identified caudally along its medial aspect. This is called the **facial colliculus** and is formed by the presence of the fibers of the facial nerve that pass over the dorsal aspect of the abducens nucleus (Fig. 11-1B). The lateral walls of the fourth ventricle are formed by the superior cerebellar peduncles that arise mainly from the cerebellum and enter the brainstem from a dorsolateral position at the level of the rostral pons.

The tegmentum of the pons also consists of nuclei and fiber pathways. Nuclear groups include groups associated with cranial nerves as well as those that are unrelated to cranial nerves but that serve important sensory, motor, autonomic, and behavioral functions. The fiber pathways in this region consist of axons that may arise in the pons and that run either dorsally or caudally. In addition, this region also contains other ascending or descending fiber pathways, which originate in the brainstem, spinal cord, other parts of the brainstem, or forebrain. Details concerning the nature of these cell groups and fiber pathways are considered in the following sections.

INTERNAL ORGANIZATION OF THE PONS

FIBER PATHWAYS

Many of the same pathways present within the medulla are also present within the pons. Two of the most prominent ascending tracts include the **medial lemniscus** and **medial longitudinal fasciculus** (MLF) (Fig. 11-3). Note that, as the medial lemniscus passes in a rostral direction within the pontine tegmentum, it becomes oriented more laterally and somewhat more dorsally until it reaches its most lateral and dorsal position in the caudal diencephalon where it synapses in the ventral posterolateral nucleus (VPL) of the thalamus (see also Chapter 9). In contrast, the MLF retains its dorsomedial position as it ascends towards the midbrain. In addition, other pathways are situated in a lateral position within the pontine tegmentum as they ascend to the midbrain and more rostral levels. These pathways include the spinothalamic and trigeminothalamic pathways that mediate somatosensory information from the body and head region to the ventral posterolateral and ventral posteromedial nuclei of the thalamus, respectively. These two pathways are sandwiched between the lateral lemniscus, a part of the auditory relay circuit, and the medial lemniscus.

The major descending pathways include the corticobulbar and corticospinal tracts (Fig. 11-3). These pathways maintain a position within the basilar aspect of the pons. Other pathways (not clearly discernible from normal sections of the pons) include the rubrospinal and tectospinal tracts. The rubrospinal tract occupies a position within the pons just dorsal to the medial lemniscus. The position of the tectospinal tract within the

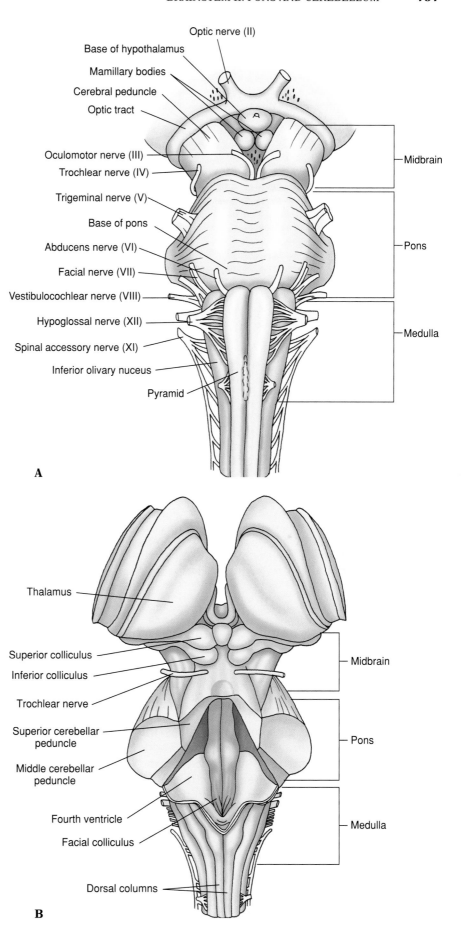

Optic nerve (II)

Base of hypothalamus

Mamillary bodies

Cerebral peduncle

Optic tract

Oculomotor nerve (III)

Trochlear nerve (IV)

Trigeminal nerve (V)

Base of pons

Abducens nerve (VI)

Facial nerve (VII)

Vestibulocochlear nerve (VIII)

Hypoglossal nerve (XII)

Spinal accessory nerve (XI)

Inferior olivary nuceus

Pyramid

Midbrain

Pons

Medulla

A

Thalamus

Superior colliculus

Inferior colliculus

Trochlear nerve

Superior cerebellar peduncle

Middle cerebellar peduncle

Fourth ventricle

Facial colliculus

Dorsal columns

Midbrain

Pons

Medulla

B

Figure 11–1 Ventral and dorsal views of the brainstem. (A) View of the ventral surface of the brainstem illustrating the position of the pons in relation to the medulla and midbrain and the loci of the cranial nerves. Note that CN VI and VII exit medially and laterally, respectively, at the level of the caudal pons, and CN V exits laterally at the level of the middle of the pons. (B) View of the dorsal surface of the brainstem looking down into the fourth ventricle illustrating the positions of the pons in relation to the medulla and midbrain. The cerebellum was removed to demonstrate the position occupied by the fourth ventricle. Note the positions occupied by the superior and middle cerebellar peduncles.

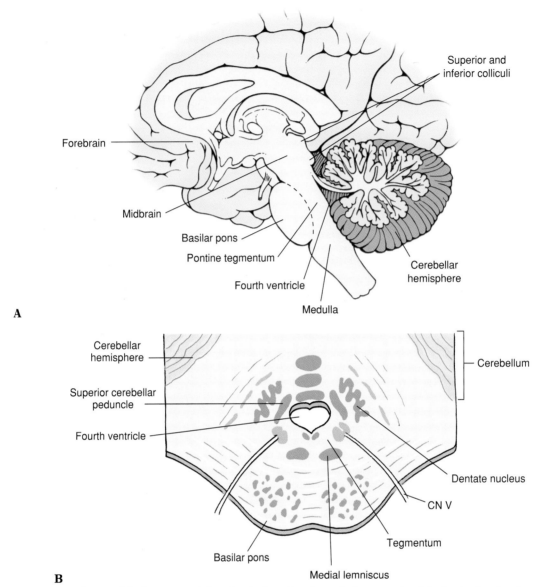

Figure 11–2 Sagittal view of the brainstem. (A) Midsagittal section through the neuraxis of the brain showing the relationship of the pons to the medulla, midbrain, cerebellum, and forebrain. Note that the pons can be divided into two regions: a ventral aspect called the basilar pons and a dorsal aspect called the tegmentum. (B) A cross section taken through the middle of the pons reveals the division of the pons into the basilar and tegmental regions.

level of the pons is similar to its position within the medulla; namely, it lies dorsomedially just ventral to the MLF. In addition, the dorsolateral aspect of the tegmentum of the pons (as well as the tegmentum of the midbrain and medulla) contains descending fibers from the limbic system and hypothalamus that project to regions of the lower brainstem that mediate autonomic functions.

MAJOR CELL GROUPS (FIGS. 11-3 TO 11-6)

Caudal Pons

A number of important nuclei, associated in part with cranial nerves, are present in the caudal

pons. These include the motor nuclei of the facial (cranial nerve [CN] VII) and abducens (CN VI) nerves, the spinal nucleus of the trigeminal CN V, the superior olivary nucleus (a relay nucleus of the auditory pathway), raphe nuclei, and pontine nuclei of the basilar pons.

Rostral Pons

The principal nuclei present in the rostral half of the pons include the main sensory, mesencephalic, and motor nuclei of CN V, the superior and lateral vestibular nuclei, and the locus ceruleus. Other cell groups, such as the pontine nuclei (of the basilar aspect) and the raphe nuclei (of the tegmentum), are also present at all levels of the pons.

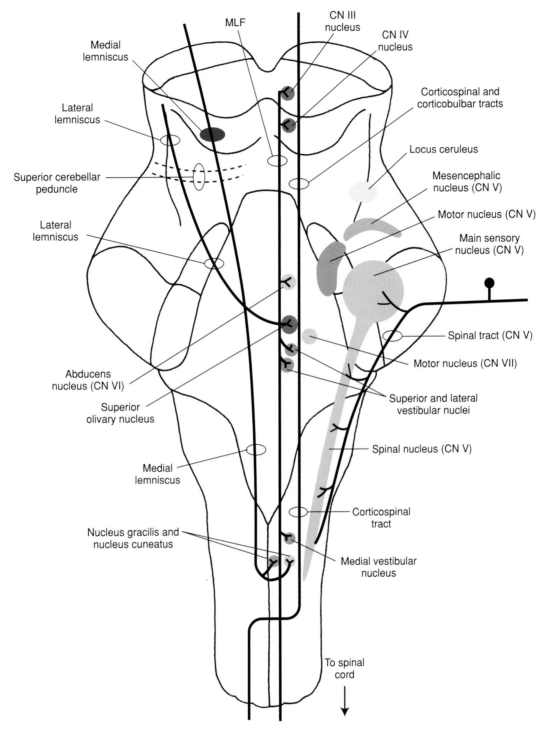

Figure 11-3 The general positions of the major nuclear groups and most prominent ascending and descending pathways that traverse the pons.

BASILAR ASPECT OF THE PONS

Throughout its entire length, the pons is divided into two distinct parts, a dorsal and a ventral region. The dorsal part is called the **tegmentum**, which is continuous with the tegmentum of the medulla and midbrain. The ventral part is called the **basilar** (or ventral) pons. The basilar pons may be viewed as a rostral extension of the ventral aspect of the medulla, which contains the pyramidal tract. However, at the level of the pons, significant morphological changes can be noted. The most characteristic feature is the marked presence of massive bundles of fibers that run transversely and coalesce as the middle cerebellar peduncle, which enters the cerebellar cortex. Interspersed among the transverse fiber bundles are large numbers of cells. These cells are referred to as **(deep) pontine nuclei**. They are important because they give rise to the **transverse pontine fibers**. The pontine nuclei, which receive significant inputs from the cerebral cortex, send their axons (the transverse pontine fibers) to the cerebellar cortex. Thus, the pathway from the cerebral cortex to the cerebellar cortex constitutes a two-neuronal arc (corticopontine and pontocerebellar fibers). The functional importance of these connections is discussed in more detail in Chapter 21.

In addition to the deep pontine nuclei and transverse pontine fibers, the basilar pons contains the corticospinal and corticobulbar tracts, which follow the longitudinal axis of the brainstem and which pass at right angles to the transverse pontine fibers. At the level of the pons, numbers of corticobulbar (also called corticonuclear) fibers exit and terminate mainly upon interneurons of the reticular formation situated near cranial nerve motor nuclei as well as nuclei of reticulospinal fibers.

PONTINE TEGMENTUM
LOWER (CAUDAL) HALF OF THE PONS (FIG. 11-4)

Within the caudal aspect of the pons, several features characteristic of the medulla are still present. The following structures are noted: the MLF and tectospinal tracts that lie in the dorsomedial aspect of the pons; the spinal nucleus and tract that lie in the lateral aspect of the pons; and the medial lemniscus, whose position at this level remains within the ventromedial aspect of the pontine tegmentum.

Important structures that appear at this level include:

1. **The abducens nucleus (nucleus of CN VI).** This nucleus lies in a dorsomedial position within the pons close to the floor of the fourth ventricle. This nucleus serves as a general somatic efferent (GSE) (lower motor neuron), which innervates the lateral rectus muscle and thus provides the anatomical basis for the lateral movement of the eye.

2. **The facial nucleus (nucleus of CN VII).** This nucleus lies in the ventrolateral aspect of the tegmentum. Its axons (special visceral efferent [SVE] fibers) follow an unusual course by initially passing in a dorsomedial direction. Where the axons approach the dorsal aspect of the pons, the fibers course laterally over the abducens nucleus, forming the facial colliculus. They then continue ventrolaterally to where the fibers exit the brain to innervate the muscles controlling ipsilateral facial expression.

3. **Superior and lateral vestibular nuclei.** These nuclei are located in the dorsolateral aspect of the pontine tegmentum and essentially replace the medial and inferior vestibular nuclei that are situated more caudally in the medulla. The superior and lateral vestibular nuclei receive direct inputs from the vestibular apparatus and contribute fibers to the MLF. In addition, axons of the lateral vestibular nucleus form the lateral vestibulospinal tract, which innervates all levels of the spinal cord. As noted in Chapters 9 and 19, the action of this tract is to facilitate extensor motor neurons.

4. **Auditory relay structures—trapezoid body (and nucleus of trapezoid body), superior olivary nucleus, and lateral lemniscus.** These nuclei are located in the ventral aspect of the pontine tegmentum. The nucleus of the trapezoid body and superior olivary nucleus receive auditory inputs primarily from the cochlear nuclei and transmit auditory signals to higher centers of the brainstem. The trapezoid body is made up of commissural fibers, which originate from either the ventral cochlear nucleus or superior olivary nucleus. The lateral lemniscus represents fibers of the cochlear nuclei and superior olivary nucleus that transmit auditory signals to the inferior colliculus. Details concerning the organization and nature of the auditory pathway are presented in Chapter 17.

5. **Superior salivatory nucleus.** This nucleus (GVE) lies in a position just ventrolateral to the abducens nucleus. It gives rise to preganglionic parasympathetic axons of CN VII, which innervate submandibular, submaxillary, and pterygopalatine ganglia. Thus, this nucleus serves to mediate lacrimation, salivation, and vasodilation. This nucleus is quite small and cannot be

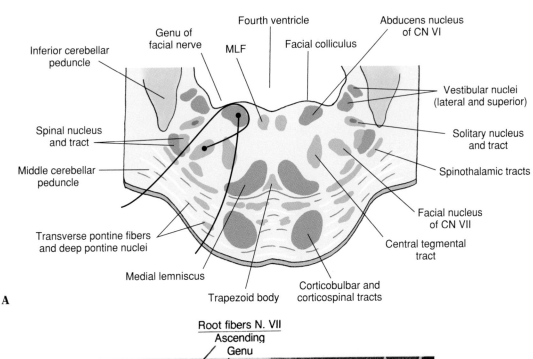

A

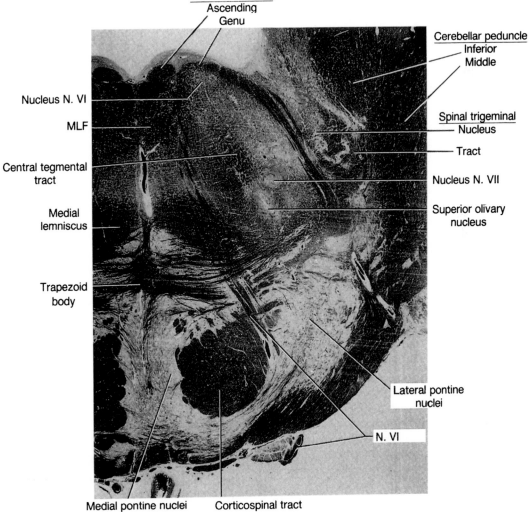

B

Figure 11–4 Caudal pons. (A) Cross section through the caudal aspect of the pons at the level of the facial colliculus of the pons. Note that the axons of CN VII pass dorsomedially around the dorsal aspect of the nucleus of CN VI, forming the facial colliculus, and then pass ventrolaterally to exit the brainstem. In contrast, the axons of CN VI pass ventrally to exit the brainstem in a relatively medial position. (B) Myelin-stained cross section through the caudal aspect of the pons. (Panel B: Reproduced with permission from Parent A: Carpenter's Human Neuroanatomy, 9th ed. Baltimore: Williams & Wilkins, 1996, p. 496.)

seen without special physiological or histological manipulations. (See Chapter 14 for details concerning functions of the cranial nerves.)

6. **Nuclei and fibers of the reticular formation.** As noted in Chapter 10, the reticular formation extends from the lower medulla to the rostral aspect of the midbrain. Three areas of the pontine reticular formation are noted: a midline region, containing **raphe nuclei**; a large-celled region situated within the medial two thirds of the reticular formation; and a small-celled region situated in the lateral aspect of the reticular formation. In brief, the raphe cells produce serotonin; these cells project to many areas of the central nervous system. The large-celled region gives rise to long ascending and descending fibers contained to a considerable extent in the central tegmental tract, and the small-celled region serves as a source of inputs to the reticular formation.

UPPER (ROSTRAL) HALF OF THE PONS

Within the rostral half of the pons, a number of structures appear for the first time. These include:

1. **Main sensory (trigeminal) nucleus [NV].** The main sensory nucleus of NV (general sensory afferent [GSA]) is a large nucleus found in the dorsolateral aspect of the tegmentum. It replaces the position occupied by the spinal trigeminal nucleus at lower levels. It contains second-order neurons for the transmission of somatosensory information from the head region as its axons project to the ventral posteromedial nucleus of the thalamus (Fig. 11-5).

2. **Motor nucleus [NV].** The motor nucleus of NV (SVE) projects its axons to the muscles of mastication and, therefore, plays a vital role in closing the jaw. It lies immediately medial to the main sensory nucleus and can be distinguished from it by the presence of trigeminal root fibers that pass between it and the main sensory nucleus (Fig. 11-5).

3. **Nucleus locus ceruleus.** This nucleus can be found in the dorsolateral aspect of the tegmentum of the upper pons at the level of the motor nucleus of NV and the region slightly rostral to it (Fig. 11-6). The locus ceruleus consists of norepinephrine-containing neurons, which project to different cell groups in the brainstem, forebrain, including the cerebral cortex, and cerebellum.

4. **Mesencephalic nucleus of NV.** The mesencephalic nucleus extends from the level of the rostral pons into the midbrain. It is located in the ventrolateral aspect of the gray matter surrounding the rostral end of the fourth ventricle and the beginning of the cerebral aqueduct (Fig. 11-6). It receives mainly muscle spindle afferents from the jaw and related areas of the face (i.e., masseter and temporalis muscles), which serve as afferents for reflex closing of the jaw.

5. **Superior cerebellar peduncle.** At the rostral aspect of the pons, the superior cerebellar peduncle, which contains the large majority of cerebellar efferent fibers to the midbrain and thalamus, forms the lateral wall of the fourth ventricle (Fig. 11-5). The superior cerebellar peduncle on each side is attached by the **superior medullary velum**, which forms the roof of the fourth ventricle. At the rostral border of the pons (Fig. 11-6), the superior cerebellar peduncle enters the pons and courses towards the midline. At the level of the caudal midbrain, these fibers will ultimately cross over to the opposite side of the brainstem.

THE CEREBELLUM

As pointed out in Chapter 1, the cerebellum plays a major role in the integration of motor functions. Damage to different parts of the cerebellum will cause such deficits as loss of balance, tremors, lack of coordination of muscles, and reduced muscle tone. The cerebellum is attached to the brainstem by three pairs of peduncles (see Fig. 1-9). The inferior cerebellar peduncle extends from the dorsolateral aspect of the upper medulla into the cerebellum. The middle cerebellar peduncle is attached to the lateral aspect of the pons and, therefore, enters the cerebellum from a lateral position. The superior cerebellar peduncle passes from the rostro-medial aspect of the cerebellum in a rostral direction and enters the brainstem at the level of the upper pons. The inferior and middle cerebellar peduncles generally contain cerebellar afferent fibers, while most fibers present within the superior cerebellar peduncle constitute cerebellar efferent fibers.

The cerebellum consists of two hemispheres continuous with a median vermal region (Fig. 11-7). The cerebellar hemispheres are divided into three lobes. The lobe closest to the midbrain is called the **anterior lobe** and is separated from **the posterior lobe** (which is the largest lobe) by the primary fissure. The smallest lobe is called the **flocculonodular lobe**. It is located most caudally and is separated from the posterior lobe by the **posterolateral fissure**.

Internally, the cerebellum consists of a cortex, white matter that lies immediately deep to the

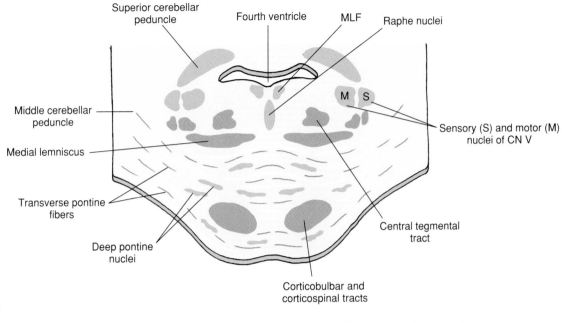

A

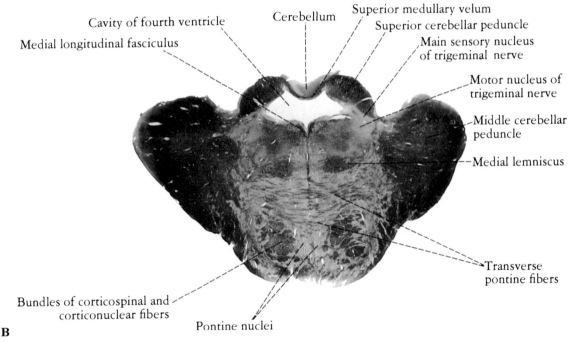

B

Figure 11–5 Middle pons. (A) Cross section through the middle of the pons at the level of the main sensory and motor nuclei of the trigeminal nerve. (B) Myelin-stained section through the same level of the pons at the level of the main sensory and motor nuclei of the trigeminal nerve. (Panel B: Reproduced with permission from Snell RS: Clinical Neuroanatomy, 5th ed. Philadelphia: Lippincott Williams & Wilkins, 2001, p. 203.)

gray matter, and a series of nuclei referred to as **deep cerebellar nuclei**. The most lateral and largest of the nuclei is called the **dentate nucleus** (Fig. 11-8). The most medial nucleus is called the **fastigial nucleus**. Between the dentate and fastigial nuclei lie two smaller nuclei, called the **emboliform** and **globose** nuclei. In humans, the globose nucleus lies medial to the emboliform

nucleus, and the **emboliform nucleus** is situated close to the hilus of the dentate nucleus. However, in lower forms of animals, such as the cat, these two nuclei are fused, and the structure is referred to as the **interposed nucleus**. The overall importance of these nuclei is that their axons constitute the primary means by which information exits the cerebellum.

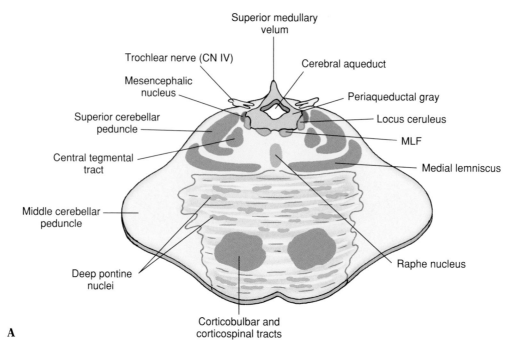

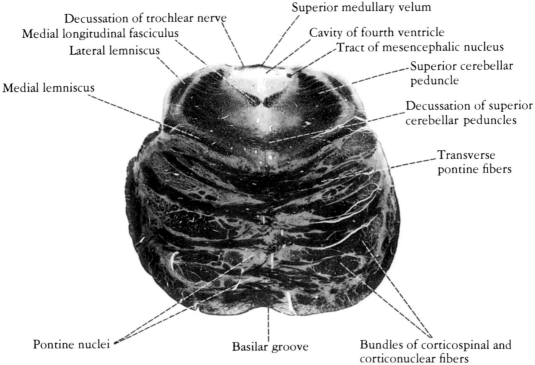

Figure 11–6 Rostral pons. (A) Diagram of a cross section through the upper pons at the level of the locus ceruleus and mesencephalic nucleus of the trigeminal nerve. (B) Myelin-stained section through the same level of the pons as the level of the nucleus ceruleus and mesencephalic nucleus of the trigeminal nerve. (Panel B: Reproduced with permission from Snell RS: Clinical Neuroanatomy, 5th ed. Philadelphia: Lippincott Williams & Wilkins, 2001, p. 204.)

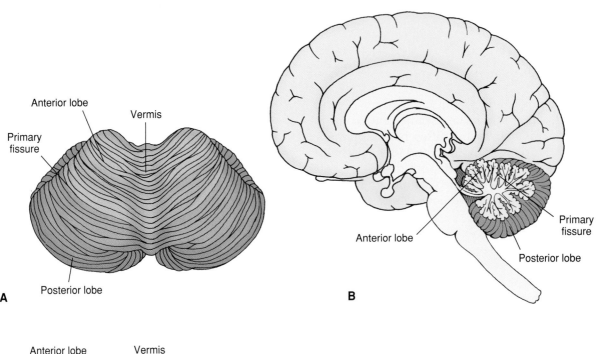

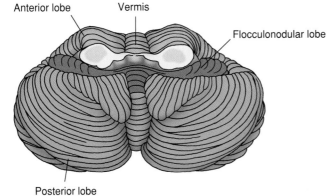

Figure 11–7   Cerebellum. Superior (A), midsagittal (B), and inferior (C) views of the cerebellum illustrating anterior, posterior, and flocculonodular lobes, as well as hemispheres and vermal regions.

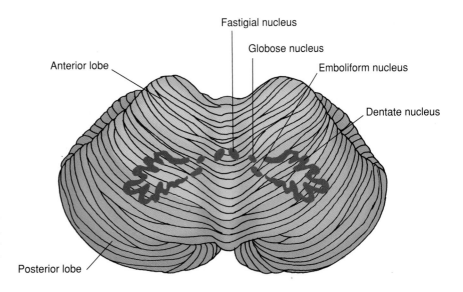

Figure 11–8   Cerebellum and deep cerebellar nuclei. This view of the cerebellum illustrates the positions occupied by the deep cerebellar nuclei. The largest nucleus, the dentate nucleus, is located laterally. The fastigial nucleus is situated medially, and the globose and emboliform (interposed) nuclei are located in an intermediate position.

A detailed analysis of the anatomy, physiology, and clinical associations of the cerebellum is provided in Chapter 21.

CLINICAL CONSIDERATIONS

As shown in Chapter 10, vascular occlusions involving different arteries target different groups of structures, thus producing different combinations of neurologic deficits. With respect to the pons, different syndromes associated with distinct regions of the pons can be identified. The more common ones are described in the following sections.

CAUDAL TEGMENTAL PONTINE SYNDROME

This syndrome, caused by occlusion of circumferential branches of the basilar artery, impacts upon structures situated within the caudal aspect of the pontine tegmentum. The major structures thus affected include the MLF, motor nuclei of CN VI and CN VII, spinal nucleus of CN V, spinothalamic tracts, and descending pathways from the hypothalamus. Therefore, deficits seen from this vascular occlusion would include ipsilateral facial nerve palsy (CN VII), lateral gaze palsy (CN VI), and Horner's syndrome (resulting from loss of descending sympathetic input to the lower brainstem). The exact nature of these deficits is a function of the extent of damage incurred by the vascular occlusion.

CAUDAL BASAL PONTINE SYNDROME

This syndrome, which is associated mainly with the paramedian branches of the basilar artery, affects mainly the descending corticospinal tract and root fibers of CN VI if the lesion extends far enough medially. The effects of such a lesion would typically produce a contralateral hemiplegia and signs of a paralysis of CN VI (loss of lateral gaze in the eye on the side ipsilateral to the lesion).

ROSTRAL BASAL PONTINE SYNDROME

Occlusion of portions of the paramedian branches of the basilar artery, which affects the rostral half of the basilar pons, will most likely affect axons of sensory and motor components of the trigeminal nerve and the corticospinal tract. The common deficits would presumably include a contralateral hemiplegia (corticospinal tract deficit) and ipsilateral loss of facial sensation and ability to chew (CN V deficits).

ROSTRAL PONTINE TEGMENTAL SYNDROME

This syndrome is associated mainly with occlusion of the long circumferential branches of the basilar artery. The structures affected include the sensory and motor nuclei of CN V, medial lemniscus, spinothalamic tracts, reticular formation, and, if the lesion extends far enough laterally, also the cerebellar afferent fibers contained in the middle cerebellar peduncle. The deficits associated with this syndrome would typically include ipsilateral loss of sensation to the face and ability to chew (CN V deficits); contralateral loss of pain, temperature, Horner's syndrome and conscious proprioception from the body (spinothalamic and medial lemniscal deficits); and possibly ataxia of movement (due to disruption of the cerebellar afferent fibers).

OTHER RELATED SYNDROMES OF THE PONS

In addition to the syndromes just described, others have been characterized, and several of them are noted here.

The Locked-In Syndrome

After a large infarct of the basilar pons, there is significant loss of functions associated with both the corticobulbar and corticospinal tracts. As a result, there is a paralysis of most motor functions, including the limbs (corticospinal loss), and functions associated with motor cranial nerves (corticobulbar loss) other than the ability to blink one's eyes and display vertical gaze. Consequently, the patient can only communicate by blinking or moving his or her eyes.

The Medial Tegmental Syndrome

If the lesion is restricted to the medial aspect of the pons, the likely targets will include the nucleus of the abducens nerve (CN VI), the fibers of the facial nerve (CN VII), which pass over the nucleus of CN VI, and possibly the medial lemniscus. The consequent loss of functions will include an ipsilateral facial paralysis, loss of lateral gaze on the side ipsilateral to the lesion, and contralateral loss of conscious proprioception and discriminative touch if the lesion extends sufficiently ventral to involve the medial lemniscus.

The One and a Half Syndrome

If there is a discrete lesion of the dorsomedial tegmentum, which involves the nucleus of CN VI, the pontine (lateral) gaze center of the paramedian pontine reticular formation (see Chapter 14), and the MLF, the patient will display a syndrome that includes a combination of lateral gaze paralysis (CN VI) coupled with an internuclear ophthalmoplegia (an inability to gaze to the side of the lesion). Thus, the patient cannot move the ipsilateral eye horizontally, and the contralateral eye can only be abducted, usually resulting in nystagmus of that eye (see Chapter 14 for discussion of nystagmus).

CLINICAL CASE

HISTORY

On an intern's first night on call in the hospital, a nurse asked the intern to come to the room of an elderly patient named Seymour, who suddenly appeared to have become comatose. Except for a history of vascular disease and an inability to stop smoking, there did not seem to be any clues to the cause of the man's coma.

EXAMINATION

The intern examining Seymour noticed that he appeared at first to stare straight ahead and blinked when the intern asked him to do so. When asked to blink twice or keep his eyes closed, he was also able to comply. However, he was unable to follow any commands involving other parts of his body. Seymour was unable to speak or move his arms or legs. He was able to move his eyes in the direction of the intern when he spoke. The intern asked Seymour to blink twice if he understood the commands but was unable to move, and he complied. His arms and legs appeared to be paralyzed, and when the lateral portion of the plantar surface of both his feet were scratched, the great toes dorsiflexed with an upward fanning of the remaining toes.

EXPLANATION

Seymour has the *locked-in syndrome*, a syndrome of infarction of the medial half of the basilar pons supplied by the basilar artery. This area contains the corticospinal and corticobulbar tracts, and infarction of this area causes paralysis of most, if not all, motor functions, including bilateral paralysis of the face and body as well as loss of voice. Often the tegmentum of the pons (i.e., reticular formation) is spared, thus preserving consciousness and sensation. Therefore, the patients who suffer an infarction of this type will appear to be comatose but remain alert. One of the first descriptions of this syndrome can be found in *The Count of Monte Cristo*, by Alexandre Dumas, written in 1844. The character, Monsieur Noirtrier de Villefort, lost the use of his voice and limbs; he was able to communicate by the use of eye blinks and went as far as to dictate a will in this manner. The condition, as described by Dumas, occurred suddenly and was probably the result of a vascular accident.

CHAPTER TEST

QUESTIONS

Choose the best answer for each question.

Questions 1 and 2. A 68-year-old woman was admitted to the emergency room after having lost consciousness at her home. Several days after regaining consciousness, a neurologic examination revealed the presence of nystagmus, deviation of the right eye medially, loss of sensation of the right side of the face and pain and temperature sensation from the left side of the body, Horner's syndrome, and some loss of coordination. The neurologist concluded that the patient had suffered a stroke.

1. Where was the most likely location of her stroke?
   a. Bilaterally, at the pontine-midbrain border
   b. In the right basilar pons
   c. In the left basilar pons
   d. In the right pontine tegmentum
   e. In the left pontine tegmentum

2. Structures affected by the stroke include:
   a. Corticospinal tract, medial lemniscus, spinothalamic tract, middle cerebellar peduncle, trigeminothalamic tracts, and reticular formation of right side of the rostral pons
   b. Spinothalamic tract, trigeminal structures, medial lemniscus, MLF, CN VIII, and middle cerebellar peduncle of right side of the caudal half of pons
   c. MLF, CN VI, middle cerebellar peduncle, reticular formation, spinothalamic fibers, and trigeminothalamic structures of right side of the caudal half of the pons
   d. Reticular formation of the right pontine tegmentum near the border with the pons
   e. Cerebellum, MLF, medial lemniscus, spinothalamic tract, main sensory nucleus of CN V, and motor nucleus of CN VII of the right side of the rostral pons

3. Examination of a patient reveals the presence of a right lateral gaze palsy and diplopia, as well as a loss of ability to express a smile on the right side of the face. The primary focus of the lesion is on:

a. The dorsal aspect of the right caudal pons
b. The dorsal aspect of the right rostral pons
c. The caudal aspect of the basilar pons on the left side
d. The rostral aspect of the basilar pons on the right side
e. The midline of the pons at the level of the main sensory nucleus of CN V

4. An elderly female patient was brought into the emergency room after suffering injuries to her head and body as a result of falling in her bathroom. A routine neurologic examination revealed that she would lose her balance when attempting to walk and would tend to fall to one side. She also showed very poor coordination in the use of her right arm and further displayed a tremor when attempting to produce a purposeful movement with that arm. The most likely locus of the lesion is:

a. Basilar pons
b. Lateral aspect of the caudal pontine tegmentum
c. Lateral aspect of the rostral pontine tegmentum
d. Cerebellum
e. Midline region of the tegmentum and basilar aspects of pons

5. A neuronal cell group that responds directly to activation of muscle spindles from the jaw is:

a. The facial motor nucleus (CN VII)
b. The spinal nucleus of CN V
c. The main sensory nucleus of CN V
d. The motor nucleus of CN V
e. The mesencephalic nucleus of CN V

ANSWERS AND EXPLANATIONS

1 and 2. Answers: 1-d, 2-c

In order for this constellation of deficits to be present, the lesion must be present in the right pontine tegmentum. The lesion has to be on the right side because the first-order sensory fibers from the head are uncrossed, whereas pain and temperature fibers from the body are crossed. The pontine tegmentum contains these sensory fibers. In addition, it also contains descending sympathetic fibers, the MLF, and the nucleus and fibers of CN VI, the damage of which would account for the loss of functions described in this case.

3. Answer: a

The loss of ability for the right eye to gaze laterally coupled with loss of control over the muscles of facial expression can only occur if the lesion is present in the region of the facial colliculus, which includes the fibers of CN VII passing over the nucleus of CN VI. Lesions in the other regions would not include both of these cranial nerve structures.

4. Answer: d

The cerebellum is concerned with the control of motor functions, and lesions of this structure can cause a variety of motor deficits, including loss of balance and coordination and tremor in attempting to move the limb. Lesions of other regions of the pons would produce different motor deficits, such as an upper motor neuron paralysis, associated with damage to the corticospinal tract.

5. Answer: e

The mesencephalic nucleus of CN V contains cell bodies of first-order neurons whose peripheral receptors are muscle spindles contained in muscles of the head, which respond to stretching of one of these muscles. The alternate choices relate to other sensory modalities (main sensory or spinal nucleus of CN V) or to structures mediating motor functions (motor nucleus of CN V or CN VII).

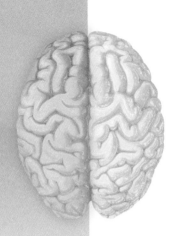

CHAPTER 12

BRAINSTEM III: THE MIDBRAIN

OBJECTIVES

In this chapter, the student is expected to:

1. Have a general understanding of the gross anatomic arrangement of the midbrain

2. Be able to identify the major cell groups that are situated at two levels of the midbrain: the inferior colliculus and superior colliculus

3. Know the organization and relationships of the major fiber pathways that either arise from or traverse the midbrain

4. Begin to understand the neural bases underlying syndromes associated with damage to different regions of the midbrain

The **midbrain** lies between the **pons** and the **forebrain** (Figs. 12-1 and 12-2). When viewed in cross section at either rostral or caudal levels of the midbrain, it is customary to divide this region of the brainstem into three anatomically distinct components (Fig. 12-3). (1) The most dorsal part is called the **tectum**. It is sometimes referred to as the **corpora quadrigemina**, which means "four bodies" (i.e., the superior and inferior colliculi appear as four rounded bodies when looking down on the midbrain). (2) The ventral aspect is referred to as the **crus cerebri**. It includes massive bundles of fibers that pass from the cerebral cortex to the brainstem and spinal cord. (3) The central part of the midbrain is called the **tegmentum**, which is continuous with the tegmentum of the pons. A cell group called the substantia nigra separates the tegmentum from the crus cerebri. The cerebral aqueduct, which is surrounded by gray matter called the **periaqueductal gray (PAG)**, separates the tegmentum from the tectum (Fig 12-3). As described in Chapter 3, the cerebral aqueduct is part of the ventricular system of the brain and serves as a conduit for the flow of cerebrospinal fluid from the third ventricle to the fourth ventricle. Some authors divide the midbrain into two parts: a tectal region, as described earlier, and a **cerebral peduncle**, which includes both the crus cerebri (located ventrally) and the tegmentum (located dorsally).

The midbrain contains two cranial nerves. The **trochlear nerve** (cranial nerve [CN] IV) emerges on the dorsal aspect of the caudal midbrain just caudal to the inferior colliculus (Figs. 12-3 and 12-4). The **oculomotor nerve** (CN III) emerges on the ventromedial aspect of the midbrain at a position just medial to the crus cerebri (Fig. 12-5). Because of the arrangement of the principal cell groups and fiber bundles, it is convenient to examine the organization of these structures at two levels of the midbrain. The caudal half includes the level of the **inferior colliculus**, and the rostral half includes the level of the **superior colliculus**.

INTERNAL ORGANIZATION OF THE MIDBRAIN

LEVEL OF THE INFERIOR COLLICULUS

Tectum

In the caudal half of the midbrain, the tectal region contains the **inferior colliculus** (Figs. 12-1, 12-3, and 12-4). The inferior colliculus consists of a large nuclear structure that represents an important relay component of the auditory pathway. It receives ascending inputs from auditory relay nuclei of the medulla and pons (i.e., cochlear and superior olivary nuclei and nucleus of the trapezoid body; see Chapter 17). These groups of neurons supply the inferior colliculus via a pathway called the **lateral lemniscus**, which ascends in the lateral aspect of the pons and caudal midbrain (Fig. 12-3). The inferior colliculus, in turn, projects its axons through a fiber bundle called the **brachium of the inferior colliculus** (to the **medial geniculate nucleus** of the thalamus) (see Fig. 12-6, which does not include the medial geniculate nucleus because it lies at a more rostral position).

Tegmentum (Including the Periaqueductal Gray Matter)

The tegmentum includes a variety of cell groups and fiber tracts. The periaqueductal gray (**PAG**), a transitional region between the tectum and tegmentum, is composed mainly of tightly packed cells that surround the cerebral aqueduct (Figs. 12-3 and 12-5). Although not typically visible through normal stained material, axons arising from both the PAG as well as from regions of the forebrain descend through different levels of the PAG to terminate either within the PAG or at lower regions of the brainstem. The PAG contains high concentrations of the neurotransmitter peptide, enkephalin (see Chapter 8). The PAG plays important roles in the regulation of autonomic functions and affective and emotional processes and in the modulation of pain impulses.

Just beneath the PAG lies the nucleus of the trochlear nerve (a general somatic efferent [GSE] nucleus). Its axons pass dorsally and caudally until they exit the brain on the contralateral side at the caudal aspect of the inferior colliculus (see Chapter 14, Fig. 14-1). These axons then innervate the superior oblique muscle, which moves the eye downward when it is displaced medially. Damage to this cranial nerve is manifest in particular in the form of diplopia when the patient tries to look downward, such as when attempting to walk down a flight of stairs. Beneath the nucleus of the trochlear nerve lies the medial longitudinal fasciculus (MLF); this serves as an afferent source to the trochlear nucleus (Fig. 12-4).

The lateral aspect of the tegmentum contains a number of important ascending sensory pathways. These pathways include the lateral lemniscus, which provides auditory inputs into the inferior colliculus from other auditory relay nuclei of the upper medulla, and the spinothalamic, trigeminothalamic, and medial lemniscal pathways (Figs. 12-1 and 12-3).

Between the medial and lateral aspects of the tegmentum lies the **central tegmental area**. The

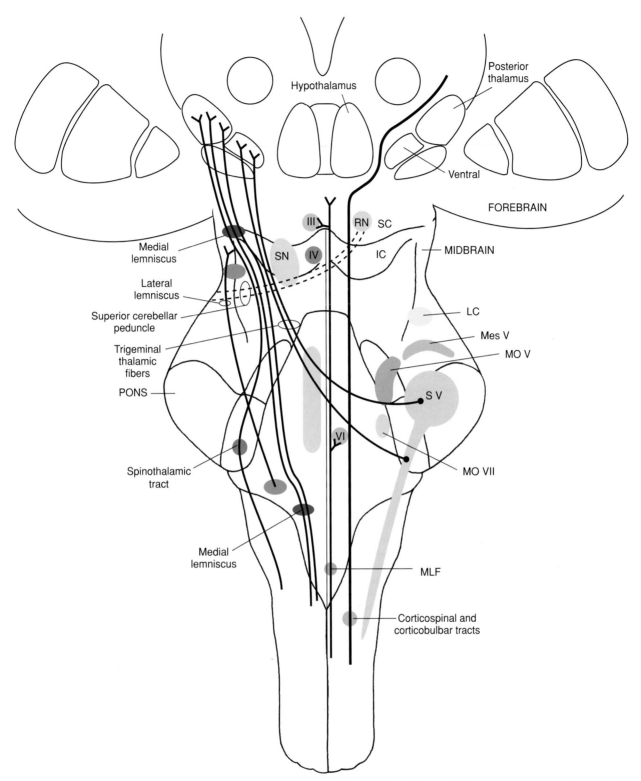

Figure 12–1 The loci of the major cell groups and fiber tracts at the level of the midbrain. Abbreviations: IC, internal capsule; LC, locus ceruleus; MLF, medial longitudinal fasciculus; Mes V, mesencephalic nucleus of CN V; MO V, motor nucleus of CN V; MO VII, motor nucleus of CN VII; RN, red nucleus; SC, superior colliculus; SN, substantia nigra; VI, nucleus of CN VI; IV, nucleus of CN IV; III, nucleus of CN III.

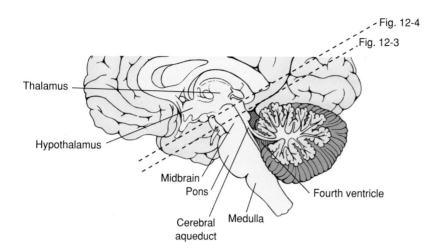

Figure 12–2 Midsagittal section of the brainstem depicting the midbrain and the levels at which the cross-sectional diagrams were taken, as indicated in Figures 12-3 and 12-4.

central tegmental area contains the reticular formation, which extends rostrally from the medulla as described previously (Fig. 12-4). At this level of the brainstem, the reticular formation contains a variety of nuclei and fiber tracts. Along its medial edge can be found raphe nuclei, which include serotonin-containing neurons that project to the forebrain and to lower regions of the brainstem. Nuclei of this region of the tegmentum also contribute to the regulation of somatomotor, autonomic, and other visceral processes.

Embedded within the tegmentum at this level of the midbrain is the decussation of the superior cerebellar peduncle (Fig. 12-4). The superior cerebellar peduncle originates from the dentate and interposed nuclei of the cerebellum and passes into

the brainstem at the level of the upper pons. At the level of the inferior colliculus, these fibers decussate as they continue to ascend to the red nucleus and ventrolateral nucleus of the thalamus, where they terminate (Fig. 12-5).

Crus Cerebri

The ventral aspect of the brainstem at this level contains the **crus cerebri** (Fig. 12-5). As described earlier, the crus cerebri contains massive bundles of descending axons from the cerebral cortex that terminate either within the brainstem (i.e., corticobulbar fibers) or within the spinal cord (i.e., corticospinal fibers). This peduncle is clearly organized in the following manner. Fibers in the lateral fifth arise from the parietal, occipital, and

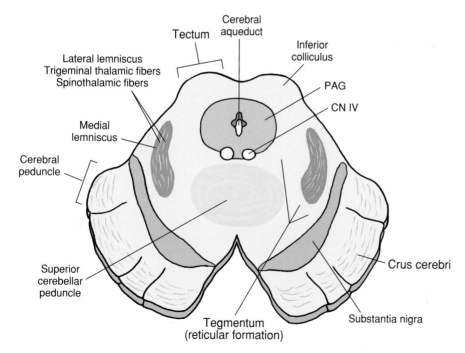

Figure 12–3 Cross-sectional diagram in which the principal structures of the midbrain at the level of the inferior colliculus are depicted. Note the basic divisions of the midbrain into the tectum, tegmentum, and crus cerebri. PAG, periaqueductal gray.

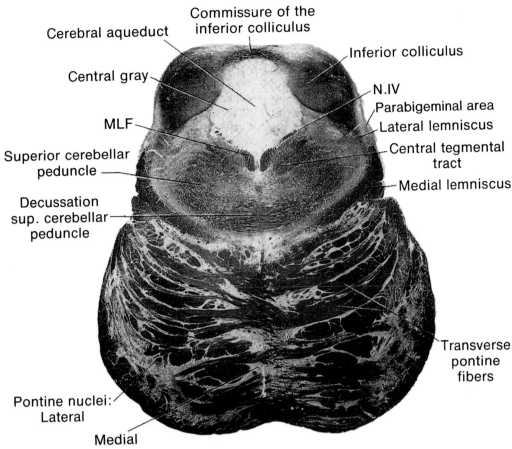

Figure 12–4 Photograph of a cross section taken at the level of the inferior colliculus (Weigert stain). (Reproduced with permission from Parent A: Carpenter's Human Neuroanatomy, 9th ed. Baltimore: Williams & Wilkins, 1996, p. 528.)

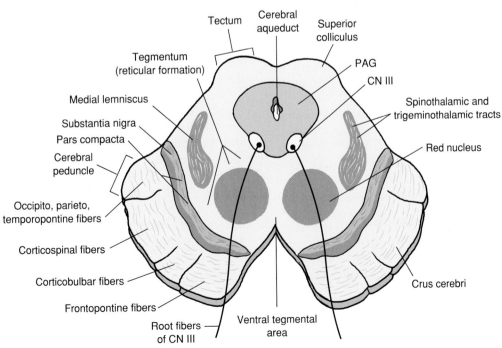

Figure 12–5 Cross-sectional diagram in which the principal structures of the midbrain at the level of the superior colliculus are depicted.

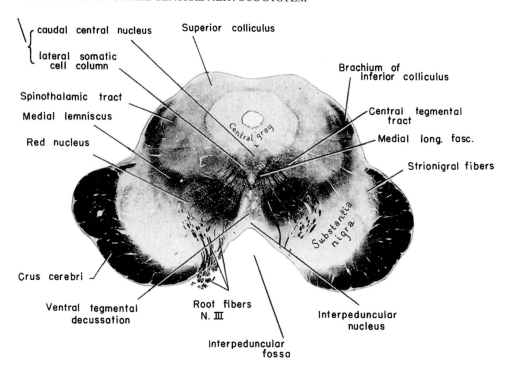

Figure 12–6 Photograph of a cross section taken at the level of the superior colliculus (Weigert stain). (Reproduced with permission from Parent, A: Carpenter's Human Neuroanatomy, 9th ed, Baltimore, Williams & Wilkins, 1996, p. 534).

temporal neocortices and terminate upon deep pontine nuclei. Fibers contained in the medial fifth also terminate upon deep pontine nuclei, but they arise from the frontal lobe. Fibers contained within the medial three fifths constitute the corticobulbar and corticospinal tracts (Figs. 12-1 and 12-5). The organization of these fibers is such that fibers associated with the head region are located medially (corticobulbar fibers); whereas fibers associated with the upper limb, trunk, and lower limbs are located laterally (see Chapters 9 and 10, Fig. 9-12).

Situated in a transitional position between the crus cerebri and the tegmentum is the **substantia nigra.** It contains two groups of cells; one group is located medially and is highly compacted (called the **pars compacta**), and one is located laterally, reticulated in appearance, and called the **pars reticulata** (Fig. 12-5). Each of these regions is important because of the neurotransmitters that they synthesize as well as their projection targets. Dopamine, for example, is associated with the pars compacta and is released onto neurons of the neostriatum. In contrast, neurons of the pars reticulata project to the thalamus, using gamma-aminobutyric acid (GABA) as a neurotransmitter. Clinically, it is known that loss of dopaminergic neurons in the substantia nigra results in a motor disorder

called **Parkinson's disease.** (A more detailed analysis of the substantia nigra and its functions is presented in Chapter 20.)

LEVEL OF THE SUPERIOR COLLICULUS

Tectum

In the rostral half of the midbrain, the tectum is formed by the superior colliculus, which has replaced the inferior colliculus (Figs. 12-5 and 12-6). The superior colliculus receives retinal inputs. Its projections to the cervical spinal cord via the tectospinal tract presumably serve to produce reflex movements of the head and neck in response to sensory inputs. It contributes to the regulation of oculomotor responses and, in particular, mediates tracking movements of objects as they move through the visual field (i.e., horizontal conjugate gaze).

Tegmentum

There are few overt morphological changes in the appearance of the PAG at the level of the superior colliculus relative to that of the inferior colliculus. Just below the PAG lies the oculomotor nuclear complex (CN III), which has now replaced the trochlear nucleus (Fig 12-5). The oculomotor nerve, which includes both GSE and general visceral efferent (GVE) components, passes through the red nucleus and exits in a ventromedial position within the midbrain. The somatomotor component includes nerve bundles that innervate the medial, inferior, and superior rectus muscles, as well as the inferior oblique and levator palpebrae muscles. Thus, the somatomotor components of this cranial nerve are essential for most vertical eye movements, medial deviation of the eyes, and elevation of the eyelid. The parasympathetic components are described in the *Crus Cerebri* section, and the functions of this and other cranial nerves are described in detail in Chapter 14.

Another major change that takes place at this level is that the **red nucleus** begins to replace the superior cerebellar peduncle. The red nucleus is present throughout the rostral half of the midbrain and extends into the caudal diencephalon (Fig. 12-5). It plays an important role in motor functions. The axons supply all levels of the spinal cord and facilitate the discharge of flexor motor neurons. The red nucleus also influences cerebellar activity by projecting its axons to the inferior olivary nucleus, which, in turn, supplies the contralateral cerebellar cortex.

An additional new feature of the tegmentum is the presence of an important source of dopaminergic fibers that supply much of the forebrain other than the striatum. These dopaminergic cells are located in the ventromedial aspect of the tegmentum, called the **ventral tegmental area**, adjacent to the position occupied by the pars compacta of the substantia nigra (Fig. 12-5).

Other features of the tegmentum remain essentially similar to those found at the level of the inferior colliculus. Ascending sensory pathways (i.e., medial lemniscus and trigeminothalamic and spinothalamic fibers) are situated in the lateral aspect of the tegmentum. Likewise, the substantia nigra remains essentially unchanged at this level. The reticular formation is also present throughout this level of the tegmentum and extends to the rostral limit of the midbrain.

Crus Cerebri

The crus cerebri appears similar at all levels of the midbrain, and the topographical arrangement of the descending fibers remains the same as described earlier for the level of the inferior colliculus.

At the far rostral aspect of the midbrain, several morphological changes begin to appear. On the dorsal aspect of this level of the midbrain, the superior colliculus is replaced by a large mass of cells called the **pretectal region**. This region constitutes part of the circuit for the **pupillary light reflex**, which is a reflex that causes constriction of the pupil when the eye is exposed to light. This reflex involves the activation of retinal fibers (in response to light) that make synaptic contact with neurons in the pretectal region, which, in turn, project to the nucleus of CN III. Preganglionic parasympathetic neurons of the **Edinger-Westphal nucleus** send their axons in CN III and then synapse with postganglionic neurons in the ciliary ganglion, which innervate the pupillary constrictor muscles of the pupil. It is via this reflex pathway that, when light is shone into the eye, the pupil constricts (i.e., pupillary light reflex).

This parasympathetic component also innervates the ciliary muscle, which when contracted, causes a release of the suspensory ligament of the lens; the result is an increase in the curvature of the lens. When this parasympathetic component, together with the somatic motor component of CN III, is activated, an **accommodation reaction** for near vision takes place.

Other morphological changes that may be noted at this level include the presence of the **posterior commissure**, which is situated just dorsal to the PAG. It contains fibers that arise from various nuclei, including the pretectal region, which synapse with cranial nerve nuclei that control extraocular eye muscles. Such connections coordinate movements of the two eyes.

Because this level of the brainstem constitutes a transitional region between the midbrain and diencephalon, it is not surprising that several structures associated with the diencephalon begin to appear in sections at this level. Three thalamic nuclei are evident that appear to sit over the midbrain like a tent. The largest of these structures is called the **pulvinar**, which is a massive nucleus that forms a large part of the posterior thalamus and which lies dorsolateral to the pretectal region and superior colliculus. Two other nuclei include: the **medial geniculate nucleus**, which is part of the auditory relay system and located lateral to the tegmentum; and the **lateral geniculate nucleus**, which is part of the visual relay pathway and located lateral to the medial geniculate nucleus. The functions of these structures are described in greater detail in Chapters 13 and 26.

CLINICAL CONSIDERATIONS

The most common disorders of the midbrain result mainly from vascular lesions of branches of the posterior cerebral artery but may also derive from tumors such as those situated in the region of the pineal gland.

WEBER'S SYNDROME

Weber's syndrome is characterized by an ipsilateral oculomotor paralysis, coupled with a contralateral upper motor neuron paralysis. The specific oculomotor deficits may include a dilated, unresponsive pupil, a drooping eyelid, and an eye that deviates downward. This disorder typically results from a vascular lesion that affects the medial aspect of the cerebral peduncle at the level of the superior colliculus and the root fibers of the oculomotor nerve.

BENEDIKT'S SYNDROME

In this disorder, the patient exhibits an ipsilateral paralysis of the oculomotor nerve as well as a tremor of the opposite limb, coupled with the possible somatosensory loss in the contralateral side of the body. This disorder also results from a vascular lesion that affects root fibers of the oculomotor nerve and the region of the red nucleus, including the superior cerebellar peduncle and adjoining portions of the medial lemniscus, and possibly the spinothalamic tracts. The tremor may result from damage to the superior cerebellar peduncle or to fibers of the basal ganglia that pass close to the red nucleus or, perhaps, even damage to the red nucleus itself. Sensory loss is likely due to damage to the medial lemniscus and spinothalamic tracts.

GAZE PALSY (PARINAUD'S SYNDROME)

This disorder results from a vascular lesion or a pineal tumor and involves the dorsal aspect of the midbrain, including the pretectal area and region of the posterior commissure. The patient presents with an upward gaze paralysis (see Chapter 14 for discussion of vertical gaze), possible nystagmus with downward gaze, light-near dissociation, large pupil, abnormal elevation of the upper lid, and paralysis of accommodation.

CLINICAL CASE

HISTORY

Mark is a 35-year-old man without prior history of any neurological dysfunction. For several days, some of his friends thought that his left pupil was somewhat dilated,

and for a day or so, he was perhaps developing a "lazy eye," in which he had difficulty in opening the eye. He ignored the comments and did not seek medical advice. While driving, he noticed that he had some difficulty seeing; he experienced double vision, and, while swerving to avoid hitting a tree that he believed suddenly "came out of nowhere," he collided with a tree that he didn't see at all on his left side. While he was waiting for the ambulance, he thought that perhaps he had hurt his right leg because he had difficulty moving it.

EXAMINATION

After arriving at the emergency room, a neurologist was called in because of the damage to Mark's left eye and right leg. The left eye was found to deviate to the left. When Mark attempted to look toward the right, his left eye remained deviated to the left and somewhat inferiorly. The pupil in that eye did not react when a flashlight was shone into it. The left side of Mark's mouth did not elevate as much as the right side when he was asked to smile, but his forehead remained symmetric when he raised his eyebrows. Both his right arm and leg were slightly weak, and when the lateral aspect of the plantar surface of his right foot was scratched, the great toe dorsiflexed and the other toes fanned upwards. When this maneuver was repeated on the left side, the toes deviated downward. Mark was immediately sent for a magnetic resonance imaging scan (MRI) of his head.

EXPLANATION

Mark has **Weber's syndrome**, a lesion involving the midbrain where the outflow tract of the third cranial nerve is compromised, as well as the corticospinal and corticobulbar tracts running through the cerebral peduncle. The MRI scan revealed an aneurysm (out-pouching of the artery, often congenital in origin) of the posterior communicating artery pressing on the left cerebral peduncle and outflow tract of the left third nerve.

CN III innervates four of the six extraocular muscles, which move the eyes. Unopposed actions of the superior oblique and lateral rectus muscles, the only two muscles that the third nerve doesn't innervate, cause the eye to remain in a "down and out" position. Pressure from the aneurysm on the third nerve fibers originating from the Edinger-Westphal nucleus causes the pupil to be nonreactive. The pressure on the cerebral peduncle causes the classic upper motor neuron findings, such as facial palsy with sparing of the forehead due to bilateral central innervation of this area, weakness, and **Babinski sign** on the right foot.

The Weber's syndrome may also occur as a stroke syndrome, resulting from occlusion of the interpeduncular branches of the posterior cerebral artery, a tumor pressing on this area, or a multiple sclerosis plaque.

CHAPTER TEST

QUESTIONS

Choose the best answer for each question.

1. A 68-year-old man fell down a flight of stairs. Although the patient was not seriously injured from the fall, he reported that he experienced double vision when he attempted to walk down the stairs. Neurologic examination failed to show any other evidence of diplopia when the patient was asked to move his eyes upward or to either side. The neurologist concluded that there was damage to:

   a. Cranial nerve III
   b. Cranial nerve IV
   c. Cranial nerve VI
   d. Ventromedial aspect of midbrain
   e. Superior colliculus

2. A patient presents with double vision, drooping of the eyelid (ptosis), dilation of the pupil, a downward abducted eye, and inability to accommodate to a near object. A staff neurologist concluded that the patient had suffered damage to:

   a. Cranial nerve III
   b. Cranial nerve IV
   c. Cranial nerve VI
   d. Superior colliculus
   e. Lateral tegmentum

3. A 47-year-old woman is admitted to the emergency room. She is diagnosed as having a vascular infarction of the brainstem, resulting in loss of conscious proprioception, pain, and temperature of both the same side of her body and face. The neurologist concluded that the affected region included the:

   a. Midbrain periaqueductal gray
   b. Tectal area
   c. Lateral aspect of midbrain
   d. Medial aspect of dorsal midbrain
   e. Ventromedial aspect of midbrain

4. A patient was admitted to the hospital and examined by a neurologist, who made the following report. When the patient was asked to look to the left, the right eye deviated to the right. Likewise, when looking straight ahead, the right eye also deviated to the right. The patient also reported having double vision and had difficulty in focusing on an object when it was placed close to him. In addition, the patient was unable to move his left arm or leg. The neurologist concluded that there was damage to the midbrain that was localized to the:

   a. Reticular formation
   b. Superior colliculus
   c. Nucleus of CN III
   d. Lateral aspect of midbrain
   e. Ventromedial aspect of midbrain

5. Specialized cells in the ventral aspect of the midbrain are a major source of:

   a. Enkephalin to the basal forebrain
   b. Serotonin to the limbic system
   c. Norepinephrine to the cerebral cortex
   d. Serotonin to the spinal cord
   e. Dopamine to the neostriatum

ANSWERS AND EXPLANATIONS

1. Answer: b

The trochlear nerve (CN IV) innervates the superior oblique muscle, whose action brings the eye downward. Damage to this nerve produces diplopia, which is most pronounced when attempting to look downward, such as when attempting to walk down a flight of stairs. The other choices are clearly incorrect. Damage to CN III and VI would produce a different constellation of deficits, most notably effects upon medial and lateral gaze, respectively. Since CN IV exits the brainstem dorsally at the pontine midbrain border, lesions of the ventromedial midbrain or superior colliculus would not affect the functions of this nerve.

2. Answer: a

The somatomotor components of the oculomotor nerve (CN III) innervate the superior, inferior, and medial rectus muscles, as well as the levator palpebrae and inferior oblique muscles. The parasympathetic components innervate the ciliary and papillary constrictor muscles. Therefore, damage to this nerve will cause lateral and downward deviation of the eye because of the unopposed actions of the superior oblique and lateral rectus muscles and will cause diplopia because the effect is on one eye, thus preventing both eyes from working together. The drooping of the eye is the result of loss of innervation of the levator palpebrae muscle; dilation of the pupil is the result of parasympathetic loss to the papillary constrictor muscles; and loss of accommodation occurred because of the combined loss of innervation to the medial rectus and ciliary muscles. CN IV and VI have no parasympathetic components; CN III passes ventrally to exit the brain through the floor of the midbrain, and thus, lesions of either the superior colliculus or lateral tegmentum would not affect basic functions of CN III.

3. Answer: c

The lateral aspect of the midbrain tegmentum contains the spinothalamic and trigeminothalamic tracts as well as the medial lemniscus. Thus, damage to the lateral tegmentum would cause loss of pain and temperature sensation to both the head and body and loss of conscious proprioception to the contralateral side of the body. The loss in each case would be contralateral to the side of the lesion because the pathways mediating these sensations have already crossed either at the spinal cord (for spinothalamic fibers) or lower brainstem (for the medial lemniscus and trigeminothalamic fibers). The other regions do not contain any of these pathways.

4. Answer: e

Lesions involving the ventromedial aspect of the midbrain at the level of CN III (and superior colliculus) would likely cause damage to both the corticospinal tracts (situated in the crus cerebri) and fibers (not nucleus) of CN III, which pass ventromedially to exit through the floor at this level of the midbrain. Therefore, damage to these structures would result in both an upper motor neuron paralysis of the contralateral limbs and an ipsilateral loss of functions associated with CN III (see explanation to question 2). Damage to the other regions of the midbrain that were provided as alternate choices would be incorrect because they don't include these two structures.

5. Answer: e

Neurons in the pars compacta of the substantia nigra, situated ventrally in the midbrain just above the crus cerebri, give rise to dopaminergic neurons that project to the neostriatum. Norepinephrine neurons are located in the pons and medulla; serotonin neurons are located in a dorsomedial position within the raphe complex of the brainstem; and enkephalinergic neurons are located in the PAG.

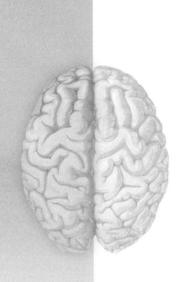

CHAPTER 13

THE FOREBRAIN

OBJECTIVES

In this chapter, the student should be able to:

1. List, diagram, and describe the major nuclear groups of the thalamus

2. List, diagram, and describe the major nuclei of the hypothalamus and the neural pathways that traverse the hypothalamus

3. List, diagram, and describe the structures that comprise the limbic system and the principal neural pathways that are most closely associated with them

4. List, diagram, and describe the structures that comprise the basal ganglia

5. Describe and diagram the internal capsule, anterior commissure, and their anatomical properties

The forebrain constitutes all parts of the brain that lie rostral to the midbrain and are derived from the prosencephalon. It includes the diencephalon (i.e., thalamus, subthalamus, epithalamus, and hypothalamus), basal ganglia, limbic system, internal capsule, anterior commissure, and cerebral cortex. These structures mediate a wide variety of functions, which include sensory, motor, autonomic, and complex behavioral and visceral processes. These functions will be discussed separately in detail in subsequent chapters. Likewise, since the topography of the cerebral cortex was previously discussed in Chapter 1 and will be considered in detail in Chapter 26, discussion of this subject will also be omitted in this chapter.

DIENCEPHALON

The diencephalon consists of two major regions called the **thalamus** and **hypothalamus** and two additional but smaller areas called the **epithalamus** and **subthalamus**. The boundaries of the diencephalon include the following: (1) the rostral boundary is the anterior commissure and the lamina terminalis (i.e., the rostral limit or wall of the third ventricle); (2) the caudal boundary is the posterior commissure, which divides the diencephalon from the midbrain; (3) the dorsal boundary is the roof of the diencephalon; (4) the ventral boundary is the base of the hypothalamus; (5) the lateral boundary is the internal capsule that divides it from the lenticular nuclei (i.e., globus pallidus and putamen); and (6) the third ventricle constitutes its medial limits (Figs. 13-1 through 13-3).

THALAMUS

The **thalamus** constitutes the largest component of the diencephalon. It appears as an oval-shaped region and is bounded rostrally by the anterior commissure and caudally by the posterior commissure. Its dorsal limit is the roof of the thalamus (subarachnoid space in the form of the transverse cerebral fissure), and it extends ventrally to the level of the hypothalamic sulcus (of the third ventricle) (Fig. 13-1). It is composed of a variety of nuclei that serve diverse functions. In general, these nuclei serve as relays by which information is transmitted from different regions of the central nervous system (CNS) to the cerebral cortex. Details concerning the input-output relationships of these thalamic nuclei and their functional properties will be considered in Chapter 26.

The major nuclear divisions of the thalamus, called **thalamic nuclei**, include anterior, medial, and lateral nuclei (Fig. 13-3B). The **anterior nucleus** forms a rostral swelling of the thalamus (Figs. 13-4 and Fig. 13-5A). It has anatomical connections with the hippocampal formation, cingulate gyrus, and mammillary bodies. Since the hippocampal formation and cingulate gyrus play a role in selective aspects of memory function, it is likely that the anterior thalamic nucleus also is involved with some aspects of memory function as well. Previously, it was believed this nucleus was also associated with the regulation of emotional behavior.

Posterior to the anterior nucleus lies a large structure called the **dorsomedial nucleus** (Figs. 13-5B and 13-6), which extends from its border with the anterior nucleus posteriorly to the level of the

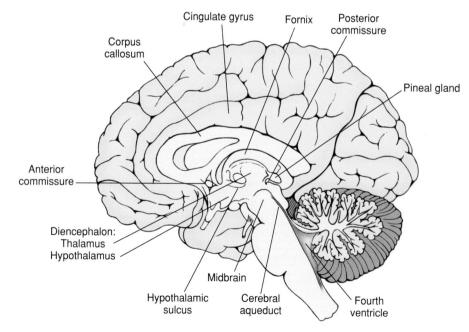

Figure 13–1 Mid-sagittal section of the brain depicting the medial aspect of the forebrain. Note that the diencephalon is bounded on its rostral end by the anterior commissure and at its caudal end by the posterior commissure. Within the diencephalon, the thalamus is separated from the hypothalamus by the hypothalamic sulcus.

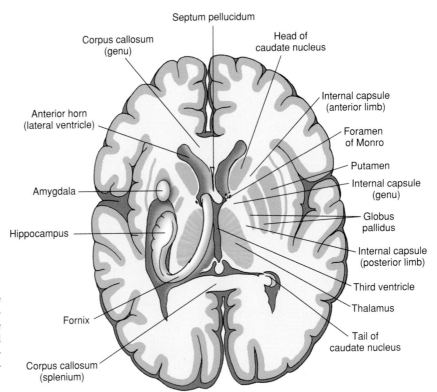

Figure 13–2 Horizontal section of the brain depicting: (1) on one side, the relationships of the internal capsule to the lateral ventricles, thalamus, and basal ganglia; and (2) on the other side, the positions occupied by the hippocampal formation, fornix, and amygdala.

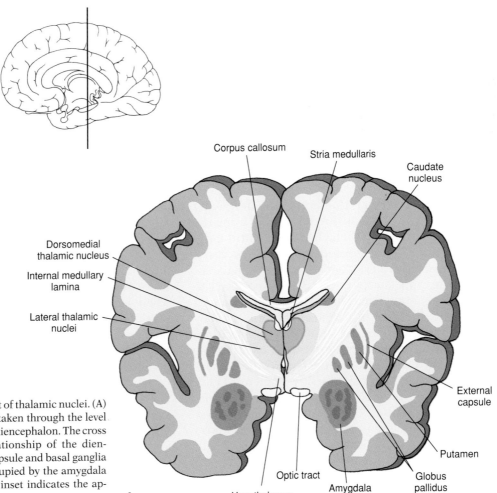

Figure 13–3 Arrangement of thalamic nuclei. (A) Cross section of the brain taken through the level of the anterior third of the diencephalon. The cross section indicates the relationship of the diencephalon to the internal capsule and basal ganglia as well as the position occupied by the amygdala in the temporal lobe. The inset indicates the approximate cut of the section.

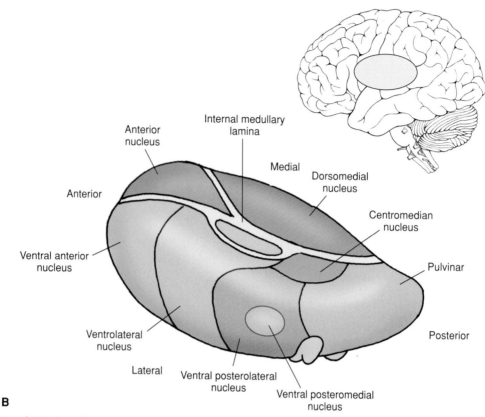

B

Figure 13–3 *Continued* (B) The relative positions of the thalamic nuclei to one another and the position of the thalamus within the brain.

posterior thalamus. The dorsomedial nucleus is separated from the lateral thalamus by a thin plate of myelinated fibers called the **internal medullary lamina** (Figs. 13-3 and 13-6). It is associated with mediation of affective processes and emotional behavior.

Within the **lateral thalamus**, the following structures can be identified beginning from the most anterior level of thalamus. The **ventral anterior nucleus (VA)** is situated at approximately the same anterior-posterior (rostro-caudal) plane as the anterior nucleus (Fig. 13-3B). Just posterior to the ventral anterior nucleus lies the **ventral lateral nucleus (VL)**. Both the VA and VL are intimately involved in the control of motor functions. At the level of VL, a second structure can be identified. It lies just off the dorsolateral aspect of the VL and is called **the lateral dorsal nucleus (LD)**. Functions of the LD are not well understood. Posterior to the VL is the **ventral basal complex**. The ventral basal complex consists of two nuclei called the **ventral posterior lateral (VPL)** and **ventral posterior medial (VPM) nuclei** (Fig. 13-

6). Both the VPL and VPM serve as relay nuclei for the transmission of somatosensory information from the body and head, respectively, to different regions of the postcentral gyrus. Adjoining the dorsolateral surface of the ventrobasal complex is the **lateral posterior nucleus (LP)**. This nucleus may be associated with integration of different modalities of sensory inputs and cognitive functions associated with them.

Within the posterior aspect of the thalamus lie three important (lateral) thalamic nuclei adjacent to the rostral midbrain; they can usually be detected when sections of the rostral midbrain are taken (Fig. 13-7). The largest of the structures is the **pulvinar nucleus**. It is relatively massive in size and appears to be associated with cognitive functions involving auditory and visual stimuli. The other two structures include the **medial geniculate nucleus**, which serves as an important relay for the auditory system, and the **lateral geniculate nucleus**, which lies ventrolateral to the medial geniculate nucleus and which serves as a key relay of visual impulses to the visual cortex from both retinas.

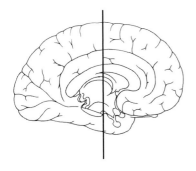

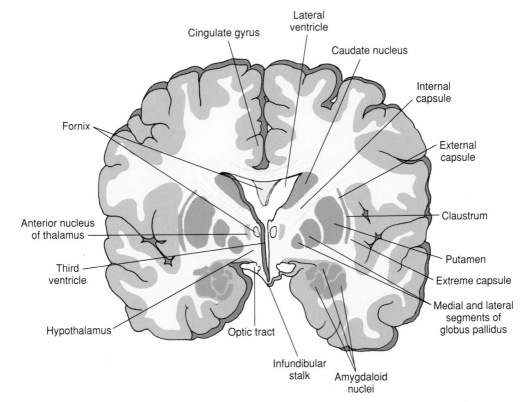

Figure 13–4 Cross section of the brain depicting the position occupied by the anterior thalamic nucleus in the anterior aspect of the thalamus. The inset indicates the approximate cut of the section.

In addition to the major nuclei of the medial and lateral thalamus, which have significant inputs into the cerebral cortex, there is another class of neuronal groups that lie either along or near the midline of the thalamus (i.e., midline thalamic nuclei) or along the lateral margin of the thalamus (i.e., **reticular nucleus**; Fig. 13-6) or are enclosed by the internal medullary lamina (i.e., called intralaminar nuclei, the most important of which is the **centromedian nucleus**; Fig. 13-3B, see also Fig. 13-8). These nuclei modulate the activity of the major projection nuclei of the thalamus and have wideranging effects upon cortical neurons throughout the cortex. Accordingly, these neurons are classified as **nonspecific thalamic nuclei**. Their functions will be considered in greater detail in Chapter 26.

EPITHALAMUS

Forming the roof of the diencephalon are a series of structures called the **epithalamus**. These structures include the **habenular complex**, the **stria medullaris**, and the **pineal gland**.

Habenular Complex and Stria Medullaris

The habenular complex consists of two sets of nuclei, a lateral and medial nucleus Fig. 13-8), which are connected anatomically on each side by a commissure called the **habenular commissure** (not shown on Fig. 13-8). Two pathways are associated with these nuclei. One arises from the medial nucleus and projects to the ventral aspect of the midline of the tegmentum (i.e., principally the interpeduncular nu-

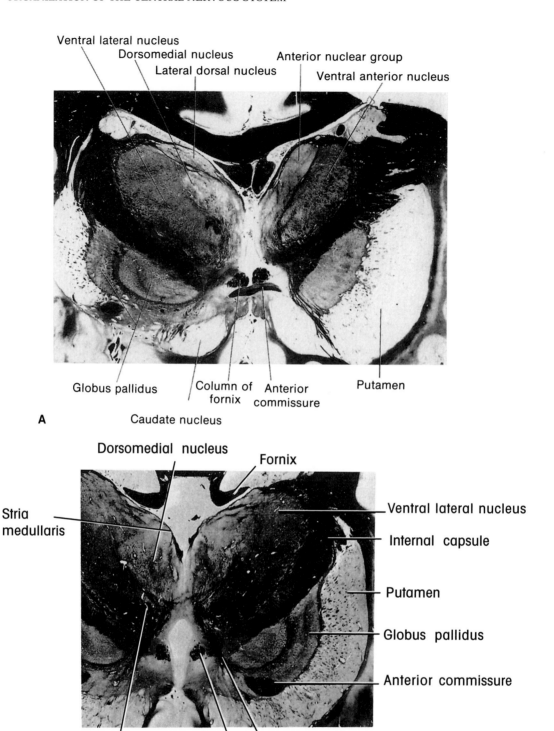

Figure 13–5 Two levels of the thalamus. (A) Photograph of an asymmetrical section taken through the level of the rostral aspect of the thalamus (on the right side) in which the anterior nucleus and ventral anterior nucleus are clearly shown. (B) Photograph of a cross section taken through the middle third of the thalamus in which the dorsomedial nucleus is clearly shown. Note also the positions occupied by the ventrolateral thalamic nucleus and stria medullaris. (Reproduced with permission from Parent A: Carpenter's Human Neuroanatomy, 9th ed. Baltimore: Williams & Wilkins, 1996, pp. 643–644.)

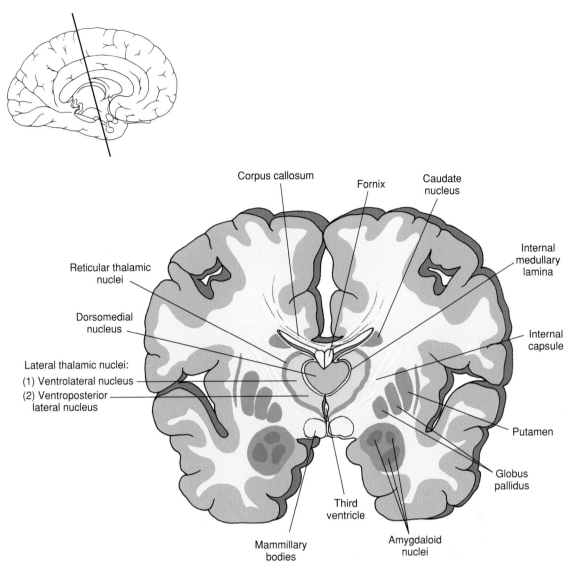

Corpus callosum

Fornix

Caudate nucleus

Internal medullary lamina

Reticular thalamic nuclei

Internal capsule

Dorsomedial nucleus

Lateral thalamic nuclei:
(1) Ventrolateral nucleus
(2) Ventroposterior lateral nucleus

Putamen

Globus pallidus

Third ventricle

Mammillary bodies

Amygdaloid nuclei

Figure 13–6 Cross section of the brain depicting the position occupied by the dorsomedial thalamic nucleus situated in the middle third of the thalamus. Note that the medial and lateral nuclei of thalamus are separated by an internal medullary lamina. The inset indicates the approximate cut of the section.

cleus) and is called the **habenulopeduncular tract** (sometimes called the **fasciculus retroflexus**; Fig. 13-8). Although the habenulopeduncular tract can be easily visualized in sections taken through the mid-brain-diencephalic juncture, its functions remain obscure. The second pathway, called the **stria medullaris** (Fig. 13-5B), contains principally habenular afferent fibers. Sources of afferent and efferent fibers linking the habenular nuclei with the lateral hypothalamus, preoptic region, **substantia innominata** (i.e., the region that lies immediate lateral to the preoptic region), septal area, and the anterior thalamic nucleus pass through the stria medullaris. When viewed collectively, the habenular complex appears to serve as a possible relay by which the limbic system and hypothalamus can influence the activity of

important midbrain structures, such as the reticular formation.

Pineal Gland

The **pineal gland** is conical in shape and is attached to the roof of the posterior aspect of the third ventricle (Fig. 13-1). It should be noted that the pineal gland has no direct connections with the CNS. However, this structure receives neural inputs from the sympathetic nervous system via the superior cervical ganglia. One of a number of unique features about the pineal gland is that, in animals, it displays a circadian rhythm to light with respect to its release of several hormones. This process is most likely due to the presence of an indirect pathway beginning with light cycle information that is relayed

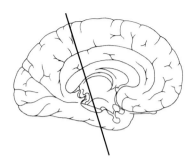

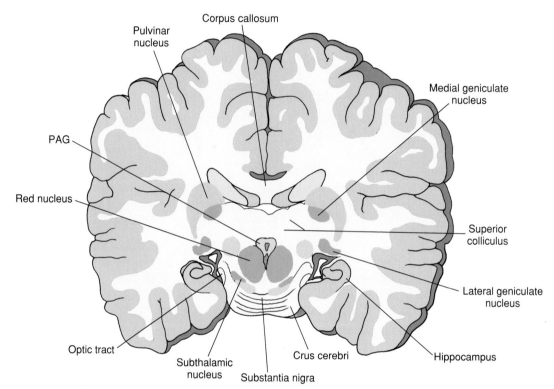

Figure 13–7 Cross section of the brain depicting the positions occupied by the pulvinar, medial geniculate, and lateral geniculate nuclei in the caudal aspect of thalamus and proximal to the midbrain. The inset indicates the approximate cut of the section.

to the **suprachiasmatic nucleus** directly from the retina. This information is then transmitted indirectly from the suprachiasmatic nucleus downstream to the intermediolateral cell column of the thoracic cord. Light cycle information is then relayed to the superior cervical ganglia, which maintains direct connections with the pineal gland.

The pineal gland also contains highly vascular connective tissue. Within the connective tissue meshwork are found specialized secretory cells called **pinealcytes**. A number of different pineal gland secretions have been identified, including biogenic amines such as melatonin (synthesized within the gland from serotonin), serotonin, and norepinephrine. High concentrations of hypothalamic-releasing hormones, such as **thyrotropin-**releasing hormone, **somatostatin**, and **luteinizing hormone-releasing hormone**, have also been identified. The pineal gland likely affects CNS functions as a result of release of these hormones into the general circulation and into the brain through the blood-brain barrier.

SUBTHALAMUS

The **subthalamus** consists of several cell groups and fiber pathways, most of which are situated at the level of the posterior third of the diencephalon and which relate to motor functions associated with the basal ganglia. The nuclear groups include the **subthalamic nucleus** and the **zona incerta** (Fig. 13-8).

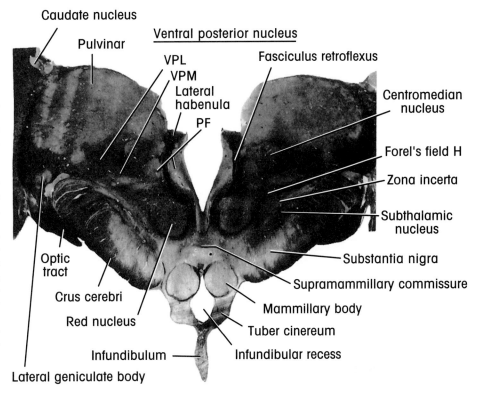

Figure 13–8 Photograph of a section taken through the caudal third of the thalamus through the level of the habenular and centromedian nucleus. Note the position of the fasciculus retroflexus, which passes around the parafascicular nucleus (PF). In this section, one can also identify several other posterior thalamic nuclei, namely the lateral geniculate nucleus and pulvinar. At this borderline region of the midbrain-diencephalic juncture, the red nucleus, H field of Forel, substantia nigra, and subthalamic nucleus can also be seen. (Reproduced with permission from Parent A: Carpenter's Human Neuroanatomy, 9th ed. Baltimore: Williams & Wilkins, 1996, p. 637.)

The **subthalamic nucleus** is oblong in shape and lies just off the ventromedial edge of the internal capsule. It maintains reciprocal connections with the globus pallidus and, therefore, plays an important role in the regulation of motor functions by the basal ganglia (see Chapter 20 for details).

On the dorsomedial aspect of the subthalamic nucleus lies the **zona incerta**, whose functions are poorly understood. The zona incerta is formed by a thin band of cells separating the lenticular fasciculus from the thalamic fasciculus (see the following sections for a description of these pathways).

HYPOTHALAMUS

The **hypothalamus** extends anteriorly from the level of the optic chiasm posteriorly to the posterior commissure (Fig. 13-9). The preoptic area, which constitutes an anterior extension of the hypothalamus, extends rostrally to the level of the lamina terminalis (anterior end of third ventricle). The dorsal limit of the preoptic zone is the anterior commissure, while the dorsal limit of the rest of the hypothalamus is the hypothalamic sulcus and ventral thalamus. On the ventral surface of the brain just caudal to the optic chiasm lies the infundibulum to which the pituitary gland is attached. The hypothalamus includes a number of distinct groups of nuclei, regions, and fiber pathways. Superficially, the descending column of the fornix divides

the hypothalamus into two basic regions, a lateral hypothalamic area and a medial region. The hypothalamus is primarily concerned with CNS regulation of visceral, endocrine, autonomic, and emotional processes. Accordingly, the hypothalamus provides central control of temperature regulation, sympathetic and parasympathetic events, endocrine functions of the pituitary, sexual behavior, feeding and drinking behavior, and affective processes such as aggression and flight. A detailed analysis of the functions of the hypothalamus is considered in Chapter 24.

Lateral Hypothalamus

The **lateral hypothalamic area**, which is present throughout the rostro-caudal extent of the hypothalamus, consists of different groups of cells and diffusely arranged cells as well as a major fiber bundle called the **medial forebrain bundle** that contains fibers that pass in both rostral and caudal directions (Fig. 13-10). The lateral hypothalamus is associated with a number of behavioral processes. These include feeding, drinking, and predation.

Medial Hypothalamus

The medial hypothalamus includes a number of significant nuclear groups as well as several fiber bundles. The medial hypothalamus contains most of the releasing hormones that control pituitary function. It also provides a mechanism that

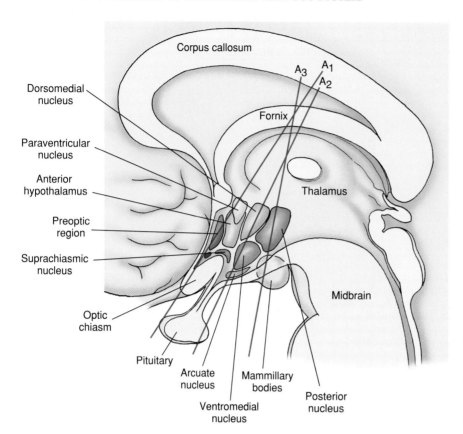

Figure 13–9 Sagittal view of the brain depicting the relative positions of the major nuclei of the hypothalamus. A1, A2, and A3 indicate the approximate levels at which the corresponding cross sections through the hypothalamus were taken in Figure 13-10.

inhibits feeding and that generates affective processes, such as rage behavior, in animals and people.

Anterior–Posterior Levels of Hypothalamus

Anterior Hypothalamus (and Preoptic Area)

Important nuclei include preoptic nuclei and suprachiasmatic, supraoptic, and paraventricular nuclei (Figs. 13-9 and 13-10). The **preoptic region** is basically divided into two regions: a lateral and medial preoptic nucleus. The medial preoptic region is principally associated with the regulation of endocrine function and temperature regulation. Functions of the lateral preoptic region are less well known. The **suprachiasmatic nucleus** is found in the ventromedial aspect of the anterior hypothalamus close to and at the preoptic area. It receives retinal inputs and is associated with diurnal rhythms for hormone release. The **supraoptic nucleus** contains large cells located near the lateral edge of the optic chiasm. The **paraventricular nucleus** lies in the dorsomedial aspect of the anterior hypothalamus adjacent to the third ventricle. Both the supraoptic and paraventricular nuclei synthesize **vasopressin** and **oxytocin**, which are then transported along their axons to the posterior pituitary. The remainder of the anterior hypothalamus consists of medial and lateral regions that are poorly differentiated anatomically.

Mid-Level of the Hypothalamus

At this level of hypothalamus, the optic chiasm has been replaced by the optic tract, which lies along the ventral surface of the diencephalon (Figs. 13-9 and 13-10). In addition, the suprachiasmatic nucleus has also been replaced by the **arcuate nucleus**, which lies in the most ventromedial aspect of the hypothalamus immediately above the **infundibular stalk**. The arcuate nucleus also lies close to the median eminence, and many of these neurons are dopaminergic. It has been suggested that these neurons may be the source of **prolactin release-inhibiting hormone**.

The **ventromedial nucleus** is a prominent structure that lies in the ventral aspect of the medial hypothalamus. The expression of rage behavior, inhibition of feeding, and endocrine control are among the functions associated with the ventromedial nucleus. Immediately dorsal to the ventromedial nucleus lies the dorsomedial nucleus, which is a region composed of relatively smaller sized cells that are situated close to the third ventricle and that share similar functions to the cells of the ventromedial nucleus. Neurons located near the third ventricle, such as the **tuberal nuclei**, release regulatory hormones (i.e., releasing or release-inhibiting hormones) that are transmitted through the portal system to the anterior pituitary gland and thus control the release of hormones from this region.

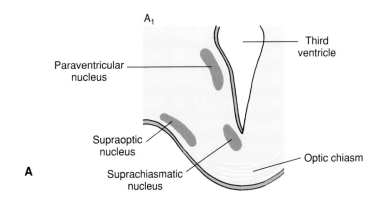

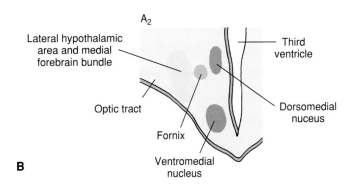

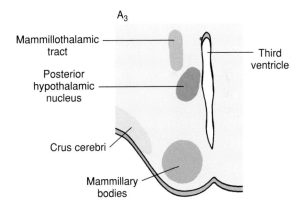

Figure 13–10 (A-C) Cross-sectional diagrams, the levels of which are depicted in Figure 13-9, illustrate the principal nuclei present at the anterior (A1), middle third (A2), and posterior (A3) aspects of the hypothalamus.

Posterior Hypothalamus

At the level of the posterior hypothalamus, the lateral hypothalamus is still present but reduced in size. The descending fibers of the fornix have terminated within the **mammillary bodies**, which have now replaced the ventromedial nucleus in the ventromedial region of the hypothalamus at this level. Although the mammillary bodies receive many fibers from the fornix, it is also the source of large numbers of axons that project to the anterior thalamic nucleus. This pathway can be seen at different levels of the hypothalamus and is referred to as the **mammillothalamic tract** (Fig. 13-10C). Functions associated with the mammillary bodies are not well understood but may be related to the functions of the **Papez circuit** (see Chapter 25).

BASAL GANGLIA

The **basal ganglia** play a key role in the regulation of motor functions. The primary components of the basal ganglia include the caudate nucleus, putamen, and globus pallidus. In addition, the substantia nigra and subthalamic nucleus are included as part of the basal ganglia because of the anatomical and functional relationships they share with the neostriatum (i.e., caudate nucleus and putamen) and globus pallidus.

PRINCIPAL COMPONENT STRUCTURES

Caudate Nucleus

The **caudate nucleus**, which was described previously in Chapter 1, is C-shaped in appearance and follows the lateral ventricle for its entire length. The largest part of the caudate nucleus is called the "head" and lies rostral to the thalamus, forming the lateral border of the anterior horn of the lateral ventricle (Fig. 13-11). The internal capsule forms the lateral and ventral borders of the caudate nucleus; and its dorsal border is the corpus callosum. As the caudate nucleus extends caudally, it becomes progressively smaller in size. The region just caudal to the head of the caudate is called the "body," and the narrowest part is called the "tail." The tail, which is situated on the dorsal aspect of the inferior horn of the lateral ventricle, follows the ventricle in its initial ventral trajectory and then rostrally toward the amygdala.

Putamen

The **putamen** is a large structure that lies between the globus pallidus and the external capsule (Figs. 13-2, 13-4, 13-5, and 13-12). The putamen and globus pallidus lie lateral to the internal capsule; in contrast, the caudate nucleus lies medial to it. The putamen extends from the level of the head of the caudate nucleus, anteriorly, to the level of the posterior third of the thalamus, posteriorly (Figs. 13-2 and 13-11). Embryologically, the anterior limb of the internal capsule grows through the striatal mass, partially separating the caudate medially and the putamen laterally. At its most rostral position, the putamen is fused with the caudate because the internal capsule is no longer present at that level. The caudate nucleus and putamen are referred to as the **neostriatum** and collectively constitute the major sites of inputs into the basal ganglia from regions such as the cerebral cortex, thalamus, and substantia nigra. The claustrum, which is a narrow group of cells separated by the external and extreme capsules, is situated immediately lateral to the putamen (Fig. 13-4). However, the functions of this region are not clearly understood, and this region is generally not included as part of the basal ganglia.

Globus Pallidus

The **globus pallidus** lies immediately lateral to the internal capsule and medial to the putamen (Fig. 13-12). The globus pallidus consists of two parts: a lateral and a medial segment, which are separated by a thin band of white matter sometimes referred to as **medial medullary lamina. A lateral medullary lamina** separates the globus pallidus from the putamen. The rostral limit of the globus pallidus extends to a

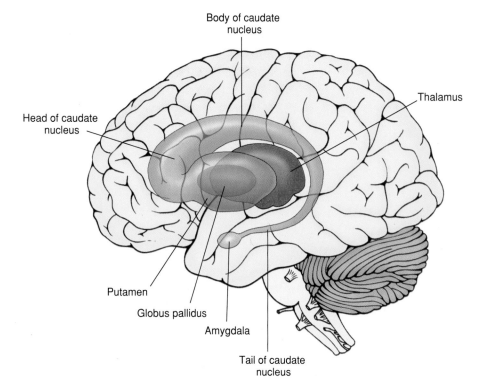

Body of caudate nucleus

Head of caudate nucleus

Thalamus

Putamen

Globus pallidus

Amygdala

Tail of caudate nucleus

Figure 13–11 The components of the caudate nucleus and their relationship to the thalamus, internal capsule, globus pallidus, putamen, and brainstem.

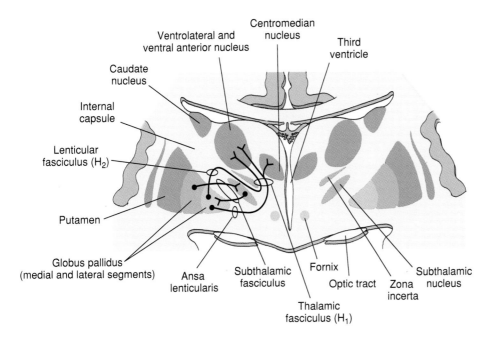

Figure 13–12 The major output pathways of the basal ganglia. The medial segment of the globus pallidus gives rise to two major efferent pathways of the basal ganglia: the ansa lenticularis and the lenticular fasciculus (H_2 field of Forel). The fibers of the ansa lenticularis and lenticular fasciculus, together with axons from the cerebellum (dentatothalamic fibers), merge en route to the thalamus and are referred to as the H_1 field of Forel.

level just beyond the anterior commissure, and the caudal limit is approximately the mid-level of the thalamus. In contrast to the neostriatum, which constitutes the primary receiving area for inputs into the basal ganglia, the globus pallidus represents the primary region for the outflow of information from the basal ganglia. Specifically, fibers, which form the ansa lenticularis and lenticular fasciculus, arise from the globus pallidus (see the following section).

FIBER PATHWAYS OF THE BASAL GANGLIA

Two pathways emerge from different parts of the globus pallidus and can be detected in a cross-sectional illustration taken through the middle of the diencephalon (Fig. 13-12). The **ansa lenticularis** emerges from the medial segment of the globus pallidus and passes in a ventromedial direction and caudally toward the midbrain (Figs. 13-8 and 13-12). The second pathway is called the **lenticular fasciculus** (Fig. 13-12). This pathway passes in a dorsomedial direction from the pallidum around the dorsal surface of the subthalamic nucleus. The fibers then curve around the dorsal aspect of the zona incerta, passing in a dorsolateral direction caudally toward the midbrain. When both the ansa lenticularis and lenticular fasciculus reach a position immediately rostral to the red nucleus, they reverse their course, turning now in a rostral direction while appearing to merge. These fiber bundles, which are joined by other fibers from the cerebellum called **dentatothalamic fibers**, are collectively referred to as the **thalamic fasciculus**. Fibers from the thalamic fasciculus ultimately terminate

mainly in the ventrolateral and ventral anterior thalamic nuclei. The region immediately in front of the red nucleus where fibers of the lenticular fasciculus and ansa lenticularis merge and course rostrally is called the **H field of Forel** (see Fig. 20-7). The H field of Forel is sometimes referred to as the pre-rubral field, a region that lies immediately rostral to the red nucleus at the diencephalic-mesencephalic juncture. The thalamic fasciculus is called the H_1 field of Forel, and the lenticular fasciculus is called the H_2 field of Forel (Fig. 13-12).

LIMBIC SYSTEM AND ASSOCIATED STRUCTURES OF THE BASAL FOREBRAIN

The term "limbic system" ("limbic" meaning border) has been used to describe a ring of structures that were originally thought to be associated mainly with olfactory functions and that lie between the neocortex and diencephalon. The primary structures that constitute the limbic system include the hippocampal formation, septal area, amygdala, and adjoining regions of cortex (i.e., **entorhinal** and **pyriform cortices**). In addition, the prefrontal cortex and cingulate gyrus are often included as well because of their anatomical and functional relationships with processes normally attributed to the limbic system.

HIPPOCAMPAL FORMATION

The **hippocampal formation** lies deep within the temporal lobe. It is an elongated structure that is oriented in an anterior-to-posterior plane along the

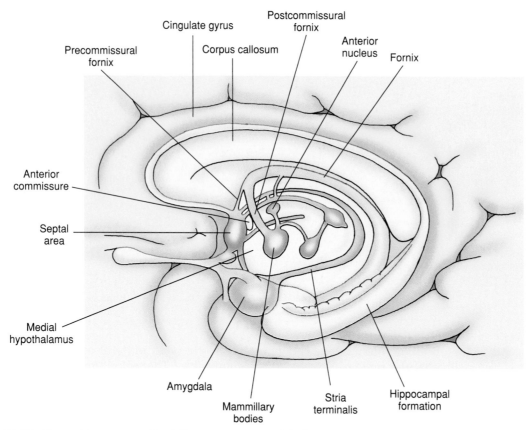

Figure 13–13 The positions occupied by different components of the limbic system. The amygdala is situated in a rostral position in the temporal lobe, and the hippocampal formation extends caudally from its rostral pole proximal to the amygdala. A major component of the fornix projects to the diencephalon (postcommissural fornix), and another component reaches the septal area (precommissural fornix). The stria terminalis projects from the amygdala to the ventromedial hypothalamus. Olfactory inputs form two fiber bundles: a lateral olfactory stria, which innervates temporal lobe structures, and a medial olfactory stria, which supplies the septal area and contralateral olfactory bulb.

longitudinal axis of the temporal lobe. It also forms the medial wall of the inferior horn of the lateral ventricle along its entire length (Fig. 13-13). In its histological appearance, the hippocampus appears as a primitive form of cortex and is therefore composed of distinct cell and fiber layers, which bear some resemblance to the neocortex.

The major outflow pathway of the hippocampal formation is the fornix (Figs. 13-2 and 13-13). The fibers of the fornix initially pass in a dorsomedial direction toward the midline of the brain until they occupy a position immediately below the corpus callosum. The fornix fibers then pass rostrally toward the front of the brain until they approach the level of the anterior commissure. Many of the fornix fibers then pass ventrally behind the anterior commissure into the diencephalon where they terminate in the anterior thalamic nucleus and mammillary bodies of the hypothalamus. The component of the fornix that is distributed to the diencephalon is called the **postcommissural fornix**. Another component of the fornix passes rostral to

the anterior commissure and is distributed to the septal area. This component of the fornix is called the **precommissural fornix** (Fig. 13-13). The hippocampal formation and septal area contribute to the central regulation of emotional behavior, motivational processes, hormonal and autonomic regulation, and memory functions.

SEPTAL AREA

The **septal area** is an important region of the limbic system because it serves, in part, as the relay nucleus of the hippocampal formation to the medial and lateral hypothalamus (Fig. 13-14). The septal area is a primary receiving area for fibers contained within the precommissural fornix that arise from the hippocampal formation. The septal area, in turn, projects many of its axons to different regions of the hypothalamus. Accordingly, the septal area may be viewed as a functional extension of the hippocampal formation.

In animals, including nonhuman primates, the septal area consists of two regions: a dorsal and a ventral division (Fig. 13-15). The dorsal division occupies a position in the anterior aspect along the midline of the forebrain rostral to the anterior commissure, thus forming the medial wall of the anterior horn of the lateral ventricle. The dorsal septal area in lower forms of animals is cell rich and, therefore, provides a thickness to this structure not seen in higher forms. The ventral region contains many cells of a relatively large size that are situated adjacent to the medial edge of the basal forebrain. Moreover, the cells lie parallel to the medial edge of the brain and extend ventrally to the base of the brain. At the base of the brain,

this group of cells then shows a horizontal (or lateral) orientation for a short distance. The cells present within the ventral division of the septal area are referred to as the **diagonal band of Broca**. In humans, the dorsal septal area is virtually absent and contains only a septum pellucidum, which is devoid of nerve cells. Instead, the septal area is relegated to the ventral region (Fig. 13-15).

There are other cells groups of the basal forebrain that are of functional importance and that lie close to the septal area. These include the bed nucleus of the stria terminalis and several regions of the basal forebrain (the substantia innominata and nucleus accumbens).

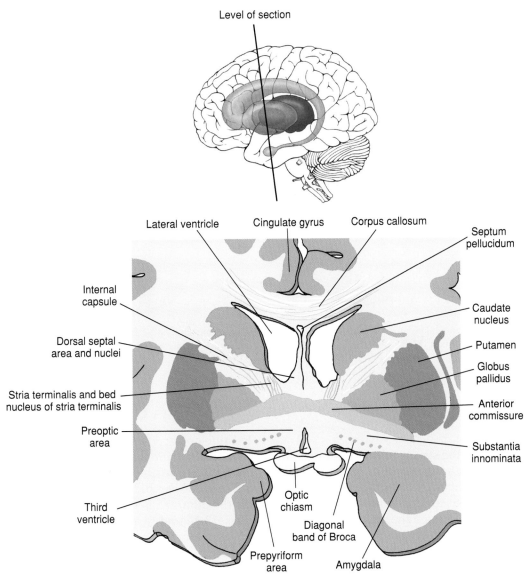

Figure 13–14 Cross section taken through the forebrain at the level of the anterior commissure. Note the positions occupied by the septal nuclei, bed nucleus of the stria terminalis, and preoptic region. The inset indicates the plane of the section.

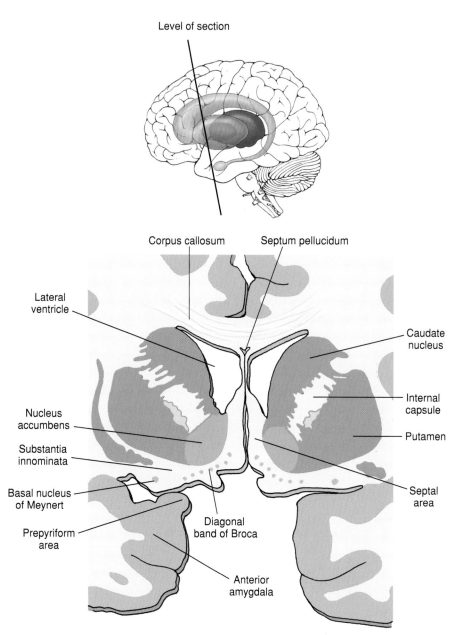

Figure 13–15 Cross section taken through the forebrain at a level rostral to that shown in Figure 13-14. Key nuclei of the basal forebrain include the diagonal band of Broca and substantia innominata. The inset indicates the plane of the section.

BED NUCLEUS OF THE STRIA TERMINALIS

The bed nucleus of the stria terminalis lies in a position immediately ventrolateral to the column of the fornix as it is about to enter the diencephalon at the level of the anterior commissure (Fig. 13-14). It receives many fibers from the amygdala and contributes fibers to the hypothalamus and autonomic centers of the brainstem. The stria terminalis is believed to regulate autonomic, endocrine, and affective processes normally associated with the amygdala.

NUCLEUS ACCUMBENS

The **nucleus accumbens** is found at the level of the head of the caudate nucleus. Its ventral border is the **substantia innominata**, the medial border is the septal area, and its lateral and dorsal borders are the putamen and caudate nucleus, respectively (Figs. 13-14 and 13-15). The nucleus accumbens receives a large dopaminergic projection from the brainstem and other inputs from the amygdala and parts of the hippocampal formation. In turn, it projects its axons to the substantia innominata, substantia nigra, and ventral tegmental area. The nucleus accumbens is believed to integrate the sequencing of motor responses associated with affective processes.

SUBSTANTIA INNOMINATA

The substantia innominata, which is sometimes identified as part of extended amygdala, is located at the level of the septal nuclei immediately below the striatum. Its medial border is the **diagonal band of Broca** and **preoptic region**. The substantia innominata extends laterally to a position where its cells appear to merge with those of the **prepyriform area**. Its ventral border is the base of the brain (Figs. 13-14 and 13-15).

Near the base of the brain can be found a large-celled region called the **basal nucleus of Meynert**. The unique feature of these cells is that they project their axons to wide regions of the cerebral cortex and to limbic structures such as the hippocampal formation and amygdala. Moreover, these cells have been shown to be cholinergic. In Alzheimer's patients, there is a loss of cholinergic inputs to the cerebral cortex coupled with degeneration of these cells, suggesting that damage to the basal nucleus of Meynert may contribute to the etiology of Alzheimer's disease. The substantia innominata shares reciprocal connections with the amygdala, and projects its axons to the lateral hypothalamus as well. In this manner, the substantia innominata might also serve as a relay of signals from parts of the amygdala to the **lateral hypothalamus**.

AMYGDALA

The amygdala is a prominent structure that lies deep within the temporal lobe at a level immediately rostral to the anterior limit of the hippocampal formation (Figs. 13-2 and 13-13). It consists of a lateral, central, basal, and medial nucleus (Fig. 13-16). Details concerning the functions, morphological organization of these nuclei, and their afferent and efferent projections are considered in Chapter 25. One of the primary functions of the amygdala is to modulate processes normally associated with the hypothalamus and midbrain periaqueductal gray (PAG) matter. Examples of these functions include rage and aggression, flight and other affective processes, feeding behavior, endocrine and hormonal activity, sexual behavior, and autonomic control.

Modulation of these processes is achieved by virtue of major inputs from the amygdala to the hypothalamus and midbrain PAG. The most significant pathway of the amygdala is the **stria termi-**

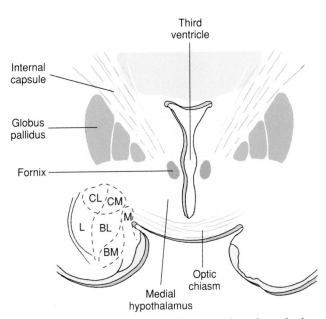

Figure 13–16 Cross-sectional diagram taken through the amygdala of the cat illustrating the principal nuclei of the amygdala. Abbreviations: BL, basolateral nucleus; BM, basomedial nucleus; CL, centrolateral division of the central nucleus; CM, centromedial division of the central nucleus; L, lateral nucleus of amygdala; M, medial nucleus of amygdala.

nalis. It arises from the medial amygdala and passes caudally and dorsally around the posterior thalamus as it follows the tail of the caudate nucleus to its subcallosal position adjoining the lateral ventricle (Fig. 13-13). The fibers then continue to follow the tail of the caudate nucleus in a rostral direction in which the strial fibers come to occupy a position just ventromedial to that of the caudate nucleus. At the level of the anterior commissure, the strial fibers descend in a ventromedial direction through the bed nucleus of the stria terminalis into the medial hypothalamus.

OTHER MAJOR PATHWAYS OF THE FOREBRAIN

INTERNAL CAPSULE

The **internal capsule** contains descending fibers from the cerebral cortex to the brainstem and spinal cord as well as ascending fibers from the thalamus to the cerebral cortex. As noted previously, the fibers contained within the internal capsule play critical roles in sensorimotor functions. It should be recalled that, when viewed in a horizontal section (Fig. 13-2), the internal capsule has three components: an anterior limb, posterior limb, and genu. The frontopontine fibers are contained within the anterior limb; the corticobulbar fibers are contained within the genu; and the corticospinal fibers are present within the posterior limb. The internal capsule also serves as an important anatomical landmark, separating the thalamus from the globus pallidus and the caudate nucleus from the putamen (Fig. 13-2).

ANTERIOR COMMISSURE

The anterior commissure, which lies just rostral to the descending column of the fornix (Fig. 13-1), contains olfactory fibers that pass from the anterior olfactory nucleus to the contralateral olfactory bulb as well as some fibers that originate in parts of the temporal lobe, including the amygdala. Details concerning the anatomical and functional properties of the olfactory system will be considered in Chapter 18.

CLINICAL CONSIDERATIONS

Vascular and other lesions of the forebrain are considered in all of the succeeding chapters that relate to discussion of forebrain structures. For this reason, disorders of different regions of the forebrain are discussed only briefly at this time.

THALAMUS

As a result of a thalamic infarct, frequently involving its posterior aspect, the patient feels a very painful and unpleasant sensation. When the pain persists generally as a burning sensation, it is referred to as a **thalamic pain syndrome**.

HYPOTHALAMUS

Because the hypothalamus mediates a variety of autonomic, visceral, and emotional responses, damage to different groups of hypothalamic nuclei can result in disorders in eating, endocrine function, temperature regulation, and aggression and rage and sympathetic dysfunction. An example of one such disorder is diabetes insipidus, which results from damage to vasopressin neurons located in the supraoptic or paraventricular nuclei and is characterized by the flow of large amounts of urine coupled with the drinking of large quantities of fluids.

BASAL GANGLIA

Diseases of the basal ganglia are characterized by abnormal, involuntary movements at rest, referred to collectively as **dyskinesia** and by abnormal changes in muscle tone. **Parkinson's disease**, an example of a hypokinetic disorder, is associated with tremor, rigidity, and akinesia. The disorder results from a loss of dopamine released from the substantia nigra that supplies the neostriatum. Other disorders include **chorea**, which is a hyperkinetic disorder associated with a loss of gamma-aminobutyric acid (GABA) in the striatum and characterized by brisk involuntary movements of the extremities, and **hemiballism**, which involves damage to the subthalamic nucleus, resulting in abnormal flailing movements of the arm and leg on the contralateral side of the body.

LIMBIC STRUCTURES

Because of their relationships with the hypothalamus and midbrain PAG, disruptions of limbic structures resulting from vascular lesions or tumors frequently are associated with marked changes in emotional behavior, irritability, impulsivity, and rage. Structures most closely associated with these effects include the amygdala, hippocampal formation, and the prefrontal cortex. Other disorders include loss of short-term memory functions particularly after damage to the hippocampal formation, a decrease in cognitive ability and flatness in emotional responsiveness after damage to the prefrontal cortex, and seizure disorders associated most commonly with damage to temporal lobe structures.

CEREBRAL CORTEX

The varieties of dysfunctions associated with the cerebral cortex are considered in detail in Chapter 26. In brief, some of these disorders are mentioned here and usually result from tumors or vascular lesions. These disorders include: (1) an upper motor neuron paralysis associated with damage of the precentral and premotor cortices; (2) several forms of **aphasias** (inability to express or understand language) associated with damage to the ventrolateral aspect of the premotor region or borderline region of the temporal and parietal lobes; (3) **apraxias** (inability to produce a motor act correctly even though sensory and motor circuits are intact) associated with damage to the premotor cortex or to the posterior parietal cortex; (4) loss of somatosensory and auditory discrimination ability after damage to the postcentral and superior temporal gyri, respectively; and (5) partial blindness after damage to the region of the calcarine fissure of the occipital cortex.

CLINICAL CASE

HISTORY

John is a 36-year-old man who had fallen forwards off a tractor at the age of 10 years, sustaining a blow to the front of his head. Ever since then, John suffered behavioral problems. In school, he had difficulty concentrating and paying attention. His behavior toward other students was often inappropriate, with the inability to suppress impulsive actions with lack of emotional reaction. Although he was ultimately promoted every year, he was given a diagnosis of attention deficit disorder and learning disability. Methylphenidate (Ritalin) and behavioral therapy did not make a major impact on his behavior, but he was able to advance in school and graduate.

As he reached adulthood, John had more difficulty controlling his impulsive behavior. He lacked appropriate social inhibition as well as awareness of the abnormal behavior. For example, after a woman rejected his advances, he drove to her house and washed her car in her driveway for 4 hours, until she finally called the police. He also became involved with meaningless activities such as collecting small objects. He often made inappropriate comments, causing him to lose several jobs. John was unable to respond appropriately to emotional situations, such as laughing upon hearing that his father suffered a serious injury.

EXAMINATION

When evaluated by a neuropsychologist, John was found to be somewhat emotionally bland. He further made comments about the examiner, which lacked appropriate inhibition, such as, "Only a stupid person would administer this test." When asked to describe situations observed in standardized drawings, he described the literal meaning of the drawing, while missing the more conceptual or abstract aspect of the meaning. For example, when asked what was wrong with a picture of two children pouring water on the floor of a kitchen and throwing eggs on the floor, he described the picture as showing these actions. However, when asked if there was something wrong with what they were doing, he stated that the materials were on the floor, but there was nothing wrong with the children's behavior. He was noted to have slight groping responses and had a tendency to imitate the examiner. John was referred for a magnetic resonance imaging (MRI) scan to determine if there were any new problems since his original injury.

EXPLANATION

John's case is an example of bilateral frontal lobe dysfunction. Frontal lobe lesions, especially those of the inferior and prefrontal regions, tend to result in disorders of initiative, apathy, abulia (lack of motor activity), primitive grasp responses like those seen in infants, inappropriate behavior, and lack of social inhibition. If the lesion is sufficiently posterior to involve the motor cortex, upper motor neuron weakness may also be observed. These properties were noted in patients who had undergone prefrontal lobotomies for mental illness in earlier periods of the 20th century and are the reason why this procedure was abandoned.

In John's case, the MRI showed atrophy (shrinkage) of the anterior frontal lobes bilaterally, which provided evidence that the initial injury remained. Subsequent MRI scans could be used to determine if this condition was indeed progressive. However, usually they are not necessary due to easy clinical evaluations.

CHAPTER TEST

QUESTIONS

Choose the best answer for each question.

1. A patient was admitted to the emergency room complaining of headaches. Further examination revealed certain motor dysfunctions characterized by involuntary movements at rest. Analysis indicated that the patient had a tumor located near the lateral wall of the anterior horn of the lateral ventricle. The deficit caused was most likely due to impingement of the tumor on the:
   a. Globus pallidus
   b. Putamen
   c. Caudate nucleus
   d. Corpus callosum
   e. Septum pellucidum

2. A patient reported a sudden loss of all forms of sensation on the left side of the body. Following a neurologic examination, it was concluded that the patient had a lesion of the:

a. Right lateral hypothalamus
b. Right medial hypothalamus
c. Right putamen
d. Right lateral thalamus
e. Right cingulate cortex

3. A patient admitted to the emergency room presented with a small pupil associated with some ptosis on one side, as well as a loss of sweating on the same side of the face. This patient was diagnosed as having a lesion limited to the:

a. Hypothalamus
b. Thalamus
c. Caudate nucleus
d. Globus pallidus
e. Hippocampal formation

4. After an automobile accident that resulted in a severe head injury to the driver, the driver was taken to the emergency room in an unconscious state. Soon after he regained consciousness, the patient showed signs of being abusive, short tempered, and subject to exhibiting explosive-like emotional responses to innocuous events. He was given an MRI and referred to a psychiatrist for further evaluation. It was concluded that the head injury resulted in trauma to the:

a. Corpus callosum
b. Caudate nucleus
c. Subthalamic nucleus
d. Amygdala
e. Internal capsule

5. The major efferent pathway of the amygdala is the:

a. Stria medullaris
b. Stria terminalis
c. Ansa lenticularis
d. Anterior commissure
e. Medial forebrain bundle

ANSWERS AND EXPLANATIONS

1. Answer: c

In this case, the tumor was located in the lateral aspect of the anterior horn of the lateral ventricle, which impinges upon the head of the caudate nucleus. Damage to this region results in motor dysfunctions such as involuntary movements at rest. The globus pallidus and putamen are situated away from the ventricle and would not likely be affected by the tumor. The septum pellucidum and corpus callosum do not have any relationship to motor functions. In addition, the septum pellucidum lies along the midline region, dividing the left and right lateral ventricles.

2. Answer: d

The lateral thalamus contains an important relay nucleus, the ventral posterior lateral (VPL) nucleus, which transmits somatosensory information from the contralateral side of the body to the postcentral gyrus. Disruption of this pathway results in somatosensory loss on the contralateral side of the body. The other choices include regions that do not transmit somatosensory information to the cortex.

3. Answer: a

This is an example of Horner's syndrome. It is characterized by a small pupil, ptosis, and loss of sweating, all of which are due to disruption of descending sympathetic fibers. The hypothalamus constitutes an important region that gives rise to such fibers. The other regions play little or no role in mediating autonomic transmission in the CNS.

4. Answer: d

The amygdala plays an important role in the regulation of emotional behaviors such as aggression, rage, and fear. Frequently, head injuries affect temporal lobe structures of which the amygdala is a component. Because the amygdala provides significant inputs into the hypothalamus, which mediates these emotional forms of behavior, damage to the amygdala would disrupt this regulatory mechanism, thus leading to the condition seen in this patient. The other choices include structures not known to be associated with emotional behavior.

5. Answer: b

The stria terminalis is the major efferent pathway of the amygdala. It projects principally to the medial hypothalamus and thus regulates hypothalamic functions via transmission over this pathway. The stria medullaris is a pathway associated with the habenula nucleus (epithalamus); the ansa lenticularis is associated with the basal ganglia, the anterior commissure is associated primarily with the olfactory bulb, and the medial forebrain bundle is associated with the hypothalamus.

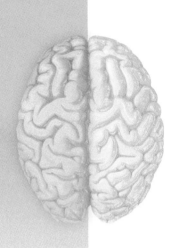

CHAPTER 14

THE CRANIAL NERVES

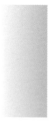

OBJECTIVES

In this chapter, the student should be able to list and describe the functional classification(s) of each of the cranial nerves including:

1. The origin of the relevant cell bodies of the first-, second-, and third-order neurons (where appropriate) for each of the cranial nerves

2. The peripheral and central distributions of each of the cranial nerves

3. The functions of each of the components of the cranial nerves

4. The reflex actions associated with different groups of cranial nerves

5. The dysfunctions associated with damage to each of the cranial nerves

INTRODUCTION

Cranial nerves are peripheral nerves associated with the brain and thus provide sensory, motor, and autonomic innervation to the head and parts of the body. They share many similarities with peripheral nerves that emerge from the spinal cord. Most cranial nerves exit the central nervous system (CNS) at the level of the brainstem (Fig. 14-1). Two cranial nerves (i.e., the olfactory [I] and optic [II]) enter the CNS at the level of the forebrain. Only one cranial nerve, the accessory nerve (cranial nerve [CN] XI), does not emerge from the brain. Instead, it emerges from the spinal cord. Several cranial nerves, such as the hypoglossal nerve (CN XII), are associated only with motor functions. Others are associated with only specific sensory functions, such as the optic nerve (CN II), and still others are associated with a combination of functions. With respect to the latter, such nerves may include both sensory and motor functions (e.g., trigeminal nerve [CN V]); a combination of sensory, motor, and autonomic functions (e.g., glossopharyngeal nerve [CN IX]); or even a combination of somatic motor and autonomic functions (e.g., oculomotor nerve [CN III]). The anatomical and functional properties of each of the cranial nerves (except CN I, II, and VIII for which separate chapters are dedicated) will be discussed in this chapter.

The overall strategy employed in this chapter is to first characterize cranial nerves in terms of the established and accepted classification scheme that has been in use in the literature for many years. This approach should enable the student to begin to learn which nerves have sensory, motor, and/or autonomic components. After analysis of this classification scheme, the anatomy, functions, and clinical correlations associated with each of the cranial nerves is considered separately. While the rationale underlying the order of presentation of cranial nerves may be viewed as somewhat arbitrary, cranial nerves in this chapter are presented beginning with the CN XII and ending with CN I. One reason for this approach is that the important medial-to-lateral columnar anatomical relationships (see *Anatomical Organization of the Cranial Nerves Within the Brainstem*, and Figs. 14-2 and 14-3) of sensory, motor, and autonomic components of cranial nerves are best observed at the level of the medulla and pons. Because this relationship can best be demonstrated with CN V to CN X and CN XII, it was accordingly deemed useful to begin with a discussion of these cranial nerves. A second reason is that this approach enables us to "work our way up" the CNS in a manner parallel to the order of presentation of the anatomy of the brainstem and forebrain. It is our belief that the consistency of this approach will further aid in the learning of this complex subject.

CLASSIFICATION OF THE CRANIAL NERVES

In Chapter 2, the general classification scheme used for the description of the functional components of

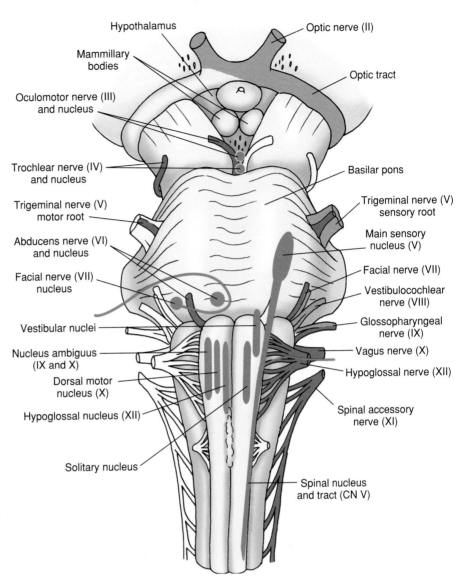

Hypothalamus

Optic nerve (II)

Mammillary bodies

Optic tract

Oculomotor nerve (III) and nucleus

Basilar pons

Trochlear nerve (IV) and nucleus

Trigeminal nerve (V) sensory root

Trigeminal nerve (V) motor root

Main sensory nucleus (V)

Abducens nerve (VI) and nucleus

Facial nerve (VII)

Facial nerve (VII) nucleus

Vestibulocochlear nerve (VIII)

Vestibular nuclei

Glossopharyngeal nerve (IX)

Nucleus ambiguus (IX and X)

Vagus nerve (X)

Dorsal motor nucleus (X)

Hypoglossal nerve (XII)

Hypoglossal nucleus (XII)

Spinal accessory nerve (XI)

Solitary nucleus

Spinal nucleus and tract (CN V)

Figure 14–1 View of the ventral surface of the brain depicting the sites of entry or exit of most of the cranial nerves. Note that the olfactory (CN I) nerve is not shown in this illustration and that the trochlear nerve exits the brainstem on the posterior surface and then passes along the exterior of the lower midbrain to enter the cavernous sinus along with CN VI.

peripheral nerves in general and cranial nerves in particular was briefly noted. At this time, it is appropriate to review this classification scheme in more detail and to indicate the categories of classification to which each of the cranial nerves are associated.

EFFERENT NERVES (FROM THE CENTRAL NERVOUS SYSTEM)

General Somatic Efferents

A **general somatic efferent** (GSE) fiber is one whose cell body lies within the brainstem or spinal cord and whose axons innervate skeletal muscle. These neurons innervate skeletal muscle derived from somites. The following cranial nerves, which include GSE components, are derived from the neural tube and are associated with specific somites: oculomotor (CN III), trochlear

(CN IV), abducens (CN VI), and hypoglossal (CN XII).

Special Visceral Efferents

A **special visceral efferent** (SVE) fiber is functionally identical to nerves categorized as GSE. Essentially, this kind of nerve arises from the brainstem and innervates skeletal muscle. The only reason for the change in classification of these cranial nerves is that these neurons innervate skeletal muscle derived from the mesenchyme of the branchial arches. The term "visceral" is based on the fact that, in less developed animals such as fish, the branchial arches are associated with nerves that synapse on postganglionic neurons that then innervate smooth muscles or glands. Cranial nerves that include SVE components are: trigeminal (CN V), facial (CN VII), glossopharyngeal (CN IX), vagus (CN X), and the spinal accessory (CN XI).

General Visceral Efferents

A **general visceral efferent** (GVE) fiber is one whose cell body lies within the central nervous system and whose fibers innervate smooth muscles or glands. The following cranial nerves include GVE components: oculomotor (CN III), facial (CN VII), glossopharyngeal (CN IX), and vagus (CN X).

AFFERENT FIBERS (TO THE BRAIN)

General Somatic Afferents

A **general somatic afferent** (GSA) fiber is one whose cell body (usually termed "pseudounipolar" neuron) lies outside the CNS. The peripheral limb of this nerve typically innervates skin, skeletal muscle, tendons, or joints. The receptors associated with such nerves mediate sensations of pain and temperature, conscious (and nonconscious) proprioception, touch, and pressure. The central limb of the nerve innervates specific nuclei within the brainstem. The primary cranial nerve associated with GSA information is the trigeminal (CN V) nerve. Several other cranial nerves also contribute GSA inputs to the brainstem. They include the vagus (CN X), glossopharyngeal (CN IX), and facial (CN VII) nerves, which are all associated with the skin of the ear.

Special Sensory Afferents

Special sensory afferent (SSA) fibers are similar to GSA fibers except that they convey information to the brain from very highly specialized kinds of somatic receptors. The cranial nerves with SSA fibers include the optic (CN II) and auditory-vestibular (CN VIII) nerves.

Special Visceral Afferents

Special visceral afferent (SVA) fibers are similar to SSAs in that they also serve special senses and have specialized receptors. However, SVA nerves are distinguished from SSAs on the basis of the receptor mechanisms. SVA nerves utilize chemoreceptors (i.e., receptors that respond to changes in their chemical environment), while receptors associated with SSA nerves utilize other kinds of mechanisms (such as light or mechanical perturbation) to become activated. Chemoreceptors include those receptors that respond principally to olfactory and taste signals. Olfaction is mediated by the olfactory (CN I) nerve, and taste is mediated by the facial (CN VII), glossopharyngeal (CN IX), and vagus (CN X) nerves.

General Visceral Afferents

General visceral afferent (GVA) fibers have their receptors located principally in the serous linings or muscle layers of the body viscera. The receptors may include Pacinian corpuscles, free nerve end-ings, or even nerve endings that are poorly encapsulated. The conscious sensations of visceral pain are generally not specific and are poorly localized. The afferent fibers associated with these sensations convey such signals as thirst, hunger, visceral pain, and general unpleasant feelings. Most of the fibers linked with these sensations do not directly involve cranial nerves. GVA components of cranial nerves convey signals associated primarily with changes in blood pressure. Some authors also include chemoreception as well (see discussion below concerning chemoreception and CN IX and X). Cranial nerves associated with GVA inputs into the brain include the glossopharyngeal (CN IX) and vagus (CN X) nerves.

ANATOMICAL ORGANIZATION OF THE CRANIAL NERVES WITHIN THE BRAINSTEM

The developmental basis for the anatomical organization of the cranial nerves within the brainstem was presented in Chapter 2. As a brief review, this material is presented here and depicts the anatomical positions of cranial nerve nuclei within the brainstem of the cranial nerves (Fig. 14-2) as well as positions with respect to functional lines (Fig. 14-3). Of significance is the relationship between the locations of cranial nerve nuclei and the cell columns with which they are associated.

The relationship between cranial nerve nuclei and the sulcus limitans is the key point to note. Recall that the sulcus limitans separates motor from sensory structures. Those structures that lie medial to the sulcus limitans are derived from the basal plate, and those found lateral to the sulcus limitans are derived from the alar plate. This relationship closely resembles that described previously for the spinal cord in which the ventral horn, which is derived from the basal plate, is associated with motor functions, while the dorsal horn, which is derived from the alar plate, is associated with sensory functions. The region near the sulcus limitans is associated with autonomic functions.

Thus, cranial nerves situated medial to the sulcus limitans have motor functions; those located lateral to the sulcus limitans have sensory functions; and cranial nerve nuclei that lie near the sulcus limitans carry out autonomic functions. As shown in Figure 14-3, the GSE and SVE columns are both located medial to the GVE column and close to the sulcus limitans. Concerning sensory structures, the SSA and GSA cell columns are located in a far lateral position, while the SVA and GVA cell columns lie close to the sulcus limitans. This arrangement of sensory, motor and autonomic nuclei remains relatively constant throughout the brainstem, and knowledge

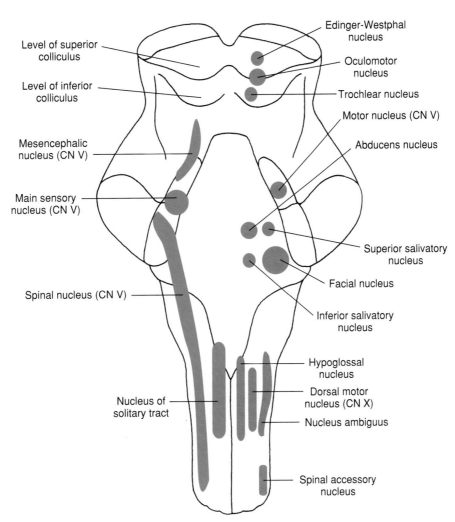

Figure 14–2 Longitudinal view of the brainstem depicting the position and arrangement of the sensory, motor, and autonomic cell groups that comprise first- and second-order neurons associated with cranial nerves. Motor nuclei of CN III, IV, VI, and XII are classified as GSE and are located near the midline. Motor nuclei of CN V, VII, IX, X (nucleus ambiguus for nerves IX and X), and XI are classified as SVE and are located slightly lateral to GSE neurons. Autonomic nuclei (GVE) are derived from CN III (Edinger-Westphal nucleus), VII (superior salivatory nucleus), IX (inferior salivatory nucleus), and X (dorsal motor nucleus) and are situated slightly more laterally. Sensory neurons lie lateral to motor neurons. GVA neurons include CN IX and X. CN I (not shown in figure), VII, IX, and X include SVA components (involving the nucleus of the solitary tract [solitary nucleus] for each of these nerves except for CN I). GSA and SSA components lie lateral to GVA and SVA components. GSA components are found among CN V (main sensory nucleus of CN V), IX, and X (spinal nucleus of CN V receives inputs from CN IX and X). Cranial nerves that are classified as SSA include CN II (optic) and VIII (auditory-vestibular), which are not shown in this illustration.

of this organization serves as a useful aid in identification of cranial nerve nuclei.

CRANIAL NERVES ASSOCIATED WITH THE LOWER BRAINSTEM AND ADJOINING REGIONS OF THE SPINAL CORD

Hypoglossal Nerve (CN XII)

Component: GSE—Origin, Distribution, and Function

The hypoglossal nerve is mainly a motor nerve (but contains some muscle spindle afferents). Because it innervates muscles derived from somites, it is classified as a GSE nerve.

1. **Origin and distribution:** The hypoglossal nerve originates from the hypoglossal nucleus, which is located within the dorsomedial aspect of the lower medulla (Figs. 14-1 and 14-4). Axons of the hypoglossal nucleus pass ventrolaterally and exit the brain between the pyramids and the inferior olivary nucleus. The hypoglossal nerve exits the brain through the hypoglossal canal and innervates both extrinsic (the styloglossus, hyoglossus, and genioglossus, which control the shape and position of the tongue) and intrinsic muscles (which control the shape of the tongue).

2. **Function:** The general functions of the hypoglossal nerve are to control the shape and position of the tongue by virtue of its innervation of

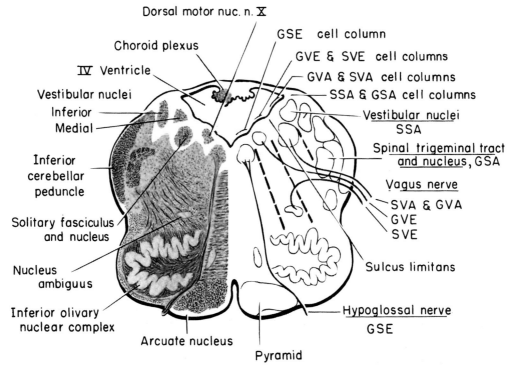

Figure 14–3 Frontal section taken through the middle of the medulla depicting the loci of the different cell columns that comprise the various components of the cranial nerves. Although this illustration is taken through the medulla, this arrangement applies for other parts of the brainstem as well. Note that the motor nuclei of cranial nerves are located medial to those of sensory nuclei. The GSE motor column is located in the most medial position; next to the GSE column lies the SVE and GVE columns. On the lateral side of the sulcus limitans lie the sensory columns, the most medial of which give rise to GVA and SVA neurons. In the far lateral column lie the SSA and GSA columns. Abbreviations: nuc., nucleus; n., nerve. The embryonic basis for this organization is discussed in detail in Chapter 2. (Reproduced with permission from Parent A: Carpenter's Human Neuroanatomy, 9th ed. Baltimore: Williams & Wilkins, 1996, p. 438.)

the extrinsic and intrinsic muscles. Contraction of the genioglossus muscle on each side causes the tongue to protrude.

Clinical Disorders

A hypoglossal paralysis can occur if either the cell bodies of the hypoglossal nucleus or axons that form the hypoglossal nerve are damaged. When an individual who has unilateral hypoglossal nerve damage attempts to protrude his tongue, it will deviate to the side of the lesion. This occurs because the genioglossus muscle on the intact side will attempt to pull the half of the tongue, which it innervates forward, while the genioglossus muscle on the affected side cannot do so. In other words, the genioglossus muscle on the affected side serves as a pivot with respect to the actions of the genioglossus muscle of the intact side.

A paralysis of the tongue, called **supranuclear paralysis**, may also result from a cortical lesion involving the region of the precentral gyrus, which supplies axons to the hypoglossal nucleus. Because many of the cortical fibers that supply the hypoglossal nucleus are crossed, the contralat-

eral hypoglossal nucleus and nerve are affected. Therefore, when asked to protrude the tongue, it will deviate to the side contralateral to the lesion.

Spinal Accessory Nerve (CN XI)
Component: SVE

Our understanding of the nature of this nerve has been clouded by several controversies. Early anatomists believed that the spinal accessory nerve had two components: a cranial portion and a spinal portion. Later studies revealed that the cranial portion represents aberrant fibers of the vagus nerve. A second issue concerns the embryological origin of the nerve—namely, whether the fibers should be classified as SVE or GSE. Most authors believe that SVE is more appropriate since the developmental features of this nerve resemble more closely those of other SVE neurons rather than GSE neurons. The important point to remember is that this nerve is a purely somatic motor nerve and contains no other components.

The spinal accessory nerve arises from ventral horn cells of the first 5 to 6 cervical segments. Fibers from these cells are initially directed later-

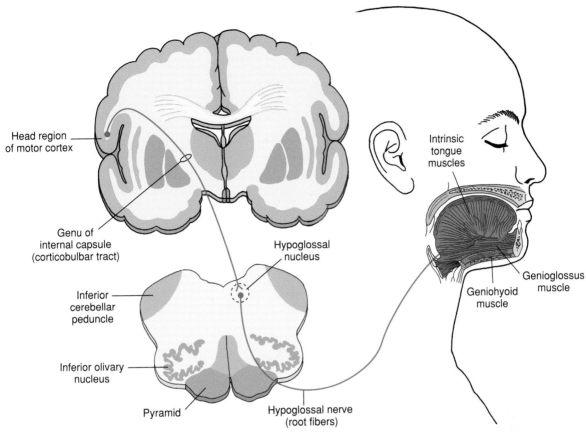

Figure 14–4 Diagram illustrates the origin and distribution of the hypoglossal nerve (CN XII) [GSE] with its innervation of the muscles of the tongue. Also shown in this illustration is the corticobulbar projection to the hypoglossal nucleus, which, for this cranial nerve, is crossed and uncrossed. In some patients, however, lesions of this corticobulbar pathway produce contralateral weakness.

ally, exit the spinal cord, ascend for a short distance within the vertebral canal into the skull, and then exit the skull through the jugular foramen. The root fibers then innervate the trapezius and sternomastoid muscles (Fig. 14-5).

The basic functions of the sternomastoid and trapezius muscles are to cause contralateral turning and lifting of the head.

Clinical Disorders

Lesions of the sternomastoid muscle may produce difficulty in movement of the head to the opposite side, while lesions of the trapezius muscle result in a lowering of the shoulder on the affected side. The scapula will appear to be lower on the affected side with its medial border situated more laterally than normal. However, reports of the effects of such lesions have not been entirely consistent because some authors have reported difficulty in movement of the head to the ipsilateral rather than the contralateral side.

Patients are tested for spinal accessory nerve damage involving the sternomastoid by being asked to raise their head from a pillow if they are lying on their back, or, if the patients are standing, they are asked to press their head forward against resistance. The muscles on both sides are then compared. As mentioned earlier, damage to fibers innervating the trapezoid muscle is evident by sagging of the shoulder and outward and downward rotation of the scapula. Damage could also be determined by asking the patient to shrug one shoulder and to compare the resistance on each side of the body.

Supranuclear palsy also can occur with CN XI. Corticospinal fibers that innervate spinal accessory neurons are contralateral in origin. Therefore, the part of the body affected will be on the side *contralateral* to the cortical lesion. Such lesions would produce a paresis or paralysis of the sternomastoid and trapezius muscles.

Vagus Nerve (CN X)

Components: SVE, GVE, GVA, SVA, GSA

Because it contains both sensory and motor neurons, by definition CN X is a mixed nerve. Its complexity is due to the fact that it contains two types of **motor** components: (1) a somatic motor component that is classified as SVE because it

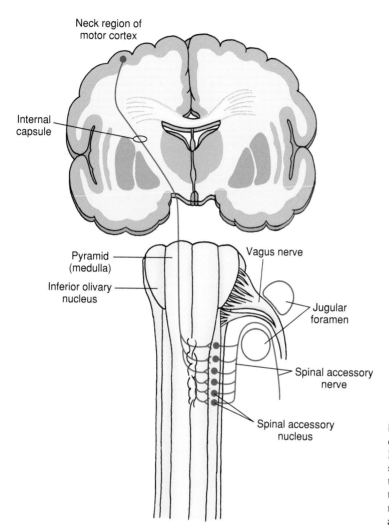

Neck region of motor cortex

Internal capsule

Pyramid (medulla)

Inferior olivary nucleus

Vagus nerve

Jugular foramen

Spinal accessory nerve

Spinal accessory nucleus

Figure 14–5 Diagram illustrates the origin and distribution of the spinal accessory (CN XI) nerve. Note that the cell bodies of origin are within the spinal cord, and the nerve fibers innervate the trapezius and sternomastoid muscles. Also shown in this illustration is the upper motor neuron for this nerve. The cell bodies of origin for this nerve receive a projection from the cortex that is crossed.

innervates muscles derived from the fourth and fifth branchial arches; and (2) a GVE component whose axons innervate wide areas of the body viscera. There are three kinds of **sensory** components: (1) a small GSA component conveying somesthetic impulses from the back of the ear; (2) a GVA component that conveys, in part, signals concerning changes in blood pressure to the brain; and (3) SVA components conveying taste impulses and changes in blood oxygen levels to the brain.

SVE Component: Origin, Distribution, and Function

The SVE component of the vagus nerve originates from the nucleus ambiguus. Axons from the nucleus ambiguus pass in a ventrolateral direction to the lateral margin of the brain and exit the skull through the jugular foramen. Peripherally, there are several branches of the SVE component of the vagus nerve. One branch, the pharyngeal nerve, constitutes the main motor branch that innervates

the pharynx and soft palate. A second branch, the superior laryngeal nerve, descends near the pharynx and breaks into further branches to supply the inferior constrictor muscle, cricothyroid muscle, and superior cardiac nerve. The third branch, the recurrent laryngeal nerve, supplies the muscles of the larynx (Fig. 14-6).

The SVE component allows the muscles of the pharynx and intrinsic muscles of the larynx to contract. Normal contractions play an important role in speech.

GVE Component

Fibers classified as GVE arise from the dorsal motor nucleus, which is located near the floor of the fourth ventricle and which extends somewhat more caudally beyond the fourth ventricle into the region of the closed medulla. Axons arising from the dorsal motor nucleus pass laterally, exiting the brain and joining the vagus nerve as preganglionic parasympathetic fibers. Preganglionic parasympa-

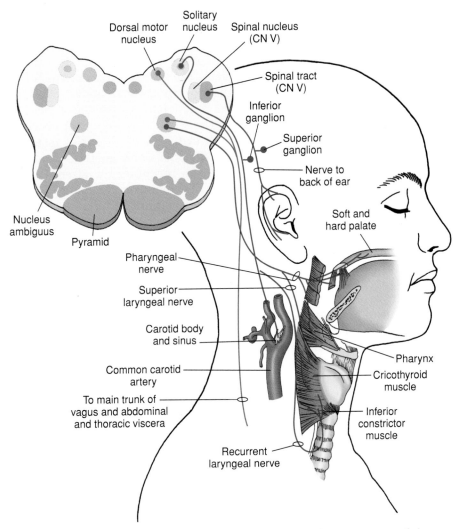

Figure 14–6 Diagram illustrates the origin, course, and distribution of all the components of the vagus (CN X) nerve. The distribution of the autonomic component of the vagus nerve is also indicated in this diagram.

thetic fibers of the vagus nerve innervate many structures within the body viscera. These include the trachea, lungs, heart, kidney, esophagus, stomach and intestines, pancreas, spleen, and liver.

With respect to the origin of the GVE component, there appear to be phylogenetic variations. Most authors agree that, in humans, the GVE component of the vagus nerve arises from the dorsal motor nucleus. Nevertheless, a variety of studies conducted in other animals, such as rodents, have indicated that, in such less-developed species, the nucleus ambiguus contributes preganglionic parasympathetic fibers that innervate the heart. Accordingly, the precise origin of the parasympathetic projection to the heart in humans remains somewhat controversial.

The main actions of the descending fibers of the vagus nerve are to cause bronchoconstriction, a speeding up of peristalsis, a slowing of the cardiac cycle, and increases in secretions of the bronchi, stomach, pancreas, and intestines.

GVA Component

GVA fibers that form afferent branches of the vagus nerve travel with GVE fibers. Therefore, these sensory fibers originate from the same regions of the viscera that receive GVE terminals. These include such regions as the plexus around the abdominal and thoracic viscera, mucosal linings of the larynx, pharynx, soft palate, and esophagus.

GVA fibers also arise from the aortic arch. Stretch receptors in the aortic arch serve as baroreceptors, sensing changes in blood pressure. GVA fibers from the aortic arch as well as other parts of the body viscera have their cell bodies located in the inferior (sometimes called the nodose) ganglion. Central processes of these neurons then enter the medulla and synapse within the solitary nucleus.

Most sensory inputs into the CNS in association with GVA of the vagus do not reach conscious levels of awareness with the exception of some vague negative or positive feelings, such as those of thirst, hunger, or satiety. These sensory inputs do serve another purpose, such as to provide afferent sources for a variety of reflexes, which ultimately involve activation of the dorsal motor nucleus of the vagus nerve. Several of these reflexes include peristalsis of the stomach and intestines, vomiting, gastric and bronchial secretions (which produce coughing), and changes in the lumen of the lungs. One reflex of considerable importance is the baroreceptor reflex. In this reflex, increases in blood pressure within the aorta activate receptors in the aortic arch. Fibers arising from the aortic arch and whose cell bodies lie in the inferior ganglion transmit signals associated with these changes in aortic pressure to the solitary nucleus. The solitary nucleus, in turn, signals the dorsal motor nucleus of the vagus and the nucleus ambiguus, which then transmit signals to the heart. The result is a lowering of heart rate. However, decreases in blood pressure result in the opposite effects, which are mediated through the same pathway. Note that the glossopharyngeal nerve also contributes to this reflex by relaying visceral sensory signals to the same region of the brainstem from receptors located in the carotid sinus (see discussion on pages 233–234). In this manner, parts of the lower brainstem serve to produce homeostatic regulation of cardiovascular processes. Further discussion concerning several of the other basic neural mechanisms of the lower brainstem that control the cardiovascular system is presented in Chapters 22 and 23.

SVA Component

There are two functional components of SVA fibers. One component is associated with **respiratory functions**. Receptors that are situated in the aortic body are chemoreceptors that can detect changes in oxygen and carbon dioxide as well as in pH levels within the blood. Therefore, this sensory component of the vagus nerve is classified here as an SVA because the defining property of an SVA neuron is that its receptors are chemoreceptors.[1] Similar to GVA neurons, SVA neurons arising from the aortic

body have their cell bodies located in the inferior ganglion. Central processes of these neurons enter the lower medulla and synapse upon neurons of the reticular formation located near the solitary nucleus. See the discussion on the SVA component of the glossopharyngeal nerve (page 234) concerning the functional significance of these SVA inputs.

The second group of SVA neurons is associated with **taste**. Small groups of taste buds located in the epiglottis and posterior wall of the pharynx serve as receptors for afferent fibers contained with the vagus nerve. Again, cell bodies for these fibers lie within the inferior ganglion, and central processes of this component of the vagus nerve enter the lower brainstem and synapse within the caudal aspect of the solitary nucleus.[2] Fibers from the solitary nucleus mediating taste signals ascend to the ventral posteromedial nucleus (VPM) of the thalamus, which, in turn, transmits this information to the ventrolateral aspect (i.e., head region) of the postcentral gyrus. Details concerning the nature of the organization and mechanisms of the taste system are considered in Chapter 18.

GSA Component

The vagus nerve also includes a very small GSA component. Receptors (for pain and temperature, pressure, and tactile stimuli) of this component lie in the skin of the back of the ear and external auditory canal. Central processes for this component have their cell bodies located in the superior (sometimes called the jugular) ganglion (Fig. 14-6) of the vagus nerve and enter the lower medulla with the vagus nerve. However, after entering the CNS, these fibers terminate on neurons in the spinal trigeminal nucleus and, thus, from a functional perspective, become part of the trigeminal system in which these signals are transmitted to the cerebral cortex via projections to the VPM of the thalamus (see discussion of pathways of the trigeminal system).

Clinical Disorders

Damage to the SVE Component. Lesions of the nucleus ambiguus or of peripheral aspects of the vagus nerve cause paralysis of the laryngeal muscles and paresis of the pharynx. The uvula is

---

[1]However, it should be noted that, since these receptors are located along the walls of blood vessels, it would be equally logical, instead, to classify these neurons that mediate information associated with changes in levels of blood oxygen as GVA. Indeed, many authors have chosen to categorize these neurons accordingly. Although either classification scheme is acceptable, the respiratory component of the vagus (and glossopharyngeal) nerve is classified as SVA in this text to maintain consistency with respect to the defining characteristic of SVA neurons.

[2]The solitary nucleus receives sensory afferent fibers from CN VII, IX, and X that mediate taste impulses to the brain and sensory afferent fibers from CN IX and X that transmit signals from baroreceptors to the brain. Each of these inputs is directed to different neuronal groups within the solitary complex. Therefore, the solitary nucleus may be viewed as a highly complex structure and one that serves, in part, as a sensory relay for transmission of taste impulses to higher regions of the CNS; the solitary nucleus may also be viewed as a regulatory mechanism for neural control of the cardiovascular and respiratory systems.

often deviated toward the normal side, as is the pharynx. Such lesions frequently produce hoarseness and difficulty in swallowing. If the lesions are bilateral, both vocal cords remain in an abducted position, which results in aphonia (loss of voice) and, more importantly, asphyxia, which can be fatal because of constriction of the laryngeal muscles.

Damage to the GVE Component. Hyperactivity of the vagus nerve may result in increased stomach secretions and ulceration of the stomach. Unilateral lesions of the GVE component of the vagus nerve are generally not very noticeable, with the exception of an ipsilateral loss of the carotid sinus baroreflex (see discussion concerning reflex activity on page 232).

Concerning supranuclear influences, both the dorsal motor nucleus and nucleus ambiguus receive inputs from the cerebral cortex bilaterally. Therefore, unilateral damage of these corticobulbar fibers is generally not noticeable.

Damage to the GVA Component. Lesions of the vagus nerve invariably affect both sensory and motor nerves. Therefore, it is difficult to state the precise effect of lesions limited only to sensory branches of the vagus nerve. However, it is reasonable to conclude that disruption of sensory fibers would certainly alter the cough reflex, vomiting, swallowing, mucous secretions of the gastrointestinal and respiratory tracts, and regulation of respiratory and cardiovascular functions. The presence of a tumor on part of the vagus nerve may have stimulation-like properties and thus cause reflex vomiting, coughing, increased secretions within the respiratory pathways, and even fainting.

Glossopharyngeal Nerve (CN IX)
Components: SVE, GVE, GVA, SVA, GSA

The glossopharyngeal nerve is highly similar to the vagus nerve both in its anatomical as well as functional relationships. It is also highly complex and contains the same number of components as the vagus nerve. It has two kinds of **motor** components. One component innervates the stylopharyngeus muscles, which are derived from mesenchyme (i.e., third branchial arch), and is therefore classified as SVE. Axons from this branch innervate the (stylopharyngeus) muscles of the pharynx. The second component, a GVE, is a preganglionic parasympathetic neuron that is associated with the process of salivation. Of the three **sensory** components, the GVA division transmits information from carotid sinus baroreceptors to the medulla; the SVA division transmits changes in blood gases and pH sensed by the carotid body and taste signals from the posterior tongue to the

medulla; and the GSA component transmits somatosensory inputs from the back of the ear to the medulla (Fig. 14-7).

SVE Component

The rostral half of the nucleus ambiguus contains the cell bodies of origin of the SVE component of the glossopharyngeal nerve in contrast to the caudal half of the nucleus ambiguus, which gives rise to vagal efferent fibers (Fig. 14-7). SVE fibers of the glossopharyngeal nerve pass laterally from the nucleus ambiguus to exit the brain. They exit the skull through the jugular foramen and innervate the stylopharyngeus muscle. Upon contraction, this muscle elevates the upper part of the pharynx, which occurs during speech and swallowing.

GVE Component

The GVE component of the glossopharyngeal nerve arises from the inferior salivatory nucleus, which is located within the reticular formation of the medulla (Fig. 14-7). These are preganglionic parasympathetic neurons that innervate the otic ganglion. The otic ganglion gives rise to short postganglionic parasympathetic neurons that innervate the parotid gland. Thus, the function of the GVE component is to stimulate the parotid gland to release saliva.

GVA Component

Baroreceptors constitute the GVA component of the glossopharyngeal nerve and are located in the carotid sinus. Like those found in the aortic arch in association with the vagus nerve, these glossopharyngeal afferents respond to changes in blood pressure. The cell bodies for these sensory fibers lie in the inferior (sometimes called the petrosal) ganglion, and the central processes enter the brainstem and synapse within the solitary nucleus.[3]

As noted earlier, the solitary nucleus synapses with the dorsal motor nucleus of the vagus nerve and nucleus ambiguus. In this manner, increases in blood pressure activate a reflex mechanism similar to that described earlier for the vagus nerve. Here, stretch receptors in the carotid sinus trigger impulses along the GVA component of the glossopharyngeal nerve, which then causes neurons in the solitary nucleus to discharge. Stimulation of the solitary nucleus causes activation of neurons in the dorsal motor nucleus of the vagus and nucleus

---

[3]Similar to CN X, CN IX also has two ganglia, an inferior (petrosal) and superior ganglion. The cell bodies for visceral afferents are contained within the inferior ganglion; those associated with somatic afferents are contained within the superior ganglion.

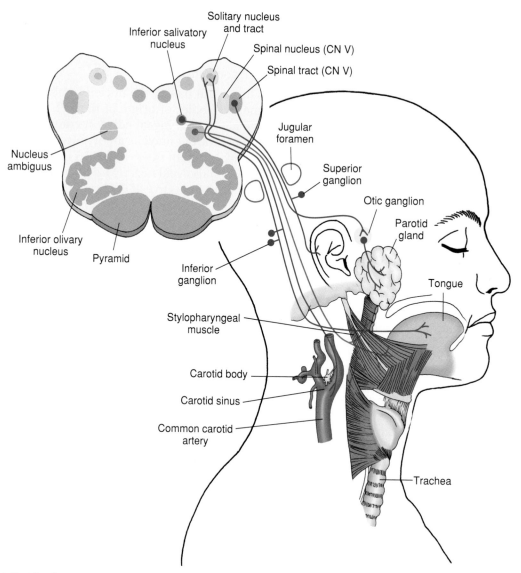

Figure 14–7 The diagram illustrates the origin and distribution of sensory, motor, and autonomic branches of the glossopharyngeal nerve. The diagram also illustrates the anatomical arrangement of the inferior and superior ganglia associated with the peripheral sensory fibers that enter the brain through the glossopharyngeal (CN IX) and vagus (CN X) nerves. Cross section of the medulla shown in the "face" illustrates the principal sensory and motor nuclei associated with the glossopharyngeal nerve.

ambiguus, thus resulting in a vagal slowing of the heart. This is called the **carotid sinus baroreflex**.

SVA Component

Similar to the vagus nerve, the glossopharyngeal nerve contains two functionally different types of SVA fibers. The receptors for one group of fibers are located in the carotid body. They are chemoreceptors and respond to changes in blood levels of carbon dioxide and oxygen and pH. Such changes are conveyed by first-order sensory afferents toward the brainstem. The cell bodies lie in the inferior ganglion and their central processes enter the brainstem and synapse in caudal parts of the solitary nucleus. When there is an increase in carbon dioxide levels within the blood, afferent fibers

within the glossopharyngeal nerve discharge and ultimately activate reticulospinal neurons within the reticular formation. These fibers descend to the spinal cord and synapse upon ventral horn cells of the cervical cord (C3–C5) whose axons form the phrenic nerve, which innervates the muscles of the diaphragm. Thus, activation of SVA afferents of the glossopharyngeal nerve can cause reflex contraction of the diaphragm, which results in increased respiratory frequency and reduction in the levels of carbon dioxide within the blood. This reflex is called the **carotid body (chemo) reflex** and functions in concert with similar receptor mechanisms associated with the vagus nerve. Again, further discussion of this subject is presented in Chapters 22 and 23.

A second group of SVA fibers are associated with taste sensation from the posterior third of the tongue. Activation of taste receptors in this region of the tongue results in a discharge along the afferent limb of the glossopharyngeal nerve whose cell bodies lie in the inferior ganglion. These axons, which synapse within the solitary nucleus, cause activation of an ascending pathway to the VPM nucleus of the thalamus, which, in turn, activates neurons within the taste-receiving areas of the postcentral gyrus (see Chapter 18).

GSA Component

GSA afferents arise from the tympanic membrane and skin of the external ear, posterior third of the tongue, eustachian tube, tonsil, and upper part of the pharynx. These afferents have their cell bodies located in the superior ganglion and convey somatosensory information, including pain sensation, to the brainstem and ultimately to the cerebral cortex. Similar to the GSA afferents of the vagus nerve, glossopharyngeal GSA afferents synapse within the spinal nucleus of the trigeminal nerve, and thus, these somatosensory inputs are conveyed to the thalamus and cortex via the trigeminothalamic pathways (see discussion on pages 237–238 for details of this pathway).

Clinical Disorders

Damage to the glossopharyngeal nerve can result in a variety of symptoms. Concerning **sensory** functions, damage to this nerve bilaterally may result in loss of taste and perhaps somesthetic sensation from the posterior third of the tongue. Glossopharyngeal neuralgia (i.e., severe pain in the region of the distribution of this nerve) may also occur in patients after chewing or swallowing.

With respect to **motor** functions, damage to this nerve would result in a weakness of the muscles of the pharynx and would impair reflexes dependent upon these muscles such as the gag, uvular, and palatal reflexes. In fact, glossopharyngeal function may be tested by determining whether the gag reflex can be elicited in response to stroking of the pharynx wall. Damage to this nerve would also affect its GVE component, resulting in a loss of secretion from the parotid gland. Since the descending corticobulbar fibers provide bilateral innervation to the motor neurons in the brainstem, unilateral lesions of the cerebral cortex have little effect upon reflex functions of the glossopharyngeal nerve.

Vestibulocochlear Nerve (CN VIII)

This nerve, which enters the brainstem at the level of the cerebellopontine angle of the upper medulla, is classified as an **SSA** because the receptors are highly specialized in that they convey auditory and vestibular signals to the CNS. The nature of the receptors, central connections, and functional mechanisms are discussed in detail in Chapter 17.

CRANIAL NERVES OF THE PONS AND MIDBRAIN

Facial Nerve (CN VII)

Components: SVE, GVE, SVA, GSA

The facial nerve is also a mixed nerve. It contains two types of motor components and two types of sensory components. Because this is the nerve of the second branchial arch and innervates muscles derived from the mesenchyme of this arch, it is classified as an SVE. The GVE components serve as preganglionic parasympathetic neurons that are associated with a number of different processes such as salivation, lacrimation, and secretion of mucous membranes within the nasal cavity. The SVA component is associated with the transmission of signals from the tongue to the brain, and the GSA component conveys somesthetic inputs to the brain from the region of the back of the ear and external auditory meatus.

SVE Component

The motor nucleus of the facial nerve is found in the ventrolateral aspect of the tegmentum of the lower pons. Its axons take an aberrant course to exit the brainstem. They initially ascend in a dorsomedial direction to the region of the floor of the fourth ventricle. They then pass laterally over the abducens nucleus (CN VI) and descend in a ventrolateral trajectory, exiting the brainstem at the level of the caudal border of the pons (Fig. 14-8). Upon exiting the brain, fibers of the facial nerve enter the internal acoustic meatus and petrous portion of the temporal bone. The fibers then continue along and through the facial canal and ultimately exit the skull through the stylomastoid foramen. SVE fibers divide into a number of branches and supply the muscles of facial expression (i.e., buccinator muscle [region of the cheek] and frontalis and orbicularis oris muscles [upper part of face]) as well as the auricular, posterior belly of the digastric, stylohyoid, platysma, and stapedius muscles.

The major function of the SVE component is to control the muscles of facial expression. Several other actions include reflex closing of the eyelids upon touching the cornea (see discussion of trigeminal reflexes on pages 238 and 240), and reflex contraction of the stapedius muscle following a loud noise.

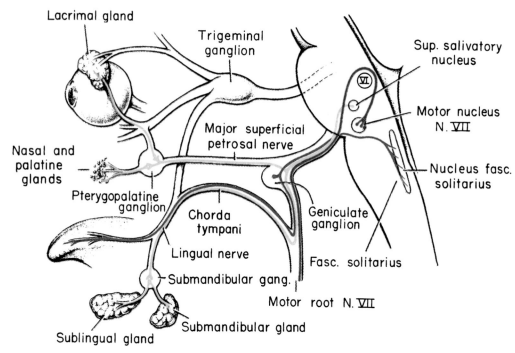

Figure 14–8 Diagram illustrates: (1) the special visceral afferent (SVA) pathway for taste inputs to the brain from the anterior two thirds of the tongue via the facial (VII) nerve; and (2) general visceral efferent (GVE) pathway to the lacrimal, pterygopalatine, nasal, palatine, and salivary glands from CN VII. Not shown is the distribution of fibers to the muscles of facial expression contained in the motor root for the special visceral efferent component (SVE) of CN VII. Abbreviations: Sup., superior; fasc., fasciculus. (Reproduced with permission from Parent A: Carpenter's Human Neuroanatomy, 9th ed. Baltimore: Williams & Wilkins, 1996, p. 495.)

GVE Component

The GVE component of the facial nerve arises from the superior salivatory nucleus located in the reticular formation of the lower pons (Fig. 14-8). Preganglionic neurons exit the brain in the intermediate nerve, which emerges between the facial and auditory-vestibular nerves. The nerve breaks into two divisions. One branch joins the chorda tympani and then the lingual nerve and ultimately synapses in the submandibular ganglion. Postganglionic parasympathetic fibers arise from the submandibular ganglion and supply the submandibular and sublingual glands. Other preganglionic fibers in the intermediate nerve join the major petrosal nerve and terminate in the pterygopalatine ganglion. From this ganglion, postganglionic parasympathetic fibers arise and supply the lacrimal, nasal, and palatine glands.

Activation of the GVE components induces salivation from the submandibular and sublingual glands and secretion from the lacrimal and mucous glands of the nasal and oral cavities. Lesions of the intermediate nerve frequently produce disturbances in secretion of saliva and lacrimal secretion.

SVA Component

SVA neurons convey taste sensation from the anterior two thirds of the tongue to the CNS. The cell bodies for these neurons lie in the geniculate ganglion, and the peripheral processes run in the lingual and chorda tympani nerves. Centrally, they pass into the brainstem through the intermediate nerve and terminate in the rostral half of the solitary nucleus. Taste information is transmitted from the solitary nucleus to the nucleus VPM of the thalamus and from the VPM to the taste-receiving regions of the lateral parts of the postcentral gyrus.

GSA Component

As indicated earlier, the facial nerve also contains a small GSA component, which conveys cutaneous sensation from the back of the ear and external auditory meatus.[4] The cell bodies lie in the geniculate ganglion, and the central processes enter the CNS through the intermediate nerve. Once these fibers have entered the CNS, they then enter the spinal tract of the trigeminal nerve and synapse upon neurons of the spinal trigeminal nucleus. In this manner, cutaneous sensation originating from the facial nerve is transmitted to the cerebral cortex via the trigeminal system in a manner similar to that

---

[4]Note that somatosensory information from the anterior two thirds of the tongue passes through the mandibular branch of the GSA component of the trigeminal nerve to the brainstem.

described earlier for GSA inputs from the vagus and glossopharyngeal nerves.

Clinical Disorders

I. Upper Motor Neurons. Corticobulbar fibers provide bilateral inputs into the dorsal half of the motor nucleus of the facial nerve. However, inputs into more ventral aspects of this nucleus, whose axons innervate facial muscles below the forehead, are from the contralateral cerebral cortex. Therefore, the muscles of the forehead (i.e., frontalis and orbicularis oculi) are generally not affected by a frontal cortical lesion. Such individuals can typically wrinkle their forehead and close their eyes after unilateral lesions of the cerebral cortex. On the other hand, as a result of supranuclear lesions, patients will not be able to raise the corners of their mouths or move their lips contralateral to the lesions. Thus, this distinction is characteristic of an upper motor neuron lesion with respect to the facial nerve and clearly different from a lower motor neuron lesion of this cranial nerve (described in the following section).

II. Lower Motor Neurons. A lower motor neuron paralysis may result from damage to the facial nerve, its peripheral branches, or the facial nucleus. The patient shows little or no facial expression. If muscle tone is lost, the affected side of the face may take on the appearance of an empty, smooth-like expression. The angle of the mouth on the affected side may also droop and, when attempting to display their teeth, patients cannot bring the angle of the mouth laterally. Speech may also be affected, and patients are unable to whistle. These patients also cannot close the affected eye, and the eye-blink reflex is lost. Moreover, lesions of the facial nerve can also produce hyperacusis, which is an increase in sensitivity to sounds on the side of the lesion, because of a paralysis of the stapedius muscle. These effects are frequently due to an external blow to the face or overexposure to cold weather and affect peripheral branches of the facial nerve after the nerve exits the skull. These disorders are commonly referred to as **Bell's palsy**.

The effects of damage to the facial nerve upon sensory systems include primarily loss of taste sensation from the anterior two thirds of the tongue and loss of general sensation from the back of the ear and external auditory meatus.

Trigeminal Nerve (CN V)
Components: GSA, SVE

The trigeminal nerve is very large and can be easily seen upon its emergence at the level of the middle of the pons near the position of emergence of the middle cerebellar peduncle. It contains a massive GSA component, which provides most of the somatosensory inputs from the region of the anterior two thirds of the head (i.e., pain, touch, pressure, temperature) to the CNS. The SVE component, which innervates skeletal muscle from the mesenchyme of the first branchial arch, is much smaller in size than the sensory branches but provides motor innervation of the muscles of mastication.

GSA: Origin, Distribution, and Function

The cell bodies of the GSA component of the trigeminal nerve are located in the trigeminal (sometimes called the gasserian or semilunar) ganglion. The ganglion itself is located on a cleft of the petrous bone lateral to the cavernous sinus. There are three principal divisions of the sensory components of the trigeminal nerve: ophthalmic, maxillary, and mandibular (Fig. 14-9A). Concerning the peripheral distribution of the **ophthalmic** division, nerve fibers supply the forehead, cornea, upper part of the eyelid, dorsal surface of the nose, and mucous membranes of the nasal and frontal sinuses. The central processes of this branch enter the skull through the superior orbital fissure. The peripheral distribution of the **maxillary** division includes the lateral surface of the nose, upper teeth, hard palate, upper cheek, and mucous membranes of the upper teeth, nose, and roof of the mouth. This division enters the skull through the foramen rotundum. The third division, called the **mandibular** division, supplies the lower jaw, lower teeth, chin, parts of the posterior cheek, temple, external ear, anterior two thirds of the tongue, and floor of the mouth. All branches of the trigeminal nerve innervate the dura. The mandibular division enters the skull through the foramen ovale.

As noted earlier, the central processes of each of the divisions of the trigeminal nerve enter the skull through different foramina. However, upon entry into the pons, these (first-order) fibers may take one of two primary directions: (1) they may synapse directly within the main sensory nucleus of CN V; or (2) the fibers may enter the tract of CN V and descend to different levels of the lower pons and medulla and then make a synapse within the spinal nucleus of CN V. Some trigeminal pain fibers associated with the posterior aspect of the face may even extend as far caudally as C2 of the spinal cord. From both the main sensory and spinal nucleus, second-order neurons arise, and their axons are distributed to the VPM nucleus of the contralateral thalamus. Fibers that arise from the spinal nucleus are distributed to the

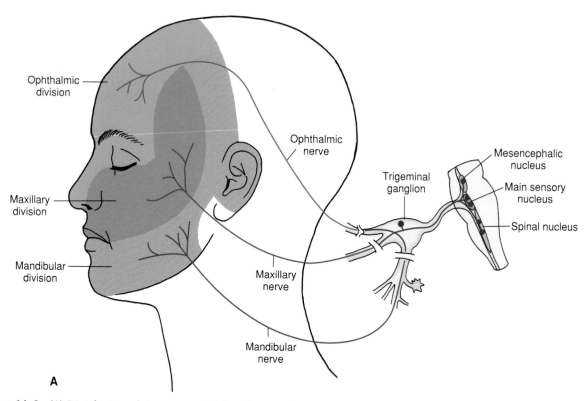

Figure 14–9 (A) Distribution of the sensory (GSA) and motor (SVE) components of the trigeminal nerve, including the sensory arrangement of the sensory divisions of the trigeminal nerve.

contralateral VPM via the ventral trigeminothalamic tract. Fibers that issue from the main sensory nucleus are distributed bilaterally to the VPM nucleus. Those fibers that pass ipsilaterally do so in the dorsal trigeminothalamic tract, while fibers passing contralaterally do so in the ventral trigeminothalamic tract. Collectively, it would certainly appear that the ventral trigeminothalamic tract is far more significant in transmitting sensory information from the trigeminal system to the thalamus. Third-order sensory fibers arising from the VPM then project to the ipsilateral face region of the postcentral gyrus (Fig. 14-9B).

Both experimental and clinical studies have revealed that the fibers mediating pain and temperature sensation are distributed to the caudal aspect of the spinal nucleus, while conscious proprioception, pressure, and tactile sensation are distributed through the main sensory nucleus and possibly parts of the spinal nucleus. Knowledge of the dissociation of pain fibers from other forms of somatosensory inputs has been applied clinically; for example, severing the sensory root fibers after they enter the spinal tract of CN V can alleviate intense forms of trigeminal neuralgia.

The receptors for some of the fibers contained within the mandibular branch are muscle spindles. These fibers mediate unconscious proprio-

ceptive signals to the brain and terminate in the mesencephalic nucleus of CN V, which represents part of the first-order sensory neuron. For this reason, the unusual feature is that the mesencephalic nucleus, which appears to be similar in appearance to cells of the Gasserian ganglion, does not lie outside the CNS but, instead, is situated within it. Although the mesencephalic nucleus is functionally similar to the dorsal root ganglion, it represents an anomaly in that it is the only sensory structure whose first-order cell bodies lie within the CNS and not in the periphery. Similar to neurons of the dorsal root ganglion, there is a second limb of the axon emanating from the mesencephalic nucleus, which transmits signals away from it to the motor nucleus of CN V. This provides the basis for a monosynaptic reflex that is sometimes referred to as the **jaw jerk reflex**. This is a stretch reflex because it occurs after stimulation of muscle spindles in the masseter muscle of the lower jaw. Afferent impulses (1a fibers) cause a discharge of neurons in the motor nucleus, which is then followed by a jaw closing response. Other fibers from the mesencephalic nucleus project to the cerebellum, thus providing the cerebellum with information concerning the status of muscles of the lower jaw.

From this discussion, it is reasonable to conclude that fibers of the trigeminal system share

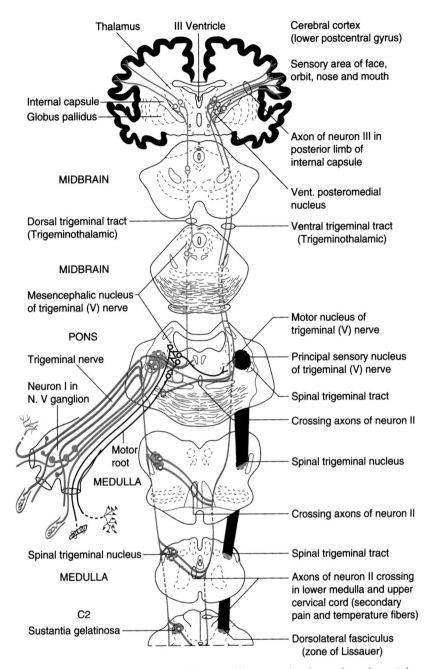

Figure 14–9 *Continued* (B) Organization and distribution of the central trigeminal pathways from the periphery to the cerebral cortex. (Used with permission from Parent A: Carpenter's Human Neuroanatomy, 9th ed. Baltimore: Williams & Wilkins, 1996, p. 505.)

parallel relationships with several of the sensory pathways of the spinal cord. For example, the pathways that mediate pain and temperature sensation from the head to the thalamus via the ventral trigeminothalamic tract can be likened to the lateral spinothalamic tract; the pathways that mediate conscious proprioception and tactile inputs to the thalamus via the dorsal trigeminothalamic tract can be likened to the medial lemniscus; and the pathway involving inputs to the mesencephalic nucleus and its projection to the cerebellum shares

similarities with the posterior spinocerebellar tract. In this manner, the same kinds of sensory inputs that reach the brain from the body region can also reach the brain from the region of the head by virtue of specific ascending pathways within the trigeminal complex.

SVE: Origin, Distribution, and Function

The motor trigeminal nucleus is located just medial to the main sensory nucleus of CN V and is separated from it by root fibers of the trigeminal nerve

(Fig. 14-9B). Axons of the motor nucleus pass in a ventrolateral direction and exit the brain at the approximate level of entry of the sensory fibers. Motor fibers exit the skull through the foramen ovale and supply the muscles of mastication (i.e., masseter, pterygoid, temporalis, and mylohyoid muscles). The main functions of these muscles are to produce chewing and biting responses (see earlier description of jaw jerk reflex on page 238). The motor nucleus receives bilateral inputs from the cerebral cortex. Therefore, motor deficits following a unilateral upper motor neuron lesion are generally not observed.

Clinical Disorders

Because the trigeminal nerve contains both motor and sensory components, dysfunctions of either component may result from lesions of this nerve. If there is a paralysis or paresis affecting the muscles of mastication, they will become flaccid after showing spasticity. Moreover, if the patient is asked to open his mouth, and the pterygoid muscles are affected, then the jaw will deviate to the affected side.

Concerning the sensory components, applying pain, tactile, or temperature stimuli to the area in question can test for damage to any of the sensory branches. Failure to recognize any of these stimuli would indicate a sensory loss to the affected area. If sensory loss includes the ophthalmic branch, then it is likely that the **corneal reflex** (i.e., blinking in response to touching the cornea, which involves reflex connections between sensory afferent fibers in the ophthalmic nerve that make synaptic connections with motor fibers of CN VII) will be lost. Severe pain can result from irritation of the trigeminal nerve by such factors as inflammation, tumor, or vascular lesion. This is called trigeminal neuralgia (sometimes called **tic douloureux**) and is often localized to a portion of one side of the face (usually associated with a specific branch of the trigeminal nerve that is subject to such irritation). Neurologic pain may also occur in association with the viral disease, herpes zoster (shingles), affecting mainly the ophthalmic division of the trigeminal nerve, called **ophthalmic zoster.**

Sensory loss does not only result from peripheral nerve damage. It may result from damage to the CNS as well. For example, a lesion resulting from an occlusion of the posterior inferior cerebellar artery involves the lateral aspect of the medulla; the ensuing disorder is the **Wallenberg syndrome.** This will produce (in addition to some problems with eating) damage to both the lateral spinothalamic tract as well as to the spinal trigeminal tract and nucleus. Accordingly, there will be a loss of pain and temperature sensation on the ipsilateral side of the face and contralateral side of the body.

CRANIAL NERVES OF THE PONS AND MIDBRAIN ASSOCIATED WITH THE CONTROL OF EYE MOVEMENTS

Abducens Nerve (CN VI)

Components: GSE

The abducens nerve is a pure motor nerve whose principal function is to move the eye laterally (i.e., abduct the eye). The cell bodies of origin of the abducens nerve lie in the abducens nucleus in the dorsomedial aspect of the posterior pons. The axons pass ventrally and exit the brain in a medial position at the pons-medulla border. The abducens nerve courses ventrally into the cavernous sinus and exits the skull through the superior orbital fissure, as do CN IV and III. Peripherally, the fibers innervate the **lateral rectus muscle** on the ipsilateral side (Fig. 14-10). Stimulation of the abducens nerve results in a contraction of the lateral rectus muscle and causes the eye to be moved laterally.

Clinical Disorders

A peripheral or central lesion involving the abducens nucleus produces a paralysis of the lateral rectus muscle. This results in a medial strabismus, which is the inability for both eyes to be focused on the same object. This is due to the fact that the affected eye cannot abduct and that the affected eye will tend to lay medially when looking forward. The resulting effect is double vision. To eliminate the double vision, the patient moves her head so that the affected eye is facing the object directly, while the unaffected eye then compensates for a change in position of the object in the visual field. The function of this nerve is tested by asking the patient to focus on an object that is placed in the lateral aspect of her visual field without moving her head. Because the affected eye cannot move beyond the midline of the visual field as a result of the unopposed action of the medial rectus muscle, the patient (with the normal eye closed) will be unable to identify the object located in the lateral aspect of her visual field, and the disorder is thus easily identified.

Trochlear Nerve (CN IV)

Components: GSE

The trochlear nerve is unique in that it is the only nerve that exits the brain dorsally and is also crossed. The cell bodies lie in a medial position just below the midbrain periaqueductal gray at the level of the inferior colliculus in proximity to the medial longitudinal fasciculus (MLF) (Fig. 14-11). The

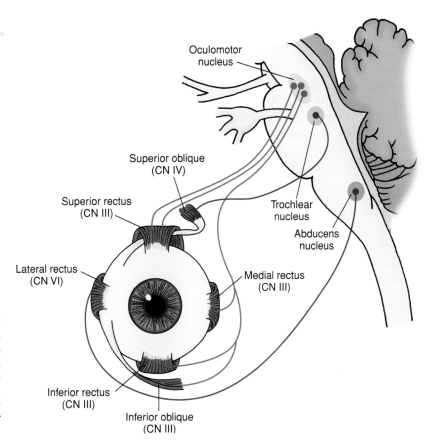

Figure 14–10 Origin and distribution of CN VI, IV, and III, which innervate extraocular eye muscles. The focus of the upper part of this figure includes the abducens (CN VI) nerve and the GSE component of the oculomotor (CN III) nerve, which are essential for horizontal gaze. The lower part of this figure depicts the muscles of the eye and their relationship with CN III, IV, and VI.

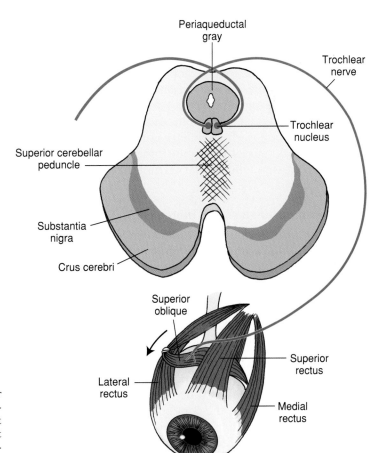

Figure 14–11 Origin and distribution of the trochlear (CN IV) nerve to the superior oblique muscle. As indicated in the cross section of the brainstem, note that this nerve exits the brain from the dorsal aspect, and it is the only nerve that is crossed. Arrow indicates direction of movement of the bulb downward and inward.

fibers pass dorsally and caudally, cross over to the contralateral side, and emerge from the brain just behind the inferior colliculus. The fibers continue anteriorly and enter the cavernous sinus. These fibers enter the orbit through the superior orbital fissure and supply the **superior oblique muscle**. The primary action of this muscle is to move the eye downward when it is located in a medial position.

Clinical Disorders

When there is a paralysis of the trochlear nerve, there is an outward rotation of the eye due to the unopposed action of the inferior oblique muscle. Therefore, when the patients attempt to look downward and inward, such as when walking down a staircase, they experience double vision and will tend to fall down. Patients will frequently compensate for this double vision by tilting their head. Tilting of the head upon downward gaze thus provides a clue of the presence of a trochlear lesion. Clinically, one could test for fourth nerve lesions by asking patients to follow an object as it is moved downward within their medial field of vision without moving their head. Again, failure to do so would indicate the likelihood of a fourth nerve lesion.

Oculomotor Nerve (CN III)

Components: GSE, GVE

The oculomotor nerve controls both skeletal and smooth muscles (via a postganglionic neuron). The GSE component of the third nerve provides innervation to all of the extraocular eye muscles (skeletal muscle) except for the lateral rectus and superior oblique muscles (Fig. 14-12). The GVE component provides preganglionic parasympathetic innervation to the pupillary constrictor and ciliary muscles (smooth muscle) through connections with postganglionic parasympathetic neurons in the ciliary ganglion.

GSE: Origin, Distribution, and Function

The oculomotor nucleus is located in a medial position just below the floor of the midbrain periaqueductal gray at the level of the superior colliculus (Fig. 12-6). The nucleus actually consists of a group of subnuclei, each of which gives rise to axons that innervate skeletal muscle or the ciliary ganglion. The nerve fibers pass ventrally in the medial aspect of the midbrain, exit the brain medial to the cerebral peduncle, pass through the interpeduncular fossa, enter the cavernous sinus, and then enter the orbit through the superior orbital fissure. The GSE component of the oculomotor nerve supplies the superior, medial, and inferior rectus muscles as well as the **inferior oblique** and **levator palpebrae superior muscles**. The action of the

medial rectus muscle is to move the eye medially; the superior and inferior rectus muscles move the eye up and down, respectively; the inferior oblique muscle elevates the eye when it is in the medial position; and the levator palpebrae superior muscle elevates the upper eyelid.

GVE Component

As described earlier, the cells that give rise to the GVE component of the oculomotor nerve, called the **Edinger-Westphal nucleus**, are located close to the GSE component and are situated around the midline (Figs. 14-13 and 14-14). Fibers from the Edinger-Westphal nucleus, which constitute preganglionic parasympathetic neurons, project to the ciliary ganglion. Postganglionic parasympathetic fibers from the ciliary ganglion then innervate the **pupillary constrictor muscles** and the **ciliary muscles**. Note that the pupillary dilator muscles of the eye receive their innervation from postganglionic sympathetic fibers that arise from the superior cervical (sympathetic) ganglion.

Contraction of the pupillary constrictor muscles results in a constriction of the size of the pupil. Likewise, constriction of the ciliary muscles causes a release of tension from the suspensory ligament of the lens, thus causing it to bulge (i.e., increase its curvature). Accordingly, the GVE component of the oculomotor nerve is capable of regulating both the size of the pupil (i.e., the amount of light that enters the eye) and the shape of the lens.

These connections provide the basis for several reflexes that are described later in Chapter 16 but that are reviewed at this time because of their relationship to functions of CN III. The first reflex is called the **pupillary light reflex**. In this reflex, light shown into one eye results in a constriction of the pupil in both eyes. Constriction of the pupil in the same eye that received the light is called the **direct light reflex**, and the constriction in the other eye is called the **consensual light reflex**. The pathway for this reflex involves afferent signals passing in the optic nerve and optic tract whose fibers terminate, in part, in the pretectal region. Fibers from the pretectal region innervate the oculomotor nucleus bilaterally (Fig. 14-15A). When the oculomotor nucleus on each side is stimulated, impulses are transmitted along the preganglionic neurons to the pupillary constrictor muscles on each side via postganglionic neurons in the ciliary ganglion.

A second reflex is called the **accommodation reflex** (Fig. 14-15B). This reflex occurs when an individual attempts to focus on a near object after looking at more distant objects. The responses that occur include: (1) pupillary constriction; (2) medial convergence of the eyes by the simultaneous ac-

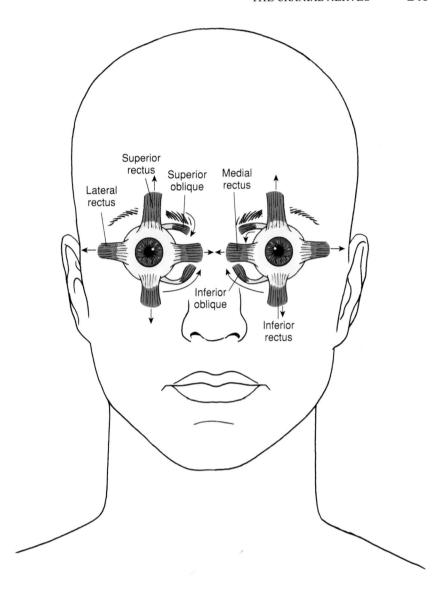

Figure 14–12 Diagram illustrating the direction of actions of the extraocular muscles of the eye (indicated by arrows). The lateral rectus muscle is innervated by the abducens nerve, the superior oblique muscle is innervated by the trochlear nerve, and the remaining muscles are innervated by the oculomotor nerve.

tions of medial recti muscles; and (3) focusing of the eyes on the near object, which requires contraction of the ciliary muscles, causing the suspensory ligament to relax and the lens to bulge. This reflex occurs by the activation of the following pathways: (1) descending cortical fibers from the occipital cortex to the oculomotor complex via a synapse in the pretectal region; (2) activation of both somatic motor fibers that cause the medial rectus muscle on each side to contract; and (3) activation of the visceral motor neurons that stimulate the ciliary ganglion, resulting in both pupillary constriction and a bulging of the lens, which allows the light rays to properly focus on the near object.

Clinical Disorders

Lesions involving the third nerve can affect both GSE and GVE components. Concerning the GSE component, lesions will produce a lower motor neuron paralysis of the extraocular eye muscles supplied by this nerve. The most common forms of deficits include: (1) the inability to move the eye inward or vertically (because of the loss of all of the recti muscles, except the lateral rectus muscle, as well as the loss of the inferior oblique muscle); (2) lateral strabismus, in which the eye on one side is now not coordinated with the opposite eye whose extraocular eye muscles are intact, causing diplopia (double vision); and (3) drooping of the eyelid (called **ptosis**), which results from damage to the nerves innervating the levator palpebrae superior muscle.

Lesions of the GVE components will produce the following autonomic effects: (1) loss of the pupillary light reflex; and (2) accommodation, which includes the convergence reactions. It is also possible that, as a result of a lesion, the pupil will remain small, but pupillary constriction will be brisk during accommodation. This disorder results

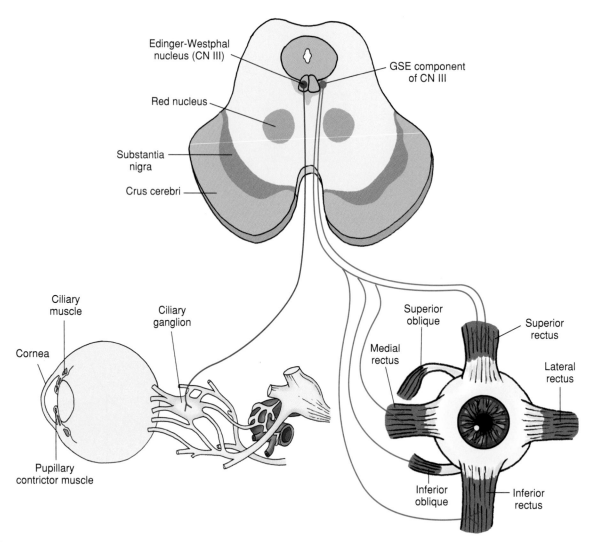

Figure 14–13 Origin and distribution of the oculomotor (CN III) nerve. The anatomical organization of the somatic (GSE) cell columns of the oculomotor (CN III) nerve complex, whose axons innervate all of the extraocular eye muscles except the lateral rectus and superior oblique muscles, is shown; the Edinger-Westphal nucleus, whose axons (GVE) serve as preganglionic parasympathetic neurons, innervate the ciliary ganglia. The postganglionic parasympathetic neurons from the ciliary ganglia (not shown in figure) innervate the constrictor muscles of the pupil and the ciliary muscle.

from syphilis and is referred to as the **Argyll Robertson pupil**, but the locus of the lesion for this disorder remains unknown.

If lesions involving the third nerve are located within the CNS rather than peripherally, it is likely that a constellation of deficits will be present. The most typical case involves a lesion located near the ventromedial aspect of the midbrain. Such a lesion invariably affects both fibers of the third nerve and corticospinal fibers contained within the crus cerebri because of the proximity of one fiber system to the other (see Chapter 12). In such a condition, the patient displays both a third nerve paralysis as well as an upper motor neuron paralysis of the contralateral limbs. This is referred to as **Weber's syndrome** or **superior-alternating hemiplegia**.

Control of Eye Movements: Role of the Pontine Gaze Center

While CN III, IV, and VI are essential for eye movements, the control of eye movements is under supranuclear control. The precise mechanisms are not totally understood, but several of the key structures have been identified. With respect to the control of horizontal gaze, they include the cerebral cortex, the region adjacent to the abducens nucleus called the **pontine gaze center**, and the vestibular nuclei.

It is likely that the motor nuclei of CN III, IV, and VI do not receive direct inputs from the cortex. Instead, cortical influences are via indirect pathways. These relationships are depicted in Figure 14-14. Briefly, the major structure for the integration

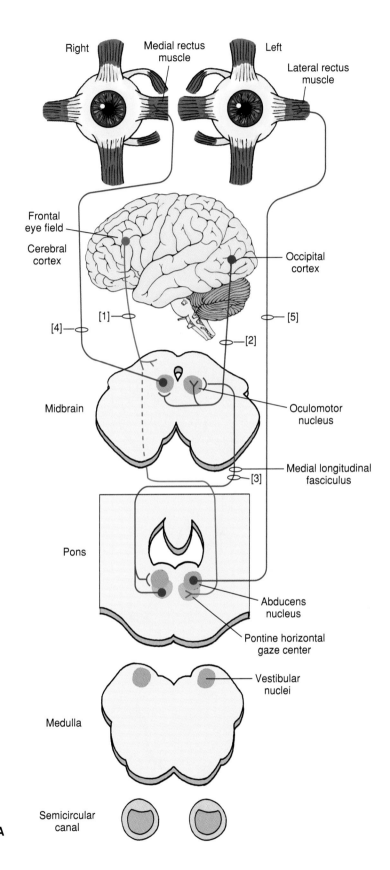

Figure 14–14 Diagram illustrating the anatomical substrates underlying conscious and unconscious regulation of conjugate gaze and the vestibular-ocular reflex. (A) Several of the key relationships revealing the connections between the cerebral cortex and the pontine gaze center as well as the linkage between CN VI and III are shown. Concerning conscious regulation of conjugate gaze, this process originates from the frontal lobe, where axons project to the contralateral horizontal gaze center (1). In this manner, activation of the left frontal eye field will result in movement of the eyes to the right because of excitation of the right abducens and left oculomotor nucleus. Involuntary regulation of conjugate gaze begins in part in the occipital cortex and projects bilaterally to CN III (2). The pontine gaze center projects ipsilaterally to CN VI and contralaterally to CN III (3). The connections of CN III (4) to the medial rectus muscle and CN VI to the lateral rectus muscle (5) are also indicated.

A

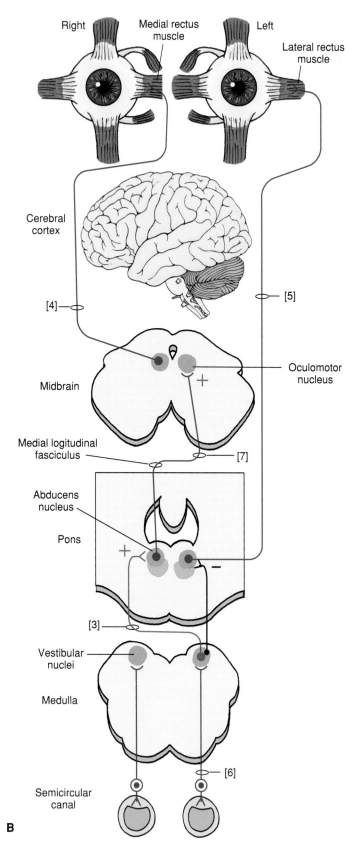

Figure 14–14 *Continued* (B) This diagram illustrates other important relationships essential for conjugate gaze and the regulation of the vestibular-ocular reflex. An essential element in this relationship includes vestibular inputs to vestibular nuclei (6). Vestibular nuclei project to the ipsilateral CN VI, which is inhibitory, and to the contralateral CN VI, which is excitatory (3). Projections from CN VI to the contralateral CN III are also excitatory (7). The MLF contains fibers passing from vestibular nuclei and the pontine gaze center to CN VI and III as well as fibers passing from CN VI to the contralateral CN III. To illustrate how these relationships function, assume that the head is rotated to the left. The net result is that the eyes are rotated to the right. In order for this to be achieved, there must be contraction of the right lateral rectus and left medial rectus muscles. Activation of these muscles is induced by initial activation of vestibular nerve fibers originating from the left horizontal semicircular canal, which project to vestibular nuclei. Projections from left vestibular nuclei to the right abducens nucleus are excitatory, causing contraction of the lateral rectus muscle of the right eye. Because the projection from the right abducens nucleus to the left oculomotor nucleus is also excitatory, activation of the right abducens nucleus results in excitation of the left medial rectus muscle. Because the projection from the left vestibular nucleus to the ipsilateral (left) abducens nucleus is inhibitory, the left lateral rectus muscle will have a greater tendency not to contract; likewise, the excitatory projection from the left abducens nucleus to the right oculomotor nucleus would not be activated because of the inhibitory input from the vestibular nuclei, therefore reducing the likelihood of excitation of the right medial rectus muscle.

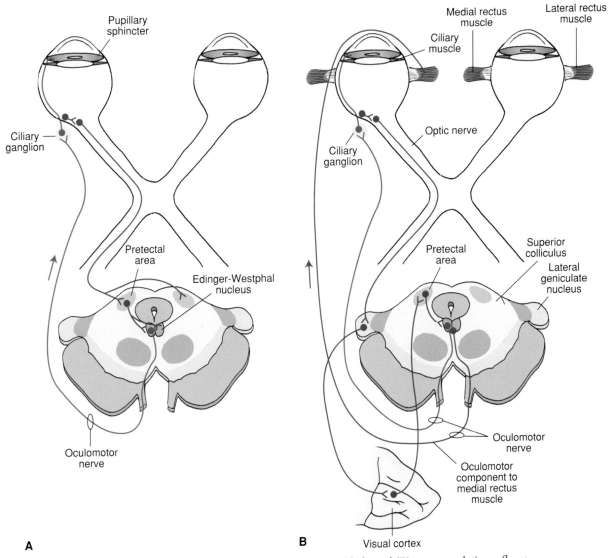

A   **B**

Figure 14–15 The pathways mediating (A) the pupillary light and (B) accommodation reflexes.

and control of horizontal gaze is the **pontine gaze center**. It receives inputs from the contralateral cerebral cortex and ipsilateral vestibular nuclei. After integrating signals from these regions, the pontine gaze center projects its axons to the nucleus of CN VI on the ipsilateral side and the nucleus of CN III on the contralateral side. In this manner, stimulation of the right pontine gaze center by either the ipsilateral vestibular nuclei or contralateral cerebral cortex will result in activation of the ipsilateral CN VI and the contralateral CN III. The effects of stimulation will thus cause the right eye to be abducted and the left eye to adduct (i.e., the eyes are directed to the right). Conversely, if there is a lesion of the right pontine gaze center, then the eyes cannot be moved to the right. However, the left pontine gaze center, which remains intact, allows the eyes to be moved to the left. Testing of the horizontal eye movement reflex is done by passively turning the head from side to side, and if the reflex is intact, the eyes will move conjugately in the direction opposite to movement. This is called the **doll's eye (oculocephalic) maneuver.** This procedure is applied when a patient is unable to perform voluntary eye movements and serves to determine whether the brainstem is intact. A lesion affecting the brainstem in the region between the midbrain and pons where vestibular and oculomotor pathways (MLF) are affected would cause the eyes to move in the same direction as the head. Further discussion of vestibular reflexes is considered in the following sections.

Cortical and Vestibular Control of Extraocular Eye Muscles

Voluntary Control of Eye Movements

As indicated in Figure 14-14, the region of the frontal cortex called the **frontal eye fields** projects to the contralateral pontine gaze center. Such a connection provides the basis for voluntary control of **horizontal eye movements**, which can even override certain reflex eye movements associated with inputs into the pontine gaze center from the vestibular nuclei (with the exception of nystagmus). However, if, for example, there is a lesion of the projection from the left cortex to the right pontine gaze center (Fig. 14-16), the ability to gaze to the right will be impaired.

Control of horizontal eye movements serves very important functions. It is used extensively in reading and in looking at stationary and moving objects within our visual field. Horizontal movements can occur quite rapidly, with the duration being less than 50 milliseconds. These are called **saccadic movements**. If an individual fixates on an object within his visual field, the movements change from saccadic to smooth pursuit movements. Such movements most likely involve utilization of primary, secondary, and tertiary regions of the visual cortex, which have connections with the frontal lobe, including the frontal eye fields.

Vestibular-Induced Reflexes

Vestibular nuclei receive direct inputs from the semicircular canals of the vestibular apparatus. The vestibular nuclei transmit these inputs to both the pontine gaze center and nuclei of CN VI, IV, and III. The relationship between the vestibular system and the nuclei of the extraocular eye muscles is a very important one. It provides the anatomical basis by which the eyes can continue to **fixate** upon a given object as the head moves in space. For example, when an individual's head is rotated to the right, the eyes will turn toward the left. This is because the inertia of the endolymph in the semicircular canals generates a force across the cupula, moving it in the opposite direction to movement (i.e., to the left), which triggers action potentials in the first-order vestibular neurons on the left side that project to the left vestibular nuclei (see Chapter 17 for details of the peripheral mechanisms governing receptor activation of vestibular neurons).

The left vestibular nuclei, via the MLF, excite the lateral gaze center and motor nucleus of CN VI on the left side and motor neurons of CN III on the right side that supply the medial rectus muscle. Other projections will inhibit the lateral gaze center on the right side and its projection targets in the right CN VI and left CN III. As the head continues to be rotated, the eyes show a smooth pursuit movement in the opposite direction to continue to fixate upon the object. Continued rotation of the head will eventually bring the object out of the individual's visual field, and he or she will attempt to fixate on another object. This attempt will result in

a rapid (i.e., saccadic) movement of the eyes in the direction in which the head is turning. The entire process results in a number of sequences where the eyes first display a slow movement in the direction opposite of the movement of the head, which is then followed by a rapid movement in the same direction in which the head is moving. This phenomenon is called the **vestibulo-ocular reflex** or **nystagmus**. It is named for the direction of the rapid component of the eye movement (i.e., if the rapid component of the movement is to the right, it is called a right nystagmus).

Nystagmus can be demonstrated experimentally by placing a normal individual in a chair (called a Barony chair) that can be rotated. The individual is then asked to focus on a given object and is spun around rapidly. When the chair stops, the individual displays a period of nystagmus in the direction opposite to that of movement. This is called **postrotary nystagmus** and is due to the fact that the endolymph continues to move (because of inertia) even after the individual has stopped moving.

Nystagmus can also occur clinically, usually in association with lesions of the MLF at levels rostral to the pontine gaze center. These lesions disrupt the mechanisms that regulate normal conjugate deviation of the eyes, and this disorder is referred to as **internuclear ophthalmoplegia**. In addition to the nystagmus, which is typically present in the abducting eye, there is a paralysis of the adducting eye when the individual attempts to look to the opposite side. For example, if a patient who has a lesion of the left MLF attempts to look to the right, her left eye cannot be adducted, although her right eye can be abducted (Fig. 14-16, lesion #2). Moreover, nystagmus is present in the left (abducting) eye.

Vertical Gaze Center

It is generally an accepted view that a region of the midbrain serves to coordinate the up and down movements of the eyes. This region is called the **vertical gaze center**. However, much less is known about the mechanisms governing the control of vertical gaze. Experimental studies have suggested that the key region for vertical gaze movements lies in the ventrolateral aspect of the rostral midbrain periaqueductal gray (the structure is called the **rostral interstitial nucleus** of the MLF). These cells discharge in response to vertical eye movements and also project their axons to the cell columns of the oculomotor nucleus that supply the extraocular eye muscles. Clinically, disorders involving vertical gaze have been reported and result, in part, from tumor formation in the region of the ventrolateral midbrain periaqueductal gray and from multiple sclerosis plaques.

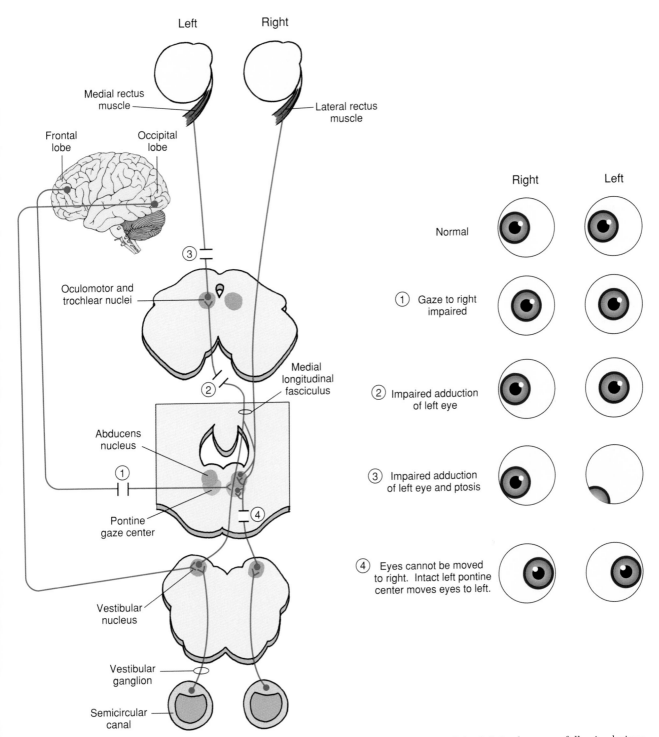

Figure 14–16 Diagram of the anatomical substrates for lateral gaze (left side of figure) and the deficits that occur following lesions at different sites along this pathway (right side of figure). For purposes of illustration, the diagram depicts the mechanisms involved in right conjugate gaze. Voluntary right conjugate gaze is initiated from pathways arising from the left frontal lobe that project to the pontine (lateral) gaze center. Involuntary pathways mediating conjugate gaze are associated with the occipital cortex. Note that the pontine gaze center projects to the ipsilateral abducens (CN VI) nucleus and contralateral oculomotor (CN III) nerve. The loci of the lesions (1–4) are shown on the left illustration. The corresponding deficits are depicted on the illustration on the right side.

CRANIAL NERVES OF THE FOREBRAIN

Optic Nerve (CN II)

The optic nerve is a highly specialized sensory cranial nerve that conveys visual signals to the CNS nervous system and is thus classified as an **SSA**. It enters the brain at the level of the preoptic region of the diencephalon. Details concerning the nature of the receptors, receptor mechanisms, and functional mechanisms are discussed in Chapter 16.

Olfactory Nerve (CN I)

The olfactory nerve is classified as an **SVA** because its receptors are chemoreceptors. The olfactory nerve enters the brain through the cribriform plate of the ethmoid bone and supplies the olfactory bulb. Details concerning the nature of the receptor mechanism, central connections of the olfactory system, and its other functional properties are considered in detail in Chapter 18.

CLINICAL CASE

HISTORY

Judy is a 29-year-old secretary who has had diabetes since childhood. One morning, she awoke feeling that the left side of her face was drooping and that she was unable to close her left eye. This eye felt dry as well, and noises seemed louder on the left than on the right side. Feeling that it was a transient condition, perhaps resulting from a sleeping position, she went to work anyway, where her supervisor told her that she should go to the emergency room because it looked as if she was having a stroke.

EXAMINATION

In the emergency room, the doctor noted a left-sided facial droop immediately. Because of this, there was some slight slurring of her speech, but there was no evidence of any problems forming sentences or understanding the content of speech. Her left eye would not close completely and appeared to droop slightly. The corneal reflex was absent on the left side. She was not able to hold air in her cheeks, and only the right side of her mouth was elevated when she was asked to smile. Only the right eyebrow became elevated when she was asked to wiggle her eyebrows. She was very sensitive to sounds on her left side, even those that were not especially loud. When sugar water was placed on the left side of her tongue, she was unable to taste it, but was able to taste it when placed on the right side. The doctor drew some blood and gave Judy some medication to take for the condition. He also patched her left eye to prevent it from becoming ulcerated.

EXPLANATION

Judy has a **Bell's palsy**, or paralysis of the seventh cranial nerve at or distal to its exit from the facial nerve nucleus in the pons. The motor deficits described on the face are typical of a lower motor neuron weakness, where much of the face is involved. This could not be an upper motor neuron disorder because when there is upper motor neuron weakness, the neurons of the facial nucleus representing the superior third of the face are bilaterally innervated from the cerebral cortex, thus preserving function in this area. This is not preserved in a lower motor neuron lesion.

The loss of taste ipsilateral to a peripheral facial nerve lesion is found when the lesion occurs proximal to the position where the chorda tympani nerve joins the facial nerve. This nerve controls taste function of the anterior two thirds of the tongue. The facial nerve sends a branch to the stapedius muscle distal to the geniculate ganglion, so a facial nerve lesion can also cause weakness of this muscle. Since the function of this muscle is to dampen the motion of the ossicles, which are the small bones within the middle ear modulating quality of sound stimuli, sounds appear louder than they normally would (hyperacusis). The corneal reflex is lost because the facial nerve serves as the efferent arm of the reflex. The result is possible damage to the cornea. Lacrimation, another function governed by the facial nerve, is also diminished and may cause further damage to the cornea.

Often, no definitive cause can be found for most cases of Bell's palsy. Some causes include diabetes, a blow to the face, and infections and inflammation.

CHAPTER TEST

QUESTIONS

Choose the best answer for each question.

1. A 34-year-old man is hit in the head with a heavy object that was carelessly thrown out of a window under which he was walking. He was taken to the emergency room, given a magnetic resonance imaging (MRI) scan, and 36 hours later, regained consciousness. Several days later, the patient reported difficulty in following a moving object presented within his visual field and also felt little or no sensation of the

forehead after a mild pinprick administered to that region. The MRI provided evidence that the head injury most likely caused damage to:

a. Peripheral fibers of the facial nerve
b. Central processes of the trigeminal nerve
c. Nerve fibers in the superior orbital fissure
d. The ventral half of the midbrain
e. Processes passing through the jugular foramen

2. A 60-year-old man was admitted to the local hospital after complaining that, for the past few months, he has had difficulty in swallowing and his voice has become increasingly hoarse and, at times, little or no voice could be produced. The patient was given a neurologic and general medical examination, and an MRI was done. The examinations revealed deviation of the uvula to one side and significant reduction of gastric fluids. The MRI revealed the presence of a growing tumor. The location of this tumor is in the:

a. Ventromedial medulla
b. Dorsolateral pons
c. Internal acoustic meatus
d. Jugular foramen
e. Hypoglossal canal

3. In a lateral gaze paralysis, both eyes are conjugatively directed to the side opposite the lesion. The most likely site of the lesion is:

a. Cranial nerve III
b. Medial longitudinal fasciculus
c. Cranial nerve IV
d. Pontine gaze center
e. Cranial nerve VI

4. A patient displays an ipsilateral medial gaze paralysis coupled with a contralateral hemiplegia. The lesion is located in the:

a. Medulla
b. Caudal pons
c. Rostral pons
d. Midbrain
e. Diencephalon

5. During a routine examination, the physician attempted to elicit a gag reflex response in the patient by stroking the posterior pharynx with a cotton-tipped probe. This reflex is initiated primarily by activating the sensory endings of:

a. Cranial nerve V
b. Cranial nerve VII
c. Cranial nerve IX
d. Cranial nerve XI
e. Cranial nerve XII

ANSWERS AND EXPLANATIONS

1. Answer: c

CN II, IV, and VI exit the skull through the superior orbital fissure. In addition, the ophthalmic division of the trigeminal nerve (CN V) also exits through the superior orbital fissure. Therefore, any damage to this fissure would affect functions of these cranial nerves. In this case, there would be loss of ability to move the eyes, such as in following a moving object, and there would also be loss of pain and temperature sensation to the forehead because of damage to the ophthalmic division of the trigeminal nerve. The other choices cannot account for this constellation of deficits (i.e., the facial nerve is not involved in this disorder; central processes of the trigeminal nerve could only account for the sensory losses; damage to the ventral midbrain would affect CN III but not CN VI, IV, and V; and the jugular foramen does not contain any of these cranial nerves).

2. Answer: d

The jugular foramen contains fibers of CN IX and CN X. In particular, damage to fibers associated with CN X could account for both the somatomotor and autonomic effects described in this case. Since CN X innervates the intrinsic muscles of the larynx, damage to the nerve would affect swallowing and speech (producing hoarseness). Reduction in gastric secretions is due to damage to the parasympathetic inputs to the stomach from the vagus nerve. The other choices are not appropriate because none of them contain any fibers or cell bodies associated with CN X.

3. Answer: d

The pontine gaze center projects its axons to the ipsilateral CN VI (for lateral gaze) and the contralateral CN III (for medial gaze). Because conjugate lateral gaze requires activation of CN VI on one side and CN III on the opposite side and is controlled by the pontine gaze center, a lesion at this site will produce conjugate gaze to the side opposite the lesion due to the unopposed action of the pontine gaze center on the intact side. Lesions of CN III, IV, or VI would produce effects that would be expressed ipsilateral to the lesion, and lesions of the MLF would produce failure of adduction of the eye ipsilateral to the lesion because of loss of MLF input to CN III. MLF lesions also produce nystagmus.

4. Answer: d

Medial gaze is governed by the action of the oculomotor (CN III) nerve. This nerve passes close to the crus cerebri en route to exiting the brain.

Therefore, a lesion located in the ventromedial aspect of the midbrain can quite easily affect both the root fibers of CN III as well as the descending fibers of the corticospinal tract. Such a lesion would produce a paralysis of the limbs on the contralateral side of the body, due to the disruption of the corticospinal tract, and an ipsilateral third nerve paralysis. This constellation of deficits is called Weber's syndrome.

5. Answer: **c**

The afferent (sensory) limb of the gag reflex involves somatic afferent fibers (i.e., GSA) of the glossopharyngeal (CN IX) nerve that enter the brainstem and make a synapse with special visceral motor fibers of CN X, whose axons comprise the efferent (motor) limb of the reflex that innervates pharyngeal muscles. The other cranial nerves are not involved in this reflex.

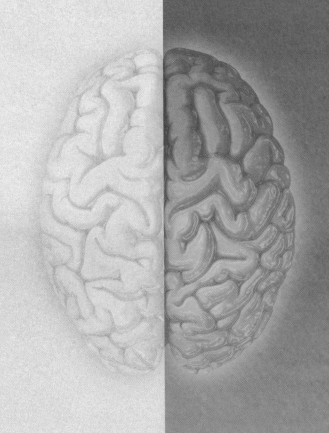

SECTION IV

Sensory Systems

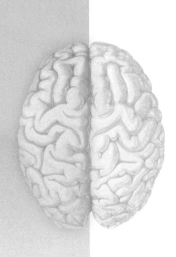

CHAPTER 15

SOMATOSENSORY SYSTEM

OBJECTIVES

After reading this chapter, the student should be able to:

1. Describe the general organization of the sensory systems

2. List, diagram, and describe different components of sensory systems

3. Describe the classification of major sensory systems

4. Describe and diagram the receptors, anatomical pathways, and physiological functions associated with the following sensations:

   a. Tactile sensations (touch, pressure, and vibration mediated by mechanoreceptors of the skin)

   b. Conscious proprioception (perception of joint position, joint movements, and direction and velocity of joint movements or kinesthesia)

   c. Nonconscious proprioception (sensations mediated by muscle spindles and Golgi tendon organs)

   d. Pain

   e. Temperature

GENERAL ORGANIZATION OF SENSORY SYSTEMS

Our knowledge of the environment around us depends on the information that we receive from peripheral receptors that are specialized nerve endings of sensory neurons. The major sensory systems include **somatic**, **visual**, **auditory**, **vestibular**, **taste**, and **olfactory** (smell) systems. In this chapter, the **somatosensory** system is described. The sensory neurons in each system project centrally, where they make synaptic contact with the second-order neurons that, in turn, project to higher order neurons. The different components of sensory systems and the terminology associated with them are described in the following sections.

SENSORY RECEPTORS

Initial contact with our environment occurs at the sensory receptors, which are specialized neural structures. The sensations experienced by the peripheral receptors include touch, position of the body, pain, sight, sound, smell, and taste. Each stimulus has the following characteristics.

Modality

Different forms of stimuli (e.g., mechanical, thermal, chemical, visual, and auditory) activate sensory receptors.

Intensity

The strength of the stimulus determines the intensity of sensation. The smallest intensity at which a particular sensation is detected is called the **sensory threshold**.

Duration

Usually, intensity of the sensation diminishes when the stimulus is continuous for an extended period of time. This is called **adaptation**.

Location

Awareness of the sensory experience includes the ability of the subject to identify the site of stimulation and the ability to distinguish between stimuli that are applied at close distances. The ability to distinguish between two stimuli applied at a close distance is determined by measuring the minimum distance between the two stimuli; this measure has been defined as **two-point discrimination**. There is a marked variation in two-point discrimination in different regions of the skin. For example, when a pair of calipers is applied to the skin on a fingertip, the sensation induced by each prong is felt even when the distance between the two prongs is very small (e.g., 5 mm). However, when the pair of calipers is applied to the forearm, the distance between the two prongs has to be at least 40 mm in order to feel sensations induced by each prong. This difference in two-point discrimination is explained by the observation that the mechanoreceptors that respond to two-point discrimination are much more numerous in the skin on the fingertips than on the forearm.

Stimulus Transduction

The sensory receptor converts a stimulus into neural activity; this conversion involves a process called stimulus transduction. A stimulus induces a generator (or receptor) potential in the receptor membrane. This local potential propagates electrotonically (for propagation of action potentials, see Chapter 6). Usually, the stimulus depolarizes the membrane by opening channels, thus selectively permitting influx of Na^+ and efflux of K^+. Specific characteristics, such as intensity and duration, are converted into specific patterns of action potentials that are called **neural codes**. For example, an increase in the intensity of the stimulus elicits an increase in the magnitude of the receptor potential, which, in turn, produces an increased rate and number of action potentials. Similarly, an increase in the duration of the stimulus usually decreases the amplitude of the generator (receptor) potential that, in turn, results in the adaptation of the response. The adaptation of the response may be rapid (e.g., Pacinian corpuscle) or slow (e.g., Merkel's receptor). These receptors are discussed later in this chapter under *Tactile Sensations*.

Receptive Field

The space in which the sensory receptor is located and where it produces the transduction of the stimuli is called the **receptive field** of the receptor.

RELAY NUCLEI

The thalamus contains a number of **relay nuclei** that serve to transmit the sensory information to different sensory receiving areas of the cerebral cortex. One exception to this general rule is that sensory information from the olfactory system can be transmitted to the prefrontal cortex through pathways that do not make a synapse in the thalamus.

CORTICAL MECHANISMS

The sensory areas of the cerebral cortex play a critical role in the perception of the sensation. Cortical mechanisms related to sensory perception are discussed in Chapter 26.

CLASSIFICATION OF NERVE FIBERS

Nerve fibers have been divided into the following four groups: (1) myelinated fibers from **annulospiral endings** of the muscle spindle (called type Ia or Aα fibers) or myelinated fibers from **Golgi tendon organs** (called type Ib or Aα fibers); (2) myelinated fibers from flower-spray endings of the muscle spindles (called type II or Aβ fibers); (3) myelinated fibers that conduct crude touch, temperature, and pain sensations (called type III or Aδ fibers); and (4) unmyelinated fibers that carry pain and temperature sensations (called type IV or C fibers). The nomenclature, diameters, and conduction velocities of these fibers are listed in Table 15-1.

SOMATOSENSORY SYSTEM

SENSORY MODALITIES

Sensations mediated by this system include tactile sensations (touch, pressure, and vibration); perception of joint position, joint movements and direction and velocity of joint movements (conscious proprioception or kinesthesia); nonconscious proprioception (sensations mediated by muscle spindles and Golgi tendon organs); pain; and temperature.

Tactile Sensations (Touch, Pressure, and Vibration)

Receptors

Skin is important for tactile sensations. There are two types of skin: hairy (e.g., skin on the back of the hand) and hairless (glabrous) skin (e.g., skin on the palms of the hand). The cutaneous and deeper subcutaneous mechanoreceptors (Table 15-2) respond to external stimuli. Different receptors mediating tactile sensations are shown in Figure 15-1 and described in the following sections.

Hair follicles. Each hair grows from a follicle, which is embedded in skin and innervated by nerve endings that surround it or run parallel to it (Fig. 15-1). When a hair is bent, a deformation of the follicle and the tissue around it activates adjacent nerve endings.

Meissner's Corpuscles. This receptor consists of stacks of horizontally flattened epithelial cells enclosed in a connective tissue sheath. One to four myelinated axons enter the capsule, the myelin sheath (in case of myelinated axons) terminates, and the axon arborizes among the epithelioid cells. Meissner's corpuscles are located beneath the epidermis (Fig. 15-1) of the fingers, palm of the hand, plantar surface of the foot, and the toes (glabrous skin). They are low-threshold, rapidly adapting mechanoreceptors and are sensitive to touch and vibration.

Merkel's Receptors (Merkel's Disks). These receptors are located in the skin below the epidermis (Fig. 15-1) especially on the lips, distal parts of the extremities, and external genital organs (glabrous skin). The receptor consists of a large epithelial cell in the basal layer of the epidermis that is in close contact with an axon. They are low-threshold, slowly adapting mechanoreceptors, and are sensitive to pressure stimuli.

Pacinian Corpuscles. These receptors are located deep in the dermis layer of both hairy and glabrous skin (Fig. 15-1). For example, these receptors are located in the skin of hands, feet, nipples, and

Table 15–1   Classification of Nerve Fibers

Nerve fiber	Numerical Nomenclature	Alphabetical Nomenclature	Fiber Diameter (μm)	Conduction Velocity (meters/sec)	Examples
Myelinated	Ia	Aα	17 (approx)	80–120	Fibers from annulospiral endings of the muscle spindle
	Ib	Aα	16 (approx)	80–120	Fibers from Golgi tendon organs
	II	Aβ	8 (approx)	35–75	Fibers from flower-spray endings of the muscle spindles; cutaneous tactile receptors
	III	Aδ	1–5	5–30	Fibers conducting crude touch, temperature, and pain sensations
Unmyelinated	IV	C	0.2–1.5	0.5–2	Fibers carrying pain and temperature sensations

Table 15–2   Mechanoreceptors

Mechanoreceptor Type	Receptor	Function
Cutaneous and subcutaneous: involved in touch, pressure, and vibration	Meissner's corpuscle (low-threshold, rapidly adapting); found in glabrous skin	Touch, vibration below 100 Hz
	Merkel's receptor (low-threshold, slowly adapting); found in glabrous skin	Pressure
	Pacinian corpuscle* (low-threshold, rapidly adapting); found in both hairy and glabrous skin	Rapid indentation of skin, e.g., the sensation caused by a high frequency vibration (100–400 Hz)
	Ruffini's corpuscle (low-threshold, slowly adapting); found in both hairy and glabrous skin	Magnitude and direction of stretch
Muscle mechanoreceptors	Muscle spindles	Limb proprioception
	Golgi tendon organ	Limb proprioception

*Pacinian corpuscle is also present in the mesentery.

mammary glands. They are also found in the walls of the mesenteries, vessel walls, periosteum, and joint capsules. Pacinian corpuscles consist of concentric lamellae of flattened cells that are supported by collagenous tissue. The spaces between the lamellae are filled with fluid. A myelinated nerve enters the corpuscle, the myelin sheath disappears, and a bare nerve terminal occupies the center of the corpuscle. These receptors are low-threshold and rapidly adapting and are sensitive to

rapid indentation of the skin caused by vibration of high frequency.

Ruffini's Corpuscles (Endings). These receptors are located in the dermis layer of both hairy and glabrous skin (Fig. 15-1) and are widely distributed. They consist of encapsulated bundles of collagen fibrils that are connected with similar fibrils of the dermis. The endings of a sensory axon ramify within the collagen fibrils. These receptors are

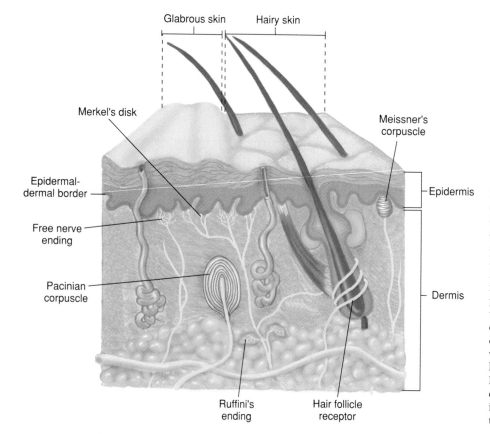

Figure 15–1   The receptors mediating tactile senses. Hair follicle: located in the epidermis and dermis. Meissner's corpuscle: sensitive to touch and vibration, located beneath the epidermis. Merkel's receptor (Merkel's disk): mechanoreceptor sensitive to pressure stimuli, located deep to the epidermis. **Pacinian corpuscle**: receptor sensitive to rapid indentation of the skin caused by vibration of high frequency, located deep in the dermis. Ruffini's corpuscle (ending): located in the dermis and provides information about the magnitude and direction of stretch.

low-threshold, slowly adapting, and sensitive to stretching of the skin. They provide information about the magnitude and direction of stretch.

Proprioception

There are two types of proprioception: conscious and nonconscious.

Conscious Proprioception

Unlike cutaneous mechanoreceptors that provide information in response to external stimuli, proprioceptors respond to mechanical forces generated *within the body* itself. In conscious proprioception, the receptors located in the joints and joint capsules (proprioceptors) provide sensory information to the cerebral cortex, which, in turn, uses this information to generate conscious awareness of kinesthesia (i.e., the joint position, direction, and velocity of joint movements).

Receptors. Conscious awareness of kinesthesia is believed to depend predominantly on joint receptors. Receptors located in ligaments and joint capsules consist of free nerve endings and encapsulated receptors. The encapsulated joint receptors are low-threshold mechanoreceptors. Some of them are slowly adapting and provide information about the *static* aspect of kinesthesia (i.e., the ability of an individual to judge the position of a joint without seeing it and without a movement). Other receptors are rapidly adapting and provide information about the *dynamic* aspect of kinesthesia (i.e., ability of an individual to perceive the movement of a joint and to judge the direction and velocity of its movement).

Anatomical Pathways. Tactile sensation and conscious proprioception are mediated by the dorsal column (dorsal or posterior funiculus)–medial lemniscus system (see Fig. 9-7) The cell bodies of sensory neurons that mediate touch and conscious proprioception are located in dorsal root ganglia. The receptors that mediate tactile sensations (Meissner's, Merkel's, Pacinian, and Ruffini) and **conscious proprioception** (receptors located in the joints and joint capsules) are specialized endings of the peripheral process of the sensory neurons located in dorsal root ganglia. The central axons of these sensory neurons travel in dorsal roots and enter the dorsal (posterior) funiculus of the spinal cord. As noted in Chapter 9, axons arising from the sensory neurons located below the sixth thoracic (T6) segment form the medial part of the dorsal funiculus (fasciculus gracilis), and axons arising from the sensory neurons located above the sixth thoracic segment form the lateral part of the dorsal funiculus (fasciculus cuneatus). Fibers in the gracile and cuneate tracts ascend ipsilaterally in the spinal cord and synapse upon the neurons located in the dorsal column nuclei (nuclei gracilis and cuneatus) of the medulla. Collectively, the axons of these second-order (dorsal column) nuclei pass ventromedially and decussate as internal arcuate fibers to form the medial lemniscus. The latter ascends through the medulla, pons, and midbrain and then projects to neurons located in the ventral posterolateral nucleus (VPL) of the thalamus. These third-order neurons in the thalamus then project to the primary somatosensory cortex of the parietal lobe in a somatotopic manner such that the head region is situated laterally, the upper limb is situated more dorsally, and the leg region is situated medially.

Deficits After Lesions in the Dorsal Column–Medial Lemniscus System. Patients with such lesions have loss of kinesthetic sensation and thus are unable to identify the position of their limbs in space when their eyes are closed and do not know if one of their joints is in flexion or extension. In addition, they cannot identify the shape, size, or texture of objects in their hands by means of touch. This deficit is called **astereognosis**. The opposite is stereognosis, which is defined as the appreciation of shape, size, or texture of objects by means of touch. These patients are unable to maintain steady posture when their eyes are closed or to perceive vibration when it is applied to their body.

Nonconscious Proprioception

The impulses arising from the proprioceptors mediating this type of sensation (muscle spindles and Golgi tendon organs) are relayed to the cerebellum rather than to the cerebral cortex. Proprioception mediated by muscle spindles is predominantly "nonconscious." These sensations are mediated by the following muscle receptors: muscle spindles and Golgi tendon organs (Table 15-2).

Muscle Spindles. **Muscle spindles** are present in skeletal (flexor as well as extensor) muscles (Fig. 15-2A). They are more numerous in muscles that control fine movements (e.g., muscles of the hands and speech organs and extraocular muscles). Different components of muscle spindles are shown in Figure 15-2B. Each spindle consists of a connective tissue capsule in which there are 8 to 10 specialized muscle fibers called **intrafusal fibers**. The intrafusal fibers and the connective tissue capsule in which they are located are oriented parallel to the surrounding skeletal muscle fibers called **extrafusal fibers**. The intrafusal fibers are innervated by spinal gamma motor neurons, whereas the extrafusal fibers receive motor innervation

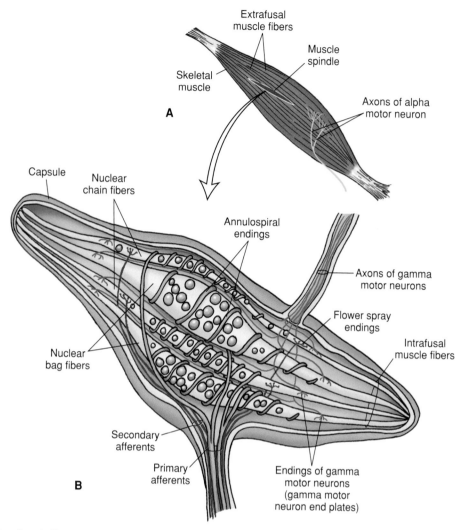

Figure 15–2 (A) Muscle spindles are located deep in the skeletal muscles parallel to the extrafusal muscle fibers, which are innervated by axons of alpha motor neurons. (B) Each spindle consists of a connective tissue capsule containing 8 to 10 intrafusal fibers (nuclear chain and nuclear bag fibers). Spinal gamma motor neurons provide efferent innervation on the ends of the intrafusal fibers. Note also the primary afferents (arising from annulospiral endings) and secondary afferents (arising from the flower spray endings) located on the intrafusal fibers. (See text for other details.)

from alpha motor neurons located in the spinal cord. There are two types of intrafusal fibers. **The nuclear chain fiber** contains a single row of central nuclei and is smaller and shorter than the nuclear bag fiber. **The nuclear bag fiber** has a bag-like dilation at the center where a cluster of nuclei is located. Efferent innervation is provided to the polar ends of both types of intrafusal fibers (i.e., nuclear bag and nuclear chain fibers) by efferent axons of gamma motor neurons that are located in the ventral horn of the spinal cord.

Two types of afferents arise from the intrafusal fibers: (1) **annulospiral endings** (primary afferents), which are located on the central part of the nuclear bag and nuclear chain fibers; and (2)

flower-spray endings (secondary afferents), which are located on both types of intrafusal fibers on each end of the annulospiral endings. Annulospiral endings are activated by brief stretch or vibration of the muscle, whereas both types of afferent endings (annulospiral and flower-spray) are activated when there is a sustained stretch of the muscle. Thus, muscle spindles detect changes in the length of the muscle.

The Stretch Reflex (Myotatic Reflex). When a muscle is stretched, the receptor endings located on the intrafusal fibers of the muscle spindle (flower-spray and annulospiral) are stimulated, impulses are initiated in the afferent nerve fibers (Ia type; see

Table 15-1), which project to alpha motor neurons located in the ventral horn of the spinal cord. The alpha motor neurons supply efferents to the extrafusal muscle fibers. Activation of these efferents results in a reflex-induced contraction of the extrafusal fibers. Thus, as a result of activation of muscle spindles, there is a rapid increase in muscle tension that opposes the stretch (see Chapter 9).

Gamma Motor Neurons. These neurons are interspersed between alpha motor neurons in the ventral horn of the spinal cord. Gamma motor neurons do not receive afferents from muscle spindles. As noted in the section on stretch reflex, when a muscle is stretched, the afferents arising from the muscle spindles are activated, which, in turn, induce a reflex contraction of the parent muscle. Contraction of the parent muscle results in a decrease in the tension of the intrafusal fibers and cessation of activity in the afferents arising from the muscle spindles. However, during voluntary movements, alpha and gamma motor neurons are activated simultaneously by higher centers so that the sensitivity of muscle spindles to stretch is maintained. The mechanism by which gamma motor neurons regulate the sensitivity of muscle spindles is as follows. When gamma motor neurons are activated, the contractile parts of the muscle spindle (intrafusal fibers) attempt to shorten, but the length of the muscle spindle does not change because it is anchored at both ends (i.e., isometric shortening of the muscle spindle occurs). A pull is generated at the equitorial region of the muscle spindle that results in a distortion of the annulospiral and flower-spray endings, and they fire. As stated earlier, muscle spindle afferents synapse on alpha motor neurons, which are activated and elicit a contraction of extrafusal fibers in the homonymous muscle.

Golgi Tendon Organ. These high-threshold receptors are located at the junction of the muscle and tendon. Golgi tendon organs are arranged in series with the muscle fibers, in contrast to muscle spindles, which are arranged parallel to the extrafusal muscle fibers. A tendon is composed of fascicles of collagenous tissue that are enclosed in a connective tissue capsule. A Golgi tendon organ consists of a large myelinated fiber that enters the connective tissue capsule of a tendon and subdivides into many unmyelinated receptor endings that intermingle and encircle the collagenous fascicles. Active contraction of the muscle or stretching of the muscle activates the Golgi tendon organs. Thus, Golgi tendon organs are sensitive to increases in muscle tension caused by muscle contraction. Unlike muscle spindles, they do not respond to passive stretch. As stated in Chapter 9, activation of the Golgi tendon organ produces a volley in the associated afferent fiber (called a Ib fiber). This afferent fiber makes an excitatory synapse with an interneuron that then inhibits the alpha motor neuron, which innervates the homonymous muscle group. The net effect is that the period of contraction of the muscle in response to a stretch is reduced. This type of response (i.e., reduction of contraction of homonymous muscle) elicited by stimulation of Golgi tendon organs is referred to as the **"inverse myotatic reflex."**

Anatomical Pathways. The sensation of limb proprioception is mediated by two pathways: the posterior (dorsal) spinocerebellar tract (see Fig. 9-8) and anterior (ventral) spinocerebellar tract (see Fig. 9-9). In both of these pathways, the cell bodies of the first-order sensory neurons, which mediate these senses, are located in dorsal root ganglia. As noted earlier, muscle spindles and Golgi tendon organs are specialized endings of the peripheral process of the sensory neurons located in dorsal root ganglia.

Dorsal (Posterior) Spinocerebellar Tract. The anatomical course of this tract is shown in Fig. 9-8, and its function is described here. The peripheral processes of the first-order neurons (located in dorsal root ganglia) innervate mainly muscle spindles and, to a lesser extent, Golgi tendon organs. The central axons of the sensory neurons of muscle spindles travel in dorsal roots and project to the ipsilateral nucleus dorsalis of Clarke in the spinal cord (i.e., the tract is uncrossed). Axons arising from these second-order neurons in the nucleus dorsalis of Clarke form the posterior (dorsal) spinocerebellar tract. This tract ascends ipsilaterally in the lateral funiculus of the spinal cord and then the lateral aspect of the medulla. It reaches the cerebellum via the **inferior cerebellar peduncle (restiform body),** conveying impulses concerning the actions of individual muscles of the trunk and lower limb.

Central axons entering the spinal cord via dorsal roots above T6 (conveying signals from the individual muscles of the upper limb) ascend to the medulla ipsilaterally and synapse on neurons located in the accessory cuneate nucleus. Axons of the second-order neurons located in the accessory cuneate nucleus form the **cuneocerebellar tract**, which reaches the cerebellum via the inferior cerebellar peduncle.

Ventral (Anterior) Spinocerebellar Tract. The anatomical course of this tract is shown in Figure 9-9. Impulses from the Golgi tendon organs travel in the dorsal root, enter the posterior horn of the spinal cord, and synapse on neurons located in the lateral part of the base and neck of the dorsal horn. The axons of these second-order neurons cross to the contralateral lateral funiculus of the spinal cord. The axons then ascend through the medulla to the pons, join the superior cerebellar peduncle (brachium conjunctivum), cross to the contralateral side, and terminate in the vermal region of the anterior lobe of the cerebellum. The cerebellum receives information regarding movement of muscle groups through this pathway.

Pain

Pain is the perception of an unpleasant sensation. Painful (noxious) stimuli (e.g., sharp pricking or slow burning) stimulate specialized receptors called **nociceptors**. The reception of signals from nociceptors by the central nervous system (CNS) is called **nociception**. Different components of the pathway mediating nociception are described in the following sections.

Nociceptors. Nociceptors are free nerve endings. There are three types of receptors activated by different noxious stimuli, and they are listed in Table 15-3 according to their functional properties. Mechanical nociceptors are activated by mechanical stimuli (e.g., sharp pricking); thermal and mechano-thermal receptors are activated by stimuli that cause slow, burning pain; and polymodal receptors are activated by mechanical stimuli as well as temperature (e.g., hot, cold, burning sensation).

Afferents Carrying Pain Sensations. Information regarding fast and acute pain sensations is conducted to the CNS by small, myelinated Aδ fibers; conduction velocity in these fibers is much faster than that of C fibers. Slow, chronic pain sensation is carried to the CNS by unmyelinated C fibers. Both types of fibers enter the spinal cord at the apex of the dorsal horn, branch, and then ascend and descend for one to three segments and then enter the dorsal horn.

Table 15–3   Types of Nociceptors

Receptor Type	Fiber Group	Sensation
Mechanical	Aδ	Sharp, pricking
Thermal and mechano-thermal	Aδ	Slow burning, sharp, pricking
Polymodal	C	Hot, burning sensation, cold, and mechanical stimuli

Anatomical Pathways Mediating Pain Sensations from the Body. The cell bodies of sensory neurons mediating pain are located in the dorsal root ganglia (first-order neurons). The nociceptors represent nerve endings of the peripheral axons of the sensory neurons located in the dorsal root ganglia. The central axons (both Aδ and C fibers) of these sensory neurons reach the dorsal horn and branch into ascending and descending collaterals, forming the **dorsolateral tract (fasciculus) of Lissauer**. In Lissauer's tract, these fibers (Aδ and C fibers) ascend or descend a few spinal segments, enter the gray matter of the dorsal horn, and synapse on neurons located in laminae I and II (substantia gelatinosa). Sensory information from laminae I and II is transmitted to second-order neurons located in laminae IV to VI. The second-order neurons in laminae IV to VI are collectively called the **principal sensory nucleus (nucleus proprius)**.

The **neospinothalamic tract** is the major ascending pathway involved in conveying pain signals to the higher centers; it arises from the nucleus proprius (principal sensory nucleus). The axons of the principal sensory nucleus, which mediate nociceptive signals, cross to the contralateral side in the anterior (ventral) white commissure of the spinal cord and form the neospinothalamic tract in the lateral funiculus. The neospinothalamic tract then ascends through the medulla, pons, and the midbrain and projects upon neurons located in the ventral posterolateral nucleus and posterior nuclei of the thalamus. Axons of the thalamic neurons project to the primary sensory cortex (see Fig. 9-10). The neospinothalamic tract gives off many collaterals and makes connections with the brainstem reticular formation (see Chapter 9).

Descending Pathways Modulating Pain Sensory Mechanisms. Pain sensation is modulated by the following descending pathways.

Pathway from the Periaqueductal Gray. The neurons located in the periaqueductal gray matter (PAG) of the midbrain project to the **nucleus raphe magnus**, which is located in the medulla. Electrical stimulation of PAG in human subjects and experimental animals is known to suppress the activity of nociceptive mechanisms (i.e., analgesia is produced). Therefore, stimulation of the PAG is believed to excite neurons in the raphe magnus, which, in turn, modulate pain sensation (see the following sections).

Pathway from the Nucleus Raphe Magnus. The anatomical course of this pathway is shown in Figure 15-3. The nucleus raphe magnus lies in the midline medulla, and many neurons located in

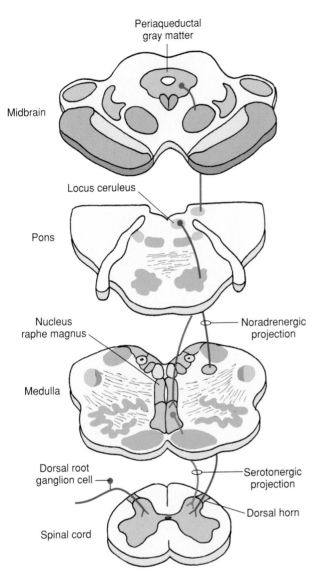

Figure 15–3 Descending pathways modulating pain sensory mechanisms. The neurons located in the periaqueductal gray matter of the midbrain project to the serotonergic neurons in the nucleus raphe magnus that is located in the midline of the medulla. Locus ceruleus noradrenergic neurons are located in the upper pons. The axons of serotonergic raphe magnus neurons and noradrenergic locus ceruleus neurons descend to all levels of the spinal cord and synapse on enkephalin-containing interneurons located in the dorsal horn.

this nucleus are serotonergic. The axons of these neurons descend to all levels of the spinal cord and synapse on enkephalin (an endogenous opioid peptide; see Chapter 8) containing interneurons located in the dorsal horn. The enkephalinergic interneurons form axo-axonal type synapses on the primary afferent terminals of pain fibers and axo-dendritic type synapses on the second-order dorsal horn neurons mediating the pain sensation. Stimulation of the descending serotonergic projections from the raphe magus excites enkephalinergic interneurons in the spinal cord. Enkephalins re-

leased from these interneurons inhibit the release of transmitter from the central processes of nociceptive dorsal root ganglion neurons. Stimulation of the enkephalinergic interneurons also inhibits the second-order spinothalamic dorsal horn neurons via a postsynaptic mechanism (see *Neurotransmitters Involved in Pain Pathways*). Thus, stimulation of the raphe magnus neurons produces analgesia by inhibiting the dorsal horn neurons from which the spinothalamic tract arises.

Noradrenergic Pathway. Axons of noradrenergic locus ceruleus neurons located in the upper pons descend through the medulla to the dorsal horn of the spinal cord. Stimulation of this descending noradrenergic pathway inhibits dorsal horn neurons that relay pain sensation by activating enkephalinergic interneurons via the mechanism described in the previous section (*Pathway from the Nucleus Raphe Magnus*).

Neurotransmitters Involved in Pain Pathways. Our current knowledge regarding various transmitters released at different sites in the neuronal circuits mediating pain sensation can be summarized as follows (Fig. 15-4). The neurotransmitters released in the dorsal horn of the spinal cord, at the terminals of central processes of first-order nociceptive neurons (located in dorsal root ganglia), are believed to be **glutamate** and **substance P**. These neurotransmitters excite second-order spinothalamic dorsal horn neurons. The axons of these second-order neurons cross to the contralateral side and form the ascending neospinothalamic tract. Opiate receptors are present on the terminals of the central processes of the first-order nociceptive dorsal root ganglion neurons (presynaptic opiate receptors) and on the dendrites of second-order spinothalamic neurons (postsynaptic opiate receptors).

The enkephalinergic interneurons located in the dorsal horn make axo-axonal and axo-dendritic synapses at the terminals of the central processes of the first-order nociceptive dorsal root ganglion neurons and dendrites of second-order spinothalamic neurons, respectively. The enkephalinergic interneurons are activated by the projections from the medullary serotonin-containing nucleus raphe magnus and pontine locus ceruleus noradrenergic neurons. Enkephalin released from terminals of enkephalinergic dorsal horn interneurons acts on the opiate receptors located on the central processes of the nociceptive neurons located in the dorsal root ganglia, reduces Ca^{2+} entry into the terminal, and decreases the release of neurotransmitters (glutamate and/or substance P). Enkephalin released from terminals of these dorsal horn in-

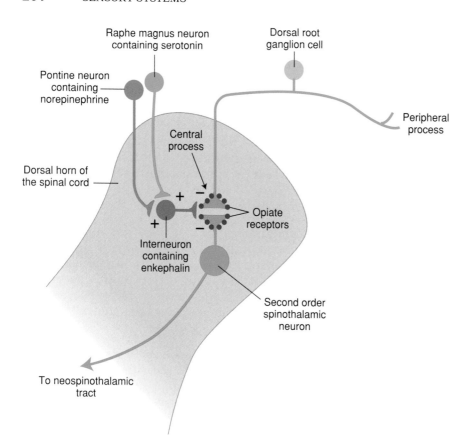

Figure 15–4 Neurotransmitters involved in pain pathways. Substance P and glutamate are released in the dorsal horn of the spinal cord in response to peripheral painful stimulus. Descending projections from the raphe magnus and locus ceruleus activate enkephalinergic interneurons in the dorsal horn. Enkephalin released from these interneurons inhibits the release of substance P and glutamate. (See text for other details.)

terneurons also activates postsynaptic opiate receptors on the dendrites of the second-order spinothalamic neurons, hyperpolarizes them by increasing K^+ conductance, and inhibits them. These actions of enkephalin attenuate the effects of nociceptive stimuli. Thus, stimulation of descending serotonergic and noradrenergic projections to the dorsal horn results in the stimulation of enkephalinergic interneurons in the dorsal horn, and enkephalin released from them inhibits second-order spinothalamic neurons by pre- and postsynaptic mechanisms.

Deficits After Injury to the Neospinothalamic Tract. Injury to the tract in the brainstem or spinal cord results in loss of pain and thermal sensation on the contralateral side below the level of the lesion. Knowledge of the anatomical and functional properties of this pathway has been applied by neurosurgeons to eliminate intractable pain by surgically interrupting the lateral spinothalamic tract (**cordotomy**) usually at the level of the spinal cord.

Anatomical Pathways Mediating Pain Sensation from the Head. The main circuits mediating pain sensation from the head are the trigeminal-thalamic pathways. The nerve endings of peripheral processes of sensory cells located in the **trigeminal**

(Gasserian) ganglion sense nociceptive stimuli from the face, oral mucosa, and the anterior two thirds of the head. The trigeminal ganglion is located in a dural cleft on the cerebral surface of the petrous bone. The central processes of the sensory cells located in the trigeminal ganglion enter the brainstem at the level of the pons and descend in the pons and medulla as the descending (or spinal) tract of the trigeminal nerve. These fibers project to the caudal aspect of the spinal trigeminal nucleus. Thus, nociceptive impulses, transmitted by the central processes of sensory neurons located in the trigeminal ganglion, eventually reach second-order neurons located in the spinal trigeminal nucleus. The axons of these neurons cross to the contralateral side and ascend as the ventral trigeminal-thalamic tract to reach the ventroposteromedial (VPM) and posterior nuclei of the thalamus. Axons of these thalamic neurons then pass to the head region of the primary somatosensory cortex in the parietal lobe.

Some Specific Pain Syndromes.

Hyperalgesia. Enhancement of the sensation of pain is called **hyperalgesia**, which results from tissue damage and the release of many endogenous chemicals. These chemicals may activate nociceptors themselves or may sensitize the nociceptors (e.g., lower their threshold). One of the endogenous substances known to sensitize nociceptors, causing hyperalgesia, is **prostaglandin E₂** (a cyclo-oxygenase metabolite of arachidonic acid). Aspirin and other nonsteroidal anti-inflammatory analgesics inhibit the enzyme cyclo-oxygenase and prevent the synthesis of prostaglandins. This effect may be responsible for their analgesic effect. Other endogenous chemicals that produce hyperalgesia are histamine, substance P, serotonin, and bradykinin.

Phantom Limb Pain. When a limb is amputated, some persons experience the sensation of pain emerging from the missing limb. This is called **phantom limb pain.** It is believed that overactivity of the dorsal horn neurons on the side of the amputated limb may create a false feeling in the person that the pain is emanating from the amputated limb.

Causalgia (Sympathetic Dystrophy Syndrome). The burning sensation in this syndrome is caused by increased sympathetic efferent activity after a peripheral nerve injury.

Neuralgia. Neuralgia is characterized by severe persistent pain in the distribution of a cranial or spinal nerve. For example, in **trigeminal neuralgia,** the pain (which comes in episodes and feels like stabbing) is precipitated by activities such as eating or brushing one's teeth and is limited to the sensory distribution of the trigeminal nerve located in the face. Surgical interruption of the trigeminal nerve or medullary spinal tract (trigeminal tractotomy) is sometimes done to reduce or eliminate trigeminal neuralgia. Oral administration of anticonvulsants (e.g., carbamazepine or phenytoin) can alleviate paroxysmal pain by limiting aberrant transmission of nerve impulses. Electrocoagulation of the trigeminal ganglion or injection of alcohol in the trigeminal nerve have also been used to alleviate trigeminal neuralgia.

Thalamic Pain Syndrome. Lesions in the posterior thalamus may cause chronic pain in some patients (see Chapter 26 for further discussion of this syndrome). The etiology of this disorder and its nature are poorly understood.

Referred Pain. Sometimes, pain arising from deep visceral structures is felt at sites on the surface of the body. For example, pain stimuli arising due to myocardial ischemia are felt radiating to the arms and wrists. This is called **referred pain.** One explanation for this phenomenon is that the same dorsal horn neuron receives afferent signals from deep visceral nociceptors as well as from cutaneous nociceptors. Higher centers involved in the perception of the pain sensation incorrectly ascribe the pain stimuli to the skin instead of a deeper visceral structure. This is because the input from the cutaneous nociceptors is more predominant than the visceral nociceptors.

Temperature

The signals from a cold stimulus are carried by small, myelinated Aδ fibers, and the impulses from warm-sensitive receptors are conducted by unmyelinated C-fiber afferents. These fibers enter the tract of Lissauer, branch, and then ascend or descend one to three segments and terminate in the dorsal horn. The anatomic pathways that mediate temperature sensations are identical to those that mediate pain sensation. The pathways mediating temperature sensation also mediate crude touch from naked nerve endings.

CLINICAL CASE

HISTORY

Annie is a 56-year-old woman who has suffered from diabetes for over 30 years. For the past few years, she has noticed that she frequently experienced numbness, tingling, and pain in her feet. However, more recently, she noticed that she was suffering from ulcers on her feet, and was frequently tripping. While carrying a large box down a steep staircase, she missed a step and fell down several steps. She called for help and was taken to the local emergency room.

EXAMINATION

At the emergency room, the examining physician noted that Annie had several large bruises on her head, back, and extremities but was alert and oriented. She had several ulcers on her feet. Although she could feel a hand placed on her feet, she was unable to tell which way her toes were moved if her eyes were closed. She was also unable to feel a vibrating tuning fork placed on her ankles but was able to feel the vibrations slightly when the tuning fork was placed on her knees. Her gait was a bit unsteady but improved when she looked down as she walked. When the doctor asked Annie to stand with her feet together and her eyes closed, she became very unsteady. Although there was a trace of knee jerk reflexes bilaterally, the ankle jerk reflexes were absent.

EXPLANATION

Annie's neurologic problem is a classic example of a peripheral neuropathy (dysfunction of the peripheral nerves without involvement of the CNS). This condition is often described as "stocking glove" in nature because of the anatomic pattern it follows in which the affected parts include the hands and feet. Diabetes is a common cause of peripheral neuropathy. The exact mechanism is unknown, but the disease preferentially affects the larger myelinated fibers, prior to the smaller motor fibers, and Aδ and unmyelinated C fibers, which govern primarily pain and temperature. Although there is a sensation of numbness, examination revealed that the primary deficits lie with position and vibratory senses. Because there is some degree of numbness, it is not uncommon for diabetics to suffer from foot ulcers, since it is difficult to recognize poorly fitting shoes. The gait described is called *sensory ataxia* and is an unsteady gait resulting from a deficiency in identifying the location of feet on the floor. When Annie walked down the stairs carrying a large box, she was most likely

mechanically unable to look down at her feet and thus could not feel their location on the stairs, causing her to trip. The ankle jerk reflexes are lost due to loss of the sensory component of the deep tendon reflex. In the **Romberg test**, the patient is asked to stand with feet together and eyes closed; it is a test of position sense. If cerebellar and motor function are normal (as we presume that they are in this case), the reason for unsteadiness is the loss of position sense. Because the same fibers carry position and vibratory sense, the latter is lost as well. In more advanced cases of diabetic neuropathy, motor function and pain and temperature sensation may be lost as well.

CHAPTER TEST

QUESTIONS

Choose the best answer for each question.

1. A 47-year-old man had complained to his physician that he had recently begun to experience some difficulty in maintaining his balance while attempting to walk and loss of ability to recognize objects placed in his hand when his eyes were closed. His internist referred him to a local neurology clinic where a battery of tests revealed the presence of a growing tumor. The tumor was most likely affecting the:

a. Anterior spinocerebellar tract
b. Posterior spinocerebellar tract
c. Dorsolateral tract of Lissauer
d. Dorsal columns
e. Neospinothalamic tract

2. A 67-year-old woman was admitted to the emergency room complaining of brief, repetitive paroxysms of excruciating pain in the face region. Following a neurologic examination, it was concluded that the patient was suffering from trigeminal neuralgia. After pharmacological approaches failed to alleviate the pain, neurosurgery was recommended. The neurosurgeon's goal was to surgically destroy a small region of the CNS. The most logical placement of this lesion was the:

a. Dorsomedial pons
b. Ventromedial aspect of midbrain
c. Lateral aspect of lower medulla
d. Substantia gelatinosa
e. Basilar pons

3. A neuroscientist wanted to design an experiment to investigate the brain mechanisms that regulate pain. This investigator discovered that, when electrical stimulation was applied to the midline of the medulla, pain sensation was attenuated. Which of the following possibilities could account for this observation?

a. Release of serotonin in the dorsal horn of spinal cord
b. Release of acetylcholine in the substantia gelatinosa
c. Release of norepinephrine from the central processes of dorsal root ganglion cells
d. Increased release of substance P from the central processes of dorsal root ganglion cells
e. Inhibition of enkephalinergic interneurons in the substantia gelatinosa

4. Which of the following receptors signal changes in muscle activity?

a. Golgi tendon organs
b. Meissner's corpuscle
c. Pacinian corpuscle
d. Merkel's receptor
e. Ruffini's corpuscle

5. The terminals of nociceptive afferents release which one of the following transmitters?

a. Substance P
b. GABA
c. Enkephalins
d. Serotonin
e. Acetylcholine

ANSWERS AND EXPLANATIONS

1. Answer: d

The dorsal columns of the spinal cord contain the fasciculus gracilis and fasciculus cuneatus. Patients with lesions in the dorsal columns have loss of kinesthetic sensation and thus are unable to identify the position of their limbs in space when their eyes are closed, and these patients also do not know if one of their joints is in flexion or extension. In addition, they cannot identify the shape, size, or texture of objects in their hands by means of touch (astereognosis). These patients are unable to perceive vibration when it is applied to their body and, therefore, cannot maintain steady posture when their eyes are closed. The posterior and anterior spinocerebellar tracts are involved in nonconscious sensation of limb proprioception. The lateral neospinothalamic tract and dorsolateral tract of Lissauer are involved in mediating pain sensation.

2. Answer: c

Trigeminal neuralgia is characterized by episodes of excruciating pain that feel like stabbing. It is precipitated by activities like eating and brushing one's teeth and is limited to the sensory distribution of the trigeminal nerve located in the face. Surgical intervention is sometimes necessary to relieve the pain. A rarely performed operation involves sectioning of the spinal trigeminal tract in the lower medulla caudal to the obex (caudal end of the rhomboid fossa, which forms the floor of the fourth ventricle). In this manner, afferent input to the caudal spinal trigeminal nucleus is interrupted, and pain is relieved. This procedure leaves the tactile sensibility intact. The nerve endings of peripheral processes of cells sensing pain in the face and the anterior two thirds of the head are located in the trigeminal (Gasserian) ganglion. The central processes of the sensory cells located in the trigeminal ganglion enter the brainstem at the level of the pons and descend laterally in the pons and medulla as the descending (or spinal) tract of the trigeminal nerve. These fibers project to the caudal third of the spinal trigeminal nucleus. Thus, interruption of

the pathway in the dorsomedial pons, ventromedial midbrain, and substantial gelatinosa of the spinal cord would not be helpful in relieving pain in this patient.

3. Answer: a

Stimulation of raphe magnus neurons in the midline medulla is expected to result in the release of serotonin at their terminals in the dorsal horn and excite (not inhibit) enkephalin-containing interneurons located in the dorsal horn. Enkephalin is released in the dorsal horn, acts on opiate receptors on the terminals of central processes of nociceptive dorsal root ganglion cells, and decreases the release of transmitters involved in nociception (glutamate and substance P). Enkephalin also inhibits the second-order spinothalamic neurons located in the dorsal horn by activating their dendritic opiate receptors. Thus, nociception is attenuated by enkephalins by presynaptic and postsynaptic mechanisms. Acetylcholine is not involved in pain-sensing mechanisms in the spinal cord. Although norepinephrine can activate enkephalin-containing interneurons, it is released by the stimulation of pontine noradrenergic neurons (not central processes of dorsal ganglion cells).

4. Answer: a

Golgi tendon organs are activated by active contraction or stretching of the muscle and provide information regarding the activity of the muscle. Meissner's corpuscles and Merkel's receptors mediate the sensation of touch. Pacinian corpuscles are sensitive to vibration. Ruffini's corpuscle senses the magnitude and direction of stretch.

5. Answer: a

The terminals of nociceptive afferents in the spinal cord release substance P and glutamate. Enkephalins and serotonin are not the transmitters released by the terminals of nociceptive afferents. These transmitters are released at different sites in the descending pain control circuits. GABA and acetylcholine are inhibitory and excitatory neurotransmitters, respectively, in the central nervous system, and they are not involved in nociception.

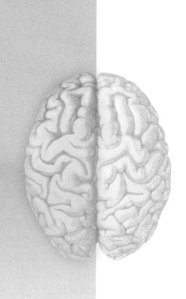

CHAPTER 16

VISUAL SYSTEM

OBJECTIVES

After reading this chapter, the student should be able to:

1. Describe and diagram the components of the eye

2. List, describe, and diagram the layers of the retina

3. Describe the structure and function of photoreceptors

4. Describe the mechanism of phototransduction

5. Describe the role of different retinal cells in relaying signals from the photoreceptors to the retinal ganglion cells

6. Describe and diagram the visual pathways

7. Describe and diagram the visual reflexes

8. Describe color vision

9. List, describe, and diagram, where appropriate, the prominent defects in vision

Vision is one of the most important sensory functions. It serves as the basis for our perception of the outside world. For example, our ability to detect forms, images, colors, and movement of objects is derived from the functions of the visual system. The initial processing of light signals received by the photoreceptors occurs in the retina. The axons emerging from the retina terminate in a relay nucleus located in the dorsal thalamus. The neurons located in the thalamic relay nucleus, in turn, project to the visual cortex where further processing occurs for visual perception. Details of different components of the visual system are described in the following section.

COMPONENTS OF THE EYE

The receptor organ for the visual system is the eye (Fig. 16-1A). Three layers of tissue enclose the eye. The outermost layer is called the **sclera** and consists of a tough white fibrous tissue. An anterior portion of the sclera, the **cornea**, is transparent and permits light rays to enter the eye.

The middle layer, the **choroid**, is highly vascularized. It is continuous with the iris and the **ciliary body**. The **iris** is the colored portion of the eye that is visible through the cornea. The iris has a central opening, which is called the **pupil**. The size of the pupil is neurally controlled via the circular and radial muscles of the iris.

The innermost layer of the eye is the **retina**. The optic nerve exits the retina at a pale circular region called the **optic disc** or **optic nerve head** (Fig. 16-1A). Blood vessels supplying the eye enter via the optic disc. Because there are no photoreceptors in the optic disc, it is called the **blind spot**. Near the lateral edge of the optic disc lies a circular portion that appears yellowish in appropriate illumination

due to the presence of a yellow pigment in the cells located in this region. This region of the retina is called the **macula lutea** (or simply macula). This part of the retina is for central (as opposed to peripheral) vision. At the center of the macula lies a depression called the **fovea**, which contains primarily cones. The layers of cell bodies and processes that overlie the photoreceptors in other regions of the retina are displaced in the fovea. A small region at the center of the fovea, known as the **foveola**, is also devoid of blood vessels. The fovea, including the foveola, represents the region of retina with highest visual acuity because there is minimum scattering of light rays due to the absence of layers of cells and their processes and blood vessels in this region. The structure and function of photoreceptors (rods and cones) and their distribution in different regions of the retina are described later in this chapter.

Different tissue layers enclosing the eye are continuous with certain structures of the eye. For example, sclera is continuous with the cornea, choroid is continuous with the iris and ciliary body, neural retina is continuous with ora serrata, and nonneural retina is continuous with epithelium of the ciliary body. Ora serrata is the serrated margin located just behind the ciliary body and represents the limits of the neural retina (photoreceptors and other cells associated with sensing and processing of light stimulus). Details of the structure of the retina and the structure and function of photoreceptors (rods and cones) and their distribution in different regions of the retina are described later in this chapter.

The space between the lens and the cornea, called the **anterior chamber**, is filled with a watery fluid called **aqueous humor**. This fluid is produced continuously by the epithelial cells of the ciliary processes that constitute the vascular component of

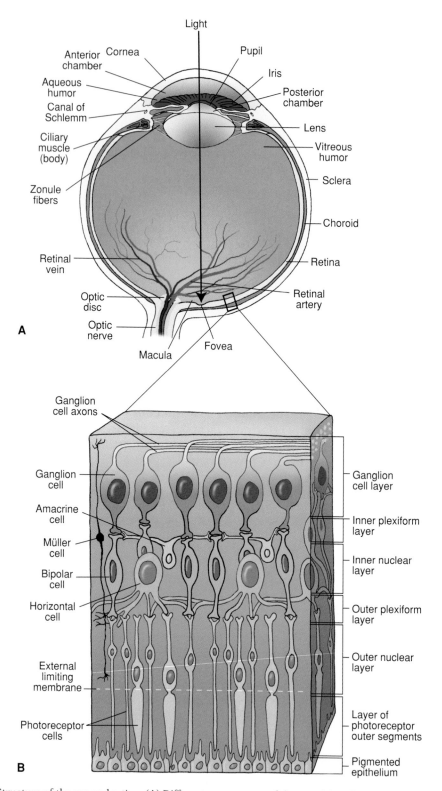

Figure 16–1 Structure of the eye and retina. (A) Different components of the eye. (B) Different layers of the human retina.

the ciliary body. The ciliary processes are located around the rim of the **posterior chamber** (the space between the lens and the iris). The aqueous humor flows into the anterior chamber through the pupil and provides nutrients to the lens and cornea. It is then reabsorbed through a specialized collection of

cells (trabeculae) into the **canal of Schlemm** (a venous channel) that is located at the junction of iris and cornea (the anterior chamber angle). Under normal circumstances, the production and uptake of aqueous humor is in equilibrium. When this equilibrium is disrupted, there is an accumulation of the aqueous humor in the anterior and posterior chambers, and the pressure in these chambers increases. Because the posterior chamber is in contact with the vitreous body (see next paragraph), an increase in the pressure within the anterior and posterior chambers is exerted within the entire eyeball. The increase in intraocular pressure reduces blood supply to the eye, causing damage to the retina. This eye disease, known as **glaucoma**, is a major cause of blindness. There are two major types of glaucoma: open-angle and closed-angle (also called narrow-angle or angle-closure) glaucoma. In **open-angle glaucoma**, the removal of aqueous humor is decreased due to reduced permeability through the trabeculae into the canal of Schlemm. In **closed-angle glaucoma**, the anterior chamber angle is narrowed by the forward movement of the iris, thus obstructing the removal of the aqueous humor. Open-angle glaucoma is a chronic condition and is treated by cholinomimetic drugs (e.g., pilocarpine, applied topically) and diuretics (e.g., dorzolamide, applied topically, or acetazolamide, administered orally). The most popular drugs for the treatment of open-angle glaucoma are prostaglandin analogs (e.g., lantanoprost) and beta-adrenergic receptor blockers (e.g., timolol) applied topically. Prostaglandin analogs increase the outflow of the aqueous humor from the anterior chamber, while beta-adrenergic receptor blockers decrease the secretion of aqueous humor from the ciliary epithelium. Acute closed-angle glaucoma is associated with a painful increase in intraocular pressure, which must be treated with drugs on an emergency basis or prevented by surgical removal of the iris (iridectomy).

As mentioned earlier, a thick, gelatinous material, called **vitreous body or vitreous humor**, fills the space between the lens and retina. It contains phagocytes that remove blood and debris in the eye under normal circumstances. In certain situations, such as aging, the debris particles are too large to be removed by the phagocytes in the vitreous humor. These floating debris particles, called "**floaters**," cast shadows on the retina.

The iris, ciliary body, and choroid constitute the **uveal tract**. Inflammation of these structures, which usually is secondary to an injury or infection, is called uveitis. Usual treatment consists of administration of atropine to relieve ciliary muscle spasm, which is the cause of pain in this condition. Topical application of steroids is usually effective in relieving inflammation.

Three pairs of extraocular muscles that move the eyeball within the bony orbit are attached to the sclera. The extraocular muscles are not visible normally because of the presence of **conjunctiva**, a membrane that folds back from the eyelids and attaches to the sclera. The neural control of extraocular muscles and prominent defects in the control of eye movements are discussed in Chapter 14.

Light rays pass through the cornea, lens, and anterior and posterior chambers and reach the **photoreceptors** (rods and cones) located in the retina. Focusing of images on the photoreceptors depends on refraction (bending) of light rays as they pass through the cornea and the lens. The change in refractive power of the lens is called **accommodation**. Radially arranged connective tissue bands hold the lens in place; these bands are called **zonule fibers** and are attached to the **ciliary muscle**. The ciliary muscle forms a ring. When it contracts, the zonule fibers relax, the tension on the lens is reduced, and its shape becomes rounder and thicker, which is suited for **near vision**. Under normal circumstances, the ciliary muscle is relaxed, the zonule fibers are stretched to exert tension on the lens, and its shape becomes thin and flat, which is suited for **distant vision**.

DIFFERENT LAYERS OF THE RETINA

The human retina consists of the following layers (Fig. 16-1B).

THE PIGMENT EPITHELIUM LAYER

The pigment epithelium layer is the outermost layer of the retina consisting of pigmented cuboidal cells that contain melanin. The bases of these cuboidal cells are firmly attached to the choroidal layer of the eye located outside the retina. The presence of tight junctions between these cuboidal cells prevents the flow of ions and plasma. The cuboidal cells have microvilli at their apical regions, which interdigitate with photoreceptors. The pigmented epithelium cells provide nutrition (glucose and essential ions) to photoreceptors and other cells associated with them. The black pigment, **melanin**, absorbs any light that is not captured by the retina and prevents it from reflecting back to the retina, which would otherwise result in the degradation of the image. Thus, the pigment epithelium layer protects the photoreceptors from damaging levels of light.

The pigmented epithelium layer develops from the outer aspect of the optic cup as a component of the choroidal layer. The rest of the retina develops from the inner aspect of the optic cup, which folds inwards and becomes apposed to the pigmented epithelium. A potential space persists between the pigmented epithelium and rest of the retina. This anatomic arrangement renders the contact between the pigmented epithelium layer and the neural retina (photoreceptors and other cells associated with the sensing and processing of light stimulus) mechanically unstable. Therefore, the pigment epithelium layer sometimes detaches from the neural retina. In this condition, known as **retinal detachment**, the photoreceptors can be damaged because they may not receive the nutrition that is normally provided by the pigment epithelium layer. Retinal detachment is now repaired by laser surgery.

THE LAYER OF RODS AND CONES

Rods and cones are photoreceptors. The structure and function of photoreceptors are described later. The light-sensitive portions of these photoreceptors are contained in this layer. In most regions of the retina, the rods outnumber the cones (there are approximately 100 million rods and 5 million cones in the human retina). One exception to this rule is the region of greatest visual acuity, the fovea (a depression in the center of the macula). The fovea contains only cones. High visual acuity at the fovea, especially in its central region called the foveola, is attributed to the presence of an extremely high density of cone receptors in this region of the retina. Other anatomical features that contribute to high visual acuity at the fovea are diversion of blood vessels away from the fovea and displacement of layers of cell bodies and their processes around the fovea. These anatomical features allow minimal scattering of light rays before they strike the photoreceptors. Disorders affecting the function of fovea, which, as mentioned earlier, is a restricted region of the retina (1.2-1.4 mm in diameter), cause dramatic loss of vision (other prominent defects in vision are described later in this chapter).

THE EXTERNAL LIMITING MEMBRANE

The photosensitive processes of rods and cones pass through this membrane in order to be connected with their cell bodies. This region also contains processes of **Müller cells** (these cells are homologous to the glial cells of the central nervous system [CNS] and are unique to the retina).

THE OUTER NUCLEAR LAYER

The cell bodies of rods and cones are located in the outer nuclear layer.

THE OUTER PLEXIFORM LAYER

The outer plexiform layer contains the axonal processes of rods and cones, processes of horizontal cells, and dendrites of bipolar cells. This is one of the layers where synaptic interaction between photoreceptors and horizontal and bipolar cells takes place.

THE INNER NUCLEAR LAYER

The inner nucleus layer contains the cell bodies of amacrine cells, horizontal cells, and bipolar cells. Amacrine and horizontal cells, sometimes called **association cells**, function as interneurons. Amacrine cells are interposed between the bipolar and ganglion cells and serve as modulators of the activity of ganglion cells. The role of horizontal and bipolar cells in the processing of signals from the photoreceptors is discussed later.

THE INNER PLEXIFORM LAYER

The inner plexiform layer contains the axons of bipolar cells, processes of amacrine cells, and dendrites of ganglion cells. This is another layer where synaptic interaction between different retinal cells takes place.

THE LAYER OF GANGLION CELLS

The cell bodies of multipolar ganglion cells are located in the layer of ganglion cells. The fovea centralis of the retina has the greatest density of ganglion cells. The final output from the retina after visual stimulation is transmitted to the CNS by the ganglion cells via their axons in the optic nerve. The ganglion cells are the only retinal cells that are capable of firing action potentials.

THE OPTIC NERVE LAYER

The optic nerve layer contains the axons of ganglion cells and processes of **Müller cells**. The axons of the ganglion cells travel towards the posterior pole of the eye and exit at the optic disc through the sclera to form the optic nerve.

The following layers of the retina are concerned with sensing and processing of light stimulus. They constitute the neural retina, which includes the layer of rods and cones, external limiting membrane, outer nuclear layer, outer plexiform layer, inner nuclear layer, inner plexiform layer, layer of ganglion cells, and optic nerve layer.

THE PHOTORECEPTORS

As noted earlier, the human retina consists of two types of photoreceptors: the rods and cones. The rods and cones consist of the following functional regions: an outer segment, an inner segment, and a synaptic terminal (Fig. 16-2A).

The **outer segment** is located toward the outer surface of the retina and is involved in phototransduction (described later). This segment consists of a stack of membranous discs that contain light-absorbing photopigments. These discs are formed by an infolding of the plasma membrane. In the rods, these discs are free floating because they pinch off from the plasma membrane. In the cones, the discs remain attached to the plasma membrane. The outer segments are constantly being renewed. The discarded tips are removed by phagocytosis by pigment epithelial cells. The **inner segment** contains the nucleus and most of the biosynthetic mechanisms. The inner segment is connected to the outer segment by a stalk or cilium that contains microtubules. The synaptic terminal makes synaptic contact with the other cells.

CONES

Cones are responsible for daylight vision. The loss of cones results in blindness. Vision mediated by cones is of higher acuity than that mediated by

rods. Cones mediate color vision, whereas rods do not. Cones have a fast response, and their integration time is short. Their conical shape makes them more sensitive to direct axial rays. As mentioned earlier, they are concentrated in the fovea.

RODS

Rods are highly sensitive and can detect dim light. They are specialized for night vision and saturate in daylight. The loss of rods results in night blindness and loss of peripheral vision. They contain more photosensitive pigment than the cones. The photosensitive pigment is responsible for the ability of rods to capture more light.

Both rods and cones, unlike ganglion cells, do not respond to light with an action potential. Instead, they respond with graded changes in

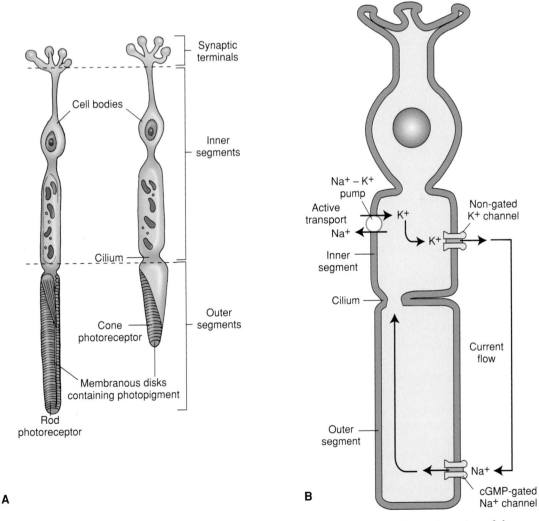

Figure 16–2 The structure of the photoreceptors. (A) Each type of photoreceptor (rods and cones) consists of three regions: an outer segment, an inner segment, and the region of synaptic terminals. (B) Note the location of cGMP-gated Na^+ channels and non-gated K^+ (leakage) channels. For details, see text.

Table 16–1 Comparison of Rods and Cones

	Cones	**Rods**
Sensitivity to light stimulus	Low	High
Photosensitive pigments	Less abundant	More abundant
Response to light stimulus	Fast	Slow
Specialized for	Day vision	Night vision
Effects of damage	Loss of cones causes blindness	Loss of rods causes night-blindness and loss of peripheral vision
Acuity of vision	Acuity of vision mediated by cones is high	Acuity of vision mediated by rods is low
Saturation	Saturate when light is very intense	Saturate in day light
Role in color vision	Mediate color vision (3 types of cone cells)	They are achromatic
Concentration in fovea	High	Absent in fovea
Relative numbers	Less numerous than rods	More numerous than cones (20:1)

membrane potential. The response of rods is slow, whereas the response of cones is fast (Table 16-1).

PHOTOTRANSDUCTION

In the outer segment membrane of the photoreceptors (rods and cones), there are cyclic guanosine monophosphate (cGMP)–gated Na^+ channels. cGMP binds directly to the cytoplasmic side of the channel, which causes it to open, allowing an influx of Na^+. During darkness, the presence of high levels of cGMP in photoreceptors results in opening of Na^+ channels, and an inward current carried by Na^+ flows into the outer segment of the photoreceptor (Fig. 16-2B). Thus, the photoreceptors remain depolarized during darkness. K^+ flows out across the inner segment of the receptor membrane through nongated K^+ (leakage) channels. Steady intracellular concentrations of Na^+ and K^+ are maintained by Na^+-K^+ pumps located in the inner segments of the photoreceptor.

A photoreceptor pigment, **rhodopsin**, is present in the rods. It consists of a protein called **opsin** that is attached with a light-absorbing component, called retinal (an aldehyde form of vitamin A). Opsin is embedded in the disc membrane and does not absorb light. In the cones, the protein is called cone-opsin, and it is attached with a light-absorbing component similar to that present in rhodopsin. The events that occur in the presence of light are shown in Figure 16-3: (1) the retinal component of rhodopsin absorbs light, which results in a change in the conformation of the photoreceptor pigment, and a G-protein (called **transducin** in rods) is stimulated, (2) the G-protein activates cGMP phosphodiesterase (PDE), (3) the activated PDE hydrolyzes cGMP and reduces its concentration, (4) a reduction in the concentration of cGMP

results in closing of the cGMP-gated Na^+ channels, and (5) the influx of Na^+ is reduced, and the photoreceptor cell is hyperpolarized. Thus, photoreceptors produce a hyperpolarizing generator (receptor) potential instead of a depolarizing generator potential, which is observed in other receptors. The photoreceptors (rods and cones) do not fire action potentials.

The rods and cones make synaptic contacts with the dendrites of bipolar and horizontal cells. The signals from rods and cones are transmitted to the bipolar and horizontal cells via chemical synapses. As mentioned earlier, vision during normal daylight depends on cones, while night-vision involves rods.

PROCESSING OF SIGNALS FROM THE PHOTORECEPTORS BY DIFFERENT RETINAL CELLS

BIPOLAR, HORIZONTAL, AND GANGLION CELLS

The cell bodies of bipolar neurons are located in the inner nuclear layer of the retina. These cells constitute the main link in the transmission of visual signals from rods and cones to ganglion cells. The **receptive field** of a bipolar cell is a circular area of the retina that, when stimulated by a light stimulus, changes the membrane potential of the bipolar cell. The receptive field of a bipolar cell consists of two parts: the **receptive field center**, which provides a *direct* input from the photoreceptors to the bipolar cells, and the **receptive field surround**, which provides an *indirect* input from the photoreceptors to the bipolar cells via horizontal cells (Fig. 16-4A). The changes in membrane potential of bipolar cells to a light stimulus upon the receptive field center and surround are opposite.

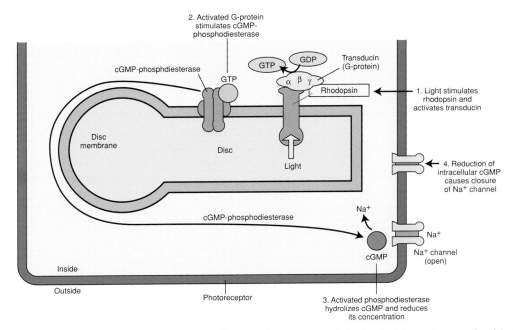

Figure 16–3 The mechanism of phototransduction in rods. The retinal component of rhodopsin (photopigment of rods) absorbs light, the conformation of rhodopsin is changed, a G-protein (transducin in rods) is activated, cGMP phosphodiesterase (PDE) is activated, hydrolysis of cGMP takes place, reducing its concentration, cGMP-gated Na$^+$ channels are closed, the influx of intracellular Na$^+$ is reduced, and the photoreceptor cell is hyperpolarized.

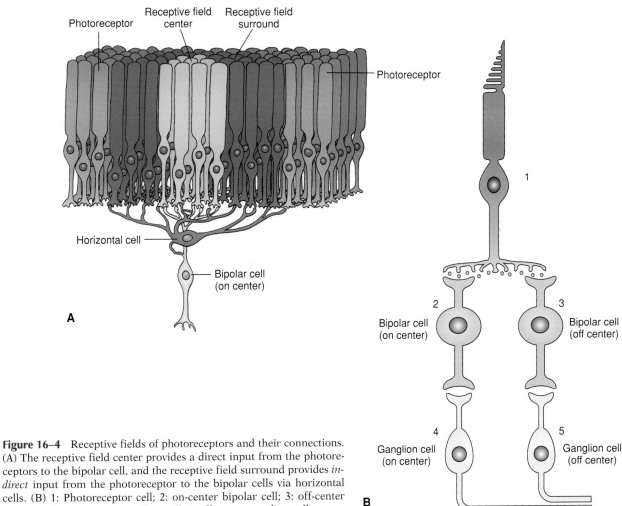

Figure 16–4 Receptive fields of photoreceptors and their connections. (A) The receptive field center provides a direct input from the photoreceptors to the bipolar cell, and the receptive field surround provides *indirect* input from the photoreceptor to the bipolar cells via horizontal cells. (B) 1: Photoreceptor cell; 2: on-center bipolar cell; 3: off-center bipolar cell; 4: on-center ganglion cell; 5: off-center ganglion cell.

The mechanism of membrane potential changes in the bipolar cells in response to light can be summarized as follows. There are two populations of bipolar cells: **"on"-center bipolar cells** and **"off"-center bipolar cells.** When stimulated, bipolar cells exhibit graded potentials rather than action potentials (see Chapter 7). Each photoreceptor cell (e.g., a cone; Fig. 16-4B, 1) synapses on an "on"-center (Fig. 16-4B, 2) and an "off"-center bipolar cell (Fig. 16-4B, 3). Each "on"-center bipolar cell, in turn, synapses with an "on"-center ganglion cell (Fig. 16-4B, 4), and each "off"-center bipolar cell synapses with an "off"-center ganglion cell (Fig. 16-4B, 5).

When the "receptive field center" is in dark (Fig. 16-5A, 1), the photoreceptors are depolarized (Fig. 16-5A, 2), and they release glutamate constantly (Fig. 16-5A, 3). Glutamate released from the photoreceptor terminals stimulates metabotropic glutamate receptors on the "on"-center bipolar cells, K^+ channels are opened, there is an efflux of K^+, the "on"-center bipolar cell is *hyperpolarized*, and the release of its transmitter (probably glutamate) is decreased (Fig. 16-5A, 4). On the other hand, glutamate released from the photoreceptor terminals stimulates ionotropic glutamate receptors on the "off"-center bipolar cells, Na^+ channels are opened, Na^+ flows into the cell, the "off"-center bipolar cell is *depolarized*, and the release of its transmitter (probably glutamate) is increased (Fig. 16-5A, 5). Hyperpolarization of "on"-center bipolar cells (Fig. 16-5A, 4) results in a decrease in the release of their transmitter, which, in turn, results in a decrease in the firing of the corresponding "on"-center ganglion cells (Fig. 16-5A, 6). Depolarization of "off"-center bipolar cells (Fig. 16-5A-5) results in an increase in the release of their transmitter which, in turn, results in an increase in the firing of the corresponding "off"-center ganglion cells (Fig. 16-5A, 7).

When the photoreceptor in the "receptive field center" receives a light stimulus (Fig. 16-5B, 1), it is

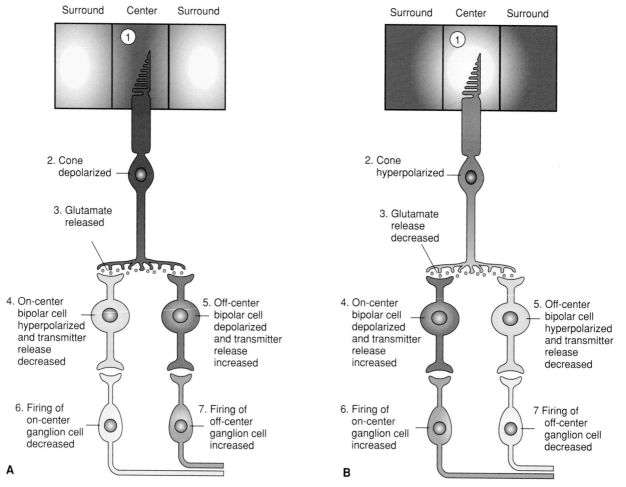

Figure 16–5 Responses of retinal bipolar and ganglion cells to darkness and illumination in the "receptive field center." (A) Changes in the electrical activity of the photoreceptor and on- and off-center bipolar and ganglion cells when the photoreceptor receptive field center is in the dark. (B) Changes in the electrical activity of the photoreceptor and on- and off-center bipolar and ganglion cells when the photoreceptor receptive field center is illuminated. See text for details.

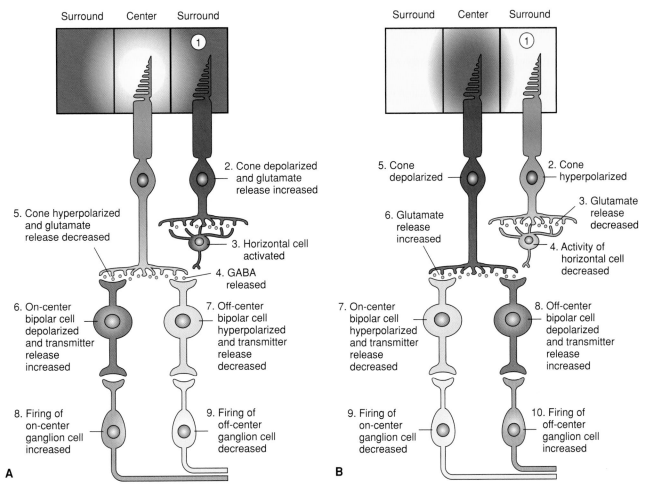

Figure 16–6 Responses of retinal bipolar and ganglion cells to darkness and illumination in the "receptive field surround." (A) Changes in the electrical activity of the photoreceptor and on- and off-center bipolar and ganglion cells when the photoreceptor receptive field surround is in the dark. (B) Changes in the electrical activity of the photoreceptor and on- and off-center bipolar and ganglion cells when the photoreceptor receptive field surround is illuminated. See text for details.

hyperpolarized (Fig. 16-5B, 2), and glutamate release from its terminals is decreased (Fig. 16-5B, 3). The reduction in the release of glutamate from the photoreceptor terminals causes depolarization of the "on"-center bipolar cell and an increase in its transmitter release (Fig. 16-5B, 4), whereas the "off"-center bipolar cell is hyperpolarized, and there is a decrease in its transmitter release (Fig. 16-5B, 5). Depolarization of "on"-center bipolar cells (Fig. 16-5B, 4) results in an increase in the release of their transmitter, which, in turn, results in an increase in the firing of the corresponding "on"-center ganglion cells (Fig. 16-5B, 6). Hyperpolarization of "off"-center bipolar cells (Fig. 16-5B, 5) results in a decrease in the release of their transmitter, which, in turn, results in a decrease in the firing of the corresponding "off"-center ganglion cells (Fig. 16-5B, 7).

Bipolar and ganglion cells elicit opposite responses when light is received at the "receptive field surround." The photoreceptors located in the "receptive field surround" of the bipolar cells are connected to photoreceptors in the "receptive field center" by interneurons called **horizontal cells**. During darkness (Fig. 16-6A, 1), the photoreceptors in the "receptive field surround" are depolarized, and there is an increase in the release of their transmitter (glutamate) (Fig. 16-6A, 2). Glutamate released from the photoreceptors activates horizontal cells (Fig. 16-6A, 3) that, in turn, release an inhibitory transmitter (probably gamma aminobutyric acid [GABA]) (Fig. 16-6A, 4) at their synapses with photoreceptors located in the "receptive field center" and cause their hyperpolarization and decrease in the glutamate release from their terminals (Fig. 16-6A, 5). This phenomenon is called **lateral inhibition**. Decrease in glutamate release from the terminals of photoreceptors in the "receptive field center" results in depolarization of "on"-center bipolar cells and an increase in the release of their transmitter (Fig. 16-6A, 6), whereas the "off"-center bipolar cells are hyperpolarized, and there is a decrease in the release of their transmitter (Fig. 16-6A, 7). As mentioned earlier, depolarization of "on"-center bipolar cells (Fig. 16-6A, 6) causes an increase in the firing of corresponding ganglion cells (Fig. 16-6A, 8), while hyperpolarization of the "off"-center bipolar cells (Fig. 16-6A, 7) causes a decrease in the firing of corresponding ganglion cells (Fig. 16-6A, 9).

When light is received at the "receptive field surround" (Fig. 16-6B, 1), the photoreceptor in this field is hyperpolarized (Fig. 16-6B, 2). There is a decrease in the release of glutamate from their terminals (Fig. 16-6B, 3), activity of horizontal cells is decreased (Fig. 16-6B, 4), GABA release at the terminals of horizontal cells is decreased, and lateral inhibition exerted by them on the photoreceptors in the "receptive field center" is decreased. Thus, the photoreceptors located in the "receptive field center" are released from lateral inhibition from horizontal cells. Consequently, the photoreceptors in the "receptive field center" are depolarized (Fig. 16-6B, 5), and there is an increase in the glutamate release from their terminals (Fig. 16-6B, 6). Subsequently, the "on"-center bipolar cells are hyperpolarized, and there is a decrease in the release of their transmitter (Fig. 16-6B, 7). The "off"-center bipolar cells are depolarized, and there is an increase in the release of their transmitter (Fig. 16-6B, 8). Again, hyperpolarization of "on"-center bipolar cells (Fig. 16-6B, 7) causes a decrease in the firing of corresponding ganglion cells (Fig. 16-6B, 9), whereas depolarization of "off"-center bipolar cells (Fig. 16-6B, 8) causes an increase in the firing of corresponding ganglion cells (Fig. 16-6B, 10).

SIGNIFICANCE OF CHANGES IN "ON"- AND "OFF"-CENTER BIPOLAR AND GANGLION CELL ACTIVITIES

As described earlier, the changes in membrane potential of "on"- and "off"-center bipolar cells and firing of corresponding ganglion cells to light stimulus to the "receptive field center" and "receptive field surround" are opposite. This mechanism renders the bipolar and ganglion cells sensitive to contrast in illumination that falls in the "receptive field center" and "receptive field surround." The sensitivity of the bipolar and ganglion cells to the contrast properties, rather than to an absolute level of illumination, renders brightness or darkness of objects constant over a wide range of lighting conditions. For example, on a printed page, the darkness of the print or white background of the page appears the same whether we look at the page inside a room or in sunlight. In experimental conditions, when "on"-center ganglion cells are damaged, the animals can still see objects that are darker than the background. However, they cannot see objects brighter than the background. These observations indicate that information about brightness and darkness of objects in a visual field is transmitted to the brain by "on"-center and "off"-center ganglion cells, respectively.

There are at least two types of retinal ganglion cells: M and P cells. P cells are more numerous than the M cells. M-type retinal ganglion cells project to magnocellular layers of the lateral geniculate nucleus located in the thalamus, while P cells project to the parvocellular layers of the same nucleus (see the section titled "Visual Pathways"). M cells have larger cell bodies, dendritic fields, and axons compared to P cells. The responses of M ganglion cells to visual stimuli are transient, while those of P ganglion cells are sustained. M cells cannot transmit information about color, while P cells can. The P cells are capable of transmitting color information because their centers and surrounds contain different types of cones. For example, the center of P retinal ganglion cells may contain cones sensitive to long wavelength light (red color), while their surrounds may contain cones sensitive to medium wavelength light (green color). These P retinal ganglion cells will be sensitive to differences in wavelengths of light falling on their center and surround regions.

COLOR VISION

There are three types of cone receptors, each of which contains a different photopigment that is sensitive to one of the primary colors (red, blue, and green). The relative frequency of impulses from each cone determines the sensation of any particular color. Besides cones, other cells in the retina that are involved in the processing of color vision include the horizontal cells (which are either hyperpolarized or depolarized by monochromatic colors) and ganglion cells (which are either turned "on" or "off" by monochromatic colors). Information following stimulation of a particular cone preferentially by a monochromatic color (e.g., green) is processed by the visual cortex and interpreted as a particular color (green in this case). If two different types of cones are stimulated equally by two different monochromatic colors (e.g., red and green), the visual cortex interprets them as a yellow color. The visual cortex contains cells that can differentiate between brightness and contrast and cells that respond to a particular monochromatic color. Processing of color vision in the visual cortex involves integration of the responses of the cones, horizontal cells, ganglion cells, and lateral geniculate body cells.

BLOOD SUPPLY OF THE RETINA

The retina receives blood supply from branches of the ophthalmic artery. One branch (central retinal artery) enters the eye at the optic nerve disc and supplies the inner portion of the neural retina. The other branch (ciliary artery) penetrates the sclera near the exit of the optic nerve and supplies a part of the choroid, called the choriocapillaris. The outer portions of retina, including the rods and cones, are metabolically dependent on the blood supply to the choroidal layer because they receive nutrients from the choriocapillaris.

VISUAL AND RETINAL FIELDS

To understand visual deficits, it is helpful first to make a distinction between the visual and retinal fields. The **visual field** of each eye is the region of space that the eye can see looking straight ahead without movement of the head. The *fovea* of each retina is aligned with a point, called the **fixation point,** in the visual field. A vertical line can divide the visual field of each eye into two halves: the **left half field** and **right half field.** A horizontal line can divide each visual hemifield into superior and inferior halves. Each half can be further divided into quadrants. The vertical and horizontal lines dividing the visual field of each eye intersect at the fixation point (Fig. 16-7A). Similarly, the surface of the retina may be divided into two halves by a vertical line drawn through the center of the fovea: a **nasal hemiretina** that lies medial to the fovea and a **temporal hemiretina** that is located lateral to the fovea. A horizontal line drawn through the center of the fovea can divide the retina into superior and inferior halves. The vertical and horizontal lines dividing the retina intersect at the center of the fovea (Fig. 16-7B). Each hemiretina is further subdivided into quadrants.

The images of objects in the visual field are right-left reversed and inverted on the retina. Accordingly, images present in the left half of the visual field of the left eye fall on the nasal hemiretina of the left eye, and images present in the right half of the visual field of the left eye fall on the temporal

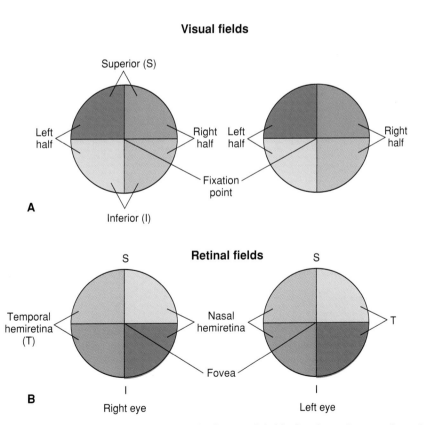

Figure 16–7 Visual and retinal fields. (A) Vertical lines divide the visual field of each eye in space into right and left halves. Horizontal lines divide the visual field of each eye into superior and inferior halves. These lines intersect at the fixation point. (B) Vertical lines divide the retina of each eye into temporal and nasal hemiretinae. Horizontal lines divide the retina of each eye into superior and inferior halves. These lines intersect at the fovea.

hemiretina of the left eye (Fig. 16-8, lines 1 and 2). Similarly, images present in the left half of the visual field of the right eye fall on the temporal hemiretina of the right eye, and images present in the right half of the visual field of the right eye fall on the nasal hemiretina of the right eye (Fig. 16-8, lines 3 and 4). A similar relationship exists between the superior and inferior halves of the visual fields of the superior and inferior hemiretinae of each eye (not shown in Fig. 16-8).

The central portion of the visual field of each eye can be seen by both retinae. This portion of full visual field is called a **binocular visual field**. In a simplified diagram of the binocular visual field (Fig. 16-8), the visual fields of the two eyes are superimposed; the left half of the binocular visual

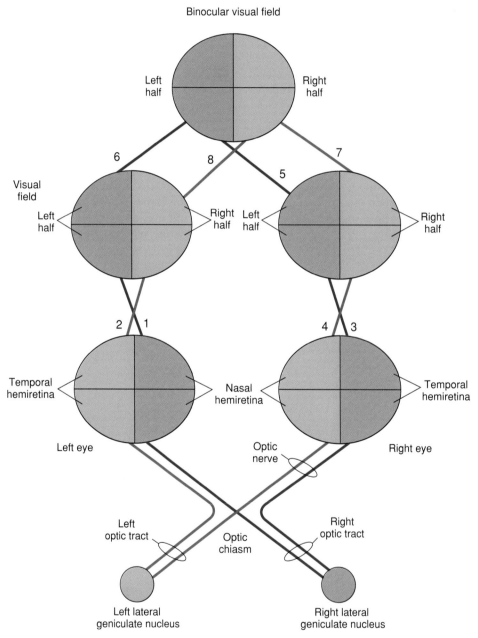

Figure 16–8 Relationship between the visual fields and retinae. 1 and 2: The nasal half of the left eye sees objects in the left half of the visual field of the left eye (*shown in blue*) and the temporal half of the left eye sees objects in the right half of the visual field of the left eye (*shown in red*). 3 and 4: Relationship between the visual fields and hemiretinae of the right eye is similar to that of the left eye. 5 and 6: When the visual fields of the two eyes are superimposed, the left halves of the two eyes coincide to form the left half of the binocular visual field (*shown in blue*). 7 and 8: When the visual fields of the two eyes are superimposed, the right halves of the two eyes coincide to form the right half of the binocular visual field (*shown in red*). Each optic nerve contains axons from the nasal and temporal hemiretinae. At the optic chiasm, the axons from the nasal hemiretinae cross to the contralateral side, while the axons from the temporal retinae remain uncrossed. The crossed and uncrossed axons on each side form the optic tracts.

field (shown in blue) represents the left half of the visual field of each eye (Fig. 16-8, lines 5 and 6), and the right half of the binocular visual field (shown in red) represents the right half of the visual field of each eye (Fig. 16-8, lines 7 and 8).

VISUAL PATHWAYS

The axons of ganglion cells travel towards the posterior pole of the eye where the optic disc is located. At this point, the axons become myelinated and exit the eye as the optic nerve. Extensions of meninges covering the brain also ensheathe the optic nerves. The optic nerves and tracts and their relationship with visual fields of the eyes are shown in Figure 16-8. When the optic nerves of the two eyes reach the brain, they join to form the optic chiasm. At this site, the fibers representing the nasal half of the retina of each eye cross to the contralateral side, while the fibers representing the temporal half of the retina of each eye remain uncrossed. After leaving the optic chiasm, the crossed and uncrossed fibers on each side join to form the optic tracts. The left optic tract contains axons from the temporal hemiretina of the left eye and the nasal hemiretina of the right eye. As mentioned earlier, the temporal hemiretina of the left eye sees objects in the right half of the visual field of the same eye, and the nasal hemiretina of the right eye sees objects in the right half of the visual field of the same eye (Fig. 16-8, lines 2 and 4). This means that the left optic tract contains fibers that convey visual information from the right half of the visual field of each eye or the right half of the binocular visual field (Fig. 16-8, lines 7 and 8).

The right optic tract contains axons from the temporal hemiretina of the right eye and the nasal hemiretina of the left eye. Recall that the temporal hemiretina of the right eye sees objects in the left half of the visual field of the same eye, and the nasal hemiretina of the left eye sees objects in the left half of the visual field of the same eye (Fig. 16-8, lines 3 and 1). Thus, the right optic tract contains fibers that convey visual information from the left half of the visual field of each eye or the left half of the binocular visual field (Fig. 16-8, lines 5 and 6). The optic tracts on each side project to the corresponding lateral geniculate nucleus of the thalamus (see next section).

THE LATERAL GENICULATE NUCLEUS OF THALAMUS

The projections of the optic tracts to the lateral geniculate nuclei are shown in Fig. 16-9A. This nucleus consists of 6 layers. The ventral layers (layers 1 and 2) are called **magnocellular layers** because they contain large cells, while the dorsal layers (layers 3, 4, 5, and 6) are called **parvocellular layers** because they contain cells of smaller size. Injury to magnocellular layers reduces the ability to detect fast-moving visual stimuli, but there is little or no effect on visual acuity or color perception. On the other hand, damage to the parvocellular layers eliminates color vision and impairs visual acuity without affecting perception of fast-moving visual stimuli. Thus, the parvocellular system seems to be concerned with color and detailed form, while the magnocellular system is concerned with location and movement. In general, the parvocellular system projects to more ventral portions (deeper regions) of the **primary visual cortex**, and the magnocellular system projects to more dorsal portions (superficial regions) of the primary visual cortex. Axons from the contralateral nasal hemiretina project to layers 1, 4, and 6, while axons from the ipsilateral temporal hemiretina project to layers 2, 3, and 5. The macular or central areas in the retina are represented to a greater extent in the lateral geniculate nucleus than are the peripheral areas of the retina.

THE GENICULOCALCARINE TRACT

Axons of the neurons in the parvocellular and magnocellular layers of the lateral geniculate nucleus project through the **geniculocalcarine tract** (also known as **optic radiations**) to the primary visual cortex located on the medial aspect of the occipital lobe of the cortex. The course of different fiber bundles in this tract is shown in Figure 16-9B. The fibers in the geniculocalcarine tract serving the inferior quadrant of the contralateral visual hemifield (via superior retina) arise from the dorsomedial region of the lateral geniculate nucleus and use a superior (dorsal) trajectory to synapse on the **superior bank of the calcarine fissure** of the visual cortex. The axons conveying information from the superior quadrant of the contralateral visual hemifield (via inferior retina) arise from the ventrolateral region of the lateral geniculate nucleus and use a relatively more inferior trajectory traveling toward the tip of the temporal horn of the lateral ventricle, looping caudally (called **Meyer's loop**) in the inferior part of the temporal lobe and terminating in the **inferior bank of the calcarine fissure** of the visual cortex. The axons conveying information from the macula (including fovea) arise from the central portion of the lateral geniculate nucleus and synapse on the caudal pole of the occipital cortex.

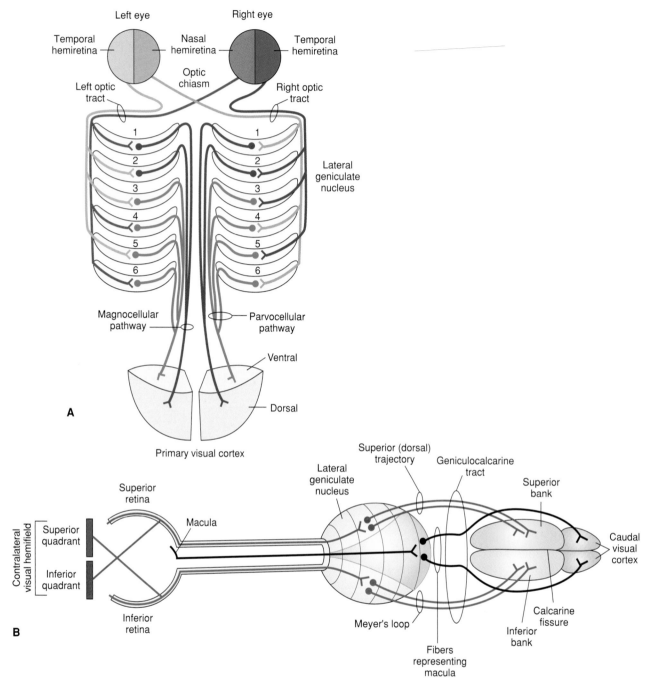

Figure 16–9 Course of axons from the retinal halves. (A) On each side, the axons from ipsilateral temporal hemiretinae in the optic tract synapse in layers 2, 3, and 5 of the lateral geniculate nucleus, and the axons from the contralateral nasal hemiretinae synapse in layers 1, 4, and 6. The postsynaptic axons emerging from the lateral geniculate nucleus on each side project to the primary visual cortex. (B) The axons from the superior retinae and inferior retinae project to the lateral geniculate nuclei. The postsynaptic neurons in the lateral geniculate nuclei receiving inputs from the inferior retinae form Meyer's loop and project to the inferior bank of the calcarine fissure. The postsynaptic neurons in the lateral geniculate nuclei receiving inputs from the superior retinae form the superior trajectory and synapse on neurons in the superior bank of the calcarine fissure. The fibers conveying visual information from the macula synapse in the central regions of the lateral geniculate ganglion, and axons from the postsynaptic neurons in the lateral geniculate nucleus project to the caudal pole of the occipital cortex. For other details, see text.

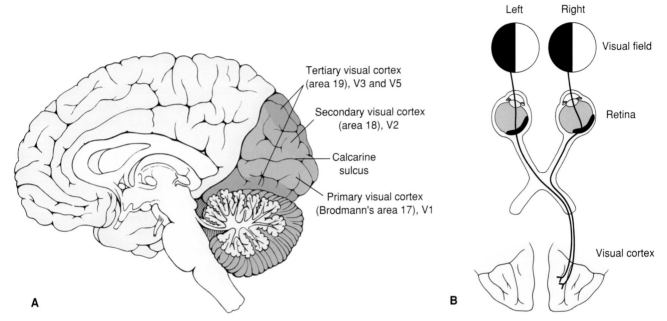

Figure 16–10 The visual cortex. (A) Note the location of the primary visual cortex (V1; Brodmann's area 17), the secondary visual cortex (V2; Brodmann's area 18), and the visual areas V3 and V5 (Brodmann's area 19). (B) Information from the nasal retina of the left eye and temporal retina of the right eye (representing the left visual field of both eyes) is directed to the right visual cortex. Likewise, information from the nasal retina of the right eye and temporal retina of the left eye (representing the right visual field of both eyes) is directed to the left visual cortex (not shown).

VISUAL CORTEX

Different areas in the primary visual cortex are shown in Figure 16-10A. The primary visual cortex (V1; **Brodmann's area 17**) is located on the superior and inferior banks of the calcarine sulcus on the medial side of the occipital lobe and receives projections from the lateral geniculate nucleus of the thalamus. The secondary visual cortex (V2; **Brodmann's area 18**) and tertiary visual cortex (V3 and V5; **Brodmann's area 19**) are located adjacent to the primary visual cortex. The secondary and tertiary visual areas are also known as **association, extrastriate, or prestriate areas**. Visual area V4 is located in the inferior occipitotemporal area (not visible in Fig. 16-10A). V3 is associated with form, V4 is associated with color, and V5 is associated with motion. The portion of area V5 that is concerned with motion of an object lies in the middle temporal gyrus. The primary visual cortex sends projections to the secondary visual cortex; from here, this information is relayed to the tertiary visual cortex. Thus, information from the nasal retina of the left eye and temporal retina of the right eye (representing the left visual field of both eyes) is directed to the right visual cortex (Fig. 16-10B). Likewise, information from the nasal retina of the right eye and temporal retina of the left eye (representing the right visual field of both eyes) is directed to the left visual cortex. The overall representation of the retina in the primary visual cortex is as fol-

lows: the macular part of the retina is represented in the posterior part of the visual cortex, the peripheral part of the retina is represented in the anterior part of the visual cortex, the superior half of the retina relating to the inferior visual fields is represented in the superior visual cortex, and the inferior half of the retina relating to the superior visual fields is represented in the inferior part of the visual cortex. Details concerning the processing of visual signals within the visual cortex are presented in Chapter 26.

THE SUPERIOR COLLICULUS

The superior colliculus controls **saccadic (high velocity) eye movements**. The superficial layers of the superior colliculus receive converging inputs related to visual processes from the retina (via the optic tracts) and from the visual cortex. The superior colliculus also receives additional inputs from somatic sensory and auditory systems. Based on information received from these three sensory systems, the deeper layers of the superior colliculus control motor mechanisms responsible for saccadic movements and orientation of the eyes towards the stimulus. The superior colliculus achieves this function by virtue of its projections to cranial nerve nuclei of III and VI, which regulate horizontal movements of the eye. In addition, descending fibers of the tectospinal tract (from the superior colliculus) reach the upper spinal cord, activate neurons controlling neck muscles, and thus produce reflex neck movements in response to visual input. Other tectal fibers innervate the cerebellum indirectly through synaptic connections in the ventral pontine and paramedian reticular nuclei. These connections enable the cerebellum to coordinate eye and head movements.

BINDING MECHANISM

Information about the form, depth, motion, and color of objects in a visual field is conveyed by separate neuronal pathways to the brain. This information is processed by different cell groups in the cortex. A mechanism, which has not yet been delineated, is believed to integrate the information processed by different cortical cell groups in order to build an image of an object that combines specific information regarding its form, depth, color, and motion. This mechanism is called the **binding mechanism.**

VISUAL REFLEXES

PUPILLARY LIGHT REFLEX

Sympathetic innervation of the eye is described in Chapter 22. Briefly, the axons of preganglionic sympathetic neurons, which are located in the intermediolateral cell column at the T1 level, synapse on neurons in the superior cervical ganglia. The postganglionic sympathetic fibers arising from the superior cervical ganglia innervate the radial (dilator) smooth muscle fibers of the iris. Activation of the sympathetic nervous system results in contraction of the radial muscles of the iris, which brings about **mydriasis** (pupillary dilatation). Interruption of sympathetic innervation to the eye results in Horner's syndrome (see Chapter 22).

The pathways involved in the parasympathetic component of the pupillary light reflex (described in Chapter 4) are shown in Figure 16-11. The axons of the retinal ganglion cells project to the pretectal area via the optic tract. The pretectal area of the midbrain is located just rostral to the superior colliculus. The cells in the pretectal area send bilateral projections to preganglionic parasympathetic neurons located in the **Edinger-Westphal nucleus, a component of the oculomotor nucleus.** The axons of the preganglionic parasympathetic neurons located in the Edinger-Westphal nucleus leave the brainstem through the **oculomotor nerve** (cranial nerve [CN] III) and synapse on the postganglionic parasympathetic neurons in the ciliary ganglion, which is located in the orbit. The postganglionic fibers from the ciliary ganglion enter the eyeball and innervate the circular smooth muscle (sphincter muscle) of the iris and the circumferential mus-

cles of the ciliary body. When the retinal ganglion cells are activated by bright light, the neurons in the pretectal area discharge, which, in turn, excite parasympathetic preganglionic cells in the Edinger-Westphal nucleus. These events finally result in an increase in the activity of parasympathetic innervation to the smooth muscle of the pupillary sphincter, which contracts to produce **miosis** (constriction of the pupil) and reduce the light entering the eye. Light shone on the retina of one eye causes constriction of pupils in both eyes. The response in the eye on which the light was directed is called the **direct pupillary light reflex**, while the response in the contralateral eye is called the **consensual pupillary light reflex**. The consensual response occurs because the pretectal area projects bilaterally to the Edinger-Westphal nuclei. Contraction of circumferential muscles of the ciliary body results in the relaxation of the **suspensory ligaments of the lens**, causing it to become more convex and thus allowing for greater refraction of the light rays, which is more suitable for near vision. These two responses (i.e., constriction of the pupil and increasing the convexity of the lens) are included in the **accommodation reflex** (described in the next section).

ACCOMMODATION REFLEX

This reflex comes into play when the eye has to focus from a distant object to a near one. The reflex involves the following three events: (1) convergence of the eyes, (2) constriction of the pupil, and (3) fixation of the lens for near vision (i.e., by making it more convex). Convergence of the eyes takes place as a result of direct or indirect cortical projections to somatic components of the Edinger-Westphal nucleus, which activate the medial rectus muscles bilaterally. As mentioned earlier, pupillary constriction, which is necessary for the near object to be in focus, results from activation of a parasympathetic pathway from the Edinger-Westphal nucleus to the ciliary ganglion and postganglionic fibers to pupillary constrictor muscles. Fixation of the lens for near vision is brought about by activation of the parasympathetic component of the third nerve. Preganglionic fibers project to the ciliary ganglion, which, in turn, send postganglionic fibers to the circumferential muscle fibers of the ciliary body. Contraction of these muscles reduces tension on the suspensory ligament, allowing the lens to become more convex.

PROMINENT DEFECTS IN VISION

In a normal eye (emmetropic eye), parallel rays of light from a distant object are focused sharply on the retina when the ciliary muscle is completely relaxed.

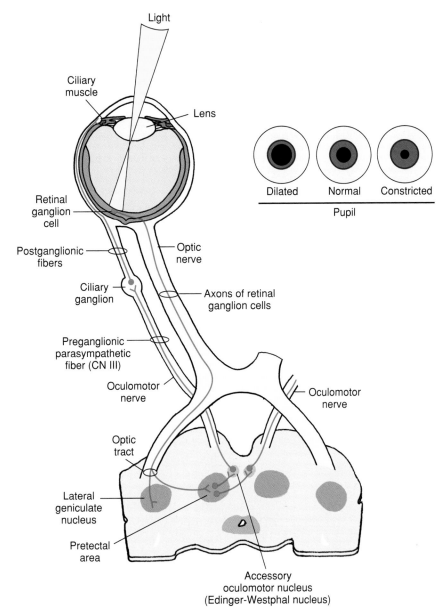

Figure 16–11 Pathways mediating the pupillary light reflex. The axons of the retinal ganglion cells project to the pretectal area. The neurons in the pretectal area send projections to the preganglionic parasympathetic neurons of the ipsilateral and contralateral Edinger-Westphal nuclei. The axons of the neurons in each Edinger-Westphal nucleus exit through the ipsilateral oculomotor nerve and project to the corresponding ciliary ganglion. The postganglionic fibers of the ciliary ganglion innervate the ciliary muscle (see text for details).

To be able to focus a near object on the retina in an emmetropic eye, the ciliary muscle must contract and accommodate for near vision (Fig. 16-12A).

HYPERMETROPIA (HYPEROPIA; FAR-SIGHTEDNESS)

In this condition, either the eyeball is too small or the lens system is too weak so that parallel light rays from an object are not bent sufficiently and are focused behind the retina when the ciliary muscle is completely relaxed (Fig. 16-12B). This condition can

be corrected by placing a convex lens of appropriate strength in front of the eye; after this correction, the parallel light rays coming from a distant object are converged and focused on the retina (Fig. 16-12C).

MYOPIA (NEAR-SIGHTEDNESS)

This condition is usually caused by the increased length of the eyeball or, occasionally, by increased power of the lens system. When the ciliary muscle is completely relaxed, the light rays coming from a distant object are focused in front of the retina (Fig.

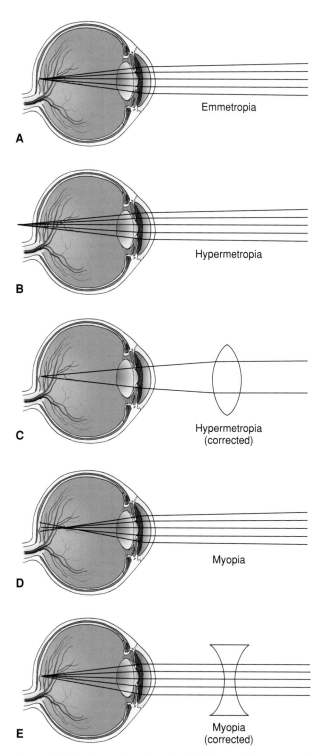

Figure 16–12 Errors in refraction. (A) Normal (emmetropic) eye. (B) In hypermetropia (hyperopia, far-sightedness), light rays are focused behind the retina when the ciliary muscle is completely relaxed. (C) Hypermetropia can be corrected by placing a convex lens of appropriate strength in front of the eye. (D) In myopia (near-sightedness), the light rays coming from a distant object are focused in front of the retina when the ciliary muscle is completely relaxed. (E) Myopia can be corrected by placing a concave lens of an appropriate strength in front of the eye.

16-12D). This condition can be corrected by placing a concave lens of an appropriate strength in front of the eye; in this manner, parallel light rays coming from a distant object are diverged by the concave lens and thus focused on the retina (Fig. 16-12E).

ASTIGMATISM

Astigmatism usually occurs when the shape of the cornea is oblong. Because of this shape, the curvature of the cornea in one plane is less than the curvature in the other plane. Accordingly, the light rays coming from an object are bent to a different extent in these two different planes, preventing the light rays from coming to a single focal point. This condition is corrected by placing a cylindrical lens in front of the eye.

STRABISMIC AMBLYOPIA

Stereoscopic vision develops as early as 3 months after birth. In some infants, the visual axes of the two eyes are not parallel; this is called **strabismus** (squint). To avoid diplopia (double vision), the infant suppresses foveal vision in the nondominant eye that is perhaps mediated from the cerebral cortex. If the axes of the eyes are corrected during the first 6 months of the development, strabismic amblyopia is reversed. Strabismus is usually treated successfully by eye muscle training exercises and by the use of glasses with prisms that bend light rays so that the abnormal position of the eyeball is compensated. In some cases, strabismus is corrected by the shortening of some of the eye muscles using careful surgical procedures.

NIGHT BLINDNESS (NYCTALOPIA)

As noted already, the photosensitive pigments are composed of a protein (opsin) and vitamin A aldehyde (retinal). Vitamin A deficiency is, therefore, likely to reduce the amount of this photosensitive pigment in rods and cones. Even though the photosensitive pigment is depleted, daylight is able to activate the remaining pigment. Therefore, daylight vision is not significantly affected. However, light level at night is insufficient to activate the depleted pigment; therefore, the person cannot see in the dark. Oral supplements of vitamin A are helpful in these conditions.

COLOR BLINDNESS

Lack of a particular color cone may render a person unable to detect a particular color. Most individuals are red-green blind, and the majority of persons are blind to green color. A minority of individuals are blue color-blind. Because red-green color blindness is inherited by an X-linked recessive gene, more males than females are afflicted with this defect.

ARGYLL ROBERTSON PUPIL

In syphilitic patients with CNS complications (tabes dorsalis or neurosyphilis), the pupils do not contract in response to light, but they do exhibit constriction as a component of the accommodation reflex. This indicates that the retina is still sensitive to light and that the pre- and postganglionic autonomic fibers innervating the eye are intact. In these patients, the pupillary light reflex is absent because the pretectal area, which receives inputs from optic fibers that are essential for eliciting this reflex, is damaged. However, the pretectal area is not essential for eliciting pupillary constriction during the time when the accommodation reflex occurs. The precise location of the lesion is not known in Argyll Robertson pupil. However, it is hypothesized that the descending pathways from the visual cortex, which mediate pupillary constriction in the accommodation reflex, bypass the pretectal area and project to the Edinger-Westphal nucleus of the third nerve. These pathways are not affected in patients with neurosyphilis. Therefore, the mechanism of pupillary constriction during the accommodation reflex remains largely intact in these patients, whereas the pupillary light reflex is absent due to damage to the pretectal area.

ADIE'S PUPIL

In Adie's pupil, there is a prolonged and sluggish constriction of the pupil to light. Following the pupillary constriction, the dilation of the pupil is delayed. Patients with this disorder have pathological changes in the ciliary ganglion.

MARCUS-GUNN PUPIL

In Marcus-Gunn pupil, one of the eyes has an optic nerve lesion. **A swinging flashlight test** is conducted to test the pupillary light reflex in such patients as follows. During this test, the patient sits in a dimly lit room, then the light source is moved quickly back and forth from one eye to another, and pupillary constrictions are noted. When light is shone on the normal eye, both pupils constrict (direct and consensual light reflexes). When the light is shone on the eye with the optic nerve lesion, lesser signals reach the Edinger-Westphal nucleus. This nucleus senses the lesser intensity of light and shuts off the parasympathetic response to the light stimulus, causing paradoxical dilation of both pupils.

WEBER SYNDROME

Weber syndrome is usually caused by an infarct that affects the rootlets of the oculomotor nerve. The symptoms include deviation of the eye downward and outward, drooping of the eyelid, and a dilated and nonresponsive pupil on the ipsilateral side, accompanied by contralateral upper motor neuron paralysis.

PARINAUD SYNDROME

Parinaud syndrome is caused by lesions in the pretectal area. The patient suffers from paralysis of upward gaze, a large pupil, and retraction of eyelids.

DEFICITS AFTER A LESION AT DIFFERENT SITES IN THE VISUAL PATHWAY

In Figure 16-13, the sites of lesion in the visual pathways are labeled by numbers (panel A), and corresponding visual field deficits are labeled by letters (a to i, in panel B).

Damage to the right optic nerve (site 1): all axons of ganglion cells emanating from the right eye are injured. Therefore, there is a total loss of vision in the right eye (Fig. 16-13B, a).

Damage to the optic chiasm (site 2): a lesion at the optic chiasm interrupts the axons from the *nasal hemiretinae of both eyes*, leaving the axons from the temporal retinae intact. Therefore, loss of vision occurs in the right half of the right visual field and left half of the left visual field. This visual defect is called **nonhomonymous bitemporal hemianopia** (Fig. 16-13B, b). The term nonhomonymous or heteronomous visual deficit indicates that the deficit is in different halves of the visual field.

Nonhomonymous bitemporal hemianopia is a frequent manifestation of a large pituitary adenoma compressing on the optic chiasm. This condition is often associated with a deficiency in circulating follicle-stimulating and luteinizing hormones, which can cause, among other actions, amenorrhea (absence of menstrual periods) in women and reduction in sperm count in men. In these patients, trans-sphenoidal microsurgery is done to remove the pituitary tumor. In some cases, irradiation is used to destroy the tumor. Pituitary adenomas can secrete prolactin or growth hormone. Dopamine, which is present in the arcuate

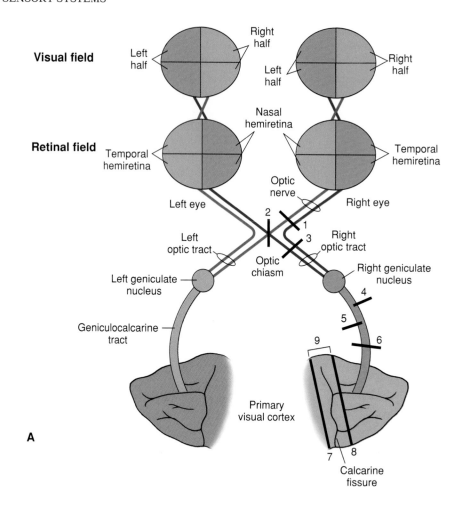

A

B

Site of Lesion	Deficit in the visual field		Name of the disorder
	Left eye	Right eye	
1			a. Total loss of vision in the right eye
2			b. Non-homonymous bitemporal hemianopia
3			c. Contralateral (left) homonymous hemianopia
4			d. Superior left homonymous quadrantanopia (pie in the sky disorder)
5			e. Inferior left homonymous quadrantanopia (pie in the floor disorder)
6			f. Contralateral (left) homonymous hemianopia
7			g. Superior left homonymous quadrantanopia (with macular sparing)
8			h. Inferior left homonymous quadrantanopia (with macular sparing)
9			i. Contralateral (left) homonymous hemianopia (with macular sparing)

Figure 16–13 Deficits after lesions in the visual pathways. (A) The sites of lesions in the visual pathways are numbered. (B) Numbers in the first column refer to the site of lesion shown in panel A; the deficits in the visual fields of both eyes are shaded in *black*; and the disorders are described on the right side and marked with lowercase letters (a-i). Macular sparing, where applicable, is shown as a notch in the center of the visual field (see text for details).

nucleus of the hypothalamus, normally inhibits the secretion of prolactin from the anterior pituitary. Therefore, administration of a dopamine receptor agonist, bromocriptine, is used to inhibit prolactin secretion if the tumor is of the prolactin-secreting type. Somatostatin, a peptide present in the hypothalamus, is known to inhibit the secretion of growth hormone from the anterior pituitary. If the pituitary tumor is a growth hormone-secreting type, a somatostatin analog, octreotide, is administered to inhibit the secretion of growth hormone.

Damage to the right optic tract (site 3): axons from the ganglion cells of the temporal retina of the right eye (which sees objects in the left visual hemifield of the same eye) and the nasal retina of the left eye (which sees objects in the left visual hemifield of the same eye) are damaged. Therefore, objects in the left half of the visual field of each eye cannot be seen. This visual deficit is called **contralateral (in this case left) homonymous hemianopia** (Fig. 16-13B, c). This is called a homonymous visual deficit because the loss of vision is in the *visual field* of the same half of each eye (in this case left visual hemifield of each eye).

Damage to the right temporal lobe (including Meyer's loop)(site 4): Vascular occlusions in the middle cerebral artery may cause lesions in the inferior portion of the temporal lobe. Recall that axons of the neurons in the lateral geniculate nucleus project through the geniculocalcarine tract (optic radiations) to the ipsilateral primary visual cortex. Because damage is in the right Meyer's loop, vision will be lost in the superior quadrant of the left visual hemifield of each eye. This disorder is referred to as a **"superior left homonymous quadrantanopia," "contralateral superior homonymous quadrantanopia,"** or **"pie in the sky visual disorder"** (Fig. 16-13B, d).

Damage to the right parietal lobe (site 5): These lesions may be caused by vascular occlusion of the middle cerebral artery. In the geniculocalcarine tract, the axons that convey information about the inferior visual hemifields pass lateral to the ventricle in the inferior portion of the parietal lobe. Therefore, vision will be lost in inferior quadrants of the left visual hemifield of each eye. This disorder is called **"inferior left homonymous quadrantanopia," "contralateral inferior homonymous quadrantanopia,"** or **"pie in the floor visual disorder"** (Fig. 16-13B, e).

Damage to entire geniculocalcarine tract (optic radiations) on the right side (site 6): the visual defect in this type of damage will be similar to that described under the damage to the right optic tract (site 3); the deficit is called **contralateral homonymous hemianopia** (Fig. 16-13B, f).

Lesion of the inferior bank of the right calcarine fissure (site 7): the fibers of Meyer's loop on the right side project to the inferior bank of the right calcarine fissure. Therefore, such a lesion will produce a superior left quadrantanopia identical to that described for Meyer's loop (Fig. 16-13B, g).

Lesion of the superior bank of the right calcarine fissure (site 8): the superior bank of the right calcarine fissure receives fibers from the lateral geniculate nucleus associated with inputs from the inferior quadrant of the contralateral visual hemifield, and the deficit will be identical to that described for damage to the parietal lobe. As mentioned earlier, this disorder is called "inferior left homonymous quadrantanopia," "contralateral inferior homonymous quadrantanopia," or "pie in the floor visual defect" (Fig. 16-13B, h).

Damage to entire right calcarine cortex (both superior and inferior banks) (site 9): the visual defect in this situation is similar to that described for damage to the right optic tract (site 3). As mentioned earlier, this visual deficit is called contralateral (or left) homonymous hemianopia (Fig. 16-13B, i).

Superior left homonymous quadrantanopia, inferior left homonymous quadrantanopia, and contralateral (in this case, left) homonymous hemianopia can occur with "macular sparing," which refers to sparing of vision in a small central area of the visual field that represents the foveal (macular) region of the retina (Fig. 16-13B, g-i). "Macular sparing" can be explained as follows. Although the entire visual cortex is supplied by the calcarine artery, caudal parts of the visual cortex also receive blood from collateral branches of the middle cerebral artery. Therefore, integrity of the caudal part of the visual cortex may be preserved despite occlusion of the calcarine artery. In this situation, visual signals coming from the macula can be processed by the caudal visual cortex because axons conveying information from the macula project via the lateral geniculate nucleus to the caudal pole of the occipital cortex (Fig. 16-9B).

CLINICAL CASE

HISTORY

James is a 32-year-old man with no significant medical problems. In the past few months, he has noticed that the vision in his right eye was deteriorating, especially in the center of the right visual field. His left eye seemed normal. He also noticed that he had been having more and more frequent right frontal headaches. If he wasn't careful, he occasionally bumped into things on his right side, although he was easily able to compensate by turning his eyes (and using his left eye) or turning his head. Since he had never had any serious visual problems before, he consulted an ophthalmologist.

EXAMINATION

Ophthalmologic examination revealed a large central scotoma in the right retina (blind area in the center of his visual field). During fundoscopic examination with an ophthalmoscope, the optic disc appeared pale. When a light was shone into his right eye, the pupil in either eye did not react. However, when light was shone into his left eye, the left as well as the right pupil (consensual response) constricted. When asked the color of a bright red pen placed into the center of the right visual field, James called it pink. The ophthalmologist recommended a magnetic resonance imaging (MRI) scan of James's head and a consultation with a neurologist.

EXPLANATION

The MRI scan of James's head revealed a right optic nerve glioma, a tumor of the glia surrounding the optic nerve anterior to the optic chiasm. Disease of the optic nerve often causes it to appear pale on fundoscopic examination.

Many of the optic nerve fibers subserve the central portion of the visual field. This includes most of the visual receptors, especially the cones, which are located in the fovea. Moreover, color vision can be affected, most often at the red end of the spectrum, causing the patient to perceive the color red as "washed out" or pink. Because of lack of adequate optic nerve function, the pupillary light reflex is lost due to loss of the afferent arm of the reflex, and there is blindness in the right eye. Such a phenomenon is often called an afferent pupillary defect. The light reflex continues to function in the left eye. Because of continued normal function of the Edinger-Westphal nucleus (i.e., autonomic) component of CN III, the efferent arm of the reflex remains intact in both eyes. The consensual reflex (constriction of the opposite pupil in response to light shone into the contralateral eye) remains intact because of the bilateral distribution of retinal fibers from the intact eye to the nucleus of CN III, thus allowing the right pupil to constrict in response to light in the left eye. However, the consensual reaction is not possible when light is shone into the right eye because no signal is transmitted in the afferent arm of the reflex with respect to this eye.

CHAPTER TEST

QUESTIONS

Choose the best answer for each question.

1. Which one of the following statements is correct regarding photoreceptors?
   a. Rods are specialized for day vision.
   b. Rods contain more photosensitive pigment than cones.
   c. Loss of cones in the retina causes night blindness.
   d. Cones outnumber rods.
   e. Rods are concentrated within the fovea.

2. Which one of the following statements is correct regarding different retinal cell types?
   a. Müller cells inhibit horizontal cells.
   b. Both rods and cones fire action potentials in response to a light stimulus.
   c. Loss of cones results in night blindness.
   d. Ganglion cells represent the output of neurons in the retina.
   e. Color is mediated by rod photoreceptors.

3. A 60-year-old man consulted a neurologist with a complaint of transient episodes consisting of light-headedness, vision disturbances, nausea, and unsteadiness. Angiographic examination revealed that the patient had a vascular occlusion of the right middle cerebral artery. A computed tomography (CT) scan revealed the presence of lesions in the inferior aspect of the right temporal lobe. The visual disorder most likely experienced by the patient is:

   a. Total loss of vision in the left eye
   b. Inability to see objects in the temporal visual fields of both eyes
   c. Inability to see objects in the left superior quadrants of both eyes
   d. Inability to see objects in the left inferior quadrants of both eyes
   e. Inability to see objects in the left visual field of both eyes

4. A 55-year-old woman with a long history of menstrual irregularity consulted with her ophthalmologist, indicating that she was experiencing visual disturbances that seemed to have worsened during the past couple of months. Her ophthalmologist referred her to a neurologist. A CT

scan of the patient's head revealed the presence of a pituitary tumor impinging on the optic chiasm. Which one of the following visual deficits is the patient likely to have?

a. Left (contralateral) homonymous hemianopia
b. Nyctalopia
c. Inferior left homonymous quadrantanopia with macular sparing
d. Nonhomonymous bitemporal hemianopia
e. Strabismic amblyopia

5. A 50-year-old woman reported to her ophthalmologist that she was experiencing visual disturbances in her right eye. A CT scan of her head revealed a lesion in her right optic nerve, and she was diagnosed as having a Marcus-Gunn pupil. Which one of the following responses was observed when the ophthalmologist performed a swinging flashlight test in this patient?

a. When light was shone on her right eye, both pupils constricted.
b. When light was shone on her right eye, both pupils dilated.
c. When light was shone on her left eye, the left pupil constricted.
d. When light was shone on her left eye, both pupils dilated.
e. When light was shone on her left eye, the left pupil dilated.

ANSWERS AND EXPLANATIONS

1. Answer: b

The photopigment is more abundant in the rods, and these photoreceptors are specialized for night vision. Loss of rods causes only night blindness, while the loss of cones causes blindness. Rods are more numerous than cones. Rods are absent in the fovea, where the concentration of cones is very high (see Table 16-1).

2. Answer: d

The ganglion cells represent the output of neurons in the retina. Their axons form the optic nerve. Müller cells are glial cells unique to the retina. The rods and cones do not fire action potentials, instead they respond to the light stimulus by graded hyperpolarizing generator potentials. It is the loss of rods that causes night blindness. Color vision is mediated by cones, not by rods.

3. Answer: c

A lesion in the inferior temporal lobe is likely to damage Meyer's loop. This loop contains fibers from the inferior halves of the retinae that carry information about the superior visual fields. Since the damage is in the right Meyer's loop, the vision will be lost in both eyes: the superior quadrant of the nasal visual field of the right eye and the superior quadrant of the temporal visual field of the left eye. This disorder is referred to as a "superior left homonymous quadrantanopia," "contralateral superior homonymous quadrantanopia," or "pie in the sky visual defect."

4. Answer: d

Nonhomonymous bitemporal hemianopia involves a loss of vision in the temporal halves of both visual fields. It occurs when there is a lesion in the optic chiasm. A large pituitary tumor frequently causes nonhomonymous bitemporal hemianopia by compressing the optic chiasm. Since the nasal retinal fibers cross in the optic chiasm, damage to the chiasm will produce a bitemporal hemianopia. Contralateral homonymous hemianopia occurs when there is damage to the optic tract on one side. Inferior left homonymous quadrantanopia with macular sparing (contralateral inferior homonymous quadrantanopia with macular sparing or pie in the floor visual defect with macular sparing) occurs due to the lesion of the superior bank of the right calcarine fissure. Strabismic amblyopia occurs when the visual axes of the two eyes are not parallel. Nyctalopia (night blindness) is caused by vitamin A deficiency that results in reduction of the amount of photosensitive pigment in rods and cones. In this situation, the level of light at night is insufficient to activate the depleted pigment; therefore, the person cannot see in the dark. Pituitary tumors are usually associated with deficiencies in circulating follicle-stimulating and luteinizing hormones. These deficiencies can result in menstrual irregularities.

5. Answer: b

Patients with Marcus-Gunn pupil have a lesion of one of the optic nerves. A swinging flashlight test to evaluate pupillary light reflex involves quick movement of the light source back and forth from one eye to another. When light is shone on the normal eye, both pupils constrict. When the light is shone on the eye with the optic nerve lesion, lesser signals reach the Edinger-Westphal nucleus. This nucleus senses the lesser intensity of light and consequently shuts off the parasympathetic response to the light, causing the paradoxical dilatation of both pupils. In Adie's pupil, there is a prolonged and sluggish constriction of the pupil to light. Subsequent to the pupillary constriction, the dilation of the pupil is delayed. In these patients, there are pathological changes in the ciliary ganglion.

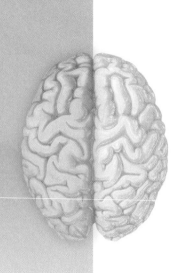

CHAPTER 17

AUDITORY AND VESTIBULAR SYSTEMS

Audition, or hearing, like vision, is one of the most important sensations. Much of human communication depends on a properly functional auditory system. For example, loss of hearing at birth can have the devastating effect of the child's inability to learn to speak. In adults, loss of hearing can also be socially debilitating.

Sound is produced by vibrations that result in the alternate compression and rarefaction of air. The pressure waves generated in the air in this manner reach the ear and are transduced into neural signals that are processed in the brain. In the first part of this chapter, the different properties of the auditory system that regulate the sensation of hearing are described. The second part of the chapter covers the vestibular system, which regulates the movement and position of the head in space in response to signals associated with angular and linear acceleration of the head as well as the gravitational pull exerted on it.

AUDITORY SYSTEM

PHYSICS OF SOUND

Auditory receptors respond to vibrations of the air that radiate from the sound source as pressure waves. The **pitch** (highness or lowness) of the sound is dependent on the frequency of the pressure wave generated by the sound. The frequency of the pressure wave is measured in cycles per second or **Hertz (Hz)**. Young humans can detect a frequency range of 20 Hz to 20 kHz. In older individuals, the range of detectable frequencies decreases to 50 Hz to 17 kHz.

The magnitude of sound is expressed as **intensity**. The range of sound intensities is large. For instance, a sound that is barely audible is about 20 μPa (micro-Pascals, which is the unit for measuring pressure), while a painful sound level is about 2×10^8 Pa. Because of this wide range of intensities, it would be tedious to express sound intensity in absolute units. The sound intensity is, therefore, expressed in terms of the logarithm of the actual sound intensity. The convention is to describe sound intensity as the logarithm of the ratio of a measured pressure to a reference pressure and is expressed in decibels. The **decibel (dB)** is a logarithmic ratio expressed by the following equation: Sound pressure (dB) = 20 $\log_{10} P_t / P_r$; where P_t = pressure of the test sound, and P_r = reference pressure 20 μPa (or 0.0002 dynes/cm^2).

COMPONENTS OF THE EAR

External Ear

The external ear, called the **pinna or auricle**, directs the sound vibrations in the air to the **external auditory canal** (Fig. 17-1A). The sound waves travel through this auditory canal and vibrate the **tympanic membrane** located at the end of the canal.

Middle Ear

Three small bones **(ossicles)**, which articulate with each other, are suspended in the cavity of the middle ear. These ossicles are the **malleus** (the cartilaginous process called **manubrium** of this bone is attached to the tympanic membrane), the **incus**, and the **stapes**. The stapes resembles a stirrup, and its footplate is bound to the **oval window** by an annular ligament. The middle ear is connected to the nasopharynx through the **eustachian tube**, which helps to equalize air pressure on the inner and outer surfaces of the tympanic membrane and to

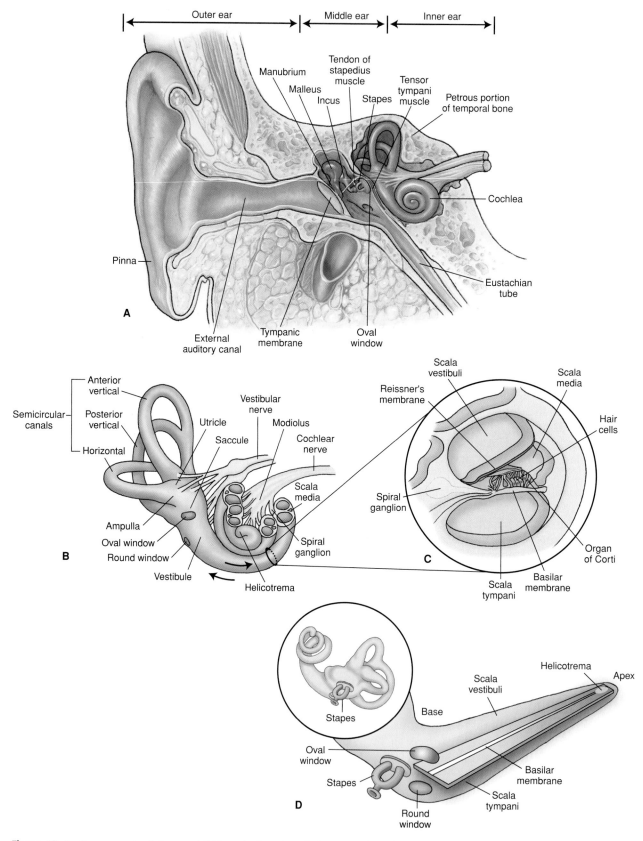

Figure 17–1 Components of the ear. (A) Note the location of the external, middle, and inner ear. The middle ear contains three small bones (the malleus, the incus, and the stapes). (B) The inner ear consists of a bony labyrinth that contains the vestibule, three semicircular (anterior, posterior, and lateral) canals, and the cochlea. (C) A cross section of cochlea reveals that the scala media is bounded by the vestibular (Reissner's) and basilar membranes, and the organ of Corti lies within the scala media (cochlear duct). (D) A diagram of an uncoiled cochlea. (Used with permission from Bear MF, et al.: Neuroscience: Exploring the Brain, 2nd ed. Baltimore: Lippincott, Williams & Wilkins, 2001, pp. 354, 358, 359.)

drain any fluid in the middle ear into the nasopharynx (Fig. 17-1A). A small muscle, the **tensor tympani**, inserts on the manubrium of the malleus; it is innervated by a branch of the trigeminal nerve (cranial nerve [CN] V). Another small muscle, the **stapedius**, inserts on the stapes ossicle and is innervated by a branch of the facial nerve (CN VII). Contraction of these muscles restricts the movement of the tympanic membrane and the footplate of the stapes against the oval window, respectively, and thus reduces the deleterious effects of loud noises on the delicate middle and inner ear structures. Therefore, the function of the middle ear and its components is to convert the sound waves in the air to waves in the fluid located in the inner ear. If the airwaves bypass the middle ear and reach the oval window directly, only about 3% of the sound would enter the inner ear. The pressure transmitted to the oval window is amplified because (1) the area of the tympanic membrane is much greater than that of the oval window, and (2) greater mechanical efficiency is provided by the ossicles (malleus and incus) because they act as levers.

Inner Ear

The inner ear consists of the bony labyrinth, the membranous labyrinth, and the cochlea containing the organ of Corti.

The **bony labyrinth** consists of a complex series of cavities in the petrous portion of temporal bone.

The bony labyrinth surrounds the inner membranous labyrinth and has three regions: a central region called the **vestibule**, three **semicircular canals**, and the **cochlea** (Fig. 17-1, A and B). The vestibule (including the saccule and utricle within it) and semicircular canals represent peripheral components of the vestibular system, which is specialized to respond to movements. The cochlea is involved in hearing and is specialized to respond to airborne sounds. All of the cavities of the bony labyrinth are filled with a fluid called the **perilymph** (a clear extracellular-like fluid containing high Na^+ and low K^+ concentrations). The three semicircular canals include anterior (superior), posterior, and lateral (horizontal) canals. The cochlea, shaped like a conical snail shell, has a central tubular conical axis, called the **modiolus**, which is surrounded by a spiral cochlear canal of two- and three-quarter turns. The cochlear canal is divided into an upper **scala vestibuli** and a lower **scala tympani** (Fig. 17-1C). The scalae tympani and vestibuli communicate with each other at the modiolar apex via a narrow slit called the **helicotrema** (Fig. 17-1D). Within the bony spiral canal of the cochlea lies the **cochlear duct**, which is a component of the membranous labyrinth. The cochlear duct is a spiral tube that runs along the outer wall of the bony cochlea and ends at its apex (cupula) (Fig. 17-2). The cochlear duct (also known as the scala media) is flanked by two channels

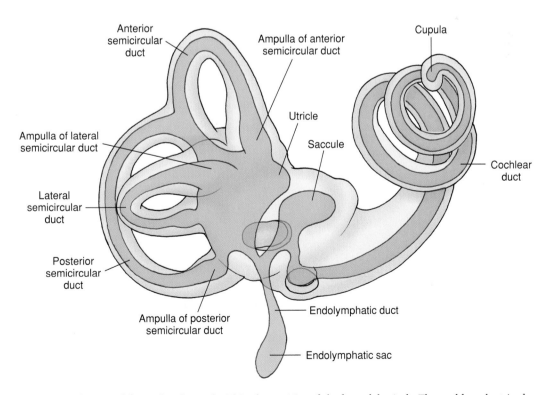

Figure 17–2 The membranous labyrinth is located within the cavities of the bony labyrinth. The cochlear duct is shown in deep blue, and the remainder of the membranous labyrinth is shown in a light green color.

within the cochlea: the scala tympani (it follows the outer contour of the cochlea) and the scala vestibuli (it follows the inner contour of the cochlea). The scala tympani ends at the round window (the secondary tympanic membrane), which separates this space from the middle ear (also known as the tympanic cavity). As mentioned earlier, the stapes (a stirrup-shaped small bone in the middle ear) is bound to the oval window by an elastic ligament. Vibrations of the stapes in response to sound waves are transmitted to the scala vestibuli via the oval window.

The **membranous labyrinth** is located within the cavities of the bony labyrinth and is filled with **endolymph** (an intracellular-like fluid containing low Na$^+$ and high K$^+$). The membranous labyrinth includes the **utricle** and **saccule** (two small sacs occupying the bony vestibule); three semicircular canal ducts, which occupy the bony semicircular canals; and the cochlear duct (already described) (Fig. 17-2). The scala media contains endolymph; and the scalae tympani and vestibuli contain perilymph. The scala media is bound by two membranes: the **vestibular membrane** (also known as **Reissner's membrane**) and the **basilar membrane** (Fig. 17-1C). These two membranes separate the endolymph contained in the scala media from the perilymph contained in the scalae tympani and vestibuli. In the lateral wall of the scala media lies the stria vascularis, which is highly vascular.

Na$^+$-K$^+$ pumps in the stria vascularis pump sodium out of and potassium into the endolymph. As noted earlier, the endolymph contains a high concentration of potassium ions and a low concentration of sodium ions.

The **organ of Corti** is the sensory area of the cochlear duct and is located on the basilar membrane. It contains **hair cells,** which are the sensory receptors for sound stimuli. It lies within the cochlear duct (the scala media) and runs along the entire length of the basilar membrane (Fig. 17-1C). The human cochlea contains two types of hair cells: inner hair cells and outer hair cells (Fig. 17-3). About 100 **stereocilia** and a single **kinocilium** (larger hair cell) are attached to the apical border of the hair cells. The stereocilia are shorter than the kinocilium, and their length increases as they approach the kinocilium. The tips of stereocilia of outer hair cells are embedded in the overlying **tectorial membrane,** which is composed of mucopolysaccharides embedded in a collagenous matrix (Fig. 17-3). Movement of the basilar membrane relative to the tectorial membrane results in displacement of the cilia that is necessary for generating afferent signals (see *Mechanism of Sound Conduction*). Inner hair cells are not attached to the tectorial membrane, and movement of their stereocilia is induced by movement of the endolymph. There are two types of supporting epithelial cells that keep the hair cells in position: the phalangeal

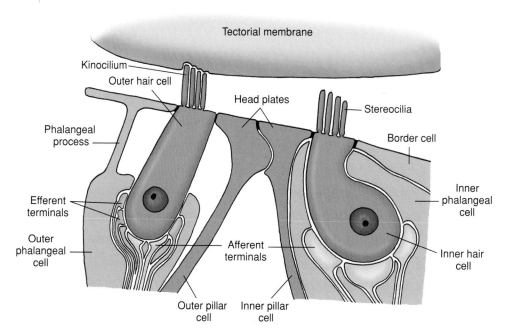

Figure 17-3 The hair cells. Note the two types of hair cells: inner and outer hair cells with stereocilia and one kinocilium present on the apical border. The tips of the cilia on only the outer hair cells are embedded in the tectorial membrane. The peripheral processes of the bipolar neurons in the spiral ganglion form the postsynaptic afferent terminals at the base of the hair cell.

cells and pillar cells. The **outer phalangeal cells (Deiter's cells)** surround the base of the outer hair cells and the nerve terminals associated with these cells (Fig. 17-3). These cells give out a phalangeal process. This process flattens into a plate near the apical surface of the hair cell and forms **tight junctions** with the apical edges of adjacent hair cells and adjacent phalangeal plates. The inner phalangeal cells surround the inner hair cell completely and do not have a phalangeal process. Similarly, there are outer and inner pillar cells whose apical processes form tight junctions with each other and with neighboring hair cells. This network of tight junctions isolates the body of the hair cells from the endolymph contained in the scala media. The **spiral (cochlear) ganglion**, located within the spiral canal of the bony **modiolus**, contains bipolar neurons. The peripheral processes of these bipolar neurons in the spiral ganglion innervate the hair cells; they form the postsynaptic afferent terminals at the base of the hair cell (Fig. 17-3). The central processes of the bipolar cells in the spiral ganglion form the cochlear division of CN VIII. The outer hair cells receive efferent fibers that arise from the superior olivary nucleus (called the olivocochlear bundle). This bundle provides a basis by which the central nervous system can modulate auditory impulses directly at the level of the receptor.

MECHANISM OF SOUND CONDUCTION

Air pressure waves cause the tympanic membrane to vibrate, resulting in oscillatory movements of the footplate of stapes against the oval window. Because the perilymph is a noncompressible fluid and the scalae tympani and vestibuli form a closed system, oscillatory movements of the stapes against the oval window result in pressure waves in the perilymph present in the scalae tympani and vestibuli. The oscillatory movement of perilymph results in vibration of the basilar membrane.

As mentioned earlier, the tips of the stereocilia (of the outer hair cells) are embedded in the tectorial membrane, and the bodies of hair cells rest on the basilar membrane (Fig. 17-4A). An upward displacement of the basilar membrane creates a shearing force that results in lateral displacement of the stereocilia (Fig. 17-4B). Mechanical displacement of the stereocilia and kinocilium in a lateral direction causes an influx of K^+ through their membranes, the hair cell is depolarized, and there is an influx of Ca^{2+} through the voltage-sensitive Ca^{2+} channels in their membranes. The influx of Ca^{2+} triggers the release of the transmitter (probably glutamate) that, in turn, elicits an action poten-

tial in the afferent nerve terminal at the base of the hair cell (Fig. 17-4C). A downward displacement of the basilar membrane creates a shearing force that results in medial displacement of the stereocilia and kinocilium (Fig. 17-4D). Mechanical displacement of the stereocilia and kinocilium in a medial direction results in hyperpolarization of the hair cell that may involve opening of voltage-sensitive K^+ channels and efflux (outward flow) of K^+. The sensory receptors (hair cells) located in the basal portion of the basilar membrane respond to high frequencies of sound, while the sensory receptors located in the apical aspect of the membrane respond to low frequencies (Fig. 17-5). This is called tonotopic distribution of responding receptors.

CENTRAL AUDITORY PATHWAYS

The central auditory pathways are shown in Fig. 17-6. The central processes of bipolar neurons in the **spiral ganglion** form the **cochlear nerve**, which joins the **vestibulocochlear nerve**, passes through the internal auditory meatus, enters the posterior cranial fossa, and reaches the medullopontine angle of the brainstem. Here the vestibulocochlear nerve splits into the vestibular and cochlear branches. Both branches enter the brainstem at the level of rostral medulla. The projections of the cochlear branch are described in the next section, whereas the projections of the vestibular branch are discussed later.

Cochlear Nuclei

The cochlear nerve contains central processes of bipolar neurons in the spiral ganglion. The spiral ganglion is located in the modiolus of the inner ear. The peripheral processes of the spiral ganglion bipolar neurons are connected to the hair cells in the organ of Corti. The axons in the cochlear nerve enter the medulla and project to dorsal and ventral cochlear nuclei located in the rostral medulla (Fig. 17-6). The axons of the cochlear nerve project to the cochlear nuclei in a tonotopic manner (i.e., the axons originating in the basal turns of the cochlea, mediating high-frequency sound, project to the deepest part of the nucleus, whereas the axons arising from the apical turns of the cochlea, mediating low-frequency sound, project to the superficial part of the nucleus). Some axons of the second-order neurons emerging from the dorsal cochlear nucleus located in the rostral medulla ascend to the pons and synapse on the ipsilateral superior olivary nucleus. Other axons from the dorsal cochlear nucleus cross to the contralateral side in the tegmentum of the pons as dorsal acoustic stria and then ascend through the rostral pons and synapse on neurons in the inferior collicu-

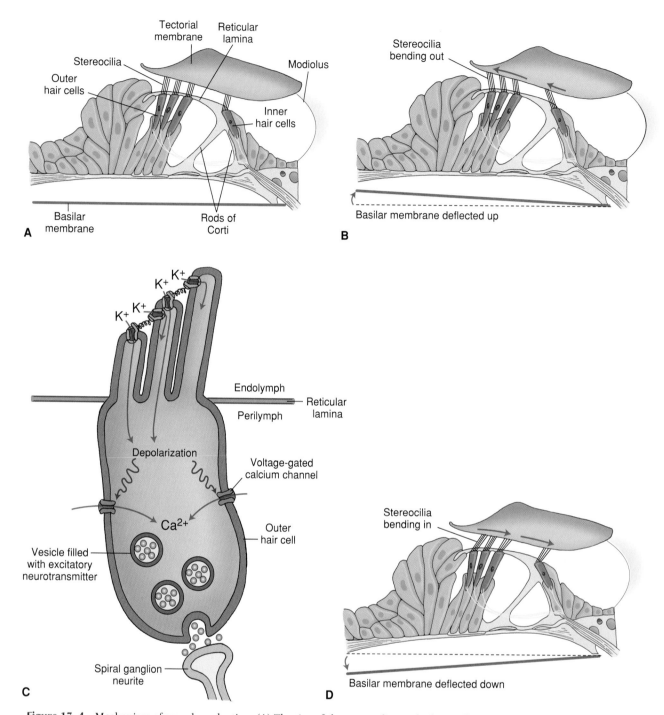

Figure 17–4 Mechanism of sound conduction. (A) The tips of the stereocilia on the hair cells are embedded in the tectorial membrane, and the bodies of hair cells rest on the basilar membrane. (B) An upward displacement of the basilar membrane creates a shearing force that results in lateral displacement of the stereocilia. (C) Mechanical displacement of the stereocilia and kinocilium in a lateral direction causes depolarization of the hair cell. (D) A downward displacement of the basilar membrane creates a shearing force that results in hyperpolarization of the hair cell. (Panels A-C were redrawn with permission from Bear MF, et al.: Neuroscience: Exploring the Brain, 2nd ed. Baltimore: Lippincott, Williams & Wilkins, 2001, pp. 363, 365.)

lus (located in caudal midbrain). Axons of both dorsal and ventral cochlear nuclei form the intermediate acoustic stria, which also cross to the contralateral side in the tegmentum of the pons, ascend through the rostral pons, and synapse on neurons in the inferior colliculus. Axons of the second-order neurons in

the ventral cochlear nucleus form the ventral acoustic stria (trapezoid body), which cross to the contralateral side in the mid-pons and synapse in the superior olivary complex (i.e., the lateral and medial superior olivary nuclei and the nucleus of the trapezoid body). Some axons of the second-order neurons

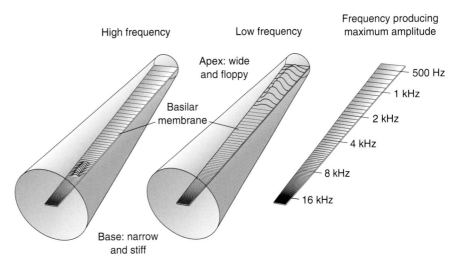

Figure 17–5 Topographical mapping of sound frequencies on the basilar membrane (tonotopy). The cochlea is depicted as an uncoiled canal. The points responding to high frequencies of sound waves are located at the base of the basilar membrane, while those responding to low frequencies are located at the apex. (Reproduced with permission from Bear MF, et al.: Neuroscience: Exploring the Brain, 2nd ed. Baltimore: Lippincott, Williams & Wilkins, 2001, p. 361.)

in the ventral cochlear nucleus synapse in the ipsilateral superior olivary complex in the mid-pons. The projections from the superior olivary nuclei are discussed in the next section.

Superior Olivary Nuclei

The superior olivary complex on either side of the brain is tonotopically organized and receives bilateral auditory inputs from the cochlear nuclei. This nuclear complex can localize sound in acoustic space by discriminating the differences in the time of arrival of the sound or the differences in the intensity of sound to each ear.

Lateral Lemniscus and Associated Nuclei

Although the axons of the third-order neurons from the superior olivary complex and nucleus of the trapezoid body ascend bilaterally in the **lateral lemniscus**, a majority of these axons ascend in the contralateral lateral lemniscus and project to the nucleus of the lateral lemniscus at the level of the pons-midbrain junction. The neurons in the nucleus of lateral lemniscus, in turn, project to the inferior colliculus (located in the caudal midbrain) (Fig. 17-6).

Inferior Colliculus

The dorsal portion of the inferior colliculus receives projections from neurons that are responding to low frequencies of sound, while the ventral portion receives projections from those neurons responding to high frequencies of sound. The auditory information is then processed and relayed by the inferior colliculus to the medial geniculate nucleus of the thalamus (located in rostral midbrain).

Medial Geniculate Nucleus

The axons of the inferior collicular neurons transmit auditory signals to the medial geniculate nucleus of the thalamus (Fig. 17-6). The medial geniculate nucleus, which is tonotopically arranged, relays precise information regarding the intensity, frequency, and binaural properties of the sound. The axons of these neurons, in turn, project to the primary auditory cortex.

Primary Auditory Cortex

In humans, this area of the cortex is located in the **transverse temporal gyri (Heschl)** of the medial aspect of the superior temporal gyrus (Fig. 17-7). Area 41 (of Brodmann; see Chapter 26) is the primary site where the auditory inputs are received. Brodmann's area 42 is the auditory association area. Together, Brodmann's areas 41 and 42 are called the **A-1 region** and receive projections from the medial geniculate nucleus (geniculotemporal fibers or auditory radiations). The tonotopic organization in the auditory relay nuclei is maintained in the auditory cortex as well. One of the secondary auditory areas includes **Wernicke's area** (Fig. 17-7), which is important for the interpretation of the spoken word (see Chapter 26 for a discussion of the clinical importance of this region).

DESCENDING PATHWAYS

The A-1 region in the cortex sends descending projections to the medial geniculate nucleus of the thalamus. The medial geniculate nucleus, in turn, sends projections to the inferior colliculus. Presumably, these descending projections provide neural feedback mechanisms within the central auditory pathways.

Other descending projections include olivocochlear efferent fibers. The axons of neurons located in the superior olivary nucleus form both the crossed and uncrossed olivocochlear bundle, travel in the cochlear nerve, and finally innervate the

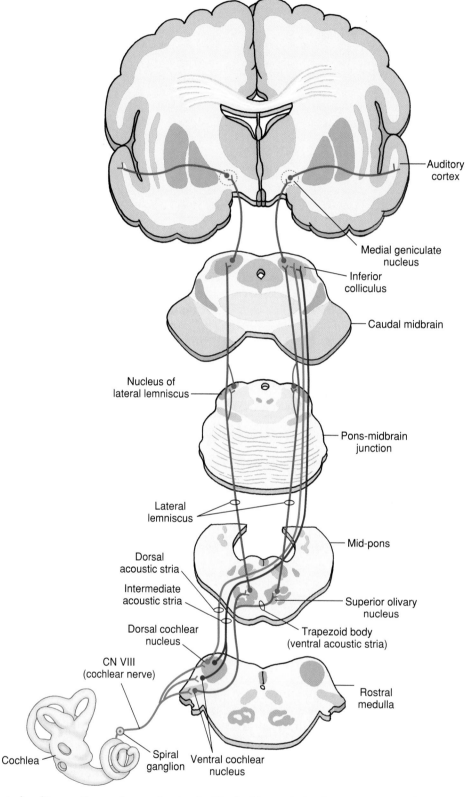

Figure 17–6 Central auditory pathways. See text for details. (Used with permission from Bear MF, et al.: Neuroscience: Exploring the Brain, 2nd ed. Baltimore: Lippincott, Williams & Wilkins, 2001, p. 369.)

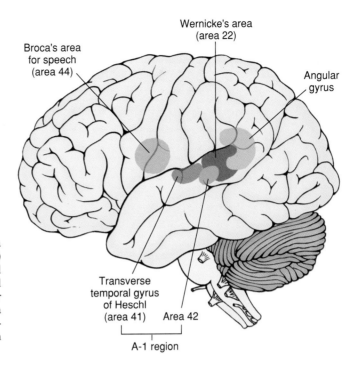

Figure 17–7 Primary auditory cortex. This area is located in the transverse temporal gyri (Heschl) of the medial aspect of the superior temporal gyrus. It receives projections from the medial geniculate nucleus (geniculotemporal fibers or auditory radiations). The secondary auditory area (Wernicke's area) is important for the interpretation of the spoken word. Other areas are shown for orientation purposes.

inner and outer hair cells of the cochlea. At the inner hair cells, uncrossed efferents make synaptic contacts with primary afferent fibers arising from bipolar neurons in the spiral (cochlear) ganglion, while crossed olivocochlear fibers enter the contralateral cochlear nerve and innervate the outer hair cells of the (contralateral) cochlea. The crossed as well as uncrossed olivocochlear efferent innervation regulates the function of hair cells by a mechanism not completely understood and modulates auditory sensitivity. The excitatory transmitters released by some of these efferents are believed to be acetylcholine, glutamate, and aspartate, while γ-aminobutyric acid (GABA) is believed to be an inhibitory transmitter released by some efferent fibers.

CLINICAL DISORDERS ASSOCIATED WITH THE AUDITORY SYSTEM

Conduction Deafness

Otosclerosis is a condition in which the bony outgrowth of the stapes impedes its movement against the oval window. Thus, the ability for efficient conversion of airborne sound waves to pressure waves in the perilymph is lost. This type of conduction deafness is currently corrected by a microsurgical procedure called **stapedectomy**. The procedure involves removing the stapes and substituting it with a prosthetic device (usually a nonmagnetic metallic wire of appropriate thickness and length). Conduction deafness can also result from chronic infection of the middle ear accompanied by fluid accumulation in the middle ear (otitis media); reduced movement of middle ear ossicles has been implicated in this condition.

Sensorineural Deafness

Pathological lesions in the cochlea, cochlear nerve, or central auditory pathways can result in this kind of deafness. Lesions of the cochlea, cochlear nerve, or cochlear nuclei elicit deafness in the ipsilateral ear. Lesions present in higher auditory nuclei may attenuate hearing; however, because of the multiple synapses and crossing and recrossing within the auditory pathways, complete deafness does not occur.

Hearing Tests

Two simple hearing tests, **Weber's test** and **Rinne's test**, are often used in an office setting. In Weber's test, the base of a vibrating tuning fork is placed at the top of the head in the midline. If the person's deafness is due to conduction disturbance in the right ear, the sound from a vibrating tuning fork will be heard louder in the same (right) ear. If the person's deafness is due to sensorineural loss in the right ear, the sound will be louder in the left ear. Rinne's test compares hearing by air conduction versus bone conduction. A vibrating tuning fork is held in the air near the affected ear, and then the base of the tuning fork is placed on the skull (usually at the mastoid process). If the sound perceived by the patient is louder when the tuning fork is

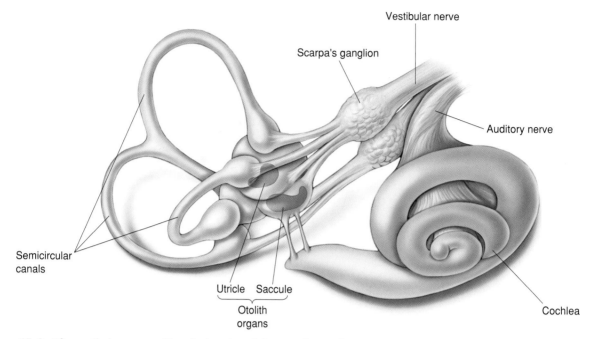

Figure 17–8 The vestibular system. Note the location of the saccule, utricle, and three semicircular canals. (Used with permission from Bear MF, et al.: Neuroscience: Exploring the Brain, 2nd ed. Baltimore: Lippincott, Williams & Wilkins, 2001, p. 386.).

placed on the mastoid process, when compared to the sound of the tuning fork held in the air, the patient is diagnosed as suffering from conductive hearing loss. If the sound perceived by the patient is louder when the tuning fork is placed in the air near the affected ear, the patient is diagnosed as suffering from sensorineural hearing loss.

Conductive hearing loss can be effectively treated by surgery (see earlier section, "Conduction Deafness"). On the other hand, sensorineural hearing loss is difficult to treat. However, during the last decade, considerable progress has been made in treating this hearing loss by cochlear implants.

Tinnitus

Tinnitus is characterized by a "ringing" noise in the ears. Its pathophysiology is not clearly understood. It is believed that damage to the cochlear and vestibular end-organs is responsible for the ringing noise in the ears. Some drugs (e.g., salicylates) induce tinnitus in toxic doses.

VESTIBULAR SYSTEM

ANATOMICAL COMPONENTS

The **vestibular system** is essential for maintaining the position of the body in space, which, in turn, is important for coordination of motor responses, eye movements, and posture. It consists of the following anatomical components: **saccule**, **utricle**, and three semicircular canals (anterior or superior, posterior and lateral, or horizontal semicircular canals). The saccule and utricle (called **otolith organs**) detect linear acceleration, while the semicircular canals detect angular acceleration (Fig. 17-8).

Saccule

The **saccule** is an ovoid sac-like structure that is connected to the cochlea (through the **canal reuniens**) and to the utricle (through the utriculosaccular duct). One of the branches of the latter duct (**the endolymphatic duct**) travels through the petrous bone and forms the endolymphatic (otic) sac in the cranium between the layers of the dura; the **endolymphatic sac** may be the site where endolymph is absorbed (Fig. 17-2). A small area containing hair cells and supporting cells is located within the saccule and constitutes the sensory organ of the saccule. This sensory organ is called the macula of the saccule. A similar area present in the utricle is called the macula of the utricle. There are two types of hair cells in the vestibular labyrinth (including those in the maculae of the saccule and utricle and ampullae of the semicircular canals). These include type I and type II hair cells (see "Vestibular Sensory Receptors"). Projecting from the hair cells are the cilia, which are embedded in a gelatinous matrix of the otolithic membrane containing **otoliths** (calcium carbonate crystals) (Fig. 17-9).

Utricle

The **utricle** is also an ovoid sac-like structure; the cavity inside is the largest in the vestibular labyrinth (Fig. 17-8). Its sensory organ, the macula of the utricle, is located in the anterolateral wall of the cavity, and the organization of its hair cells, cilia, and otolithic membrane is similar to that of the macula of the saccule. The macula of the saccule is almost at a right angle to the macula of the utricle. When the head is in an upright position, the macula of the utricle is in the horizontal plane, while the macula of the saccule is in the vertical sagittal plane.

Semicircular Canals

There are three **semicircular canals** (anterior or superior, posterior and lateral or horizontal semicircular canals) that lie in different planes and are perpendicular to each other (Fig. 17-8). Each of these canals is continuous with the utricle at each end. One of these ends is dilated, and this dilation is called the **ampulla**. Inside the ampulla, a crest (called the **crista ampullaris**) projects at a right angle to the long axis of the canal (Fig. 17-10A). The hair and supporting cells of the crista are located on this crest. A gelatinous mass (the cupula) extends from the surface of the hair cells to the roof of the ampulla. The cilia of the **hair cells** are embedded in the cupula (Fig. 17-10A).

VESTIBULAR SENSORY RECEPTORS

The receptors in the vestibular system (maculae of saccule and utricle and ampullae of semicircular canals) are the hair cells. As noted earlier, there are

two types of hair cells (type I and type II) in the mammalian labyrinth (Fig. 17-10B). The type I hair cells are goblet shaped, and the type II hair cells are cylindrical in shape. Stereocilia in large numbers project from the apical surfaces of all hair cells. A single kinocilium is present at the edge of the apical surface. The stereocilia are relatively shorter than the kinocilium, and their length increases as they approach the kinocilium. The hair cells are surrounded by supporting cells. Tight junctions are present between the hair cells and the supporting cells; this anatomic feature isolates the body of the hair cell from the endolymph, which surrounds the cilia. When the stereocilia are displaced toward the kinocilium, the hair cell is *excited*. When the stereocilia are displaced away from the kinocilium, the hair cell is *inhibited*. In the ampullae of the semicircular canals, when the head turns in the plane of one of the semicircular canals, the inertia of the endolymph generates a force across the cupula, moving it away from the direction of head movement, which results in a displacement of the hair cells within the crista (Fig. 17-10C). Displacement of the stereocilia present on the hair cells induces either depolarization or hyperpolarization of the hair cell; displacement of the cupula in the direction of the utricle results in *excitation* of the hair cell, while displacement of the cupula in the reverse direction results in *inhibition* of the hair cell. In the maculae of the utricle and saccule, linear acceleration or deceleration causes movement of the

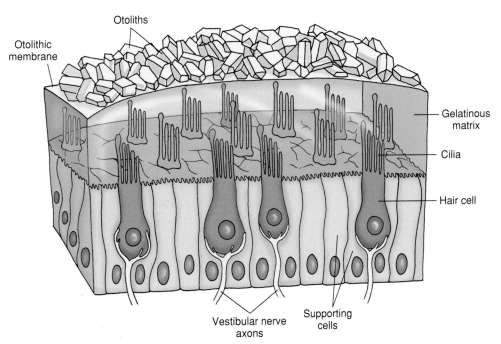

Figure 17–9 Otolithic membrane. Note that the cilia from the hair cells are embedded in a gelatinous matrix of the otolithic membrane containing otoliths that are composed of calcium carbonate crystals.

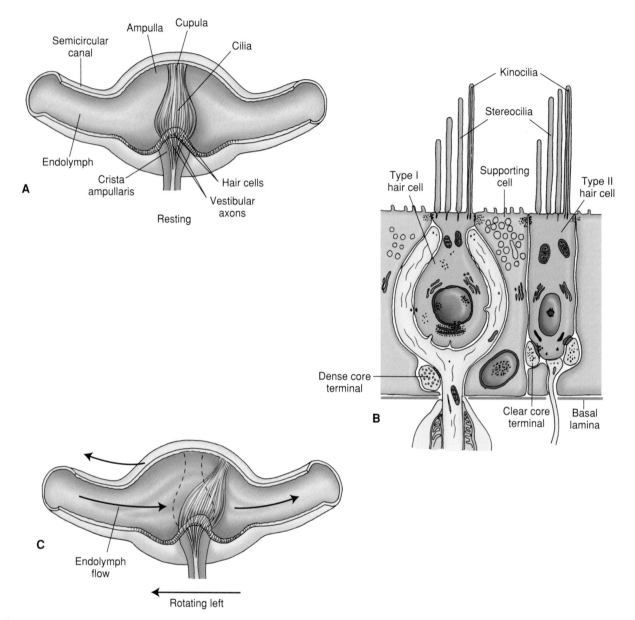

Figure 17–10 The ampulla. (A) Inside the ampulla is a crest (the crista ampullaris) on which hair and supporting cells of the crista are located. A gelatinous mass (the cupula) extends from the surface of the hair cells to the roof of the ampulla; cilia of the hair cells are embedded there. (B) Type I hair cells are goblet shaped, and type II hair cells are cylindrical. Note the stereocilia projecting from the apical surfaces of all hair cells and a single kinocilium at the edge of the apical surface. (C) Displacement of the cupula in the direction of the utricle results in excitation of the hair cell, whereas displacement of the cupula in the reverse direction results in inhibition of the hair cell.

otolithic membrane and the cilia embedded in it. This displacement causes depolarization or hyperpolarization of the hair cell. The patterns of excitation and inhibition of hair cells are processed by the central pathways and interpreted by neurons in the cerebellar and cerebral cortices for the sense of balance (equilibrium).

The mechanical movement of the cilia results in the depolarization or hyperpolarization of a vestibular hair cell, involves the influx of ions (K^+

and Ca^{2+}), and is identical to the mechanism already described for the auditory system (see "Mechanism of Sound Conduction").

CENTRAL PATHWAYS

Although the **vestibular (Scarpa's) ganglion** is referred to as a single ganglion, two vestibular ganglia are actually present (Fig. 17-8). The *peripheral* processes of the neurons located in the vestibular ganglion innervate the receptors (hair cells) in the vestibular labyrinth (maculae of the utricle and the saccule and ampullae of the semicircular canals). The *central* processes of these neurons travel in the **vestibulocochlear nerve**. The afferents from the vestibular labyrinth project to each of the vestibular nuclei located in the rostral medulla and the caudal pons. Afferents from the ampullae of the semicircular canals project to the superior vestibular nucleus (SVN) and rostral portion of the medial vestibular nucleus (MVN). Afferents from the maculae of the utricle and saccule terminate in the

lateral vestibular nucleus (LVN). Some afferents from the macula of the saccule project to the inferior vestibular nucleus (IVN) (Fig. 17-11). The excitatory neurotransmitter released at the terminals of the primary afferents from the vestibular labyrinth is believed to be glutamate or aspartate.

ASCENDING VESTIBULAR PATHWAYS

The ascending axons of the neurons located in the SVN enter the medial longitudinal fasciculus (MLF) rostral to the abducens nucleus and project

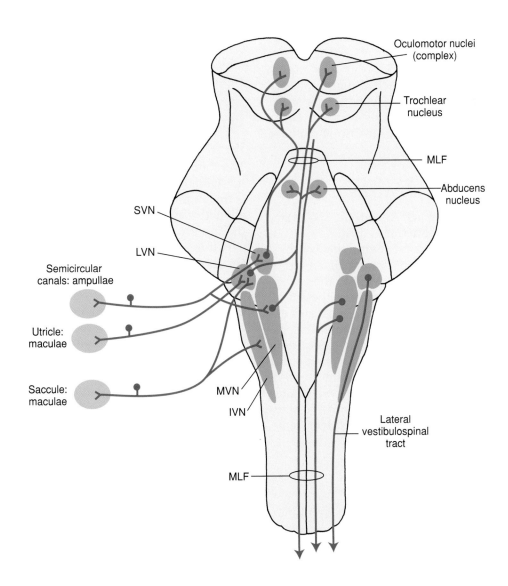

Figure 17–11 Central vestibular pathways. The afferents from the vestibular labyrinth project to each of the vestibular nuclei located in the rostral medulla and the caudal pons. Afferents from the ampullae of the semicircular canals project to the superior vestibular nucleus (SVN) and rostral portion of the medial vestibular nucleus (MVN). Afferents from the maculae of the utricle and saccule terminate in the lateral vestibular nucleus (LVN). Some afferents from the macula of the saccule project to the inferior vestibular nucleus (IVN). See text for a description of ascending and descending pathways. Abbreviation: MLF, medial longitudinal fasciculus.

ipsilaterally to the trochlear and oculomotor nuclei. Fibers from the neurons located in the medial vestibular nuclei also ascend in the MLF and project *bilaterally* to the abducens nucleus, *contralaterally* to the trochlear and oculomotor nuclei (Fig. 17-11).

CEREBELLAR AFFERENT AND EFFERENT PROJECTIONS

An important source of inputs to the cerebellum arises from the vestibular system. Afferents can reach the flocculonodular lobe directly from the vestibular apparatus (direct vestibulocerebellar fibers) or indirectly mainly from the medial and inferior vestibular nuclei. Larger numbers of fibers reach the cerebellum via this indirect route. The LVN also receives both excitatory and inhibitory signals from the cerebellum. Excitatory inputs originate from the fastigial nucleus and inhibitory inputs to the LVN arise from Purkinje cells of the anterior lobe of the cerebellar cortex (see Chapter 21 for details concerning the functions of these inputs).

VESTIBULOCORTICAL PATHWAY

It is believed that some axons from the secondary neurons located in the superior and lateral vestibular nuclei can communicate with the cerebral cortex. This may be achieved through bilateral projections of these nuclei via the MLF to the *ventrobasal complex of the thalamus*, and from these thalamic nuclei to the cortex (area 3a, which is adjacent to the primary motor cortex). This represents a possible pathway from the dorsal column–medial lemniscal system by which conscious perception of the position of the body in space and the sensation of movement is mediated. However, the precise sites in the cortex where conscious perception of vestibular sensation takes place have yet to be identified.

DESCENDING VESTIBULAR PATHWAYS

The *lateral vestibulospinal tract* (described in Chapters 9 and 19) arises from the LVN, descends through the brainstem, and terminates in the ventral horn of both cervical and lumbar levels of the spinal cord. Lateral vestibulospinal fibers descend ipsilaterally and powerfully facilitate extensor motor neurons and utilize acetylcholine as the transmitter. Projections from the MVN descend bilaterally in the MLF as the medial vestibulospinal tract, terminate in the cervical spinal cord, and

serve to adjust the position of the head and neck (Fig. 17-11).

In experimental animals, transection of the brain at the intercollicular level results in **decerebrate rigidity**. This condition is characterized by hyperactivity of extensor muscles of all four limbs. Traumatic injuries, vascular disease, or tumors in the midbrain can cause similar symptoms in humans. The corticospinal, corticorubral, corticoreticular, and rubrospinal tracts (see Chapter 26) are interrupted, whereas the facilitatory influences from the reticular formation and vestibulospinal tract on muscle tone remain intact in this situation. However, the inhibitory influences on muscle tone from the reticular formation are removed because they are dependent upon the descending impulses from higher centers. The net result of these alterations upon excitatory and inhibitory influences is an increase in the tone of antigravity muscles.

VESTIBULAR SYSTEM AND CONTROL OF EYE MOVEMENTS

The control of eye movements is described in detail in Chapter 14. Briefly, the abducens nerve (CN VI) is involved in the lateral movement of the eye (i.e., abduction of the eye). The trochlear nerve supplies the superior oblique muscle, the primary action of which is to move the eye downward when it is located in a medial position. The oculomotor nerve (CN III) innervates the superior, medial, and inferior rectus muscles as well as the inferior oblique muscles. The action of the medial rectus muscle is to move the eye medially; the superior and inferior rectus muscles move the eye up and down, respectively; and the inferior oblique muscle elevates the eye when it is in the medial position. Besides CN III, IV, and VI, other brain structures are also involved in the control of eye movements (see Chapter 14). Movements of the eyes are influenced by vestibular nuclei that send projections to cranial nerve nuclei (the abducens, trochlear, and oculomotor nuclei).

SUMMARY OF THE FUNCTIONS OF THE VESTIBULAR SYSTEM

Movements of the head (e.g., tilting activates the hair cells in the maculae of the utricle and the saccule) trigger impulses that pass centrally in primary vestibular afferents to the vestibular nuclei and monosynaptically activate these neurons. The ascending and descending vestibular projections arising from vestibular neurons serve to coordinate the movements of the eyes, neck, and trunk in response to signals from vestibular afferents. These adjustments require contraction of some antigravity muscles, relaxation of other (flexor) muscles, with modifications of the head and eyes. These effects are achieved via projections of vestibular nuclei that innervate: (1) CN III, IV, and VI, mediating appropriate adjustment of the eyes in response to change in posture; (2) ventral horn cells of the cervical cord whose axons innervate head and neck muscles, producing changes in the position of the head; (3) motoneurons of the cervical and lumbar cord, causing powerful excitation of the extensor musculature; and (4) the flocculonodular lobe of the cerebellum, producing modulation of the descending pathways from the vestibular nuclei and reticular formation, which control posture and muscle tone.

CLINICAL DISORDERS ASSOCIATED WITH THE VESTIBULAR SYSTEM

Nystagmus

Nystagmus refers to repetitive movements of the eyes produced by movements of the visual field. As indicated earlier, movements of the eyes are influenced by the vestibular nuclei (the lateral, superior, and medial vestibular nuclei) that send projections to the cranial nerve nuclei (oculomotor, abducens, and trochlear nuclei). Movement of the head in one direction results in the movement of the eyes in the opposite direction so that the eyes are fixed on an object. When the head and the body rotate, the eyes move in a direction opposite to that of the rotation. They remain fixed on an object until it is out of the field of vision. Then, the eyes move rapidly in the same direction as the rotation (called **saccadic movement**) and fix on another object until the latter is also out of the field of vision. Thus, there is an initial slow movement of the eyes in a direction opposite to that of the rotation, which is followed by a rapid movement in the direction of rotation. The slow movement of the eyes is controlled by vestibular nuclei and involves the MLF, whereas the saccadic movement is controlled by the paramedian pontine reticular formation (i.e., pontine gaze center). This pattern of eye movements is called nystagmus or the vestibulo-oculomotor reflex. Nystagmus in the absence of movements of the visual field indicates the presence of a lesion in the brainstem or cerebellum (see Chapter 14).

Nystagmus characterized by equal velocity in both directions is called **pendular nystagmus**. In **jerk nystagmus**, there is a slow phase of movement that is followed by a fast phase in the opposite direction. The direction of the fast phase of movement is used to specify the direction of the jerk nystagmus. Thus, if the movement of the fast phase is toward the left, it is referred to as leftward-beating nystagmus.

Disorders of the vestibulo-ocular pathways in patients complaining of dizziness or vertigo (see next section) is tested using a **caloric test**. For this test, first an otoscopic examination is performed to ensure that the tympanic membrane is not perforated. Then the patient is placed in a supine position, and the head is elevated 30 degrees to bring the lateral semicircular canal into the upright position. Subsequently, either warm (44°C) or cold (33°C) water is introduced into the external auditory canal for 40 seconds. The interval between the irrigation with warm and cold water is at least 5 minutes. In an individual without disorders of the vestibulo-ocular pathways, cold water produces nystagmus beating in the opposite side in which the water was introduced, while warm water produces nystagmus beating in the same side in which the water was introduced. This relationship is described by the mnemonic COWS (**c**old **o**pposite, **w**arm **s**ame; or cold water produces nystagmus beating in the opposite side, while warm water produces nystagmus beating in the same side). If there is a unilateral lesion in the vestibulo-ocular pathway, nystagmus will be either attenuated or abolished on the side ipsilateral to the lesion.

Vertigo

In this condition, the person has a *sensation of turning or rotation in space in the absence of actual rotation*. Usually, debris from the otolithic membrane, located in the saccule and utricle, accumulates at the ampulla of the posterior semicircular canal and adheres to the cupula, making it more sensitive to angular movement. Vertigo is often accompanied by nausea, vomiting, and gait ataxia. It can be caused by peripheral vestibular lesions that affect the labyrinth of the inner ear or the vestibular division of CN VIII. It can also be caused by central lesions that affect the brainstem vestibular nuclei or their connections. Vertigo due to peripheral lesions is usually intermittent, lasts for brief periods of time, and is always accompanied by unidirectional, but not vertical, nystagmus. Vertigo due to central lesions may or may not be accompanied by nystagmus. If nystagmus is present, it may be vertical, unidirectional, or multidirectional. Some H1 receptor antagonists (e.g., the piperazine derivatives, cyclizine, and meclizine) and promethazine (a phenothiazine) have proved to be beneficial in the treatment of vertigo. Promethazine has the added advantage of relieving vomiting, which often accompanies vertigo.

Motion Sickness

Afferents from the vestibular system activate their projections to the reticular formation of the pons and medulla. Subsequent activation of autonomic centers results in motion sickness.

Inflammation of the Vestibular Labyrinth

This condition is referred to as *vestibular neuronitis*. Usually, there is no hearing loss. Typical symptoms include vertigo, postural imbalance, nausea, and nystagmus. The symptoms vary in severity and last for a brief time (a few days). Treatment is the same as for Ménière's disease, which is described in the next section.

Ménière's Disease

Ménière's disease is characterized by intermittent, relapsing vertigo, which varies in severity (mild to debilitating) and duration (minutes to hours). In addition to these vestibular symptoms, the patient may suffer from hearing disorders such as tinnitus (ringing noise in the ears) and distorted hearing. The cause of this disease is unknown. Histopathological studies have shown that there is an excessive accumulation of the endolymph, edema of the spaces containing the endolymph, and damage to the hair cells. Accumulation of the endolymph is most likely caused by poor drainage of this fluid from the membranous labyrinth. Recall that endolymph is normally drained by the endolymphatic duct into the endolymphatic sac, where it is resorbed into the cerebrospinal fluid. There is no effective treatment for this disease. In some patients, administration of steroids or diuretics relieves the symptoms probably by reducing edema of the lymphatic spaces. Treatment with H1 receptor antagonists (e.g., meclizine) has also proved beneficial in this condition. In patients suffering from severe vertigo, destruction of hair cells by the antibiotic streptomycin is attempted. In other extreme cases, the affected labyrinth is surgically removed.

CLINICAL CASE

HISTORY

Francine is a 42-year-old woman without any prior medical problems. For several weeks, she believed that she had an ear infection because she had some loss of hearing and ringing in her right ear; she felt slightly unsteady and thought that her mouth was drooping slightly on the right side. She consulted her physician and was referred to a neurologist immediately.

EXAMINATION

Upon examination, the neurologist noted an asymmetry in Francine's face. Her mouth did not elevate as much on the right side as it did on the left. There was a significant hearing deficit in the right ear. When a tuning fork was placed on her forehead, she only heard the vibration in her left ear. Bone conduction, as measured by the tuning fork, was greater than air conduction in the right ear. There was rhythmic jerking laterally of Francine's right eye when she was asked to look to the right. There was also some mild insensitivity to a pin prick on the right side of her face. The neurologist ordered a magnetic resonance imaging (MRI) scan of her brain.

EXPLANATION

Francine's MRI scan revealed a right-sided acoustic neuroma, a cerebellopontine angle tumor arising from the Schwann cells of the vestibulocochlear nerve. It causes dysfunction of the vestibulocochlear nerve, including hearing loss; nystagmus (jerking of eye movements when looking laterally); and unsteadiness, usually vertigo (a spinning or falling sensation). Because the tumors are often large enough to involve other structures in the cerebellopontine angle, including the fifth and seventh nerves, there is often dysfunction of these nerves as well. This is manifested in Francine's case as a Bell's palsy or peripheral seventh nerve dysfunction including facial weakness involving the forehead. Additionally, the fifth cranial nerve is partially involved, manifesting its dysfunction as numbness on the right side of the face. The tumor may be pressing on the spinotrigeminal tract or may involve CN V directly if the tumor is large enough.

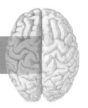

CHAPTER TEST

QUESTIONS

Choose the best answer for each question.

1. A 47-year-old woman was admitted to a local hospital after complaining of a gradual loss of hearing in one ear over time. In addition, the patient also reported some unsteadiness in balance that developed after the initial hearing loss. An MRI scan and a thorough neurological examination further revealed a facial palsy and a loss of corneal reflex on the side of the face ipsilateral to the hearing loss. The most likely cause of this disorder as revealed by the MRI and clinical evaluations was:

   a. A tumor in the region extending from the external to the middle ear
   b. An acoustic neuroma of the cerebellopontine angle affecting CN VIII
   c. A vascular occlusion affecting the medial two thirds of the basilar pons
   d. A tumor affecting the midline region of the cerebellar cortex
   e. A vascular lesion involving the MLF and adjoining regions of the dorsal pons

2. A 41-year-old man was diagnosed as having multiple sclerosis. During the course of this disorder, this patient exhibited signs of vertigo and nystagmus. The most likely explanation of these symptoms is a reduction of conduction velocity in neurons affecting the:

   a. Inner ear
   b. CN IV
   c. Cerebellum
   d. Cerebral peduncle
   e. Red nucleus

3. A 27-year-old man who had been in good health reported to his primary physician that he had episodes of dizziness. Over time, the dizziness tended to decrease, but the patient began to experience tinnitus and hearing loss, and both of these symptoms became progressively worse. A neurological examination revealed no other signs of neurological dysfunctions. The patient was treated with anticholinergics with some degree of success. The most likely basis of the disorder in this patient is:

   a. A lesion of the MLF
   b. A tumor of the cerebellum

   c. A tumor impinging on CN VIII and CN VII at the cerebellopontine angle
   d. An abnormal volume of endolymph of the inner ear
   e. A lesion of the dorsolateral pons affecting the lateral lemniscus

4. Which one of the following events is elicited by the mechanical displacement of the cochlear hair cell stereocilia towards the kinocilium?

   a. There is an influx of K^+ through the membranes of the cilia, which is followed by an influx of Ca^{2+} through the voltage-gated Ca^{2+} channels.
   b. The hair cells on which the cilia are located are hyperpolarized.
   c. Efflux of Ca^{2+} through the voltage-gated channels located in the hair cell membrane occurs.
   d. An inhibitory transmitter (probably GABA) is released by the hair cell.
   e. There is an influx of Na^+ through the membranes of the cilia, the hair cell is depolarized, and an action potential is elicited in the afferent nerve terminal.

5. A caloric test was performed on a 50-year-old man complaining of dizziness and vertigo to exclude impairment of the vestibulo-ocular pathways. Which one of the following observations would indicate normal function of vestibulo-ocular pathways in this person?

   a. Irrigation of the left external auditory canal with cold water resulted in nystagmus beating towards the right.
   b. Irrigation of the left external auditory canal with cold water resulted in nystagmus beating towards the left.
   c. Irrigation of the left external auditory canal with warm water resulted in nystagmus beating towards the right.
   d. Irrigation of the right external auditory canal with warm water resulted in nystagmus beating towards the left.
   e. Nystagmus was attenuated when the left external auditory canal was irrigated with warm water.

ANSWERS AND EXPLANATIONS

1. Answer: b

Ipsilateral hearing loss coupled with some loss of balance and with facial palsy and loss of corneal reflex on the same side as the hearing loss could only occur as a result of damage to CN VII and CN VIII. The most common place where this is likely to occur is the cerebellopontine angle, where an acoustic neuroma would affect not only CN VIII, but also CN VII because of its proximity to CN VIII. The other choices are not logically possible. A tumor of the external or middle ear could not account for the deficits due to damage to CN VII. A vascular occlusion of the medial two thirds of the basilar pons would not affect CN VIII. Damage to the cerebellum or MLF would not affect auditory functions.

2. Answer: c

Vertigo and nystagmus appear in cases of multiple sclerosis and are due to changes in conduction velocities in structures that receive inputs from the vestibular apparatus. One such structure is the cerebellum, which receives direct and indirect inputs from the vestibular apparatus. Damage to the cerebellum, and in particular, the vermal region and flocculonodular lobe, which receive vestibular inputs, results in similar nystagmus and problems with balance. The cerebral peduncle and red nucleus are unrelated to vestibular inputs. CN IV plays no role in balance, and lesions of this structure produce only deficits in eye movement (i.e., moving the eye downward when in the medial position). Likewise, an inner ear deficit would likely cause primarily a hearing loss, which was not included in the constellation of deficits described for this patient.

3. Answer: d

Because the patient experienced both auditory and vestibular symptoms but showed no other clinical signs, the site of dysfunction had to be limited to CN VIII. Such effects are typically of peripheral origin. In this case, the patient was suffering from Ménière's disease, which involves the inner ear, where the effects are likely manifested through alterations of endolymphatic homeostasis. The lesions to the other structures provided as choices do not involve the constellation of deficits indicated in this case. Cerebellar or MLF lesions would produce vestibular but not auditory deficits; damage to the dorsolateral pons involving the lateral lemniscus would affect only hearing (and perhaps somesthetic pathways); and a tumor of the cerebellopontine angle would affect both CN VIII and CN VII (see explanation to Question 1). In this case, there were no symptoms suggesting damage to CN VII.

4. Answer: a

The air pressure waves cause the tympanic membrane to vibrate which, in turn, results in oscillatory movements of the foot of the stapes against the oval window (not round window). These pressure waves in the perilymph displace only specific portions of the basilar membrane depending on the frequency of the sound stimulus. The movement of the basilar membrane with respect to the tectorial membrane results in the displacement of stereocilia. Mechanical displacement of the stereocilia (e.g., in lateral direction) causes an influx of K^+ through their membranes, the hair cell is depolarized, and there is an influx of Ca^{2+} through the voltage-sensitive Ca^{2+} channels in their membranes. The influx of Ca^{2+} triggers the release of the transmitter (probably glutamate) that, in turn, elicits an action potential in the afferent nerve terminal at the base of the hair cell.

5. Answer: a

In a normal individual, cold water produces nystagmus beating opposite to the side in which the water was introduced (remember the mnemonic "COWS"), while warm water produces nystagmus beating to the same side in which the water was introduced. Recall that the terms "leftward-beating" and "rightward-beating" indicate the direction of the nystagmus. Attenuation of nystagmus indicates a lesion in the vestibulo-ocular pathway.

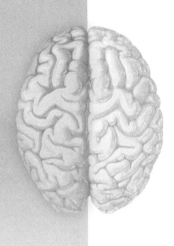

CHAPTER 18

OLFACTION AND TASTE

OBJECTIVES

After reading this chapter, the student should be able to:

1. Describe the stimuli that activate olfactory (smell) receptors

2. List, diagram, and describe the anatomical components of olfactory receptors

3. Describe transduction of olfactory stimuli

4. Describe and diagram central pathways that mediate olfactory sensations

5. List and describe clinical conditions that alter olfactory sensations

6. Describe the stimuli that activate taste (gustatory) receptors

7. List, diagram, and describe the anatomical components of taste receptors

8. Describe transduction of taste stimuli

9. Describe and diagram central pathways mediating taste sensations

10. List and describe clinical conditions that alter taste sensations

Olfaction (smell) and **gustation** (taste) constitute chemical senses. Like other sensory systems, olfactory and taste systems provide information regarding the external environment. The two sensory systems are anatomically and morphologically distinct. They are discussed together in this chapter because their specialized sensory receptors are stimulated by chemical molecules and the functions of the two systems often complement each other as special visceral afferents. For example, wine tasters often depend on the sensation of taste (flavor) and olfaction (smell) to distinguish between different wines.

OLFACTORY SYSTEM

STIMULUS

Chemicals that generate odors stimulate specialized receptors of the olfactory system. Human beings can detect these odors at very low concentrations (a few parts per trillion); thousands of such chemicals can be distinguished.

RECEPTORS

Unlike other sensory systems, the bipolar olfactory sensory (receptor) neurons are not located in a ganglion. Instead, these neurons, along with their processes, are present in the specialized olfactory mucosa of the nasal cavity just below a thin sheet of bone called the **cribriform plate** of the ethmoid bone of the skull (Fig. 18-1, A and B). The olfactory sensory neurons have single dendrites on one end that terminate in the surface of the olfactory mucosa as expanded olfactory knobs (Fig. 18-1B). A single unmyelinated axon arises on the opposite end of the sensory neuron. Collectively, these axons are called the **olfactory nerve** (cranial nerve [CN] I). The axons of olfactory sensory neurons do not form a single nerve as in other cranial nerves. Instead, small clusters of these axons penetrate the cribriform plate and synapse in the ipsilateral olfactory bulb. Supporting (**sustentacular**) cells present in the olfactory epithelium help in detoxifying chemicals that come in contact with the olfactory epithelium (Fig 18-1B).

About 10 to 20 cilia arise from the olfactory knobs (Fig. 18-1B) and spread on the surface of the mucosa. These cilia are involved in sensory transduction. The area of the olfactory mucosa is relatively small (about 5 cm^2) in humans compared with that in other animals that require and have a better sense of smell (e.g., the area of the olfactory mucosa in the dog is about 100 cm^2).

SENSORY TRANSDUCTION

A protein, called **olfactory binding protein**, is secreted by the **Bowman's glands**, which are located in the olfactory mucosa, and is more abundant around the cilia of the olfactory sensory neurons. Although the exact function of the olfactory binding protein is not known, it is believed that it carries and/or concentrates the odorant (a substance that stimulates olfactory receptors) around the cilia. The steps involved in the sensation of olfaction are shown in Figure 18-2. At least two second-messenger systems—cyclic adenosine monophosphate (cAMP) and inositol triphosphate (IP$_3$)—are involved in the transduction of olfactory signals. When an odorant molecule binds to the receptor protein on the cilia, a receptor-odorant complex is formed, which activates a G protein. The activated G protein (G$_{olf}$) combines with guanosine triphosphate (GTP), displacing guanosine diphosphate (GDP). The GTP-G$_{olf}$ complex activates adenylate cyclase, leading to the generation of cAMP, which, in turn, opens Na$^+$/Ca^{2+} channels. The influx of Na$^+$ and Ca^{2+} results in depolarizing generator potential in the cilia. In another pathway, the GTP-G$_{olf}$ complex activates phospholipase C, which generates IP$_3$. IP$_3$ activates and opens Ca^{2+} channels, causing depolarizing generator potentials. In both second-messenger pathways, an increase in intracellular Ca^{2+} concentration results in the opening of Ca^{2+}-gated Cl$^-$ channels, efflux of chloride ions, and further depolarization of the cilia. This depolarization is conducted passively from the cilia to the axon hillock of the olfactory sensory neuron. When the axon hillock reaches a threshold, action potentials are generated, which are conducted along the axons of the olfactory sensory neurons. These signals are processed in the central olfactory pathways for the sense of smell.

CENTRAL PATHWAYS

The olfactory bulb lies on the ventrorostral aspect of the ipsilateral forebrain (Fig. 18-3A). It is the first region of the central nervous system where sensory signals from olfactory sensory neurons are processed. As noted earlier, the axons of the olfactory sensory neurons travel in olfactory nerves and spread over the surface of the ipsilateral olfactory bulb, forming an **olfactory nerve layer** (Fig. 18-3B). Located near the surface of the olfactory bulb is the **glomerular layer**. Each glomerulus contains clusters of nerve terminals from olfactory sensory neurons, dendrites of the **tufted cells** (located in the **external plexiform layer** of the olfactory bulb), **mitral cells** (located in the mitral cell layer), and

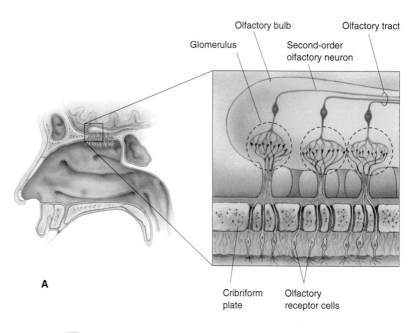

A

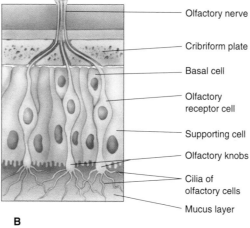

Figure 18–1 Organization of the human olfactory system. (A) The bipolar olfactory sensory neurons are present in the olfactory mucosa just below the cribiform plate. (B) Note the location of olfactory receptor cells, including their expanded ends (olfactory knobs), cilia arising from the olfactory knobs, the olfactory nerve, and supporting (sustentacular) cells. (From Bear MF, et al.: Neuroscience: Exploring the Brain, 2nd ed. Baltimore: Lippincott, Williams & Wilkins, 2001, pp. 269, 273.)

B

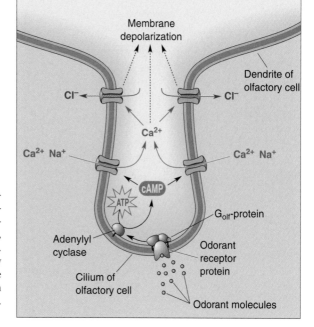

Figure 18–2 Sensory transduction in olfaction. The olfactory binding protein carries odorant molecules to the cilia of the olfactory sensory neurons. A receptor-odorant complex is formed, which activates a G-protein. Second-messenger systems are activated, Na^+/Ca^{2+} or Ca^{2+} channels are opened, and the cilia are depolarized. This depolarization is conducted to the axon hillock of the olfactory sensory neuron where action potentials are generated, which are conducted along the axons of the olfactory sensory neurons (From Bear MF, et al.: Neuroscience: Exploring the Brain, 2nd ed. Baltimore: Lippincott, Williams & Wilkins, 2001, p. 270.)

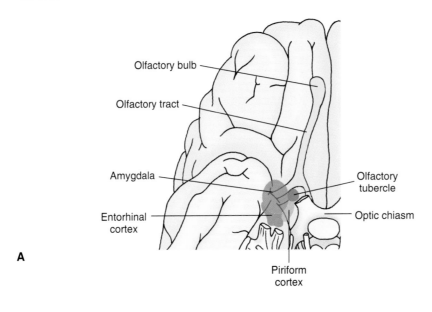

A

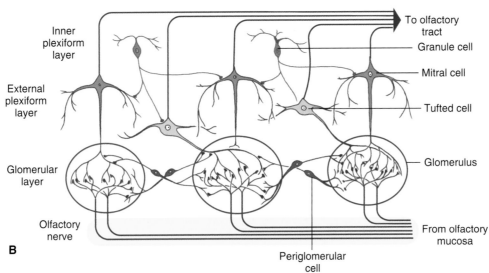

B

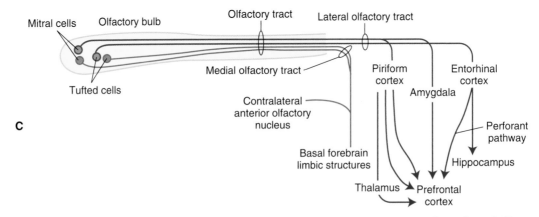

C

Figure 18–3   Central olfactory pathways. (A) The axons of the olfactory sensory neurons project to the ipsilateral olfactory bulb via the olfactory nerve. (B) The olfactory bulb contains different layers: olfactory nerve layer, glomerular layer, external plexiform layer, mitral cell layer, and inner plexiform layer. (C) The axons of mitral and tufted cells in the olfactory bulb form the olfactory tracts. The largest bundle of fibers from mitral and tufted cells exit from the olfactory bulb in the lateral olfactory tract and project to the primary olfactory cortex (piriform cortex), amygdala, and entorhinal cortex. The entorhinal and piriform cortices are located in the temporal lobe. The hippocampus lies in the medial temporal lobe. The amygdala lies just rostral to the hippocampus in the temporal lobe. The prefrontal cortex is located in the frontal lobe. Some fibers from the mitral and tufted cells exit the olfactory tract via the medial olfactory tract. For other details, see text.

γ-aminobutyric acid (GABA)-ergic interneurons called the **periglomerular cells** (located in the glomerular layer of the olfactory bulb). The terminals of first-order olfactory sensory neurons form synapses with the dendrites of the tufted, mitral, and periglomerular neurons. The transmitters released at the terminals of olfactory sensory neurons are believed to be peptides. The inner plexiform layer of the olfactory bulb contains GABAergic interneurons called granule cells. The mitral and tufted cells discharge spontaneously. They are excited by the inputs from the olfactory sensory neurons. The inhibitory interneurons (periglomerular and granule cells) modulate the activity of the mitral and tufted cells. The signals from mitral and tufted cells are then conducted to forebrain structures for further processing.

The projections of the axons of the mitral and tufted cells are shown schematically in Figure 18-3C. **Olfactory tracts**, located on the ventral (inferior) surface of the frontal lobe, arise from their enlarged ends known as the olfactory bulbs. The largest bundle of axons from the mitral and tufted cells exit from the olfactory bulb in the **lateral olfactory tract**, and their functions are mediated by the excitatory neurotransmitters, glutamate or aspartate. These axons project to the primary olfactory cortex (**piriform or pyriform cortex**), amygdala, and entorhinal cortex. The entorhinal and piriform cortices, hippocampus, and amygdala are located in the temporal lobe; the hippocampus lies in the medial temporal lobe (see Chapters 13 and 25). The prefrontal cortex is located in the frontal lobe. The neurons in the piriform cortex, amygdala, and entorhinal cortex project to the prefrontal cortex. Note that the olfactory projection system differs from other sensory systems in that the projection pathway can reach the prefrontal cortex without having to make a synapse in the thalamus first, which is typical of other sensory systems (see Chapter 26). The neurons in the entorhinal cortex also project to the hippocampus (a major limbic structure) via a fiber bundle called the **perforant pathway**. Therefore, olfactory inputs can play an important role in modulating hippocampal functions in a manner similar to that for the amygdala (see Chapter 25). Although olfactory projections can reach the prefrontal cortex without making a synapse in the thalamus, there are direct tertiary inputs from the piriform cortex to the mediodorsal thalamic nucleus, which projects to wide areas of the frontal lobe including the prefrontal cortex.

Some fibers from the mitral and tufted cells exit the olfactory tract via the **medial olfactory tract** (Fig 18-3C). These axons project ipsilaterally to basal limbic forebrain structures such as the **substantia innominata**, **medial septal nucleus**, and **bed nucleus of the stria terminalis**. Other fibers in the medial olfactory stria arise from the contralateral **anterior olfactory nucleus**. This nucleus, located in the posterior part of each olfactory bulb, receives sensory signals from mitral and tufted cells and relays them to the contralateral olfactory bulb via the **anterior commissure**.

A basic question concerns how we discriminate and become aware of different kinds of odors. While little is basically known about this process, it is believed that olfactory discrimination takes place, at least in part, within the olfactory bulb. It has been suggested that different glomeruli that are located in spatially distinct parts of the olfactory bulb respond to specific odorants. In this manner, olfactory signals become topographically organized within the olfactory bulb much the same as other sensory modalities are topographically arranged (i.e., similar to other modalities of sensation, which are tonotopically, somatotopically, and visuotopically organized for auditory, tactile, and visual sensations, respectively). This topographical arrangement, with respect to olfactory signals, provides a basis by which neuronal pools within the prefrontal cortex can receive and transform such signals into a conscious awareness of a specific odorant.

From a functional perspective, we can thus say that affective and emotional aspects of olfactory sensation are mediated by olfactory projections to the limbic system (entorhinal cortex, hippocampal formation, medial septal nuclei, and amygdala). Autonomic responses to olfactory stimuli are mediated via descending projections to the hypothalamus, midbrain periaqueductal gray, and autonomic centers of the lower brainstem and spinal cord (see Chapters 23 and 24).

CLINICAL CONDITIONS IN WHICH THE OLFACTORY SENSATION IS ALTERED

In some cases of head trauma, the olfactory bulb moves with respect to the cribriform plate, and the axons projecting from the sensory neurons (located in the olfactory mucosa) to the olfactory bulb may be damaged. This results in a loss (**anosmia**) or reduction (**hyposmia**) of olfactory function. These conditions may also result from damage to the olfactory mucosa due to infections. Loss or alteration of olfactory function may occur in Alzheimer's and Parkinson's diseases.

Seizure activity involving parts of the temporal lobe produce olfactory hallucinations of unpleasant smells (**cacosmia**). This condition is referred to as an **uncinate fit**. The neural structures affected in this condition are the **uncus**, **parahippocampal gyrus**, amygdala, and piriform and entorhinal cortices.

TASTE

STIMULUS

As mentioned in the beginning of the chapter, sensory receptors in this system are stimulated by chemical molecules. Basic sensations of taste include sweet, bitter, salty, and sour. The areas of the tongue most sensitive to different taste sensations are: tip of the tongue for sweetness, back of the tongue for bitterness, and sides of the tongue for saltiness and sourness (Fig. 18-4A).

RECEPTORS

The receptor cells that mediate the sensation of taste are located in taste buds, which are the sensory organs for the taste system. Taste buds are located in different types of papillae, which are protrusions on the surface of the tongue. The types of papillae include: **filiform, fungiform, foliate**, and **circumvallate papillae**. The filiform and fungiform papillae are scattered throughout the surface of the anterior two thirds of the tongue, especially along the lateral margins and the tip. The foliate papillae are present on the dorsolateral part of the posterior part of the tongue. The circumvallate papillae are larger than other papillae and are located in a V-shaped line, which divides the tongue into two portions: the anterior two thirds and posterior one third (Fig. 18-4B). The taste buds are located in the lateral margins of the papillae that are surrounded by a deep furrow bathed by fluids in the oral cavity (Fig. 18-4C).

Each taste bud has a pore at its tip through which fluids containing chemical substances enter (Fig. 18-4D). The taste bud contains taste receptor cells in different stages of development. The taste receptor cells live for about 10 days and have to be replaced. Small cells at the base of the taste bud (basal cells) divide to replace the taste receptor cells. Afferent nerve terminals make contact with the base of the taste receptor cells. The cell bodies of these afferent terminals are located in the ganglia of CN VII (facial), IX (glossopharyngeal), and X (vagus) (see Chapter 14).

TRANSDUCTION OF THE TASTE STIMULUS

The salivary fluids containing chemical substances enter the taste buds through the pore at the top and bathe the **microvilli**, which are located at the tip of the taste receptor cells. Interaction of the chemical molecule with the specific sites in the membrane of the microvilli brings about the depolarization of the receptor cell to produce a generator potential. This initial step of depolarization is brought about by opening or closing of different channels. For example, the transduction of **salty** taste is mediated by generation of a receptor potential due to influx of Na^+ through the amiloride-sensitive Na^+ channels (Fig. 18-5A). **Sour** taste, elicited by acids, is mediated by depolarization of the receptor cell due to closure of voltage-dependent K^+ channels (Fig. 18-5B). Other mechanisms for mediation of taste sensation involve activation of a G-protein that, in turn, activates a cascade of events resulting in transmitter release (see Chapter 8). For example, substances that generate the sense of **sweet** flavor (e.g., sugars) act on receptors that are coupled with G_s-proteins. Activation of G-proteins results in activation of adenylate cyclase (adenylyl cyclase), which increases the levels of cAMP. cAMP activates a phosphokinase that depolarizes the receptor cells by closing K^+ channels (Fig. 18-5C). **Bitter** substances activate a G-protein, which, in turn, activates phospholipase C and generates the IP_3 second-messenger system. IP_3 releases Ca^{2+} from intracellular stores (Fig. 18-5D). Activation of different second-messenger systems eventually causes opening of voltage-dependent Ca^{2+} channels and influx of Ca^{2+}, which results in transmitter release and activation of afferent nerve terminals at the base of the receptor cell.

CENTRAL PATHWAYS

The taste buds on the anterior two thirds of the tongue are innervated by the facial nerve (CN VII); taste buds on the posterior one third of the tongue are innervated by the glossopharyngeal nerve (CN IX); and the taste buds on the epiglottis and pharyngeal walls are innervated by the vagus nerve (CN X) (Fig. 18-6). The afferent terminals of the facial nerve carry sweet, bitter, and salty sensations; while those of the glossopharyngeal nerve carry sweet and bitter sensations.

Unipolar neurons mediate the sensation of taste. The unipolar neurons mediating the sensation of taste via the facial nerve (CN VII) are located in the geniculate ganglion, which is situated in the petrous portion of the temporal bone. The peripheral processes of these neurons travel in the facial nerve, which exits the cranium at the stylomastoid foramen. At this level, the peripheral processes of the sensory neurons exit from the facial nerve and form the chorda tympani nerve, which crosses the cavity of the middle ear (horizontally along the inner surface of the tympanum and over the manubrium of the malleus ossicle). The chorda tympani finally joins the lingual branch of the trigeminal

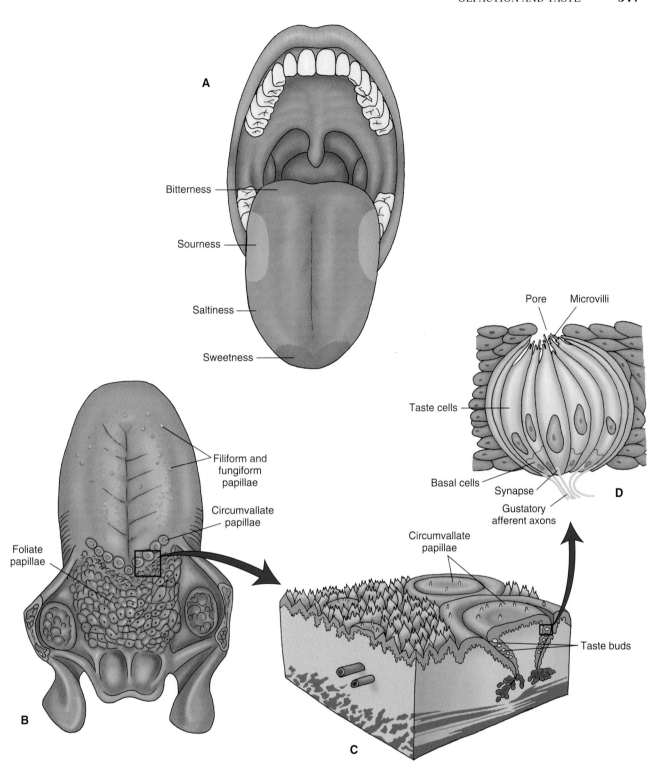

Figure 18–4 Components of the taste system. (A) The regions of the tongue that are most sensitive to different taste sensations are: the tip for sweetness, the back for bitterness, and sides for saltiness and sourness. (B) The filiform and fungiform papillae are scattered throughout the surface of the anterior two thirds of the tongue. The circumvallate papillae are located in a V-shaped line that divides the tongue into the anterior two thirds and the posterior one third. (C) The taste buds are located in the lateral margins of the papillae. (D) Each taste bud has a pore at its tip through which fluids containing chemical substances enter.

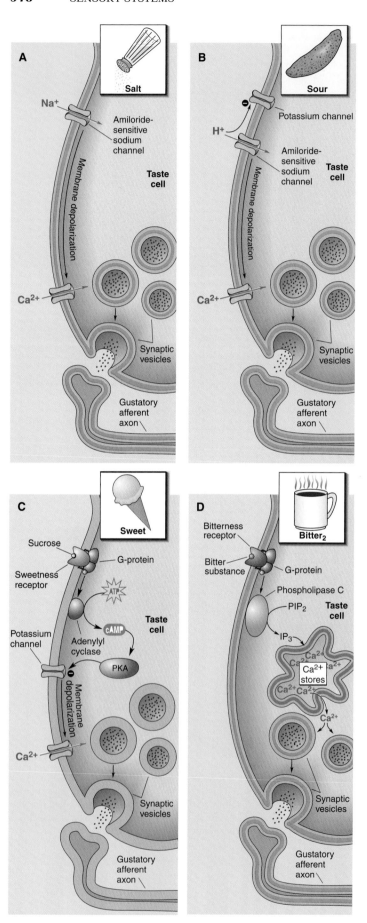

Figure 18–5 Transduction of taste stimulus. (A) The transduction of salt taste is mediated by the influx of Na^+ through the amiloride-sensitive Na^+ channels. (B) Sour taste is mediated by closure of voltage-dependent K^+ channels. (C) Sweet taste is mediated by activation of G-proteins and adenylate cyclase, which increases the levels of cyclic adenosine monophosphate (cAMP). (D) Bitter substances activate a G-protein that activates phospholipase C and generates IP_3. For other details, see text. (From Bear MF, et al.: Neuroscience: Exploring the Brain, 2nd ed. Baltimore: Lippincott, Williams & Wilkins, 2001, pp. 260–262.)

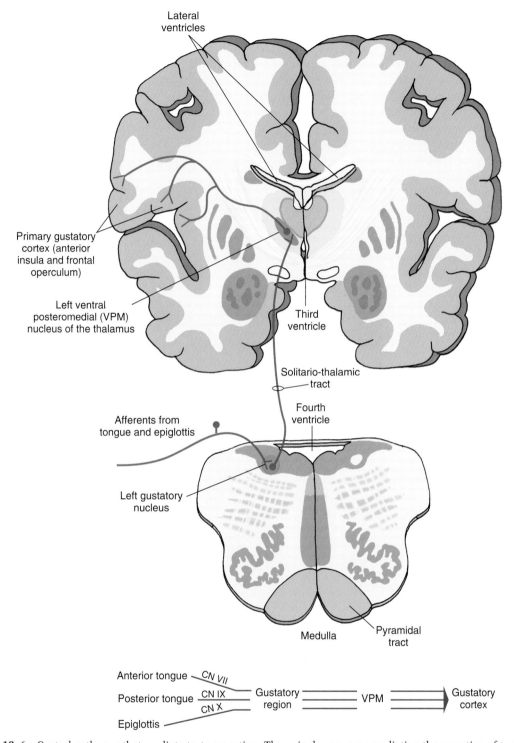

Figure 18–6 Central pathways that mediate taste sensation. The unipolar neurons mediating the sensation of taste via the facial, glossopharyngeal, and vagus nerves are located in the geniculate, inferior (petrosal), and inferior (nodose) ganglia, respectively. The peripheral processes of these neurons terminate in the rostral portion (gustatory region) of the solitary nucleus. The axons of secondary neurons located in the solitary nucleus ascend in the solitario-thalamic tract and terminate in the ventral posteromedial nucleus (VPM) of the thalamus. The neurons in VPM send their projections to the taste (gustatory) area located between the anterior insula and the frontal operculum in the ipsilateral cerebral cortex.

nerve and innervates the taste buds on the anterior two thirds of the tongue. The central processes of sensory neurons in the geniculate ganglion travel in the intermediate nerve (adjacent to the facial nerve), enter the solitary tract, and terminate in the **rostral portion (gustatory region) of the solitary nucleus** (Fig. 18-6).

The unipolar neurons mediating the sensation of taste via the glossopharyngeal nerve (CN IX) are located in the **inferior (petrosal) ganglion**, which is located in the jugular foramen. The peripheral processes of these neurons travel in the glossopharyngeal nerve and finally innervate the taste buds on the posterior one third of the tongue. The central processes of sensory neurons in the petrosal ganglion travel in the glossopharyngeal nerve, enter the solitary tract, and also terminate in the rostral portion of the solitary nucleus, which is known as the gustatory nucleus (Fig. 18-6).

The unipolar neurons mediating the sensation of taste via the vagus nerve (CN X) are located in the **inferior (nodose) ganglion**, which is located just below the jugular foramen. The peripheral processes of these neurons travel in the vagus nerve and innervate taste buds on the epiglottis. The central processes of the sensory neurons in the nodose ganglion travel in the vagus nerve, enter the solitary tract, and terminate in the gustatory nucleus (Fig. 18-6).

The axons of **secondary neurons** located in the gustatory nucleus ascend in the solitario-thalamic tract (near the medial lemniscus) and terminate in the ventral posteromedial nucleus (VPM) of the thalamus (Fig 18-6). The neurons in the VPM send their projections to the taste (gustatory) area located between the anterior insula and the frontal operculum in the ipsilateral cerebral cortex. Other fibers of the taste system pass from the solitary nucleus to the amygdala, either directly or indirectly, via connections in the pedunculopontine nucleus (i.e., pontine taste nucleus) of the reticular formation.

TASTE PERCEPTION

Our understanding of the neural basis of taste perception is incomplete. Two theories have been proposed to explain the perception of taste. One theory, called the *specific pathway* theory, states that individual taste receptors respond to a single taste stimulus (e.g., sweet taste). This information is transmitted to specific populations of neurons within the taste pathway for perception of that taste quality. The second theory is based on the concept of an across-fiber pattern coding. This theory states that individual taste receptors respond to more than one modality of taste. Therefore, the perception of a given taste may involve processing of the response patterns of many taste afferents by cortical neurons within the cortical taste area. Such a response gives us the ability to discern nuances of flavor, as in wine or other fine foods.

CLINICAL CONDITIONS IN WHICH THE TASTE SENSATION IS ALTERED

Damage to the nerves innervating the taste buds may cause **total ageusia** (loss of all taste sensation), **partial ageusia** (loss of a particular taste sensation), or **hypogeusia** (decreased sensation of taste) depending on the extent of damage.

CLINICAL CASE

HISTORY

Celia is a 32-year-old woman who had no medical problems. One day while shopping in a department store, she was admiring a dress while walking and did not notice a clothing rack rapidly being pushed in her direction. Because she was not paying attention to what was in front of her, she collided with the clothing rack, hitting her face. She immediately noticed pain in her nose and forehead. Because her nose was bleeding, she was taken to the emergency room, where skull x-rays were performed, which revealed a small fracture in the cribriform plate that was too small for any therapy. She was sent home with pain medications and told to return if there were any further sequelae.

EXAMINATION

Two weeks later, after the swelling and bleeding had subsided somewhat, while eating dinner at a restaurant, Celia noted that she was unable to smell the food. This continued with subsequent meals, so she consulted a neurologist who tested her sense of smell with several substances including coffee grounds. He concluded that her anosmia (inability to smell) was a result of her head trauma and appeared to exist on both sides of her nose.

EXPLANATION

Celia has anosmia resulting from trauma to the cribriform plate. This causes damage to the filaments of the receptor cells for smell as they pass through the cribriform plate. Depending on the extent of the injury, the sense of smell may return in approximately one third of cases in a period of days to weeks.

CHAPTER TEST

QUESTIONS

Choose the best answer for each question.

1. Olfactory information can reach the cerebral cortex by which one of the following routes?
   a. Olfactory bulb → hippocampus → anterior thalamic nucleus → prefrontal cortex
   b. Olfactory bulb → piriform cortex → amygdala → prefrontal cortex
   c. Olfactory bulb → septal area → cingulate gyrus → prefrontal cortex
   d. Olfactory bulb → bed nucleus of stria terminalis → ventroposterolateral nucleus of the thalamus → prefrontal cortex
   e. Olfactory bulb → hypothalamus → thalamus → prefrontal cortex

2. The efferent fibers from the olfactory bulb arise from which one of the following neurons?
   a. Periglomerular cells
   b. Granule cells
   c. Mitral cells
   d. Golgi cells
   e. Olfactory receptor cells

3. Which one of the following statements regarding the transduction of the taste stimulus is correct when a chemical molecule interacts with a specific membrane site on the microvilli of a taste receptor cell?
   a. The exposure of microvilli to an acid results in the depolarization of the receptor cell by opening of an amiloride-sensitive Na^+ channel.
   b. The exposure of microvilli to an acid results in the depolarization of the receptor cell by closure of K^+ channels.
   c. The exposure of microvilli to a bitter substance results in the activation of adenylate cyclase in the receptor cell.
   d. The exposure of microvilli to a sweet substance results in the activation of phospholipase C in the receptor cell.
   e. The exposure of microvilli to a salty substance results in the activation of G-protein in the receptor cell.

4. Which one of the following statements regarding the central pathways that mediate the taste sensation is correct?
   a. The central processes of sensory neurons in the geniculate ganglion terminate in the rostral solitary nucleus.
   b. The secondary neurons located in the solitary nucleus project directly to the cortical taste area.
   c. The sensory fibers innervating the epiglottis travel in the facial nerve.
   d. The taste buds located in the anterior third of the tongue are innervated by the peripheral processes of the unipolar neurons located in the petrosal ganglion of the CN IX.
   e. The secondary neurons mediating taste sensation are located in the nucleus ambiguus.

5. A 60-year-old man suffering from seizures complained that he was experiencing olfactory hallucinations of unpleasant smells (cacosmia). A magnetic resonance imaging (MRI) scan revealed the presence of a tumor in his brain. Which of the following choices is the most likely site of the location of the tumor?
   a. Postcentral gyrus
   b. Periaqueductal gray
   c. Mammillary bodies
   d. Caudate nucleus
   e. Temporal lobe

ANSWERS AND EXPLANATIONS

1. Answer: b

The signals generated by olfactory stimuli reach the olfactory bulb and are transmitted directly to the prefrontal cortex. It should be noted that there is another pathway for transmission of olfactory stimulation that involves relay of signals to the mediodorsal thalamus and then prefrontal cortex. However, the signals generated by visual, taste, and auditory stimuli must be first relayed to the thalamus.

2. Answer: c

The efferent fibers exiting the olfactory bulb are the axons of mitral and tufted cells. The periglomerular cells and granule cells are GABAergic interneurons; they have short axons that do not enter the olfactory tract. There are no Golgi cells and olfactory receptor cells in the olfactory bulb.

3. Answer: b

Sour taste, elicited by acids, is mediated by depolarization of the receptor cell due to closure of voltage-dependent K^+ channels. The following statements show that the other choices are incorrect. Bitter substances activate a G-protein, phospholipase C is activated, IP_3 is generated, and the taste receptor cell is depolarized by release of Ca^{2+} from intracellular stores. Sweet substances activate a G-protein, adenylate cyclase is activated, cAMP is generated, a phosphokinase is activated, K^+ channels are closed, and the taste receptor cell is depolarized. A salty substance depolarizes a taste receptor cell by influx of Na^+ through amiloride-sensitive Na^+ channels.

4. Answer: a

The taste buds on the anterior two thirds of the tongue are innervated by the facial nerve (CN VII); the sensory neurons mediating the sensation of taste from this region of the tongue are located in the geniculate ganglion of the facial nerve. The taste buds on the posterior one third of the tongue are innervated by the glossopharyngeal nerve (CN IX); the sensory neurons involved in the taste sensation from this portion of the tongue are located in the inferior (petrosal) ganglion of the glossopharyngeal nerve. The taste buds on the epiglottis are innervated by the vagus nerve (CN X); the sensory neurons involved in the taste sensation from the epiglottis and the pharyngeal wall are located in the inferior (nodose) ganglion of the vagus nerve. The central processes of these sensory neurons (i.e., sensory neurons located in the geniculate, petrosal, and nodose ganglia) enter the solitary tract and terminate in the rostral portion (gustatory region) of the solitary nucleus. The axons of secondary neurons located in the rostral portion of the solitary nucleus ascend in the solitario-thalamic tract (near the medial lemniscus) and terminate in the ventral posteromedial nucleus (VPM) of the thalamus. The neurons in the VPM send their projections to the cortical taste area of the postcentral gyrus.

5. Answer: e

Seizures involving parts of the temporal lobe produce olfactory hallucinations of unpleasant smells (cacosmia). This condition is also referred to as an uncinate fit. Parts of the temporal lobe include the uncus, parahippocampal gyrus, amygdala, and piriform cortex. Uncinate fits are caused when these structures are damaged. Other structures mentioned in the question are not involved in olfaction.

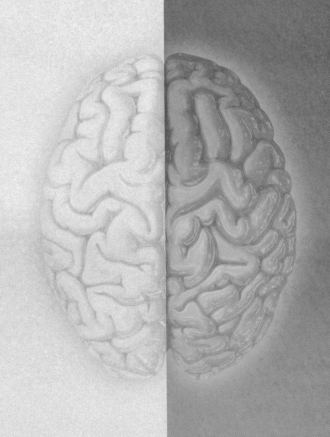

SECTION V

Motor Systems

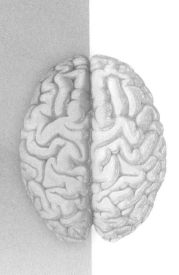

CHAPTER 19

THE UPPER MOTOR NEURONS

OBJECTIVES

In this chapter, the student should be able to:

1. Describe and diagram the origin, distribution, and somatotopic organization of the corticospinal tract

2. List and describe the functional mechanisms subserving voluntary control of movement

3. List and describe some of the basic mechanisms underlying upper motor neuron paralysis involving the corticospinal system

4. List and describe the origin, distribution, and functions of the following descending brainstem pathways in the control of movement and posture: rubrospinal, medial, and lateral vestibulospinal tracts and medial and lateral reticulospinal tracts

5. List, diagram, and describe the origin, distribution, and functions of the corticobulbar tracts

6. Define the term "upper motor neuron" and describe the nature of upper motor neuron disorders associated with damage to these tracts

The process of movement is a highly complex one. Even a supposedly simple event such as walking involves complex mechanisms regulating reflex responses, postural and voluntary motor patterns. In using walking as our model, it is important to note the patterns of movements of the legs and arms. When the left leg is extended, the right leg is normally flexed; in addition, the left arm will be extended backwards, while the right arm is flexed somewhat in a forward position. The entire sequence of events requires utilization of different regions of the central nervous system (CNS). These regions include all levels of the neuraxis, beginning with the spinal cord and extending rostrally through the brainstem, including the cerebellum, and forebrain regions of the basal ganglia and cerebral cortex.

The key structures of the CNS that relate to motor functions are illustrated schematically in Figure 19-1. As shown in this illustration, the lowest and perhaps most simple level of organization is present within the spinal cord. This level of the CNS provides the mechanisms for reflex motor functions. It also serves as the final common path for neurons that innervate skeletal muscle, which constitute the **lower motor neurons** for motor responses. It should be further noted as well that motor neurons of cranial nerves (i.e., special visceral efferent [SVE] and general somatic efferent [GSE] neurons) constitute lower motor neurons for motor functions associated with the head region.

The lower motor neurons for both the body and head region are controlled by **upper motor neurons**. Upper motor neurons are defined as those neurons of the brain that innervate lower motor neurons of the spinal cord and brainstem, either directly or through an interneuron. Therefore, an upper motor neuron may arise from the brainstem or cerebral cortex. A number of pathways arise from various levels of the brainstem and descend to the spinal cord. In doing so, these regions of the brainstem exert different influences on the activity of spinal motor neurons, resulting in directed effects upon flexor and extensor reflexes, including postural mechanisms. The pathways of importance include the medial and lateral **vestibulospinal tracts**, the medial and lateral

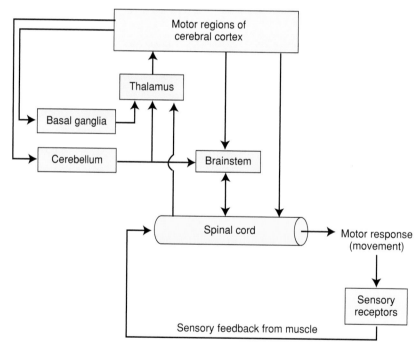

Figure 19–1 Organization of the motor systems. Spinal cord reflex mechanisms involve lower motor neurons and are subject to supraspinal control. The brain regions that have direct control over the spinal cord include the brainstem and cerebral cortex. Brainstem pathways that project to the spinal cord include the reticulospinal, vestibulospinal, rubrospinal, and tectospinal tracts. The cerebral cortex gives rise to both corticospinal and corticobulbar fibers. Corticospinal fibers are essential for voluntary control over fine movements, mainly of the distal extremities. Corticobulbar fibers contribute to the control of spinal cord indirectly, by acting on neurons of the brainstem that project to the spinal cord. Other corticobulbar fibers innervate lower motor neurons of the brainstem (cranial nerves) and provide the substrate and mechanism for voluntary movements of the head region. Two other regions, the basal ganglia and cerebellum, play important roles in motor functions. The basal ganglia affect motor systems by acting on neurons in the precentral and premotor regions that comprise the larger part of the corticospinal tract. The cerebellum affects motor function by acting on neurons in both the brainstem and the cerebral cortex that directly control motor functions of the spinal cord.

reticulospinal tracts, the **rubrospinal tract**, and the **tectospinal tract**. The tracts were described briefly in Chapter 9 and will be considered in more detail later on in this chapter.

The most significant of all the upper motor neurons are those that arise from the cerebral cortex. As indicated in previous chapters, the upper motor neurons that project to the spinal cord are called the **corticospinal tracts**, and the ones that project to lower motor neurons of the brainstem are called the **corticobulbar tracts**. They provide the anatomical substrates for voluntary control of movement. A detailed analysis of the anatomical organization, functional properties, and neurologic disorders associated with these pathways is presented later in this chapter.

Two other systems play important roles in the regulation of motor functions. These include the **basal ganglia** and **cerebellum**. The basal ganglia participate in the control of movement by receiving significant inputs from the cerebral cortex and feeding back signals to different regions of the frontal cortex involved in the initiation of movement. In this manner, the basal ganglia serve to modulate the activity of neurons of the motor regions of the cortex. The cerebellum receives inputs from most parts of the CNS that contribute to motor functions. In turn, it sends back messages to each of these regions. The presence of these feedback circuits enables the cerebellum to serve as a principal integrator of motor function by synchronizing the output messages distributed to each of these regions at any given point in time. Chapters 20 and 21 are dedicated to the analysis of the organization and functions of the basal ganglia and cerebellum, respectively.

THE CORTICOSPINAL TRACT

As noted earlier, the corticospinal tract is crucial for the expression of precise, voluntary movements. In attempting to develop an understanding of the nature of the corticospinal tract, it is important to answer the following questions:

1. From where does this tract originate?

2. What is the anatomical organization of the tract as it passes caudally through the brain to the spinal cord?

3. How are the fibers distributed within the spinal cord?

4. What are the important sources of inputs that corticospinal neurons must receive in order to function properly?

5. What are the differential contributions of the descending components of the corticospinal tact?

6. What are the clinical manifestations of lesions that affect the corticospinal tract, and how can these be understood in terms of the basic anatomical and physiological properties of this pathway?

ORIGIN OF THE CORTICOSPINAL TRACT

The corticospinal (or pyramidal) tract arises from three different regions of the cortex (Fig. 19-2). Approximately 30% of the fibers arise from the **precentral gyrus** (**area 4**, which is referred to as the primary motor cortex called MI [where I is roman numeral I]). Forty percent of the fibers arise from the postcentral gyrus (which is referred to as the **primary somatosensory cortex** [S-1] and includes areas 3, 1, and 2). The remaining 30% of the fibers originate from the region immediately rostral to the precentral gyrus (area 6, called the **supplemental motor area** [SMA] and the **premotor cortex** [PMC]). While both regions of area 6 contribute fibers to the corticospinal tract, the larger majority arises from the supplemental motor area.

Both the precentral and postcentral gyri are somatotopically organized. Electrical stimulation of the dorsal and medial aspect of the precentral gyrus in humans produces movements associated with the lower limb, while stimulation of more lateral aspects of the motor cortex produces movements of the upper limb. Moreover, stimulation of the far lateral aspect of the precentral gyrus produces movements of the face and tongue. This functional representation of the precentral gyrus is referred to as a **motor homunculus** (Fig. 19-3). A similar homunculus is also present for the primary somatosensory cortex.

HISTOLOGY OF THE MOTOR CORTEX

Based on the histological appearance of the gray matter, the cerebral cortex typically has six layers (see Chapter 26 for details). In brief, there are generally two layers of granule cells (an external and internal granule cell layer), which receive information mainly from the thalamus and other regions of the cortex, and two layers of pyramidal cells (an external and internal pyramidal cell layer), which serve as the origins of the efferent pathways of the cortex. In motor regions of the cortex, the pyramidal cell layers are of much greater size than the granule cell layers, and the reverse holds true for sensory regions. The corticospinal tracts arise from the internal pyramidal cell layer situated mainly in layer V (Fig. 19-4). Pyramidal cells lying in other cortical layers, as

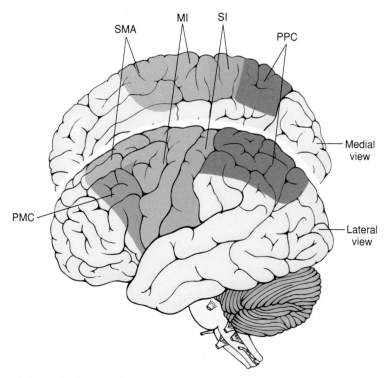

Figure 19–2 The regions of the cerebral cortex that give rise to the corticospinal tract. Abbreviations: MI, primary motor cortex; PMC, premotor cortex; PPC, posterior parietal cortex; SI, primary somatosensory receiving area; SMA, supplementary motor area. Note that the PPC does not contribute to the corticospinal tract but does modulate its activity.

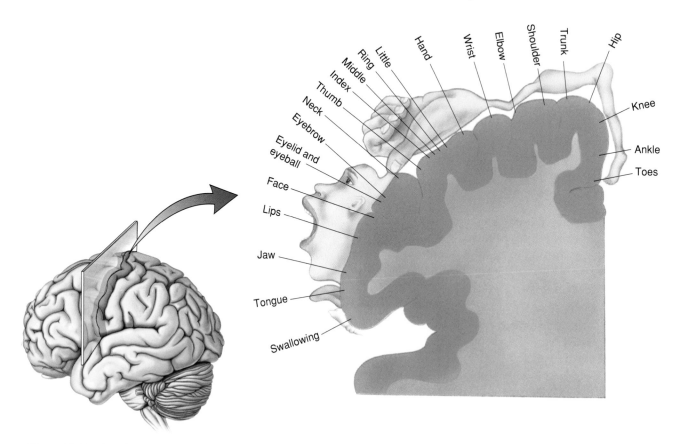

Figure 19–3 The relative homuncular representation of the primary motor cortex reveals the relative sizes of the regions of the primary motor cortex, which represent different parts of the body as determined by electrical stimulation experiments (Reproduced with permission from Bear MF, et al.: Neuroscience: Exploring the Brain, 2nd ed. Baltimore: Lippincott Williams & Wilkins, 2001, p. 474.)

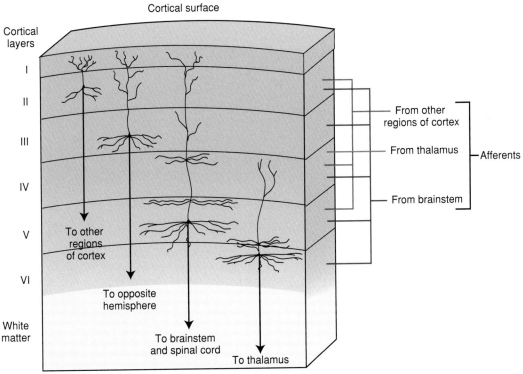

Figure 19–4 Histological appearance of the motor cortex displaying the specific layers which give rise to the varied efferent projections of this region of cortex. Afferent fibers to these layers are also shown.

well as layer V, project to different areas of the CNS. For example, the cortical pyramidal cells of layer III project to both the ipsilateral and the contralateral cortex (as axons of the corpus callosum), while pyramidal cells of layers V to VI give rise to descending fibers that reach the spinal cord, brainstem, and thalamus.

COURSE OF THE CORTICOSPINAL TRACT

Pyramidal cell axons that exit the gray matter of cortex enter the white matter and internal capsule first. Within the internal capsule and crus cerebri, pyramidal tract fibers are somatotopically organized (see Fig. 9-12). Corticospinal fibers are contained within the posterior limb, with those fibers associated with the arm region of the cortex located slightly closer to the genu of the internal capsule than those associated with the leg. Note that corticobulbar fibers are located within the region of the genu. As the fibers reach the crus cerebri of the midbrain, they become reorganized in a slightly different way (see Chapter 12). Collectively, corticobulbar and corticospinal fibers are situated within the middle three fifths of the crus cerebri. Fibers associated with the leg region are located in a more lateral position than those associated with the arm, while fibers associated with

the head region (i.e., corticobulbar fibers) are located medial to the corticospinal fibers. As the fibers reach the lower brainstem, they enter the pyramid and continue to pass caudally to the spinal cord-medulla junction. At that level, 90% of the fibers cross over to the opposite side in the pyramidal decussation and descend through the lateral funiculus of the contralateral spinal cord, largely as the **lateral corticospinal tract**. The remaining 10% of the fibers, which remain uncrossed, descend into the spinal cord, 8% as the **anterior corticospinal tract**, and 2% as the uncrossed lateral corticospinal tract. Of these 10% of fibers, 8% (anterior corticospinal tract) cross over to the contralateral side. Ulti-mately, 98% of the corticospinal tract fibers project to the contralateral spinal cord. Thus, a scant 2% of the lateral corticospinal tract remains ipsilateral over its entire course.

DISTRIBUTION OF THE CORTICOSPINAL FIBERS WITHIN THE SPINAL CORD

Fibers contained within the corticospinal tract are distributed throughout the entire rostrocaudal extent of the spinal cord. The largest components of these fibers terminate at lower cervical and lumbar levels of the cord. Within a given level of the spinal

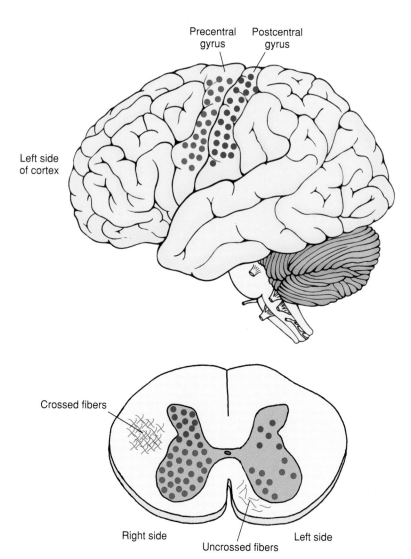

Figure 19–5 The distribution of axon terminals in the spinal cord of the monkey as determined by autoradiographic tracing procedures. Depicted also are the sites of origin of the pathway in the motor and somatosensory cortices (top). Most fibers, which are uncrossed, pass in the anterior corticospinal tract and terminate mainly in the medial aspect of the gray matter, contacting neurons that innervate axial and proximal muscles (bottom). Crossed fibers supply both the dorsal horn and the ventral horn. Fibers that issue from the postcentral gyrus (depicted in purple) supply the dorsal horn, whereas those that arise from the motor cortex (depicted in red) supply the ventral horn.

cord, corticospinal fibers terminate within both the dorsal and ventral horns as well as medial and lateral cell groups (Fig. 19-5). Anatomical and physiological studies have shown that fibers that originate from the primary motor, supplemental, or premotor cortices project primarily to interneurons of the ventral horn of the spinal cord, which then synapse upon motor horn cells; whereas fibers that arise from the primary somatosensory region of cortex project primarily to the dorsal horn of the spinal cord. Moreover, frontal lobe fibers that form the anterior corticospinal tract innervate more medial regions of the ventral gray matter, while the lateral corticospinal tract innervates more lateral cell groups of the ventral horn.

FUNCTIONS

The functional significance of these projections can be briefly summarized as follows. Recall that the ven-

tral horn is organized in such a manner that neurons located medially innervate the axial musculature, whereas neurons located more laterally innervate the distal musculature (see Chapter 9). Therefore, lateral corticospinal fibers that innervate the cervical and lumbar cord serve to control fine movements of the extremities, while axons from the anterior corticospinal tract (and elsewhere) that innervate the medial aspect of the ventral horn serve to regulate postural mechanisms. Furthermore, corticospinal neurons that innervate the dorsal horn serve to modulate primary sensory afferent information to the cerebral cortex rather than to produce movement. Further consideration of the functions of these fiber systems is discussed on pages 331–335.

Knowledge of the afferent supply to the regions of cortex that give rise to the corticospinal tract provides clues concerning the possible functions of each of these components. As such, the discussion that follows considers such inputs to provide a

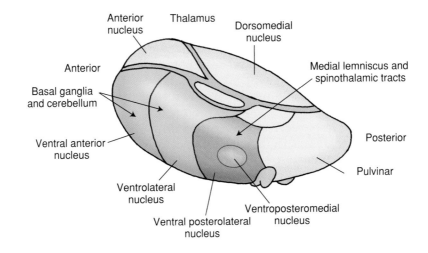

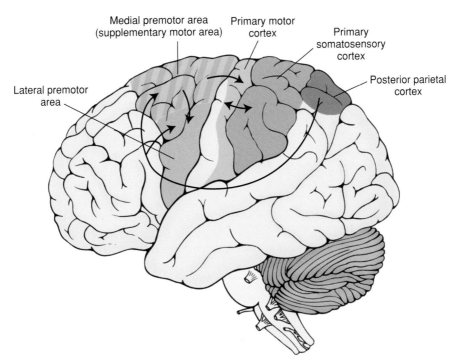

Figure 19–6 Principal afferent projections to the motor cortex. Note that the cerebellum and basal ganglia gain entry into the motor and premotor cortices via connections with the ventrolateral and ventral anterior thalamic nuclei. This diagram also illustrates several key corticocortical connections that are essential for motor functions of the cerebral cortex. These include connections from the posterior parietal cortex (areas 5 and 7) to the premotor and supplementary motor cortices, connections from area 6 (supplementary and premotor cortices) to the primary motor cortex (area 4), and connections from the primary somatosensory cortex (areas 3, 1, and 2) to the primary motor cortex.

better understanding of the functions associated with the motor regions of the cortex.

Primary Motor Cortex

The primary motor cortex receives *indirect* inputs from several important regions that are known to regulate motor activity. These include the cerebellum and globus pallidus. Each of these regions projects to the primary motor cortex via a relay in the ventrolateral nucleus (VL) of the thalamus (Fig. 19-6). These inputs do not converge upon the same cells within the VL, but instead project to different parts of the nucleus. Thus, the integration of all of these inputs occurs within the primary motor cortex rather than in the thalamus. Other studies conducted in monkeys have shown that a purposeful movement is preceded by the discharge of neurons within the basal ganglia and cerebellum, which occurs prior to neuronal discharges in the motor cortex. The neuronal discharges in the motor cortex also precede the motor response. These kinds of observations suggest that the cerebellar and basal ganglia inputs provide the motor cortex with a planning mechanism for the initiation and regulation of a given response pattern.

The primary motor cortex also receives **somatosensory afferents**. The somatosensory inputs are organized in such a manner that enables a given region of motor cortex to receive proprioceptive and tactile inputs that relate to the specific muscle groups or body parts to which the neurons in that region of motor cortex relate functionally. For example, a group of cells in the motor cortex that relate to movement of specific muscle groups of the leg will, in turn, receive proprioceptive and tactile inputs from that part of the leg. Such inputs to a specific site within the primary motor cortex likely come indirectly from a thalamic relay nucleus such as the ventral posterolateral nucleus (VPL), which is somatotopically organized, through a region of the primary somatosensory cortex that represents the same part of the body as the region of motor cortex to which it projects. This anatomical arrangement thus provides the basis for a second property of MI neurons, namely, that they discharge in response to movement. Moreover, the neurons in the cortex that respond to the action of a given muscle group are located in slightly different regions and lie close to neurons that relate to other muscle groups. Nevertheless, the neurons all generally lie within the region associated with that part of the body. Therefore, it is likely that the cortical neuronal discharge patterns indicate that the cells are responding to the synergistic actions of groups of muscles rather than to isolated muscle contractions of an individual muscle. Thus, when viewed collectively, the combination of signals from the basal ganglia, cerebellum, and sensory pathways provides the necessary inputs by which MI can produce a precise response of the appropriate force.

The fibers of the primary motor cortex project to the ventral horn at all levels of the cord but project most prominently to the lumbar and cervical levels. The corticospinal neurons make synaptic contact mainly with short interneurons that synapse upon alpha and gamma motor neurons in that region. Thus, activation of descending fibers of the primary motor cortex can directly produce muscle contractions of individual muscles as well as control the spindle mechanism associated with the tone of those muscles.

Primary Somatosensory Cortex

The primary inputs to the somatosensory cortex are from the VPL of the thalamus, which receives its afferent supply from the dorsal column-medial lemniscal system and spinothalamic pathways (Fig. 19-6). These inputs involve conscious proprioception, position sense, pain, and tactile information. However, as noted earlier, descending pyramidal tract fibers originating from somatosensory cortex project to sensory regions and not to motor neurons. The primary projection targets include the cells of the dorsal horn of the spinal cord and the dorsal column nuclei of the lower medulla.[1]

What is the significance of these descending fibers? The answer to this question resides in the fact that sequences of movements require the transmission of "positive" sensory feedback to the regions of motor cortex associated with those movements. What do these signals signify? Basically, they are involved in the regulation of sensory transmission through the nuclei of the dorsal columns and may respond to one or more of the following aspects of movement: (1) alteration of the position of the limb, (2) rate of change of the position of the limb, (3) magnitude of the muscular contraction in relation to the force exerted upon an object, and (4) a combination of force as well as rate of change.

Consider for a moment what the effect would be if, while attempting to walk, there was a loss of sensation concerning the position of either foot at any point in time. Under these circumstances, there would be a significant loss of precision to those movements. They would become awkward and ataxic. This, indeed, does occur with lesions involving the dorsal columns (see Chapter 9). The important point to remember here is that transmission of appropriate positive (sensory) feedback signals to the region of motor cortex associated with that movement requires the simultaneous filtering of other irrelevant sensory signals. Such filtering takes place at the levels of the dorsal column nuclei and dorsal horn by the inhibitory actions of the descending corticospinal fibers that arise from somatosensory cortex. Loss of this inhibitory feedback mechanism would deprive the cortical motor neurons in question from responding appropriately to the positive feedback signals.

---

[1]In a strict sense, fiber projections from the cerebral cortex to the dorsal column nuclei are referred to as *corticobulbar fibers* because they do not innervate the spinal cord. However, they are included in the discussion of the distribution of the corticospinal tract because their functions are parallel to those descending fibers that innervate the dorsal horn of the spinal cord and that originate from the same general regions as the corticospinal neurons.

Supplementary and Premotor Area Cortices

Area 6, which contributes 30% of the fibers to the corticospinal tract, consists of two secondary motor regions: a **supplemental motor area (SMA)** and a **premotor (PMC)** area. There are several highly significant inputs into these regions that should be noted. The first input is from the basal ganglia, which is directed mainly to the SMA. The primary route for this input to the cortex is through the thalamic nuclei (Fig. 19-6). Although some of the data obtained from various studies remains in conflict, the overall patterns seem to indicate that portions of both the VL and ventral anterior (VA) nuclei of thalamus, which receive inputs from the basal ganglia, project to area 6. Another source of inputs into area 6 includes the cerebellum. Here, cerebellar efferent fibers first synapse upon relay neurons in the VL, which then relay these signals primarily onto the premotor cortex (PMC). A third source of inputs is the **posterior parietal cortex (PPC)**. This region of cortex provides integrated somatosensory and visual information to area 6, which is necessary for the programming of motor sequences. Details concerning the posterior parietal cortex are described in the next section.

The most significant functional aspect of the SMA is its role in coordinating voluntary movements. It governs postural adjustments, and the associated deficits that occur after damage to this region are further evidence of its role in motor functions. Electrical stimulation of the supplemental (as well as premotor) cortex requires higher currents for the elicitation of motor responses. The motor responses are of a more complex pattern than those elicited from the primary motor cortex. Motor cortex stimulation frequently produces discrete twitching of one or several muscle groups. In contrast, stimulation of the supplementary and premotor cortices can elicit postural adjustments, body orientation, or closing or opening of the hands. The responses may be unilateral or bilateral.

The SMA can affect both the axial and the distal musculature through at least two important projections. This region of cortex controls the distal musculature by virtue of its projections upon primary motor neurons of area 4 (primary motor cortex). Its influence upon the axial musculature is by descending axons of neurons of the SMA found in the corticospinal tract that affect (through an interneuron) motor horn cells located in the ventromedial aspect of ventral gray of the spinal cord.

Patients who have lesions of the SMA display **apraxia**. Apraxia refers to the inability to initiate specific, purposeful movements, even though the sensory and motor pathways for the execution of the movement remain intact. There are several different types of apraxia. One type of apraxia is called **ideomotor apraxia**. It refers to the inability to execute a movement upon request. An example is the failure of a patient to be able to brush his hair or tie his shoelaces. **Ideational apraxia** is the inability to conceptualize the movements, and the patient is unable to identify the sequences of movements that are necessary for carrying out the response in question. Frequently, the apraxia becomes evident when the patient is asked to perform, simultaneously, different movements of both arms. On the other hand, if asked to perform the same sequence of movements with both arms simultaneously, the patient is often successful.

In a manner similar to that described earlier for the SMA, neurons of the PMC can activate, both directly and indirectly, spinal cord neurons that supply the axial and distal musculature. Corticospinal fibers arising from the PMC innervate medial and lateral ventral horn cells, directly or indirectly, by descending fibers that supply reticulospinal fibers (see page 336 and Chapter 23). (Recall that those neurons located medially in the ventral horn of the spinal cord innervate the axial musculature, and neurons located laterally innervate the distal musculature).

The premotor area plays an important role in movements that require visual guidance. Here, the inputs from the posterior parietal cortex are essential. Lesions of the PMC in humans can produce apraxia (similar to the apraxia described in the next section with lesions of the posterior parietal cortex [PPC]). With lesions of the PMC, the patient is unable to coordinate the movement of both arms at the same time. In addition, the patient may also have loss of strength in the proximal muscles of the contralateral arm or leg and have difficulty in raising or abducting that limb.

Role of the Posterior Parietal Cortex

As indicated earlier, an important source of inputs to area 6 is derived from the **posterior parietal cortex (PPC)** (areas 5 and 7) (Figs. 19-2 and 19-6). Somatosensory inputs from the postcentral gyrus as well as vestibular inputs are directed to area 5, while area 7 is concerned with visual signals. In addition, area 7 receives inputs from area 5, thus indicating that this region of the cortex integrates both somatosensory as well as visual signals.

Different groups of neurons located in the posterior parietal cortex discharge in response to exploratory hand movements or in preparation for a goal-directed response, such as reaching out to grab an object. Appropriate movements used for a given motor task require that an individual pay attention to the spatial arrangements of the objects in its visual field and to integrate that information

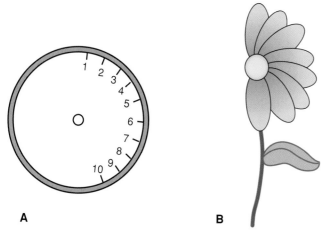

Figure 19–7 Drawings made by a patient with a lesion of the *right* posterior parietal cortex, indicating sensory neglect on the left side. The patient was asked to fill in numbers on the face of the clock (A) and to draw a flower (B).

with proprioceptive and other somatosensory signals. It is generally believed that the posterior parietal area carries out this function.

Perhaps the most interesting findings concerning functions of the posterior parietal area come from the clinical literature. Patients with lesions of the right posterior parietal cortex show two types of disorders. The first is apraxia. The second type of disorder is called **sensory neglect** (or **anosognosia**). In this disorder, the patient denies the disease condition or is unaware of it. For example, a female patient with a right hemispheric lesion may deny or ignore the fact that she cannot move her left leg. Moreover, if this patient is asked to draw the numbers on a clock, she will draw them all on the right-hand side of the clock, while ignoring the left-hand side (Fig. 19-7).

Collectively, the physiological and clinical findings suggest the posterior parietal cortex executes an important function in motor activities. This function is to generate integrated somatosensory and visual inputs to area 6, which provides the programming mechanism for the execution of complex motor responses.

SUMMARY OF THE COMPONENTS AND FUNCTIONS OF THE CORTICOSPINAL TRACT

There are three principal components of the corticospinal tract. The first includes those fiber bundles that arise from the **primary motor cortex** (area 4). This pathway is responsible for voluntary control over precise movements that affect primarily (but not exclusively) the distal musculature. The

actions of this fiber system are upon the ventral horn cells (via short interneurons) at all levels of the spinal cord. Appropriate neuronal responses in the primary motor cortex are heavily dependent on feedback signals from several regions. These include ascending inputs that signal the position of the distal musculature related to the movements associated with the primary motor cortical regions in question as well as other messages from the basal ganglia and cerebellum.

The second component involves fiber pathways that arise from the **primary somatosensory cortex** (areas 3, 1, and 2) that project to the dorsal column nuclei and dorsal horn of the spinal cord. The purpose of this component is to serve as a sensory filtering mechanism. This mechanism allows specific sensory signals, such as the position of a limb or digit of the hand and the force of contraction of a muscle or group of muscles, to reach the relevant regions of the primary motor cortex while preventing sensory signals irrelevant to the movement in question from reaching the cortical neurons critical for that response sequence. This mechanism likely operates by providing excitatory foci and inhibitory surrounds (analogous to the visual system) with respect to different motor neurons within area 4.

The third component includes area 6, the supplementary and premotor cortices, which serve to provide the programming mechanism for the sequencing of response patterns that are essential for producing movements such as lacing up one's shoes and walking. These regions of area 6 project directly to the spinal cord and send signals to the primary motor cortex. In this way, the actions of the descending pathways upon different groups of neurons within the ventral horn of the spinal cord are synchronized with the actions of area 6 neurons upon the primary motor cortex. Finally, the actions of area 6 neurons can only occur if they receive integrated somatosensory and visual signals from the posterior parietal cortex (areas 5 and 7).

THE CORTICOBULBAR TRACTS

The **corticobulbar tracts** arise from the lateral aspect of the primary motor cortex (i.e., depicted as the head or face region in Fig. 19-3) and function in a similar manner to the corticospinal tract. Essentially, these descending fibers of the corticobulbar tracts serve as upper motor neurons to the cranial nerve motor nuclei onto which they make synaptic contact. They closely follow the descending trajectory of the corticospinal tracts (Fig.

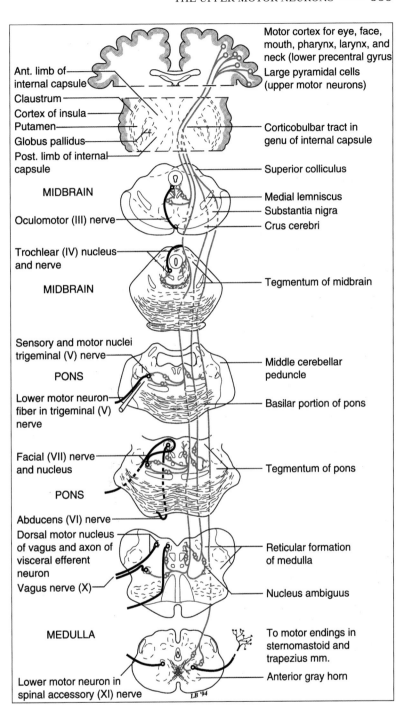

Figure 19–8 Projections of corticobulbar fibers to motor nuclei of cranial nerves. (Used with permission from Parent A: Carpenter's Human Neuroanatomy, 9th ed. Baltimore: Williams & Wilkins, 1996.)

19-8) and make direct or indirect synaptic contact (via interneurons in the reticular formation) with all motor cranial nerves (Fig. 19-8). These upper motor neurons thus serve as the anatomical substrate for voluntary control of the muscles of facial expression, eye movements, jaw opening and closing, and movements of the tongue.

However, there are several differences between the corticobulbar and corticospinal tracts that should be noted. The first is that most corticobulbar fibers that are directed toward cranial nerve motor nuclei innervate these neurons bilaterally (see Chapter 14). The exceptions include contralateral innervation of ventral cell groups of the motor nucleus of cranial nerve (CN) VII, which supply muscles of the lower quadrants of the face (below the eyes) such as the orbicularis oris muscle, and the hypoglossal nucleus (CN XII), which supplies the genioglossus muscle. It is also widely believed that the supranuclear innervation of the neurons of the spinal accessory nerve (CN XI) is mainly contralateral.

LESIONS OF CORTICOBULBAR FIBERS THAT SUPPLY NUCLEI OF CRANIAL NERVES

As indicated earlier, most of the inputs to motor nuclei of cranial nerves from the motor cortex are bilateral. A lesion of the cortex will not produce a paralysis of the muscles of the face and head. Instead, it will produce mild forms of weakness in the affected muscles (referred to as **central facial palsy**). Weakness in muscles that regulate breathing, swallowing, speech, and chewing is referred to as **pseudobulbar palsy**. If the lesion involves only the corticobulbar fibers and not corticospinal neurons, then there would be no paralysis of the upper or lower extremities. Because the neurons that innervate the muscles of facial expression of the lower quadrants of the face and those that effect protrusion of the tongue receive mainly a contralateral input, damage to the upper motor neurons will result in a more marked weakness involving the affected muscles on the side contralateral to the lesion. Such effects are manifested by a deviation of the jaw and tongue (upon protrusion) to the side contralateral to the site of the lesion. Similarly, damage to the corticobulbar fibers projecting to the hypoglossal nucleus will produce a deviation of the tongue to the side opposite the lesion. Further discussion of the effects of supranuclear lesions on cranial nerve function is considered in Chapter 14.

OTHER PROJECTIONS OF THE CORTICOBULBAR TRACTS

To Sensory Relay Nuclei

As noted earlier, one of the components of the corticospinal tract arises from areas 3, 1, and 2 (the primary somatosensory cortex situated on the postcentral gyrus). Many of the fibers project to the dorsal horn, and others project to dorsal column nuclei. Both groups of fibers essentially perform the same functions; namely, they serve to filter the flow of sensory information to the sensorimotor cortex. However, as previously indicated, the projections from areas 3, 1, and 2 to the dorsal column nuclei, strictly speaking, are called corticobulbar fibers. Other fibers from somatosensory cortex project to the sensory nuclei of the trigeminal system. These fibers also function in a parallel manner

to the descending cortical fibers that supply the dorsal horn and dorsal column nuclei. The projection to the sensory trigeminal nuclei serves as a filtering mechanism for sensory inputs associated with the head region.

Corticoreticular Fibers

Considerable quantities of fibers that arise from the sensorimotor cortex (i.e., the precentral, postcentral, and premotor cortices) also project to different regions of the reticular formation of the brainstem. Although these projections are relatively extensive, there are several projections that should be noted. Fibers originating from the precentral gyrus project to neurons of the pons and medulla, which give rise to descending bundles that comprise reticulospinal fibers (i.e., the lateral and medial reticulospinal tracts). The functions of these tracts and the corticoreticular inputs are considered later in this chapter and in Chapter 23. Other groups of fibers of the sensorimotor cortex project to the paramedian and reticular nuclei of the reticular formation of the pons and medulla, respectively, which supplies the cerebellum. These projections thus enable the cortex to provide additional influences on motor functions at the levels of both the spinal cord and cerebellum. Still other groups of cortical fibers project to regions of the reticular formation that give rise to long ascending fibers to the forebrain. One of the functions of the long ascending fiber projections of the reticular formation is to produce cortical arousal (see Chapter 23). The cortical projections to the regions that give rise to these ascending projections may provide the anatomical basis for a feedback mechanism for the regulation of cortical arousal functions.

Cortical Projections to the Red Nucleus

Studies, based mainly on cats, have shown that fibers that arise from the primary and premotor cortices also project ipsilaterally to the red nucleus. This projection is somatotopically organized. Fibers from the upper limb region of the precentral gyrus project to the dorsal part of the red nucleus, while fibers from the lower limb region of the precentral gyrus project to the ventral aspect of the red nucleus. The dorsal and ventral regions of the red nucleus project to the cervical and lumbar regions of the spinal cord. Thus, the projection to the red nucleus represents still another way by which the cerebral cortex can control motor functions of the spinal cord. Functions of this system are described in the *Rubrospinal Tract* section. However, in humans, it is believed that the descending projections of the red nucleus to the spinal cord (i.e., rubrospinal tract) are considerably diminished, with few fibers descending beyond the cervical level.

DESCENDING MOTOR SYSTEMS FROM THE BRAINSTEM

There are six descending fiber pathways from the brainstem to the spinal cord that are of importance: the **medial and lateral reticulospinal tracts**, the **medial and lateral vestibulospinal tracts**, the **rubrospinal tract**, and the **tectospinal tract**. The reticulospinal and vestibulospinal tracts innervate neurons of the ventral horn that are associated with the axial musculature, while rubrospinal (similar to corticospinal) fibers supply mainly the neurons that innervate the distal flexor musculature. Because these fiber systems have already been described in Chapter 9, only a brief review will be presented here.

RETICULOSPINAL TRACTS

There are two reticulospinal tracts; one arises from the medulla (the **lateral reticulospinal tract**), and the other arises from the pons (**medial reticulospinal tract**) (see Fig. 9-15). The medial reticulospinal tract arises from large cells located in the medial part of the reticular formation (called the **nucleus reticularis pontis oralis** and **nucleus reticularis pontis caudalis**) and descends to all levels of the spinal cord where it synapses either directly upon both alpha and gamma motor neurons or indirectly through interneurons. The primary motor function is to facilitate voluntary or cortically induced movements and to increase muscle tone because of its actions on gamma motor neurons. The lateral reticulospinal tract arises from cells called the **nucleus reticularis gigantocellularis** and other large (magnocellular) neurons located in the medial two thirds of the medulla. Axons of these cells descend to all levels of the spinal cord. The actions of this pathway are opposite to those of the medial reticulospinal tract. Activation of this pathway inhibits voluntary movements and cortically induced movements and reduces muscle tone by further inhibiting muscle spindle activity through its effects on gamma motor neurons.

VESTIBULOSPINAL TRACTS

There are two vestibulospinal tracts. One arises from the medial vestibular nucleus, and the other arises from the lateral vestibular nucleus (see Fig. 9-14), and both convey impulses to the spinal cord from the labyrinth. The **medial vestibulospinal tract** arises from the medial vestibular nucleus and projects as the descending component of the me-

dial longitudinal fasciculus (MLF) to reach cervical levels of the spinal cord bilaterally. The importance of these fibers is that they activate lower motor neurons associated with the spinal accessory nerve. In this manner, activation of the medial vestibulospinal tract can cause rotation and lifting of the head as well as rotation of the shoulder blade around its axis. Such movements are important in producing an appropriate orientation of the individual in response to forces that cause changes in posture and balance. The **lateral vestibulospinal tract** arises from the lateral vestibular nucleus and projects to all levels of the spinal cord. Stimulation of this pathway powerfully facilitates alpha and gamma motor neurons that innervate extensor motor neurons. Similar to the medial vestibulospinal tract, the lateral vestibulospinal tract also plays an important role in the maintenance of posture by exciting neurons that innervate extensor (i.e., antigravity) muscles mainly of the lower limbs. The lateral vestibulospinal tract is modulated by activation of the vestibular apparatus or cerebellum, which provides it with its major afferent supply.

RUBROSPINAL TRACT

The rubrospinal tract arises from the red nucleus. As soon as the axons emerge from the red nucleus, they cross over to the contralateral side in the ventral tegmental decussation and descend to the spinal cord (see Fig. 9-13). In less advanced animals, such as the cat, the fibers have been shown to descend to both cervical and lumbar levels. However, in higher forms, the primary projection to the spinal cord is directed to cervical levels. Thus, in humans, the primary action of the rubrospinal tract is to facilitate motor neurons that innervate flexor muscles. As noted earlier, the red nucleus receives major inputs from the primary and premotor cortices, and the entire pathway from the cortex to the spinal cord is somatotopically organized. In this manner, this system may be referred to as a cortico-rubro-rubrospinal pathway. This pathway may thus be thought of as a functionally parallel system to that of the corticospinal tract. The reasons for this conclusion are that: (1) both systems originate from the same general regions of cortex, (2) both systems are somatotopically organized, and (3) both systems act primarily on the flexor motor system. In particular, by innervating flexor muscles of the upper extremity, both corticospinal and rubrospinal neurons excite muscles that act against gravity (in humans) and that are involved in the fine control of movement. It should also be noted that, in humans, where the overall size of the rubrospinal tract is diminished, there is an increase in the size of the descending projections of the red nucleus to the cerebellum via the inferior olivary nucleus (i.e., rubro-olivary fibers), suggesting the presence of a more potent influence of the red nucleus on cerebellar function in primates. The importance of this pathway is considered in Chapter 21.

TECTOSPINAL TRACT

The tectospinal tract arises from the superior colliculus of the midbrain and soon crosses over to the contralateral side in the dorsal tegmental decussation. The fibers descend to cervical levels of the spinal cord where they terminate (see Fig. 9-13). Although little is known about the functions of this tract, it is believed that it serves to produce postural changes in response to visual stimuli that reach the superior colliculus.

THE UPPER MOTOR NEURON SYNDROME

The upper motor neuron syndrome was described initially in Chapter 9, but it is useful to review and provide further analysis of this syndrome. This syndrome is the result of disruption of central motor pathways that arise from the cerebral cortex. The lesion may occur in the cortex, internal capsule, crus cerebri, lower medulla, or even lateral funiculus of the spinal cord. Typically, however, the most common sites of damage include the internal capsule and cerebral cortex. It should be pointed out that the upper motor neuron syndrome likely reflects damage not only to corticospinal neurons, but also to other descending fibers from the cortex to the brainstem, which synapse upon descending pathways to the spinal cord. Examples of such connections include cortical projections to the reticular formation (i.e., to reticulospinal neurons) and the red nucleus (i.e., rubrospinal neurons). In fact, these connections help to account for some of the clinical signs characteristic of the upper motor neuron syndrome. Thus, it may be concluded that, while all corticospinal neurons are upper motor neurons, not all upper motor neurons are corticospinal neurons.

The most classic signs of upper motor neuron syndrome include: (1) paralysis or weakness (paresis) of movement of the affected muscles; (2) a marked increase in muscle tone (hypertonia) coupled with spasticity (i.e., resistance to movement in a single direction); (3) the presence of abnormal reflexes, such as the **Babinski reflex** (i.e., extension and fanning out of the big toe; also referred to as an **extensor plantar response**), after stroking along the sole of the foot with a sharp object (Fig. 19-9); and (4) the diminution of some reflexes such as the abdominal reflexes. However, immediately after damage (usually from a stroke) to the cerebral cortex or internal capsule, a flaccid paralysis of the contralateral limb appears with a hypotonia and loss of myotatic reflexes. Nevertheless, the condition becomes reversed after a period of time, and the hypotonia is replaced by a hypertonia. The myotatic reflexes reappear and are highly pronounced (i.e., hyperreflexia), with continued loss of function of the distal musculature.

There are several aspects to upper motor neuron syndrome. The **paralysis of movement** of the distal

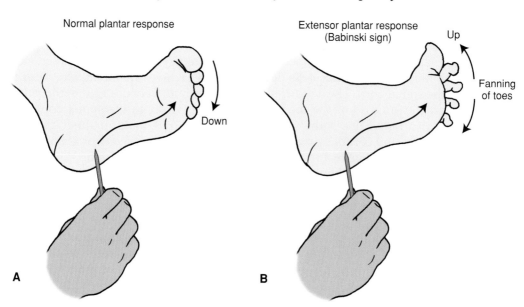

Normal plantar response

Down

Extensor plantar response (Babinski sign)

Up

Fanning of toes

A

B

Figure 19–9   Illustration of a Babinski test. The sole of the foot is stroked with a sharp object from front to back. This kind of stimulation typically produces flexion of the foot (A). However, a patient who has an upper motor neuron paralysis will show extension of the large toe coupled with a fanning out of the other toes (B).

musculature can easily enough be accounted for in terms of our understanding of the anatomical relationships between the upper and lower motor neurons. Specifically, the sequencing of discharge patterns of different groups of ventral horn cells at a given time for a purposeful movement to occur requires command signals from corticospinal fibers. The loss of such input to the ventral horn of the spinal cord would obviously prevent those neurons from discharging in a meaningful sequence. Hence, such a loss would result in paralysis of movement.

The second feature of this disorder is **spasticity** and **hypertonia**, which is still poorly understood. Several hypotheses have been advanced to attempt to account for this phenomenon. One logical possibility is that corticospinal fibers make contact with both interneurons that excite motor horn cells as well as several types of inhibitory interneurons. Such inhibitory interneurons might include Renshaw cells that, when stimulated, produce recurrent inhibition of neurons innervating an antagonist muscle group, or they might include inhibitory interneurons associated with 1b afferents from tendon organs. The loss of input to these inhibitory interneurons could result in increased levels of excitability of neurons that innervate antagonists such as extensor groups of the lower limbs and flexors of the upper limbs. The difficulty with this hypothesis is that "pure" pyramidal tract lesions of restricted regions of area 4 or at the level of the lower brainstem, which only destroy corticospinal tract fibers, do not necessarily produce spasticity. In fact, when such experimental lesions were carried out in monkeys, the resulting effect was described as a **hypotonia**.

An alternative interpretation for the presence of spasticity is that lesions of the internal capsule or cerebral cortex destroy not only corticospinal fibers, but also corticobulbar fibers. One such group of fibers of significance is the corticoreticular fibers that innervate neurons that give rise to the reticulospinal tracts. It is known that the medullary reticulospinal fibers powerfully inhibit spinal reflexes and, in particular, the actions of the gamma motor system. In contrast, the pontine reticulospinal system is facilitatory to spinal reflexes and the gamma motor system. This hypothesis proposes that the medullary reticulospinal neurons require cortical inputs to discharge, while those reticulospinal neurons located in the pons receive other kinds of afferent fibers and have less of a requirement for cortical inputs in order for them to discharge. Therefore, after damage to the cerebral cortex or internal capsule, there is a loss of inhibitory input to the spinal cord from the medullary reticular formation, while the excitatory regions of the pontine reticular formation continue to affect spinal motor neurons.

Such a condition would result in an imbalance between excitatory and inhibitory influences upon spinal motor neurons from the reticular formation; in which case, the excitatory inputs remain largely intact. Since the reticular formation acts to a great extent on the gamma motor system, the resulting changes would cause spasticity.

CLINICAL CASE

HISTORY

Jane, a 75-year-old secretary who still works for an academic physician, has a history of hypertension but was doing relatively well until she received an important phone call that relayed news regarding a poor score on a National Institutes of Health grant application submitted by her boss. Her boss grabbed the telephone from her after noting that she suddenly developed weakness in her right arm, leg, and face and that she was slurring her speech on the telephone. She needed to be helped by some of the ancillary staff to the emergency room because she continually fell to the right.

EXAMINATION

The physician who saw her in the emergency room noted that, when asked to smile, her mouth elevated only on the left side. Other than slurred speech, there were no problems with speech syntax or the construction of sentences. The right side of Jane's mouth drooped, and water dribbled from her mouth when she attempted to drink. Her right eye drooped, and did not close completely. When asked to raise her eyebrows, her eyebrows raised symmetrically. Her right arm and leg were weak, and when the doctor scratched the lateral plantar surface of her foot, the right great toe dorsiflexed, and the remainder of her toes flared. When the same procedure was performed on the left side, the toes curled downward.

EXPLANATION

Jane has an example of a left-sided cerebral vascular accident. It is unlikely that this stroke involves the cerebral cortex because of the lack of cortical signs, such as aphasia or speech dysfunction. The equal involvement of the arm, leg, and face imply that this occurred in a location where the pathways mediating these functions travel closely together, such as the internal capsule or the crus cerebri. Additionally, sensory signs were found, implying a smaller region of dysfunction. A magnetic resonance imaging (MRI) scan was obtained in the emergency room, which revealed a new internal capsule infarct that extended from the posterior limb into the genu. Note that the corticospinal fibers are contained in the posterior limb, and corticobulbar fibers are present in the genu. Thus, both of these fiber systems were damaged, which accounted for the deficits observed in this patient.

CHAPTER TEST

QUESTIONS

Choose the best answer for each question.

1. A 67-year-old man was taken to the emergency room after collapsing in a movie theater. The patient regained consciousness and, several days later, displayed a right-side paralysis with pronounced spasticity. The neurologist concluded that the stroke might have involved:
   a. Ventral horn cells
   b. Cerebellum
   c. Internal capsule
   d. Postcentral gyrus
   e. Pontine tegmentum

2. A patient presented with paralysis of the left side of the limbs and left side of the lower face and deviation of the tongue to the left with no atrophy and with no loss of taste sensation. This constellation of deficits most likely resulted from a lesion of the:
   a. Left internal capsule
   b. Right internal capsule
   c. Left pontine tegmentum
   d. Ventromedial medulla on the right side
   e. Ventromedial medulla on the left side

3. A 35-year-old man suffered a stroke that did not cause paralysis. However, he discovered that he was unable to perform complex learned movements. The region of the cerebral cortex most likely affected by the stroke was the:
   a. Precentral gyrus
   b. Postcentral gyrus
   c. Premotor cortex
   d. Temporal neocortex
   e. Prefrontal cortex

4. An investigator designed an experiment to characterize how neurons in the lower brainstem respond to administration of a specific neurotoxic substance. To effectively carry out this study, it was necessary to use a decerebrate preparation in which the region of the brain rostral to the pons was disconnected from the brainstem and spinal cord. Following this surgery, the investigator noted that the animal displayed marked rigidity of the limbs, which was most pronounced in the hind limbs. When the student of this investigator asked why there was such pronounced rigidity, the investigator should have provided which of the following answers:
   a. Direct loss of inhibitory neurons from the motor cortex to the spinal cord
   b. Damage to the red nucleus with preservation of the reticulospinal tracts and cerebellar cortex
   c. Preservation of the lateral vestibulospinal tract with loss of cortical inputs to reticular formation
   d. Loss of hypothalamic inputs to the brainstem, which normally have excitatory effects on inhibitory pathways of the brainstem
   e. Selective loss of input from the cerebral cortex to the pontine reticular formation and medial reticulospinal tract

5. During what appeared to be routine surgery for a torn ligament, a middle-aged man suffered a stroke. After a few days, the patient showed some recovery because he was able to walk with some difficulty and, in addition, sensory functions seemed normal. However, a neurologic evaluation revealed a weakness in muscles that regulate breathing, speech, swallowing, and facial expression. A subsequent MRI indicated that the stroke was limited but primarily affected the:
   a. Premotor cortex
   b. Medullary pyramids
   c. Posterior limb of internal capsule
   d. Genu of internal capsule
   e. Anterior limb of internal capsule

ANSWERS AND EXPLANATIONS

1. Answer: c

An upper motor neuron paralysis results in a paralysis or paresis of the contralateral limb(s), Babinski sign, spasticity, and hypertonicity. The most common sites where lesions produce this syndrome include the motor regions of cerebral cortex, internal capsule, and other regions that contain the descending fibers of the corticospinal and corticobulbar tracts, such as the basilar pons and lateral funiculus of the spinal cord. A lower motor neuron paralysis is characterized by a flaccid paralysis of the affected limbs and results from a lesion of the ventral horn cells that innervate the muscles in question directly. Regions such as the cerebellum, postcentral gyrus, and pontine tegmentum do not produce paralysis and spasticity when damaged. They do produce other deficits, such as movement disorders with respect to the cerebellum, coma with respect to the pontine tegmentum, and somatosensory deficits with respect to the postcentral gyrus, which are described in later chapters.

2. Answer: **b**

The right internal capsule contains corticospinal and corticobulbar fibers that project to the contralateral spinal cord and to the brainstem. The corticobulbar fibers that project predominantly to the contralateral side include those fibers that innervate motor nuclei of cranial nerves VII (lower facial muscles) and XII (hypoglossal). Therefore, a lesion of the right internal capsule will result in a paralysis of the limbs on the left side, a deviation of the tongue to the left side (i.e., side opposite to the lesion), and a paralysis of the right side of the lower face. A lesion of the right ventromedial medulla is too far caudal to affect corticobulbar fibers that supply the facial nucleus. Since the defects are on the left side, all of the choices that involve a lesion on the same (i.e., left) side are incorrect because lesions of the corticospinal and corticobulbar fibers result in motor deficits that are manifested on the contralateral side.

3. Answer: **c**

The premotor area is extremely important in providing sequencing or programming mechanism for learned movements. The most significant inputs come from the posterior parietal cortex. The premotor cortex then signals the appropriate groups of neurons in the spinal cord (and/or brainstem) to respond in a particular set of sequences. Therefore, damage to this region would result in loss of the sequencing mechanism that is so necessary for the occurrence of complex learned movements. The resulting disorder is called apraxia. Damage to the postcentral gyrus will produce a somatosensory loss. Damage to the precentral gyrus will produce an upper motor neuron paralysis. Damage to the temporal cortex will produce an auditory loss; and damage to the prefrontal cortex will produce different kinds of intellectual deficits, none of which include apraxia.

4. Answer: **c**

The lateral vestibular nucleus gives rise to the lateral vestibulospinal tract, which projects to all levels of the spinal cord. The tract passes in the ventral funiculus of the cord and innervates alpha and gamma motor neurons of extensors and provides powerful excitation of these neurons. A decerebrate preparation leaves this pathway intact, while other inhibitory inputs are lost, in particular, to the reticular formation and its descending motor pathways. Collectively, this allows for unopposed excitatory actions of the lateral vestibulospinal tract on extensor motor neurons. The other choices are incorrect. The influence of the motor cortex on the spinal cord is generally excitatory. The red nucleus excites flexor motor neurons, and its loss would not account for decerebrate rigidity. In addition, reticulospinal pathways (in particular, the lateral reticulospinal tract) are dependent on inputs from the cerebral cortex, and thus, their effects on spinal motor neurons would not be preserved. The medial reticulospinal tract facilitates extensor motor tone. Accordingly, the rigidity could not be accounted for by postulating a selective loss of cortical inputs to this pathway because it would imply that such loss would achieve just the opposite of rigidity. The hypothalamus has no known influences on extensor motor tone.

5. Answer: **d**

The symptoms described in this case reflect a "pseudobulbar palsy," which is characterized by weakness in the muscles of the head and face. It involves corticobulbar pathways that innervate, in part, cranial nerve motor nuclei. These fibers are contained in the genu of the internal capsule. Damage to the premotor cortex would produce a form of apraxia. Damage to the medullary pyramids is too low to affect corticobulbar fibers, which supply the facial nerve. The posterior limb of the internal capsule contains corticospinal fibers, which have no influence on brainstem cranial nerve activity. The anterior limb of the internal capsule contains frontopontine fibers, which synapse with pontine nuclei in the basilar pons and, thus, constitute part of a circuit linking the cerebral and cerebellar cortices. Accordingly, this pathway is not related to functions of cranial nerve motor nuclei.

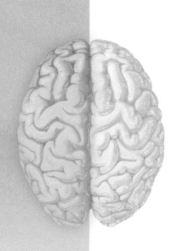

CHAPTER 20

THE BASAL GANGLIA

OBJECTIVES

After reading this chapter, the student should be able to:

1. List, diagram, and describe the anatomical structures that comprise the basal ganglia

2. List the primary afferent sources of the basal ganglia and describe how those projections are distributed to different parts of the neostriatum

3. Diagram the flow pathways through the basal ganglia

4. List and describe the principal neurotransmitters associated with the circuits within the basal ganglia and their functions

5. List, diagram, and describe how information is transmitted from the basal ganglia to the cerebral cortex

6. Describe the overall functions of the basal ganglia

7. List and describe the various neurologic disorders associated with the basal ganglia and their underlying anatomical and neurochemical bases

In Chapter 19, we pointed out the importance of the cerebral cortex in organizing and integrating signals from both the sensory and motor regions of the brain. We further indicated that highly precise, complex, and purposeful voluntary movements result from the transmission of signals passing through the corticospinal tract to the spinal cord where they act on lower motor neurons of the spinal gray matter, which produce movements by virtue of their actions on different muscle groups. If the production of movement and sequences of movements are due to the actions of the cerebral cortex and its descending axons of the corticospinal tract, then it is possible to consider that the basal ganglia provides a postural platform off of which purposeful movement can be made.

The primary function of the basal ganglia is to provide a feedback mechanism to the cerebral cortex for the initiation and control of motor responses (Fig. 20-1). Much of the output of the basal ganglia, which is mediated through the thalamus, is to reduce or dampen the excitatory input to the cerebral cortex. When there is a disruption of this mechanism, disturbances in motor function ensue. In general, it may be stated that when the discharge patterns of the basal ganglia become excessive, the effect on motor systems is to produce abnormal slowing of movements. More often, however, lesions of the basal ganglia produce a reduced output, the result of which is the presence of abnormal, involuntary movements that occur during periods of rest. This form of disorder is called **dyskinesia**. To understand how the basal ganglia functions as a feedback mechanism, it is essential to know the following: (1) the nature of the afferent supply to the basal ganglia; (2) the internal circuitry; (3) the efferent projections of the basal ganglia; and (4) the functional role of the neurotransmitters in the basal ganglia.

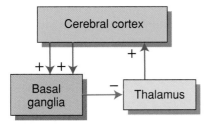

Figure 20–1 The feedback circuit between the cerebral cortex and basal ganglia. Cortical inputs into the basal ganglia are excitatory (+), and the outputs of the basal ganglia back to the cortex are mediated through the thalamus. Because the outputs of the thalamus to the cortex are generally excitatory (+), the inhibitory inputs into the thalamus from the basal ganglia (−) serve to dampen thalamic excitation of cortical neurons.

COMPOSITION OF THE BASAL GANGLIA

The anatomical organization of the basal ganglia and their output pathways were described in detail in Chapter 13. As a brief review, the basal ganglia consist of the neostriatum (caudate nucleus and putamen), paleostriatum (globus pallidus), and two additional nuclei, the subthalamic nucleus and substantia nigra, which are included with the basal ganglia because of their anatomical connections (made with different nuclei of the basal ganglia) (Fig. 20-2). The primary regions of the basal ganglia that serve as afferents (receiving areas) are the caudate nucleus and putamen. The major outputs of the basal ganglia arise from neurons located in the medial pallidal segment. These neurons give rise to two fiber bundles, the ansa lenticularis and lenticular fasciculus, which supply thalamic nuclei (see Fig. 13-12).

AFFERENT SOURCES OF THE BASAL GANGLIA

The largest afferent source of the basal ganglia arises from the cerebral cortex. In fact, most regions of the cortex contribute projections to the basal ganglia. These include inputs from motor, sensory, association, and even limbic areas of the cortex. While the **caudate nucleus** and **putamen** serve as the primary target regions of afferent projections from the cortex, the source of cortical inputs to these regions of the basal ganglia differ. The principal inputs from the primary motor, secondary motor, and primary somatosensory regions of cortex are directed to the putamen. These inputs to the putamen are somatotopically organized, which means that different regions of the putamen receive sensory and motor inputs that are associated with different parts of the body. The caudate nucleus, on the other hand, receives inputs from cortical association regions, frontal eye fields, and limbic regions of cortex (Fig. 20-3). Thus, the putamen appears to be concerned primarily with motor functions, while the caudate nucleus, which appears to receive more varied and integrated cortical inputs, is likely involved with cognitive aspects of movement, eye movements, and emotional correlates of movement (relegated to the ventral aspect of the neostriatum).

The **neostriatum** also receives an indirect source of cortical input. The source of this input is the **centromedian nucleus** of the thalamus. This nucleus receives afferent fibers primarily from the motor cortex and projects its axons topographically to the putamen as **thalamostriate fibers**. An additional

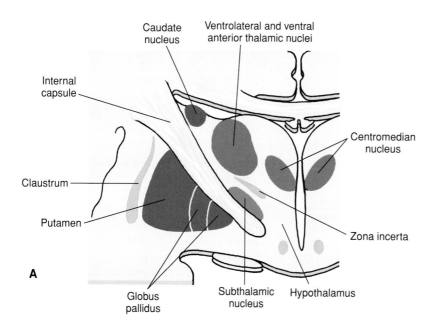

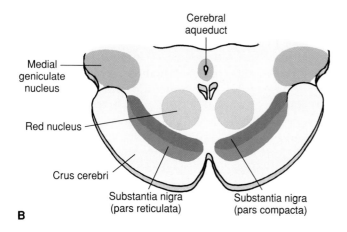

Figure 20–2 The anatomical structures that comprise the basal ganglia. (A) The principal components of the basal ganglia situated within the forebrain: the caudate nucleus, putamen, globus pallidus, and the subthalamic nucleus, which is linked to the basal ganglia by its connections with the primary structures comprising the basal ganglia. (B) The position of the substantia nigra within the midbrain, which is also linked to the basal ganglia because of its connections with the neostriatum (see text).

but highly important source of dopaminergic inputs to the neostriatum is the substantia nigra. The function of this afferent source to the neostriatum is considered later in this chapter.

The modular organization of the neostriatum is as follows. The projections from the neocortex and thalamus are not distributed uniformly to the neostriatum. Instead, the projections end in compartments within different parts of the neostriatum. The smaller of these compartments is referred to as a patch or **striosome** and is surrounded by a larger compartment referred to as a **matrix**. These two compartments are distinguished from each other because they have different neurochemical properties, contain different receptors, and receive inputs from different cortical regions. The matrix is acetylcholinesterase rich. The striosomes, however, are

acetylcholinesterase poor but contain peptides such as somatostatin, substance P, and enkephalin. The striosomes receive their inputs mainly from limbic regions of cortex, and neurons from this region preferentially project to the substantia nigra. In contrast, the neurons of the matrix receive inputs from sensory and motor regions of cortex, and many of them project to the globus pallidus. The overwhelming majority of projection neurons from both of these compartments of the neostriatum are γ-aminobutyric acid (GABA)-ergic. Their significance is considered in the following paragraph.

The presumed role of the neostriatum in motor functions can be illustrated by the following example. During active movement of a joint of a finger, the cells within a certain striosomal or matrix compartment become active, while neurons embedded

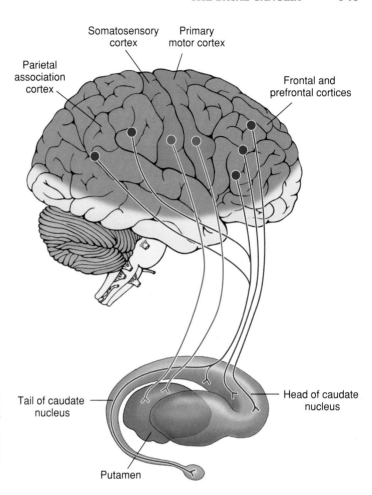

Figure 20–3 Relationship of the cerebral cortex to the putamen and caudate nucleus. The diagram illustrates that the putamen receives fibers from motor regions of the cerebral cortex, while the caudate nucleus receives inputs from association regions (temporal and parietal lobes) as well as inputs from other regions of the frontal lobe, including the prefrontal cortex.

within other compartments become active only after there is passive movement of the same joint. This would suggest that the neurons embedded within given compartments function in a similar manner to those present in functional homogenous regions of the cerebral cortex with respect to movement (i.e., specific regions of motor cortex can be subdivided into distinct functional columns in which the neurons in one column respond to one feature of movement of a limb, whereas those neurons situated in an adjoining column respond to a different feature of movement of that limb; see Chapter 26 for discussion of cortical columns).

INTERNAL CONNECTIONS OF THE BASAL GANGLIA

The anatomical relationships between different components of the basal ganglia are extensive. The most salient of the connections include the following: (1) the projections from the neostriatum to the globus pallidus; (2) the reciprocal relationships between the neostriatum and substantia nigra; and (3) the reciprocal relationships between the globus pallidus and the subthalamic nucleus. In examining these relationships, the overall role of the basal ganglia in motor functions should be kept in mind. Namely, as signals are transmitted through the basal ganglia in response to cortical inputs, they ultimately result in a distinct response transmitted back to the motor areas of the cerebral cortex. Moreover, the circuits within the basal ganglia by which signals are transmitted back to the cerebral cortex may be direct or indirect. The differences between the direct and indirect routes are discussed in the following section.

CONNECTIONS OF THE NEOSTRIATUM WITH THE GLOBUS PALLIDUS

There are two basic projection targets of the neostriatum: the globus pallidus and the substantia nigra. The neostriatum projects to two different regions of the globus pallidus: the medial (internal) pallidal segment and the lateral (external) pallidal segment (Fig. 20-4). GABA mediates the pathway from the neostriatum to the medial pallidal segment;

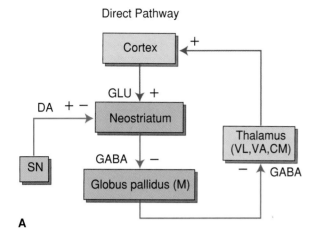

Direct Pathway

A

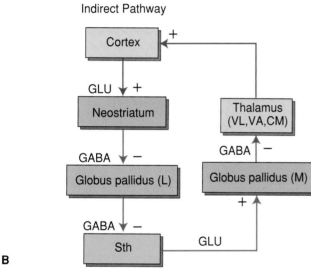

Indirect Pathway

B

Figure 20–4 The detailed anatomical and functional nature of the input, internal, and output circuits of the basal ganglia. Note the distinction between the direct and indirect pathways. (A) The direct pathway involves projections from the neostriatum to the medial (internal) pallidal segment, which in turn, projects to the thalamus and then to the cerebral cortex. (B) The indirect pathway involves projections from the neostriatum to the lateral pallidal segment (L), which in turn, projects to the subthalamic nucleus. The subthalamic nucleus then projects to the medial pallidal segment (M), and the remaining components of the circuit to the cerebral cortex are similar to that described for the direct pathways. *Red* arrows depict inhibitory pathways, and *blue* arrows indicate excitatory pathways. The *green* pathways represent dopaminergic projections to the neostriatum, which have opposing effects on D_1 and D_2 receptors (see Fig. 20-5), and the excitatory projection from the subthalamic nucleus (Sth) to the medial pallidal segment. When known, the neurotransmitter for each of the pathways is indicated. Abbreviations: DA, dopamine; GLU, glutamate; CM, centromedian nucleus; VA, ventral anterior nucleus; VL, ventrolateral nucleus; +, excitation; −, inhibition.

likewise, the pathway *from* the neostriatum to the lateral pallidal segment also primarily uses GABA as a likely neurotransmitter.

Each of these projections forms the initial links of two different circuits within the basal ganglia. Because the primary output of the basal ganglia is from the internal pallidal segment, the projection (neostriatum → globus pallidus (internal) → thalamus → neocortex) is called the **direct pathway** (Fig. 20-4). In contrast, the external segment of the globus pallidus shares reciprocal projections with the subthalamic nucleus. Thus, this circuit of the basal ganglia can be outlined as follows: neostriatum → globus pallidus (external) → subthalamic nucleus → globus pallidus (internal) → thalamus → neocortex). Because this circuit involves a loop through the subthalamic nucleus, it is called the **indirect pathway** (Fig. 20-4). The neurotransmitters involved in the reciprocal pathway between the globus pallidus and subthalamic nucleus and the overall functional significance of these pathways are discussed later in this chapter.

CONNECTIONS OF THE NEOSTRIATUM WITH THE SUBSTANTIA NIGRA

The substantia nigra has two principal components: a region of tightly compacted cells, called the **pars compacta**, and a region just ventral and extending lateral to the pars compacta, called the **pars reticulata** (Fig. 20-2B). Fibers arising from the neostriatum project to the pars reticulata. Transmitters identified in this pathway are GABA and substance P. The pathway from the substantia nigra to the neostriatum arises from the pars compacta and uses dopamine as its neurotransmitter (Fig. 20-5). The pars reticulata also gives rise to efferent fibers (which are likely inhibitory) that project to the thalamus, superior colliculus, and locally to the pars compacta. In this manner, the pars reticulata and internal pallidal segment appear to be functionally analogous because both regions provide outputs to the cerebral cortex via the thalamus. Additional functions of these pathways are discussed later in this chapter.

CONNECTIONS BETWEEN THE GLOBUS PALLIDUS AND SUBTHALAMIC NUCLEUS

As noted earlier, the globus pallidus shares reciprocal connections with the subthalamic nucleus. The lateral segment of the globus pallidus (which receives GABAergic and enkephalinergic inputs from the neostriatum) projects to the subthalamic

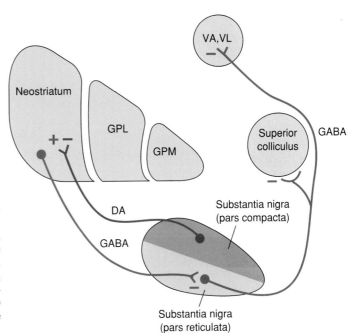

Figure 20–5 Key relationships of the substantia nigra. The pars reticulata of the substantia nigra receives an inhibitory (*red line*) GABAergic input from the neostriatum. In turn, there are two important outputs of the substantia nigra. The first is a dopaminergic (DA) projection to the neostriatum (which is excitatory when acting through D_1 receptors and inhibitory when acting through D_2 receptors). The second is an inhibitory GABAergic projection from the pars reticulata to the ventral anterior (VA) and ventrolateral (VL) thalamic nuclei as well as to the superior colliculus. +, excitation; −, inhibition.

nucleus. GABA also mediates this pathway. In turn, the subthalamic nucleus projects back to the medial segment of globus pallidus. This pathway, however, is mediated by **glutamate**.

OUTPUT OF THE BASAL GANGLIA

As indicated earlier, the basal ganglia influence motor functions primarily by acting on motor neurons of the cerebral cortex via relay nuclei of the thalamus. The output pathways of the basal ganglia achieve this. As noted in Chapter 13, two pathways arise from the medial pallidal segment and supply the ventral anterior, ventrolateral, and centromedian nuclei of the thalamus (Fig. 20-6). The first pathway, the ansa lenticularis, arises from the ventral aspect of the medial pallidal segment. It passes caudally towards the red nucleus and then turns rostrally to enter the thalamus. The second pathway, the lenticular fasciculus, which arises from the medial pallidal segment, exits the pallidum dorsally. As the fibers run caudally in the direction of the midbrain (adjacent to the red nucleus), they pass between the subthalamic nucleus and zona incerta. As the fibers approach the red nucleus, they also abruptly turn rostrally and enter the thalamus (Fig. 20-7).

In addition to the internal pallidal segment, the basal ganglia can also influence motor functions through the output pathways of the substantia nigra. We have already noted the important dopaminergic pathway from the pars compacta to the neostriatum. The pars reticulata contributes at least two pathways. One pathway projects to the ventral anterior and ventrolateral nuclei of the thalamus, and its effects upon thalamic neurons are mediated by GABA. Thus, the overall influence of the pars reticulata on motor functions of the cerebral cortex is made possible by the synaptic connections between nigral fibers and these thalamic relay nuclei. A second pathway projects to the superior colliculus. Because the superior colliculus is involved in the integration of saccadic eye movements and tracking, this pathway can influence motor functions related to reflex and voluntary control of eye movements. The efferent pathways of the substantia nigra are summarized in Figure 20-5.

FUNCTIONAL MECHANISMS OF THE BASAL GANGLIA

POSSIBLE ROLE OF INTRINSIC CIRCUITS

The information presented thus far has enabled us to identify the major circuitry of the basal ganglia. This includes the primary input pathways and the internal circuitry of the basal ganglia and their output pathways. In terms of the functional properties of this system, they may be best understood by following the flow-through relationships beginning with the inputs from the cerebral cortex.

As noted earlier, there are both direct and indirect pathways from the striatum to the thalamus, and the functional effects of each are different. Concerning the *direct* pathway, cortical inputs have excitatory effects on the neostriatum, and the neurotransmitter is glutamate. Excitation of the neostriatum by the cortex results in **disinhibition** of

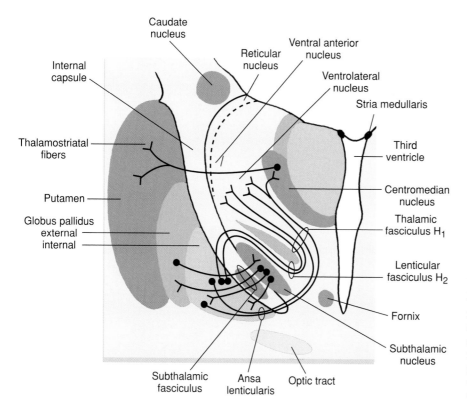

Figure 20–6 Efferent projections of the pallidum. Note that the fibers of medial pallidal segment use two pathways to supply the ventrolateral, ventral anterior, and centromedian nuclei (the ansa lenticularis and the lenticular fasciculus or H_2 field of Forel). The region where fibers of the ansa lenticularis, lenticular fasciculus, and cerebellothalamic merge is referred to as the H_1 field of Forel (see Chapter 13). The subthalamic fasciculus represents reciprocal connections between the globus pallidus and subthalamic nucleus and serves as the anatomical substrate for the indirect pathway.

thalamic nuclei. This can be understood in terms of the following relationships. The projection from the neostriatum to the medial pallidal segment is inhibitory, and likewise, the projection from the medial pallidal segment to the thalamus is also inhibitory. GABA mediates both inhibitory pathways. In this manner, activation of the cortex causes the neurons in the medial pallidal segment to be inhibited by the GABAergic projection from the neostriatum. When the neurons of the medial pallidal segment are inhibited, the thalamic neurons that project to motor regions of the cortex are then released from the inhibition normally im-

posed on them by the medial pallidal segment. Because the projections from the thalamus to cortex are direct and excitatory, movement is then facilitated by the actions of the thalamocortical projection, which excites motor regions of cortex and their descending pathways to the brainstem and spinal cord. Thus, this feedback circuit can be interpreted to mean that movement follows activation of the neostriatum by the cortex. The functional relationships of the overall circuit for the direct pathway could now be summarized as follows, with (+) indicating excitation and (−) indicating inhibition (Fig. 20-8A): cerebral cortex

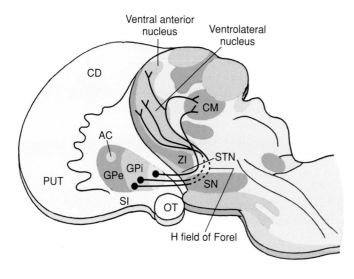

Figure 20–7 Outputs of the basal ganglia and their trajectories. The origins and trajectories of the major outputs of the globus pallidus (GP) to the thalamus are diagrammed. Note that the pathways initially pass caudally toward the red nucleus of the midbrain before reversing their course (at a position called the H field of Forel) to pass rostrally into the ventrolateral, ventral anterior, and centre median (CM) thalamic nuclei. Abbreviations: AC, anterior commissure; CD, caudate nucleus; GPi, globus pallidus internal; GPe, globus pallidus external; OT, optic tract; PUT, putamen; SN, substantia nigra; STN, subthalamic nucleus; ZI, zona incerta.

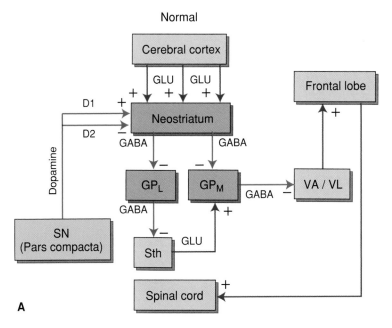

Normal

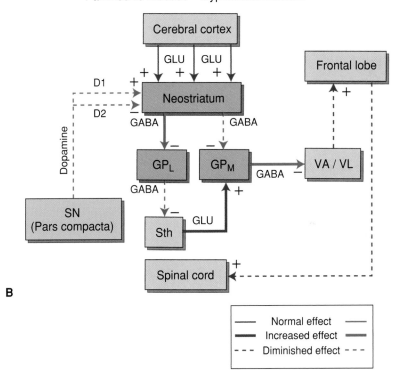

Parkinson's Disease – Hypokinetic Disorder

——	Normal effect ——
——	**Increased effect ——**
- - -	Diminished effect - - -

Figure 20–8 Schematic diagram depicting the possible mechanisms for hypokinetic and hyperkinetic disorders. (A) Normal input-output relationships of the basal ganglia. Abbreviations: GLU, glutamate; GP_L, lateral pallidal segment; GP_M, medial pallidal segment; SN, substantia nigra; Sth, subthalamic nucleus; VA, ventral anterior; VL, ventrolateral. (B) **Hypokinetic disorder (Parkinson's disease)**. This model proposes that the hypokinetic effect is manifested by the reduced quantities of dopamine released, which act on dopamine D_1 and D_2 receptors in the neostriatum. Dopamine acting through D_1 receptors in the neostriatum is excitatory to GABAergic neurons, which project to the GP_M (direct pathway). Moreover, dopamine acting through D_2 receptors in the neostriatum inhibits GABAergic neurons, which project to the GP_L segment (indirect pathway). When there is diminished dopamine in the neostriatum released onto D_1 receptors (*dotted line*), the resulting inhibitory output of the neostriatum on the GP_M is diminished. This allows for an enhancement of the inhibitory output of the GP_M to the thalamus to be increased (*thicker arrow*). Because the thalamus normally excites the cortex, greater inhibition on the thalamic nuclei by the GP_M will cause a weakened input onto motor regions of the cortex. Likewise, the projection from the neostriatum, acting through D_2 receptors, is inhibitory to the GP_L. In turn, the GP_L is normally inhibitory to the Sth. Thus, the diminished inhibitory input into the GP_L from the neostriatum allows the GP_L to exert greater inhibition on the Sth. Because the Sth normally excites the GP_M via a glutamatergic mechanism, the reduced amount of inhibition on the Sth would allow it to exert a greater excitatory effect on the GP_M. Therefore, the combined effects of reduced dopaminergic inputs into the neostriatum affect both the direct and indirect pathways in such a way as to allow for enhancement of the inhibitory outputs of the GP_M on the thalamic projection nuclei and their target regions in motor cortex, causing the hypokinetic movement disorder.

Huntington's Disease – Hyperkinetic Disorder

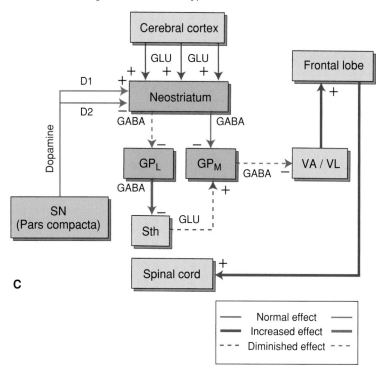

Figure 20–8 *(continued)* (C) **Hyperkinetic disorder (Huntington's disease).** Inhibitory influences mediated from the caudate and putamen to the external segment of the globus pallidus are diminished. Because of a reduction in GABA in the neostriatum, tonic inhibition mediated from the GP_L to the Sth is enhanced, thus reducing the excitation from the Sth to the GP_M. The diminished excitatory input to the GP_M results in increased excitation to the VA and VL thalamic nuclei as well as the cortical receiving areas of these thalamic nuclei. The overall effect mediated on the motor regions of the cerebral cortex is an increase in excitation and greater (inappropriate) motor activity.

(glutamate) → (+) neostriatum (GABA) → (−) internal pallidal segment (GABA) → (−) thalamus → (+) the motor regions of cortex. The net effect is excitation of the motor regions of cortex.

In contrast, activation of the *indirect pathway* has a different effect on cortical neurons. The indirect pathway involves the following elements: (1) a GABAergic projection from the neostriatum to the external pallidal segment; (2) a GABAergic projection from the external pallidal segment to the subthalamic nucleus; and (3) a glutamatergic projection from the subthalamic nucleus to the internal pallidal segment. In this circuit, cortical activation initially results in activation of a GABAergic pathway from the neostriatum to the external pallidal segment, which inhibits neurons in this region. Because the pathway from the external pallidal segment to the subthalamic nucleus is also GABAergic and inhibitory, activation of striatal neurons results in inhibition of the (inhibitory) output pathway from the external pallidal segment to the subthalamic nucleus. As a consequence of activation of this circuit, the subthalamic nucleus is released from inhibition and can then provide a heightened glutamate-mediated excitatory input to the internal pallidal segment. Activation of the internal pallidal segment results in inhibition (via a GABAergic pathway) of the thalamic nuclei to which the neurons of the internal pallidal segment project. Thus, when this circuit is stimulated, the

overall effect is to cause thalamic relay neurons to be inhibited, resulting in the reduction of excitation to the motor regions of cortex. Therefore, activation of the indirect pathway results in just the opposite effect (i.e., inhibition) on cortical motor neurons compared with the direct pathway. The functional relationships of the indirect pathway can now be summarized as follows, with (+) indicating excitation and (−) indicating inhibition: cerebral cortex (glutamate) → (+) neostriatum (GABA) → (−) external pallidal segment (GABA) → (−) subthalamic nucleus (glutamate) → (+) internal pallidal segment (GABA) → (−) thalamus → (+) motor regions of cortex. The net effect is inhibition of the motor regions of the cortex.

MODULATORY ROLE OF DOPAMINE

In addition to the direct and indirect pathways that significantly influence motor functions of the cortex, other modulatory systems are present as well. The most prominent of these systems is the *dopamine pathway* from the substantia nigra to the neostriatum. Current research suggests that the dopamine pathway has opposing effects on the direct and indirect pathways (i.e., activation of the dopaminergic pathway excites the direct pathway but inhibits the indirect pathway). As indicated earlier, the direct pathway causes excitation of the motor regions of the cortex and thus facilitates movement, but the indirect pathway inhibits cortical-induced movement. Therefore, the action of dopamine is to facilitate movement because it excites the facilitatory (direct) pathway via its excitatory effects on dopamine D_1 receptors in regions of the neostriatum that project to the medial pallidal segment, while inhibiting the inhibitory (indirect) pathway that projects initially to the lateral pallidal segment because of the inhibitory effects on dopamine D_2 receptors in the neostriatum. The result is diminution of excitation from the glutamate-mediated pathway from the lateral to the medial pallidal segment. In this manner, the overall output of the medial pallidal segment to the thalamus is diminished, resulting in greater excitation of the motor regions of cortex, the consequences of which is an increase in movement. From an overall perspective, we may speculate that purposeful movement requires a sequence of directed responses balanced by other responses, which are appropriately inhibitory. It may be that the direct pathway potentiates normally directed movements, whereas the indirect pathway enhances inhibitory sequences.

DISEASES OF THE BASAL GANGLIA

The circuitry described in the previous sections suggests the presence of a highly sophisticated and delicate set of functional mechanisms that are present within the basal ganglia for the regulation of motor functions. Thus, any disruption of a component of these mechanisms, such as the balance between direct and indirect pathways, will result in significant changes in the signals transmitted to motor regions of the cerebral cortex. Such changes are likely to result in compensatory response mechanisms within the overall circuitry, which will manifest as several kinds of movement disorders. These disorders include involuntary movements during periods of rest (called **dyskinesia**), slowness of movement (called **bradykinesia**), or even a lack of movement (called **akinesia**). In certain disorders, motor activity is also characterized by hypertonia or rigidity. The following discussion considers the various diseases of the basal ganglia, their relationships with specific neurotransmitter systems, and elements of the circuits within the basal ganglia with which they are likely associated.

In general, **hypokinetic** disorders involve *impaired* initiation of movement, bradykinesia, and increased muscle tone. They are accounted for, in part, by the loss of dopamine inputs into the part of the striatum that (1) excites the direct pathway through D_1 receptors and (2) inhibits the indirect pathway through D_2 receptors. The reduced excitation of the direct pathway (which normally inhibits

the internal pallidal segment) results in greater excitation of neurons in the internal pallidal segment, which, in turn, provides further inhibition of thalamic neurons and neurons of the motor and premotor areas. This effect is amplified because, at the same time, there is also an increase in excitation of neurons in the external pallidal segment (i.e., indirect pathway) by virtue of reduced inhibition on the GABAergic inhibitory neostriatal projections to this segment (due to the reduction of dopamine on the D_2 receptors, whose activation inhibits these neostriatal neurons). The result is an increase in excitation of neurons in the internal pallidal segment because of enhanced release of the excitatory transmitter, glutamate, from the **subthalamic nucleus** onto this segment of pallidum. These relationships are described in the flow diagram shown in Fig. 20-8B.

In contrast, **hyperkinetic** disorders involve *excessive* motor activity characterized by marked involuntary movements and decreased muscle tone. These disorders are accounted for by a diminished output through the indirect pathway to the external pallidal segment. Here, a diminished inhibitory input from the neostriatum on the external pallidal segment presumably results from a reduction in the numbers of GABAergic neurons in the neostriatum, which project to the external pallidal segment. This will result in a greater (GABAergic) inhibitory output from the external pallidal segment on the subthalamic nucleus, and the net effect is a reduced excitatory output from the subthalamic nucleus on neurons of the internal pallidal segment. Reduced excitation of the internal pallidal segment will result in reduced inhibition of the thalamus and motor regions of cortex, thus leading to excessive motor activity (Fig. 20-8C).

PARKINSON'S DISEASE

Parkinson's disease is characterized by a variety of symptoms. The patient displays involuntary movements at rest. The movements are typically rhythmic tremors at approximately 3 to 6/sec, often appearing as a "pill-rolling" tremor involving the fingers, hands, and arm. Interestingly enough, the tremor disappears when the patient begins a voluntary movement. The patient also displays a reduced number of spontaneous movements (akinesia) (e.g., reduction in spontaneous facial expressions and eye blinking) as well as a bradykinesia (i.e., slowness of movement). Postural adjustments are awkward. Patients display slower than normal movements, especially in walking, where they take short steps in a shuffling (propulsive) manner. Other characteristic symptoms include loss of facial expression (i.e., mask-like face), monotonous speech, and marked increases in muscle tone to both the flexors and extensors of the same limb, producing rigidity.

Parkinson's disease is now known to result from a loss of the dopamine-containing neurons of the pars compacta of the substantia nigra. The loss of these neurons leads to reduced quantities of dopamine content in the neostriatum, while other neurotransmitters within the neostriatum, such as acetylcholine and glutamate, appear to be unaffected. It should be noted, however, that a patient with Parkinson's disease might also exhibit reduced amounts of norepinephrine and serotonin elsewhere in the brain. Such observations indicate the heterogeneity of this disease with respect to behavioral and neurochemical variations present in different patients.

Because of the known association between reductions in dopamine content within the neostriatum and the onset of symptoms of Parkinson's disease, several lines of treatment therapies have been developed. One form of treatment involves the administration of the drug, L-3, 4-hydroxyphenylalanine (L-DOPA) (see Chapter 8). L-DOPA passes through the blood-brain barrier, and as a precursor of dopamine, it is converted to dopamine in the brain. Thus, this treatment helps to replenish the reduced amounts of dopamine present in the neostriatum of the patient with Parkinson's disease. This form of drug therapy has also been supplemented with the drug, **carbidopa**, which is a dopamine-decarboxylase inhibitor. A drug containing both L-DOPA and carbidopa is called Sinemet. Thus, the use of Sinemet has enabled more L-DOPA to reach the neostriatum. Early studies with L-DOPA were shown to be highly successful. However, difficulties have arisen with this form of therapy. Because L-DOPA is administered systemically, it can also result in increased quantities of dopamine in other parts of the brain where dopamine receptors are present. One location is the hypothalamus, which is associated with such functions as feeding, sexual behavior, and control of blood pressure. Consequently, administration of L-DOPA has had such side effects as reducing appetite, causing nausea, heightening sexual interests, and reducing the control of blood pressure. Moreover, because dopamine neurons in the substantia nigra continue to die over time, these forms of drug therapy only work temporarily.

While the etiology of Parkinson's disease remains unknown, a discovery was made in 1982 that relatively young drug abusers developed signs of Parkinson's disease after taking synthetic forms of heroin. The drug that was used was toxic and included 1-methyl-4-phenyl-1, 2, 3, 6-tetrahydropyridine (called MPTP). Because MPTP resulted in Parkinson's disease, it was suggested that it was toxic to dopamine neurons and that environmental toxins may play a role in the development of this disorder. Research has indicated that MPTP has to be converted by monoamine oxidase to 1-methyl-4-phenylpyridinium (MPP^+). This is a pyridinium ion. Thus, it was suggested that blockade of monoamine oxidase would raise dopamine levels and thus slow the progress of Parkinson's disease. Consistent with this view was the observation that a monoamine oxidase inhibitor, L-deprenyl, selectively inhibited monoamine oxidase in the central nervous system (CNS) and retarded the development of Parkinson's disease in humans. An important positive outcome of the discovery that MPTP can induce Parkinson's disease is that it provided investigators with an important experimental tool by which this disorder can be studied in a systematic manner. The use of this toxin as an experimental tool has allowed investigators to confirm the fact that Parkinson's disease results from loss of dopamine neurons in the pars compacta of the substantia nigra, with a consequent loss of dopamine levels in the neostriatum, and has led to other important findings concerning this disorder.

A second form of possible therapy for Parkinson's disease is transplantation. This procedure remains in the early stages of experimentation. Here, embryonic tissue containing dopamine neurons are transplanted directly into the neostriatum. These dopamine-containing cells then grow sprouts, synthesize, and release dopamine onto neostriatal neurons, where they serve to increase dopamine levels. Embryonic cells (in suspension) are used because there appears to be little or no evidence of rejection from such tissue. While this procedure has met with some preliminary success, difficulties remain. In particular, it is not possible to implant embryonic cells in all regions of the neostriatum. Because it is not clear which regions of the neostriatum are most critical for replenishment of dopamine levels, the effectiveness of this approach remains questionable. Another major problem is the difficulty in obtaining sufficient quantities of embryonic tissue to carry out the required procedures. The inherent legal and ethical issues remain formidable ones.

A related developing strategy is to graft **stem cells** into regions where neurons have undergone degeneration as a result of a disease process. Stem cells constitute the master cells of the organism that are capable of differentiating into different cell types. There are two types of stem cells: embryonic and adult. It has been argued that embryonic cells have several advantages. They can be obtained in large numbers and have the capacity of becoming all cell types that can easily be grown in culture. These features are not as clearly present with adult stem cells. Nevertheless, the hope is that stem cells, whether embryonic or adult, can be implanted into the appropriate brain loci and that these cells can be differentiated into dopamine neurons. In this way, this approach may serve as a method for replenishment of dopamine in the regions affected by the destruction of dopamine neurons in the substantia nigra. Recent studies using this approach in animals have provided data that has been promising.

At least three other approaches have been used. For reasons that we have just indicated, a reduced dopaminergic input to the neostriatum results in a hypokinetic disorder of which Parkinson's disease is a prime example. There are many cholinergic neurons in the neostriatum, which are excitatory to neostriatal projection neurons that supply the external pallidal segment (indirect pathway). Therefore, it is possible that the hypokinetic disorder occurs in part because of the actions of these cholinergic neurons, whose effects become more pronounced by the reduced inhibitory actions of dopamine acting through D_2 inhibitory receptors in the neostriatum (Fig. 20-8B). This line of reasoning represents the rationale for an approach that involves the use of anticholinergic drugs to reduce the imbalance between dopamine and acetylcholine levels in the neostriatum. This treatment results in a reduction in the excitatory effects generated by acetylcholine and has met with some success in patients.

Alternatively, some success has been reported in patients subjected to thalamotomy involving the ventrolateral and perhaps the ventral anterior nuclei. However, the rationale for this approach, which is to reduce the aberrant signals transmitted to the motor regions of the cortex from the basal ganglia, is conceptually difficult to understand because there already is a reduced output of the thalamocortical projections in Parkinson's disease. Other problems exist with this procedure, such as the difficulty in making accurate lesions in the appropriate region of the thalamus that eliminate symptoms of the disorder. Moreover, the placement of such lesions is also questionable because it is not known with any certainty which regions are the critical ones.

Another therapeutic approach has been electrical stimulation to parts of the basal ganglia and related structures, such as the pallidum, subthalamic nucleus, and ventral anterior and ventral lateral nuclei of thalamus. In this procedure, a stimulating electrode is implanted into one of these structures and, when current is passed through the tip of the electrode, involuntary movements are suppressed. This method is quite new, so the overall effectiveness and pitfalls of this approach have yet to be adequately determined.

CHOREA (HUNTINGTON'S DISEASE)

In general, **Chorea** is characterized by wild, uncontrolled movements of the distal musculature, which appear as abrupt and jerky. Huntington's disease is an inherited autosomal dominant illness with the genetic defect located on the short arm of chromosome 4. The gene encodes a protein referred to as **huntingtin**. In the mutated form, it includes a much longer patch (than normal protein) of glutamine residues. Specifically, the DNA segment (CAG) that encodes glutamine is repeated more than 60 times in the mutated gene as opposed to approximately 20 repeats in the normal gene. Although it is not clear how the mutant gene causes cell death, one hypothesis is that the Huntington protein causes an induction of apoptosis in the nucleus of the cell. Perhaps this occurs by the alteration of protein folding due to the increased amounts of glutamines, causing dysfunction and ultimately the death of the cell.

Degeneration is quite extensive. It involves the neostriatum, where there is significant loss of GABA. As the disease becomes more progressive, it also involves the cerebral cortex and, in particular, the frontal and prefrontal regions, as well as a number of other structures. Damage to these regions causes not only motor damage, but also loss of intellectual functions. The disease is progressive with an onset in the fifth and sixth decades of life. There is also a juvenile form of the disease; individuals usually die before the age of 21 years.

The manifestation of the hyperkinetic motor effects inherent in Huntington's disease may be understood in terms of the effects of the loss of GABAergic neurons in the neostriatum on the indirect pathway. It is believed that there is a preferential loss of GABAergic neurons that project to the subthalamic nucleus from the external pallidal segment compared with the GABAergic neurons that project elsewhere. As a result of the loss of inhibitory GABAergic inputs to the external pallidal segment from the neostriatum, this segment of the pallidum can now generate greater inhibition on the subthalamic nucleus. This will lead to a consequent loss of excitatory input from the subthalamic nucleus onto the internal pallidal segment. Since the internal pallidal segment normally inhibits the thalamic projection nuclei to the motor regions of the cortex, loss of subthalamic excitatory input to the internal pallidal segment will result in a consequent reduced inhibitory input onto these thalamic nuclei (Fig. 20-8C). This would ultimately result in excess excitation of the motor regions of the cortex, causing the choreiform movements seen in Huntington's disease.

HEMIBALLISM

Violent involuntary ballistic movements of the limbs contralateral to the lesion characterize **hemiballism**. The proximal musculature is typically involved, but choreiform (irregular, jerky) movements of the distal musculature usually in the upper extremity (which may also involve the lower extremity) may also be present. In hemiballism, the lesion has been found to be discrete and localized within the subthalamic nucleus, perhaps as a result of a discrete stroke. Since activation of the subthalamic nucleus excites inhibitory neurons from the internal pallidal segment that project to the thalamus, lesions of the subthalamic nucleus would cause a significant reduction of these inhibitory influences on the thalamus. Thus, this sequence will result in an increase in movement of the proximal and distal musculature on the side of the body opposite the lesion. (Recall that the corticospinal tract is crossed; therefore, activation of one side of the cortex will result in movement of the contralateral side of the body.)

ATHETOSIS AND DYSTONIA

Athetosis is a variant of choreiform movement. It involves slow, writhing movements of the extremities. **Dystonia** is characterized by sustained muscle contractions of the limb, axial, or cranial voluntary muscles, resulting in abnormal postures and repetitive or twisting movements. If the movements produce severe torsion of the neck or shoulder girdle, causing an appearance of a rhythmic shaking of the head, this form of dystonia is referred to as **torsion tremor**. Both athetosis and dystonia are believed to be associated with damage to the neostriatum and possibly the cerebral cortex.

TARDIVE DYSKINESIA

Involuntary movements of the tongue and face characterize tardive dyskinesia. There are repetitive chewing movements, and the tongue irregularly moves in and out of the mouth. It is not induced by lesions but, instead, is induced by the administration of antipsychotic drugs, such as haloperidol (Haldol), that block dopaminergic transmission. It is believed that such blockade results in dopamine D_2 receptor hypersensitivity. Because these dopa-

mine receptors within the neostriatum become more sensitive, dopaminergic transmission to the neostriatum becomes more potent, leading to an alteration in the balanced relationship between dopaminergic, cholinergic, and GABAergic neuronal systems. However, more recent research has suggested that this disorder may be more closely associated with depletion in GABA and its synthesizing enzyme, glutamic acid decarboxylase, in the neostriatum after treatment with antipsychotic drugs. Such compensatory changes produce movements characterized as tardive dyskinesia. Several of the treatments for this disorder include tapering down of the antipsychotic drug, administering dopamine-depleting drugs, or administering clozapine, which interferes with binding of dopamine receptors. However, after prolonged use of haloperidol, the resulting tardive dyskinesia does not disappear after cessation of drug use.

CLINICAL CASE

HISTORY

Peter is a 67-year-old man who has been having difficulty moving for the past 10 years. His family noticed that he had a slow shuffling gait and had difficulty getting out of a chair. Once he was able to get out of a chair, after an initial slow gait, his gait would become progressively faster. Although in the past he had been a jovial, expressive man, his face appeared to be masked, with very few eye blinks and with little spontaneous emotional reactions. He spoke with a slow monotonous voice, which often became softer as he spoke. After having several fainting spells, his family brought him to a neurologist.

EXAMINATION

During the neurological examination, it was noted that Peter's limbs were stiff, and he exhibited a slow, pill-rolling tremor. When he attempted to write, his handwriting started out as small and became progressively smaller. His family told the neurologist that they thought that he was forgetting progressively more appointments, and they felt that he might be depressed. They also indicated that Peter's sleep had become increasingly disrupted and that he exhibited leg movements at night.

EXPLANATION

Peter is displaying symptoms of **Parkinson's disease**, a degenerative disease caused by a progressive loss of dopaminergic cells from the substantia nigra. The substantia nigra is a component of the basal ganglia, whose functions provide refinement and feedback to cortical motor systems. The net effect of this system results in movements that are smooth and whose goals are reached efficiently. One manifestation of dysfunction of the substantia nigra includes cogwheel rigidity, where there are catches during passive movement of a rigid limb. Another classic manifestation is a pill-rolling tremor of the hand at a rate of approximately 3 to 6 Hz, which is slower than most other tremors. Patients with Parkinson's disease have difficulty when initiating movement, especially in gait and rising from a chair. Spontaneous facial expression is markedly diminished, and masked faces with paucity of movements are a hallmark of Parkinson's disease. Handwriting is often affected; it may begin with near-normal amplitude, but as the writing progresses, it becomes smaller and smaller, which is a phenomenon called micrographia.

CHAPTER TEST

QUESTIONS

Choose the best answer for each question.

Questions 1 and 2. A patient presents with violent involuntary ballistic-like movements that are jerky and irregular and mainly involve the upper extremity on one side of the body.

1. The lesion was most likely located in the:
   a. Neostriatum
   b. Paleostriatum
   c. Subthalamic nucleus
   d. Pars reticulata of the substantia nigra
   e. Claustrum

2. The motor dysfunctions characteristic of this disorder can best be accounted for in terms of loss of:
   a. Inhibitory input to the caudate nucleus
   b. Excitatory input to the medial (internal) pallidal segment
   c. Dopaminergic input to the caudate nucleus and putamen
   d. GABAergic input to the lateral (external) pallidal segment
   e. Glutamatergic input to the caudate nucleus

Questions 3 and 4. A patient presents with reduced facial expression, spontaneous movements (slower than normal) that are revealed most clearly when walking, monotonous speech, an increase in muscle tone in the arms, and a rhythmic tremor (4 to 7/sec) in the fingers, including a pill-rolling tremor.

3. This disorder can be directly linked to loss of:
   a. Glutamatergic inputs from neocortex to the neostriatum
   b. GABAergic input to the lateral (external) pallidal segment
   c. Glutamatergic input to the medial (internal) pallidal segment
   d. Dopaminergic inputs to the neostriatum
   e. Cholinergic inputs to the neostriatum

4. Which of the following pharmacological treatment strategies would be most appropriate for this patient:
   a. Cholinergic (muscarinic) agonist (Pilocarpine)
   b. GABA$_A$ agonist (Muscimol)
   c. L-DOPA plus a dopamine-decarboxylase inhibitor (Sinemet)
   d. Serotonin re-uptake inhibitor (Prozac)
   e. GABA$_B$ agonist (Baclofen)

5. A 55-year-old man was recently diagnosed with Huntington's disease. This disorder may best be understood in terms of the loss of which substance with which result?
   a. Serotonin in the globus pallidus, increased excitation of ventral anterior thalamic nucleus
   b. Substance P in the neostriatum, increased inhibition in the medial pallidal segment
   c. GABA in the neostriatum, reduction of neostriatal inhibition on the lateral (external) pallidal segment
   d. Acetylcholine and GABA in the neostriatum, reduction of inhibition on the medial (internal) pallidal segment
   e. Dopamine in the neostriatum, a reduction of neostriatal inhibition on the medial pallidal segment

ANSWERS AND EXPLANATIONS

1 and 2. Answers: **1-c, 2-b**

Hemiballism is associated with a discrete lesion of the subthalamic nucleus. It consists of wild, uncontrolled movements of the distal musculature (limb) on the side contralateral to the site of the lesion. It is believed to constitute a 'release' phenomenon in which the pallidal-thalamic fibers, which are inhibitory to ventral anterior and ventrolateral nuclei of thalamus, are prevented from discharging due to the loss of excitatory input from the glutamatergic fibers that arise from the subthalamic nucleus and that project to the medial pallidal segment. The other choices for question 1 are not correct for the following reasons. Lesions of the neostriatum are associated with Huntington's disease and other forms of choreiform movements, which can affect both the upper and lower limb. Lesions of the paleostriatum (globus pallidus) have not been associated with hemiballism; likewise, lesions of the pars reticulata of the substantia nigra have also not been associated with hemiballism. The claustrum is not linked to motor functions.

3 and 4. Answers: 3-d, 4-c

The patient described for these questions has Parkinson's disease. It is a hypokinetic disorder characterized by a reduction in spontaneous movements and facial expression, tremor (4 to 7/sec), pill-rolling tremor, and monotonous speech. This disease results from a reduction or loss of dopaminergic input into the neostriatum from the pars compacta of the substantia nigra. One pharmacological approach used for the treatment of Parkinson's disease has been to administer a drug called Sinemet, which consists of a mixture of L-DOPA, the precursor of dopamine, coupled with a dopamine-decarboxylase inhibitor. This drug serves as a means of providing dopamine to brain regions, such as the neostriatum, in place of the dopamine that would normally be provided from the pars compacta of the substantia nigra to the neostriatum.

5. Answer: c

The lateral segment of the globus pallidus projects GABAergic fibers to the subthalamic nucleus. This connection represents the first limb of the indirect pathway connecting the striatum, subthalamic nucleus, and thalamus. In turn, the subthalamic nucleus provides an excitatory, glutamatergic input to the medial pallidal segment; and the medial segment inhibits the ventrolateral and ventral anterior nuclei of thalamus (which normally excite motor regions of cortex) by virtue of its GABAergic projection. Thus, when the inhibitory GABAergic input to the lateral pallidal segment is lost, as is the case in Huntington's disease, the GABAergic input into the subthalamic nucleus from the lateral pallidal segment is more pronounced. Consequently, there is a weaker excitatory input into the medial pallidal segment from the subthalamic nucleus, resulting in less inhibition from the medial pallidal segment on the thalamic nucleus and motor regions of cortex. Hence, the loss of neostriatal GABA is manifested in the form of a hyperkinetic effect on motor responses. The other choices are incorrect for the following reasons. The role of serotonin in the globus pallidus is unknown and, therefore, not likely to play any significant role in this structure related to a hyperkinetic disorder. Substance P is excitatory and, therefore, could not be related to inhibitory processes. Acetylcholine is an excitatory transmitter whose loss would not produce a reduction in inhibition. Loss of dopamine in the neostriatum is associated with a hypokinetic rather than a hyperkinetic disorder.

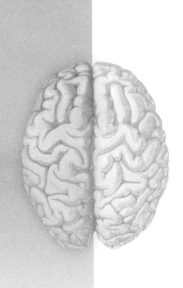

CHAPTER 21

THE CEREBELLUM

OBJECTIVES

The student should be able to:

1. Describe, diagram, and label the morphological features of the cerebellum

2. List the afferent sources of the cerebellum from: (1) the spinal cord, (2) brainstem, and (3) cerebral cortex

3. Characterize the functional properties of these afferent sources of the cerebellum

4. Describe and label the internal circuitry of the cerebellar cortex and how the neurons interact with one another

5. List the efferent projections of the cerebellum and describe their functional relationships

6. Characterize the feedback pathways that link the cerebellum with: (1) the spinal cord, (2) motor regions of the brainstem, and (3) motor regions of the cerebral cortex

7. Describe the anatomical bases of cerebellar disorders. Why are cerebellar disorders ipsilateral with respect to the cerebellum?

The cerebellum is concerned with at least three major functions. The first function is *an association with* movements that are properly grouped for the performance of selective responses that require specific adjustments. This is also referred to as **synergy of movement**. The second function includes the maintenance of upright posture with respect to one's position in space. The third function concerns the maintenance of the tension or firmness (i.e., tone) of the muscle.

If one were to analyze what is required neurophysiologically to complete even the simplest movements, such as walking or lifting a fork to one's mouth, it would be apparent that they are indeed complex acts. To be able to complete either of these responses, the following elements are required: (1) contraction of a given muscle group or groups of muscles; (2) simultaneous relaxation of antagonist set(s) of muscles; (3) specific level of muscle contraction for a precise duration of time; and (4) the appropriate sequencing of contraction and relaxation of the muscle groups required for the movement in question. The numbers of muscle fibers activated determines the extent of the muscle contraction. In turn, the numbers of muscle fibers that contract at a given time (i.e., the force or strength of contraction) are a function of the numbers of alpha motor neurons that are activated. The duration of contraction is determined, to a large extent, by the duration of activation of the nerve fibers that innervate the muscles required for the specific act.

For precise and effective execution of purposeful movements as well as the presence of appropriate posture in association with standing and with movement, a region of the brain must be able to integrate and organize the sequence of events associated with the response. Such a region should be able to both receive inputs from all the regions of the central nervous system (CNS) associated with motor function and, consequently, send "feedback" responses back to these regions. Thus, such a region must function as a computer does, to integrate sensory and motor signals, and consequently, it must have the necessary computer-like or integrative properties for analysis of the afferent signals and possess the reciprocal connections to form a series of "feedback" pathways to its afferent sources. The region of the brain possessing all of these characteristics is the **cerebellum**. It receives inputs from all regions of the CNS associated with motor functions and sensory regions mediating signals about the status of a given muscle or groups of muscles (Fig. 21-1). It also has the capacity to send back messages to each of these regions. Moreover, the cerebellum possesses the machinery for integrating each of these afferent signals. The remainder of this chapter is designed to document how the cerebellum carries out these functions.

GROSS ORGANIZATION OF THE CEREBELLUM

A description of the gross anatomical characteristics of the cerebellum is presented in Chapter 11, and the student is referred to that chapter for details concerning morphological characteristics. This material is briefly summarized here. The **cerebellum** is attached to the brainstem by three peduncles. The inferior and middle cerebellar peduncles are mainly cerebellar afferents, while the superior cerebellar peduncle contains mainly cerebellar efferent fibers. The inferior cerebellar peduncle emerges from the dorsolateral medulla and enters the cerebellum on its inferior aspect. The middle cerebellar peduncle emerges from the

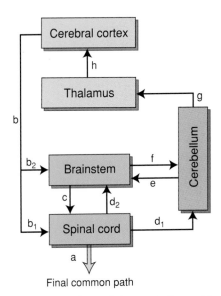

Figure 21–1 Relationships of the cerebellum with other regions of the CNS. In this scheme, the final common path (a) for the expression of motor responses is mediated through the spinal cord. These motor responses require inputs to the cerebellum from the cerebral cortex (b) via the brainstem (b_2 and f) as well as through internal reflex mechanisms contained within the spinal cord (more directly from b_1 and d_1 or indirectly from b_1, d_2, and f). The appropriate "feedback" from the cerebellum to the structures that provide input to it include outputs to the spinal cord through brainstem structures (e + c) and to the cerebral cortex (g + h).

lateral aspect of the pons and enters the cerebellum from a lateral trajectory. The superior cerebellar peduncle emerges from the superior and medial aspects of the cerebellum and enters the brainstem at the level of the upper pons (Fig. 21-2).

The cerebellar cortex consists of three lobes. Each lobe consists of two bilaterally symmetrical hemispheres separated from each other by a midline structure called a vermis (Fig. 21-3). The lobes are identified as the **anterior, posterior,** and **flocculonodular** lobes. The anterior lobe is separated from the posterior lobe by the primary fissure, and the posterior lobe is separated from the flocculonodular lobe by a posterolateral fissure. Phylogenetically, the flocculonodular lobe is the most primitive. It receives major inputs from the vestibular system and is, accordingly, referred to as the **vestibulocerebellum**. The anterior lobe and adjoining parts of the vermal region of the posterior lobe receive major spinal cord inputs. Therefore, this is referred to as the **spinocerebellum**. Because the anterior lobe evolved at a later time than the posterior lobe, it is sometimes also called the **paleocerebellum**. The largest and most recently (from a phylogenetic viewpoint) evolved region of the cerebellum is the posterior lobe. It is linked most closely with the cerebral cortex. Accordingly,

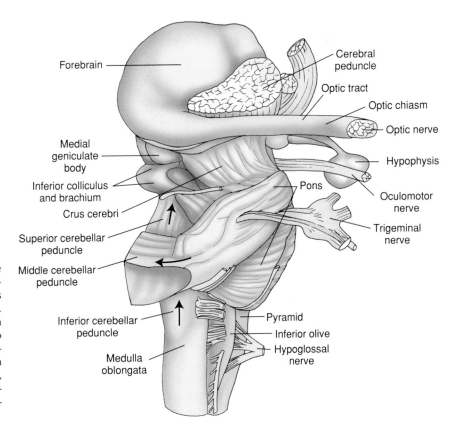

Figure 21–2 Lateral view of the brainstem indicating the relationships of the cerebellar peduncles to the brainstem and cerebellum. Arrows denote the general direction of information flow with respect to the cerebellum. The inferior and middle cerebellar peduncles contain mostly cerebellar afferent fibers, while the superior cerebellar peduncle contains mainly cerebellar efferent fibers.

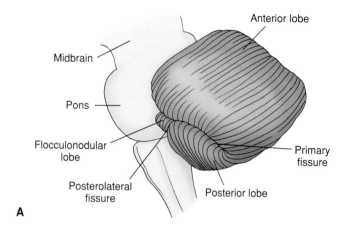

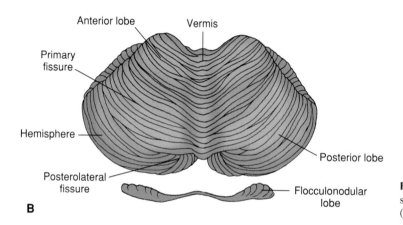

Figure 21-3 The cerebellum. Note the general fissures and divisions of the vermis as illustrated in (A) sagittal and (B) dorsal representations.

it is also called the **neocerebellum**. Thus, one can see that the cerebellar cortex can be divided into three different functional regions. Their significance will be discussed later.

Deep to the cerebellar cortex is a large expanse of white matter that separates the cortex from the underlying deep cerebellar nuclei. There are three deep cerebellar nuclei represented bilaterally. The medial structure is called the **fastigial nucleus**. The lateral structure is the **dentate nucleus**, and the nuclei that lie between the dentate and fastigial nuclei are called the **interposed nuclei** (see Fig. 11-8). The interposed nuclei consist of two relatively small nuclei; the medial structure is called the **globose nucleus**, and the lateral one is called the **emboliform nucleus**. Each of these deep cerebellar nuclei mediates different functions, which relate to their input-output properties. The functions of these nuclei are discussed later in this chapter.

AFFERENT CONNECTIONS OF THE CEREBELLUM

The cerebellar cortex receives inputs from regions of the CNS associated with the regulation of motor functions, as well as direct and indirect sensory

inputs associated with the status of individual muscles, groups of muscles, and other inputs that include tactile impulses, cutaneous afferents, and high-threshold joint afferents. The following sections elaborate on the sources, distribution, and functional nature of the afferent supply to the cerebellar cortex.

SPINAL CORD (SPINOCEREBELLUM)

The inputs from the spinal cord provide the cerebellum with essential information (i.e., the status and position of individual as well as groups of muscles) with which it can control both muscle tone and the execution of movements. The pathways most critical for supplying such inputs to the cerebellum include the dorsal spinocerebellar tract, ventral spinocerebellar tract, cuneocerebellar tract, and the rostral spinocerebellar tract (the latter identified in the cat). The projections of these pathways to the cerebellum are somatotopically organized and are directed primarily to the vermis and regions around the vermis (paravermal region) of the anterior lobe and adjacent portions of the posterior lobe. Therefore, these receiving areas are referred to as the spinocerebellum.

Dorsal (Posterior) Spinocerebellar Tract

The dorsal spinocerebellar tract and the other cerebellar afferent tracts described in the following sections were considered in Chapter 9. Therefore, the key features of these tracts will be briefly summarized at this time.

The dorsal spinocerebellar tract, which conveys signals mainly from muscle spindles and Golgi tendon organs concerning the status of individual muscles to the cerebellar cortex from the lower limbs, passes through the inferior cerebellar peduncle and terminates mainly in the medial part of the ipsilateral anterior lobe and adjacent portions of the posterior lobe (Fig. 21-4, A and B).

Ventral (Anterior) Spinocerebellar Tract

The ventral spinocerebellar tract conveys signals from the Golgi tendon organ (i.e., detecting whole limb movement) and flexor reflex afferents[1] through the superior cerebellar peduncle to the anterior lobe of cerebellum close to the regions where dorsal spinocerebellar fibers terminate (see Figs. 21- 4A and 9-9).

Cuneocerebellar Tract

The cuneocerebellar tract, the upper limb equivalent of the dorsal spinocerebellar tract, conveys inputs from muscle spindles of the upper limb to the upper limb regions of the anterior lobe and adjoining regions of the posterior lobe (Fig. 21-4C). This pathway thus provides the spinocerebellum with inputs concerning mainly the status of individual muscles of the upper limb.

Rostral Spinocerebellar Tract

An upper limb equivalent of the ventral spinocerebellar tract not yet identified in humans, the rostral spinocerebellar tract arises from the cervical cord and supplies the anterior lobe of the cerebellum, conveying whole limb movement (from the Golgi tendon organ) to the anterior lobe from the upper limb.

BRAINSTEM

A number of brainstem nuclei contribute inputs to the cerebellum. These structures include the inferior olivary nucleus, vestibular nuclei, several

groups of nuclei within the reticular formation, and deep (or ventral) pontine nuclei. The nature and functions of these cerebellar afferent fibers from each of these brainstem nuclei vary and are considered in the following sections.

Inferior Olivary Nucleus

The largest component of the inferior cerebellar peduncle is associated with fibers arising from the inferior olivary nucleus. The inferior olivary nucleus receives two different kinds of inputs. One type of input is from the spinal cord, and the second is from the cerebral cortex.

Fibers from the spinal cord convey information from cutaneous afferents, joint afferents, and muscle spindles to the inferior olivary nucleus. From this structure, axons pass to the contralateral cerebellar cortex via the inferior cerebellar peduncle, terminating somatotopically within the anterior and posterior lobes of the cerebellar cortex (Fig. 21-5).

The second kind of input relates to the sensorimotor cortex and includes motor fibers that descend from the cerebral cortex directly and indirectly via the red nucleus. In humans, the rubro-olivary fibers are much more extensive than in other species of animals. In this manner, the inferior olivary nucleus appears to transmit an integrated signal from the spinal cord and cerebral cortex to the cerebellar hemispheres via the climbing fiber system (see page 366).

Brainstem Structures Associated with Posture and Balance

As pointed out in Chapter 19, both the vestibular system and reticular formation play important roles in the regulation of motor processes that primarily affect extensor muscles and that relate to the control of balance and posture. Both of these regions also contribute significant inputs to the cerebellum.

Vestibular System

The cerebellum receives signals from the otolith organ (i.e., macula of saccule and utricle) and semicircular canals of the vestibular system. Fibers arising from the vestibular apparatus may enter the cerebellar cortex via a monosynaptic or disynaptic pathway. The monosynaptic pathway (called the **juxtarestiform body**) involves first-order vestibular neurons that terminate within the ipsilateral flocculonodular lobe. The second route involves primary vestibular fibers that synapse in the vestibular nuclei and second-order neurons that project chiefly from the inferior and medial vestibular nuclei to the same region of cerebellar cortex (Fig. 21-5). In this manner, the cerebellum

---

[1]Flexor reflex afferents refer to signals from cutaneous receptors, group II and group III muscle afferents, and high-threshold joint afferents to the spinal cord. These impulses can reach the brainstem and cerebellum over several ascending pathways. At the spinal cord level, they play a role in segmental reflexes and, therefore, likely indicate to the cerebellum the activity and status of interneurons within the spinal cord.

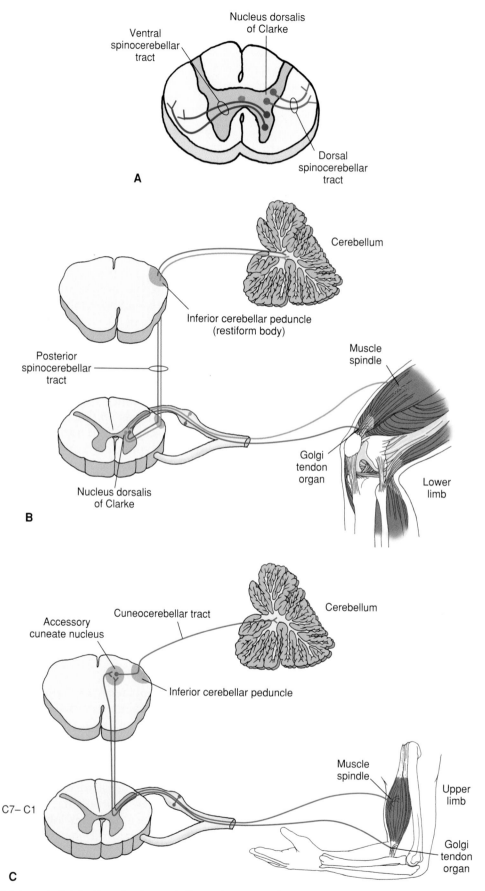

Figure 21–4 Origin and distribution of spinocerebellar and cuneocerebellar tracts. (A) The origins of the dorsal and ventral spinocerebellar tracts within the spinal cord. (B) Origin, course, and distribution of the posterior spinocerebellar tract and (C) cuneocerebellar tract.

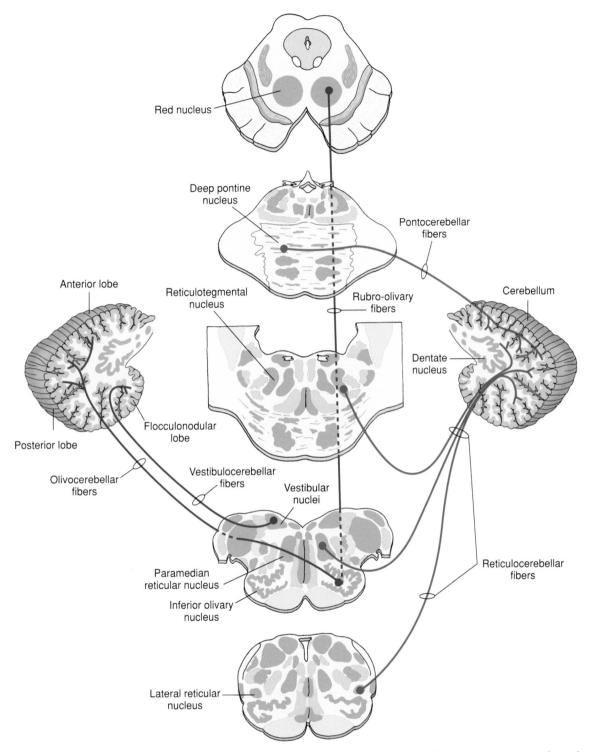

Figure 21–5 The afferent pathways to the cerebellar cortex from the brainstem. These include pathways arising from the red nucleus (shown in blue), deep pontine nuclei (shown in red), vestibular nuclei, and reticular formation (shown in blue and green, respectively).

receives important information concerning the position of the head in space at any given point in time as well as the status of those vestibular neurons that regulate extensor motor neurons (via the vestibulospinal and reticulospinal tracts). There is a further differentiation of function within the cerebellar cortex in that the flocculonodular lobe represents the specific receiving area for vestibular inputs, and the anterior lobe is the primary receiving area for spinal cord afferents.

Reticular Formation

The **reticular formation** also powerfully modulates spinal reflexes, acting, in part, on the gamma motor system (principally of extensor muscles). This important component of motor systems provides a key input to the cerebellum that presumably relates to the manner in which reticular neurons regulate extensor motor tone at any given point in time. The fibers that project to the cerebellar cortex from the reticular formation arise from the **lateral** and **paramedian reticular nuclei** of the medulla and from the **reticulotegmental nucleus** of the pons. These fibers are distributed mainly to the vermal region of the anterior and posterior lobes. Much of the information transmitted from the reticular formation is not modality specific. However, it is believed that the lateral reticular nucleus may transmit tactile impulses from the anterolateral funiculus to the cerebellar cortex. For this reason, the reticulocerebellar projection may contribute to the spinocerebellar system. Moreover, because the lateral reticular nucleus receives inputs from the spinal cord and cerebral cortex, in effect, it is also capable of sending an integrated signal to the cerebellar hemispheres (through the mossy fiber system) in a manner parallel to that of the inferior olivary nucleus (Fig. 21-5).

It should also be noted that several of the nuclei of the reticular formation that project to the cerebellum also receive significant inputs from the sensorimotor cortex. This indicates that the reticular formation also serves as a relay for cerebral cortical inputs to the vermal and paravermal regions of the anterior and posterior lobes of the cerebellar cortex. This circuit thus provides the cerebral cortex with the neural substrate for both coordination of movements and movements that govern equilibrium and maintenance of an erect posture.

CEREBRAL CORTEX

The **cerebral cortex** is concerned with the coordination, planning, and execution of movements. As indicated earlier, there are several ways by which the cerebral cortex can transmit such information to the cerebellar cortex. One way involves a multisynaptic pathway whose initial link is from the cerebral cortex to the red nucleus; the second limb is from the red nucleus to the ipsilateral inferior olivary nucleus; and the final limb includes a projection from the inferior olivary nucleus to the contralateral cerebellar hemisphere (Fig. 21-6). The other ways include projections to relay nuclei located in the basilar part of the pons and reticular formation.

While the major inputs to the cerebellar cortex from the reticular formation are directed to the vermal and paravermal regions, the projections from the red nucleus (via the inferior olivary nucleus) and deep pontine nuclei to the cerebellar cortex are directed mainly to the cerebellar hemispheres. One point to be noted is that there appear to be "patches" of somatotopically organized regions of cerebellar cortex restricted mainly to the vermal and paravermal regions. Specifically, evidence supports the view that the axial musculature is represented mainly in the vermal region, while the distal musculature is represented more laterally in the paravermal regions of the hemispheres. Overall, the pathways from the cerebral cortex to the deep pontine nuclei and red nucleus represent the substrates by which the cerebral cortex can coordinate movements associated mainly with the distal musculature.

Red Nucleus

We have indicated that the red nucleus serves, in part, as a relay from the sensorimotor cortex to the spinal cord (via the rubrospinal tract) that activates the flexor motor system. In a similar manner, the sensorimotor cortex can provide signals to the cerebellar cortex through relays in the red nucleus and inferior olivary nucleus (Fig. 21-5). Through this circuit, the status of neurons in the red nucleus (and indirectly, those of the motor regions of the cerebral cortex) is transmitted in a somatotopic manner to the cerebellar cortex. The red nucleus communicates with the cerebellar cortex through the following pathway: red nucleus → inferior olivary nucleus (crossed olivocerebellar fibers) → contralateral anterior and posterior lobes of cerebellar cortex.

Deep Pontine Nuclei

The primary route by which the cerebral cortex communicates with the cerebellar cortex is via a relay in the basilar (ventral) pons. Fibers arising from all regions of the cerebral cortex project through the internal capsule and crus cerebri, making synaptic connections upon deep pontine nuclei. The deep pontine nuclei give rise to axons called **transverse pontine fibers** that enter the contralateral middle cerebellar peduncle and are distributed to the anterior and posterior lobes of the cerebellum (Fig. 21-6).

The largest component of the projection to the cerebellar cortex arises from the frontal lobe. This provides the primary substrate by which motor regions of the cerebral cortex can communicate with the cerebellar cortex. However, sensory regions of the cerebral cortex also contribute fibers to the cerebellar cortex. These include parietal, temporal, and

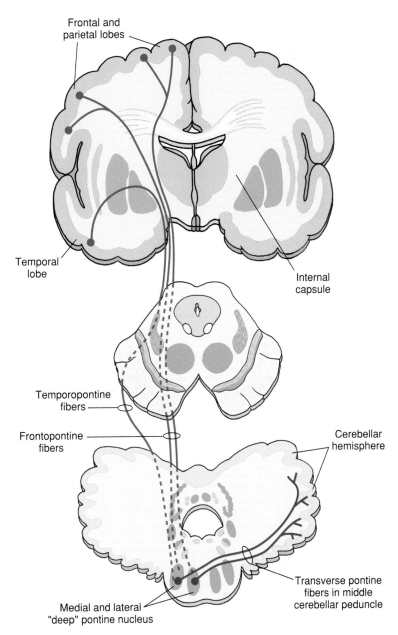

Figure 21-6 The disynaptic pathway from the cerebral cortex to the cerebellar cortex with a synapse in the deep pontine nuclei. Corticopontine fibers are shown in red, and pontocerebellar fibers are shown in blue.

visual cortices. The posterior parietal cortex provides the cerebellum with information concerning the planning or programming signals that are transmitted to the motor regions of the cerebral cortex. Temporal and occipital cortices provide the cerebellar cortex with signals associated with auditory and visual functions. In particular, the connection from the visual cortex may signal such events as moving objects in the visual field. Visual and auditory signals may also reach the cerebellar cortex from the tectum (see "Tectum" section). Somatosensory signals also reach the cerebellar cortex from the cerebral cortex. Evidence suggests that fibers from the sensorimotor cortex are somatotopically arranged within the vermal and paravermal regions of the cerebellar cortex in a manner that corresponds to the somatotopic organization associated with spinal cord inputs. However, there is little evidence that the lateral aspects of the hemisphere of the posterior lobe are somatotopically organized.

OTHER INPUTS TO THE CEREBELLAR CORTEX

Tectum

In addition to the inputs from the occipital and temporal neocortices, fibers arising from both the superior colliculus and inferior colliculus also provide visual and auditory information, respectively, to the cerebellar cortex (Fig. 21-7). They do so by projecting to the pontine nuclei, which, in turn,

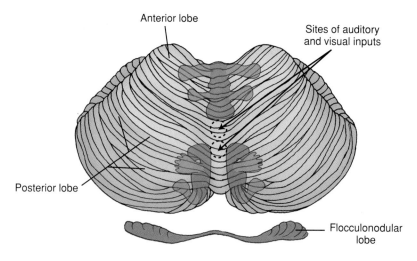

Anterior lobe

Sites of auditory
and visual inputs

Posterior lobe

Flocculonodular
lobe

Figure 21–7 Homunculi illustrating the somatotopic organization of the cerebellar cortex. Note that the body is represented on the cerebellar cortex more than once and that the axial musculature is represented in a medial position, while the distal musculature is represented more laterally. The neuronal regions associated with regulation of the distal musculature are shown in green, and the regions associated with the axial musculature are shown in red.

project through the middle cerebellar peduncle to the cerebellar cortex.

Trigeminal System

Secondary proprioceptive fibers associated with muscle spindle activity of muscles of the face and jaw reach the cerebellum chiefly from the mesencephalic trigeminal nucleus. Other (tactile) sensory fibers arising from trigeminal nuclei have been shown to project to mainly the vermal and paravermal regions of the cerebellar cortex. Their distribution to the cerebellar cortex is directed to the head regions depicted by the homunculus shown in Figure 21-7.

Monoaminergic Systems

Brainstem neurons contribute noradrenergic and serotonergic fibers to wide areas of the cerebellar cortex. The noradrenergic fibers arise mainly from the locus ceruleus, and the serotonin fibers arise from the raphe complex. Both groups of fibers function as modulators of the activities of cerebellar cortical neurons.

THE ANATOMICAL AND FUNCTIONAL ORGANIZATION OF THE CEREBELLAR CORTEX

MOSSY AND CLIMBING FIBERS

There are two kinds of afferent fibers that convey impulses to the cerebellar cortex. They are identified on the basis of their morphology and are referred to as **mossy** and **climbing fibers** (Fig. 21-8).

Mossy Fibers

Mossy fibers are found widely throughout the cerebellum. As they course through the granular layer, they give rise to many branches in this layer. These branches terminate by forming **mossy fiber rosettes**, which are held by claw-like dendrites of the granule cells (Fig. 21-9). Thus, impulses traveling along a single mossy fiber can activate many granule cells. The mossy fiber rosettes form the focus of a **cerebellar glomerulus**, which consists of the synaptic relationships between mossy fiber axons and both granule cell dendrites and Golgi cell axon terminals. Specifically, the cerebellar glomerulus consists of: (1) a mossy fiber rosette, (2) dendrites of many granule cells, (3) the proximal aspect of Golgi cell dendrites, and (4) terminals of Golgi cell axons. Mossy fibers are excitatory and arise from all regions of the CNS that project to the cerebellar cortex with the exception of the inferior olivary nucleus. The neurotransmitter released from the endings of mossy fibers is believed to be glutamate.

Climbing Fibers

Climbing fibers arise from the inferior olivary nucleus and ascend through the granular and Purkinje cell layers to reach the molecular layer. Within the molecular layer, they make synapse by climbing up the branches of the dendrites of the Purkinje cells (Fig. 21-8). In contrast to the arrangement of a single mossy fiber that can excite many granule cells, the climbing fiber maintains a one-to-one relationship with the Purkinje cell (i.e., one climbing fiber excites a single Purkinje cell). The neurotransmitter released from the endings of climbing fibers is believed to be aspartate.

An important fact to remember is that both mossy and climbing fibers, which excite their target neurons in the cerebellar cortex, also provide excitatory inputs from collaterals to the deep cerebellar nuclei (Fig. 21-10).

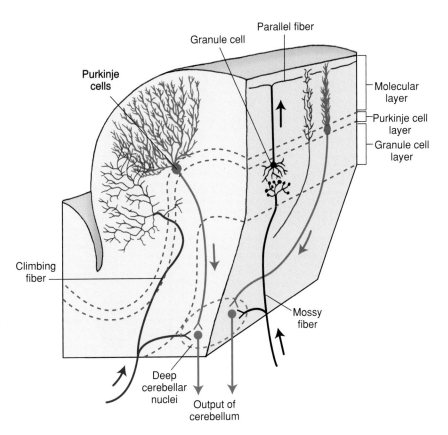

Figure 21–8 Diagrammatic representation of a folium of the cerebellar cortex illustrating the different types of cells and fibers found within the three cell layers of the cortex. Climbing fibers (cerebellar afferent fiber) are shown in blue; mossy fibers (cerebellar afferent fiber) and granule cells and their parallel fibers are shown in black; Purkinje cells and their axons (output of cerebellar cortex) are shown in red; and output of the cerebellum to other regions of the brain from deep cerebellar nuclei are shown in green.

CEREBELLAR CORTEX

HISTOLOGY

The histological appearance of the gray matter is virtually identical throughout the entire cerebellar cortex. The gray matter forms folds (folia) that are arranged transversely within the long axis of the hemisphere (Figs. 21-8 and 21-11). Deep to the gray matter of each fold lies a massive region of white matter, which contains afferent and efferent axons of the cerebellar cortex.

The arrangement of the cells and fibers within the cerebellar cortex has important functional utility. For example, individual axons within the

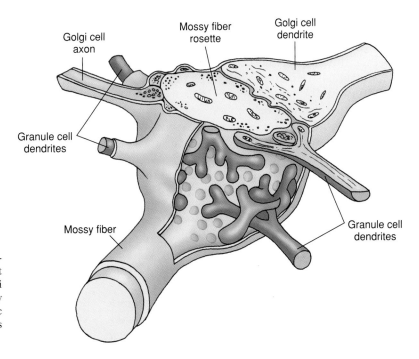

Figure 21–9 Diagram of a cerebellar glomerulus. It consists of one mossy fiber rosette (light pink), granule cell dendrites (purple), and Golgi cell axons and their dendrites (green). Mossy fiber axon terminals make numerous synaptic contacts with granule cell dendrites as well as with dendrites and axons of Golgi cells.

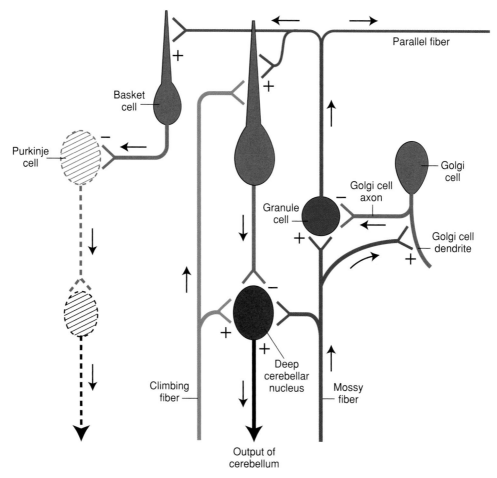

Figure 21–10 Diagram illustrating the most significant connections within the cerebellar cortex. Cells shown in red are inhibitory neurons. All other neurons shown in this figure are excitatory. Arrows indicate direction of transmission along the axon. The dotted appearance of the Purkinje cell in the left side of the figure indicates that it is present outside the plane of the section. (+), excitatory synapse; (−), inhibitory synapse.

cerebellar cortex can affect many cells over wide areas of the cortex. Such an arrangement can provide the basis by which the cerebellum influences wide regions of the body musculature at a given time. Another function of the cerebellum is to provide precise signals to distant structures in the form of excitatory-inhibitory sequences. Accordingly, the neurons within the cerebellar cortex must be arranged in such a manner that these signals can be appropriately transmitted to distal structures.

The cerebellar cortex consists of three cell layers (Fig. 21-8). The innermost layer is called the *granular cell* layer. The middle layer is the *Purkinje cell* layer; and the most superficial layer is called the *molecular* layer, which is almost devoid of cells. The anatomy and functions of the cells situated in these layers are described in the following sections.

Granular Cell Layer

The primary cell found in this layer is the **granule cell**. This cell type contains three to five dendrites, which are arranged in a claw-like appearance to receive mossy fiber cerebellar afferents. The axon of the granule cell ascends toward the surface of the cortex and, as it enters the molecular layer, it ends by bifurcating and forming axons that pass in opposite directions within the molecular layer parallel to the surface of the cortex. These fibers are called **parallel fibers**. By passing along the long axis of the folium, the parallel fibers run in a direction perpendicular to the dendrites of Purkinje cells. Accordingly, this arrangement allows individual parallel fibers to make synaptic contact with many Purkinje cell dendrites. Parallel fibers serve to excite Purkinje cells, and these actions are believed to be mediated by glutamate. Furthermore, collaterals of parallel fibers make synaptic contact with dendrites of Golgi cells.

The other cell type found in the granular cell layer of the cerebellar cortex is the **Golgi cell**. It is an inhibitory, γ-aminobutyric acid (GABA)-ergic neuron. The cell body is typically found near the border of the Purkinje cell layer. In addition to receiving afferents from parallel fibers, the Golgi cell

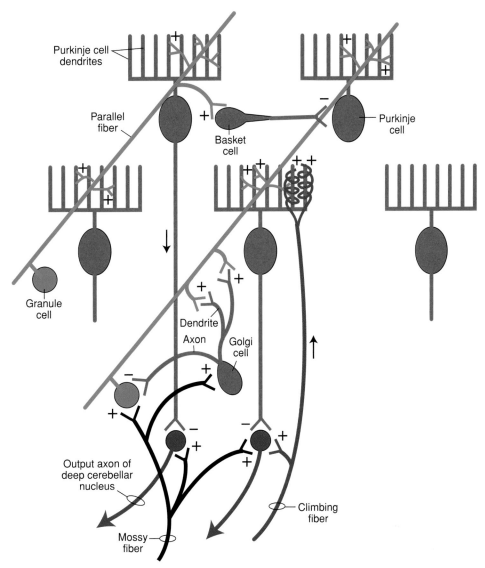

Figure 21–11 This figure shows some of the principal connections of the cerebellar cortex similar to those shown in Figure 21-10. This figure further illustrates how parallel fiber activation can lead to a beam of excitation within the plane of the parallel fiber and the Purkinje cell neurons with which they make synaptic contact and inhibition along adjacent beams of Purkinje cell neurons. The parallel fiber excites basket cells, which are inhibitory and make synaptic contact with Purkinje cells located in adjacent planes. This provides the basis for inhibition along the beam of Purkinje cells adjacent to the beam of excitation of Purkinje cells induced from the parallel fiber. The diagram also illustrates the relationship of the Golgi cell in inhibiting granule cell activity, as well as the inputs into the deep cerebellar nucleus, which constitutes the output neuron of the cerebellum. Such inputs include excitation from mossy and climbing fiber collaterals and inhibition from the Purkinje cells. Mossy fibers also excite granule cells, and climbing fibers excite Purkinje cells.

axon is short and makes synapse with dendrites of granule cells. Dendrites of Golgi cells also make synaptic contact with axon terminals of mossy fibers (Fig. 21-10).

Purkinje Cell Layer

The Purkinje cell layer contains one cell type, the **Purkinje cell**, and is, consequently, one cell in thickness. The cell body is flask-shaped, with the neck ascending vertically toward the molecular layer. Dendrites emerge from the neck, and thick dendritic trees are directed into the molecular layer

(Fig. 21-8). The axon emerges from the bottom of the cell body and descends through the granular cell layer and white matter and terminates in one of the deep cerebellar nuclei. Purkinje cells located in the vermal region project to the fastigial nucleus; Purkinje cells located in the hemispheres project to the dentate nucleus; and Purkinje cells located in the paravermal region project to the interposed nuclei. Purkinje cell axons from the anterior lobe also project to the lateral vestibular nucleus. The Purkinje cell is inhibitory and uses GABA as a neurotransmitter.

Molecular Layer

The **molecular layer** contains the dendrites of Purkinje cells, parallel fibers (i.e., axons of granule cells), and two other cell types referred to as **basket cells**. The basket cells receive inputs from parallel fibers and make inhibitory axosomatic contacts with Purkinje cells (Fig. 21-10).

FUNCTIONAL PROPERTIES OF THE CEREBELLAR CORTEX

As shown in Figure 21-10, stimulation of either the mossy or climbing fibers will result in activation of their target neurons. Consider first the flow of information through the cerebellar cortex after stimulation of the mossy fiber system. Mossy fibers excite granule cells, which, in turn, excite Purkinje cells. Within this circuit lies the Golgi cell, which can be activated in two ways. The first involves the parallel fiber, which makes synaptic contact with the dendrites of the Golgi cell. Alternatively, the mossy fiber can directly contact the dendrites of the Golgi cell. Golgi cell activation results in inhibition of the granule cell. Thus, inhibition of the granule cell can come about by either: (1) **feed forward inhibition** [mossy fiber → (+) Golgi cell → (−) granule cell], or (2) **feedback inhibition** [mossy fiber → (+) granule cell → (+) Golgi cell → (−) granule cell]. The net effect of this component of the overall circuit is that the granule cell discharge is limited by the coactivation of the Golgi cell following stimulation of the mossy fiber. In essence, this cerebellar circuit displays an "on-off" feature. Specifically, the mossy fiber turns on the granule cell, which then turns on the Purkinje cell. The granule cell is then turned off by the action of the Golgi cell. Since the granule cell is now turned off, the Purkinje cell and the Golgi cell are also turned off (called **disfacilitation** of the Purkinje and Golgi cells) because action potentials at this time are not conducted along the parallel fiber.

Concerning other elements of the cerebellar circuit, we have just indicated that parallel fiber activation, which is limited by the action of the Golgi cell, results in direct excitation of Purkinje cells that lie in a row within a given plane of the parallel fiber. The parallel fiber also can activate **basket** and **stellate cells**, which are inhibitory neurons. However, these neurons do not inhibit Purkinje cells that lie in the plane of excitation of the activated parallel fiber. Instead, these interneurons typically inhibit Purkinje cells that lie in an adjacent plane to that of the Purkinje cell excited by the parallel fiber (Fig. 21-11). Therefore, the overall process produces a beam of "excitation-inhibition"

along a given plane of Purkinje cells, with a consequent inhibition of rows of Purkinje cells lying in adjacent planes. The net effect of this process is to sharpen the signals transmitted by the beam of Purkinje cells excited by the parallel fiber.

The action of the climbing fiber on the Purkinje cell is direct and involves no interneurons. The climbing fiber affects the discharge properties of Purkinje cells differently than mossy fibers. Because a climbing fiber makes many synaptic contacts with a Purkinje cell, the effect of the climbing fiber is to produce a powerful depolarization of the Purkinje cell. Voltage-sensitive Ca^{2+} channels propagate the ensuing action potentials in the Purkinje cell axon. As a result of the activation of the climbing fibers, the sensitivity of the Purkinje cell to other types of inputs becomes altered. Specifically, parallel fibers become less effective in causing excitation in the Purkinje cell for a significant period of time (1 to 3 hours). These long-term changes are most likely the result of initiation of second-messenger activity in the Purkinje cell.

It should be pointed out that the only way that signals can leave the cerebellar cortex is through the Purkinje cell axon, which is inhibitory to the deep cerebellar nucleus. How, then, does information get out of the cerebellar cortex? In answer to this question, recall that both mossy and climbing fibers send collaterals to the deep cerebellar nuclei. Therefore, mossy or climbing fiber activation results in an immediate excitation of the deep cerebellar nucleus. This excitation is then followed by inhibition mediated by the Purkinje cell that becomes excited after climbing or mossy fibers are activated. Because the duration of excitation of the parallel fiber is limited by the action of the Golgi cell, the excitatory input to the Purkinje cell from the parallel fiber is also of short duration. When that excitation ceases, there is a consequent increase in excitation in the deep cerebellar nucleus because the Purkinje cell is no longer excited (to produce inhibition on the deep cerebellar nucleus). This release of inhibition is referred to as **disinhibition**. Thus, the signals transmitted by the deep cerebellar nucleus to its target neurons in the brainstem or thalamus after mossy or climbing fiber stimulation would consist of initial excitation, followed by inhibition, which is then followed by disinhibition. This pattern of discharge then becomes the coded message transmitted from the cerebellum to distal targets as a part of an overall feedback response pattern. It should be pointed out that, although the output of the cerebellar cortex is inhibitory, the output of the cerebellum as a whole is excitatory. Inasmuch as the actions of the deep cerebellar nuclei on their target neurons are excitatory, these coded messages are further transmitted faithfully from the deep cerebellar nuclei to their target structures in the brainstem and thalamus and ultimately to the spinal cord and motor cortex.

EFFERENT PROJECTIONS OF THE CEREBELLAR CORTEX: THE FEEDBACK CIRCUITRY

As noted earlier in this chapter, the functional anatomical organization of the cerebellum may be divided into three categories: the **vestibulocerebellum** (i.e., flocculonodular lobe), **spinocerebellum** (anterior lobe), and **cerebrocerebellum** (lateral hemispheres mainly of posterior lobe). The vestibulocerebellum is concerned with the status of the head region (in particular, control of the eyes and position of the head). The spinocerebellum is concerned with the status of the axial musculature (muscle tone) as well as its degree of flexion or extension at any given point in time. The cerebrocerebellum is concerned with the planning, organizational, and coordinating aspects of motor responses.

The cerebellar cortex transmits its signals to the deep cerebellar nuclei via the Purkinje cell axon, which is inhibitory. The inhibitory input from the Purkinje cell (which itself undergoes modification) thus alters the initial signal that the deep cerebellar nucleus receives from the mossy or climbing fiber and serves to sculpt the coded message transmitted to distant structures. The key point to remember is that the organization of the Purkinje cell projections to the deep cerebellar nuclei are topographically arranged. Purkinje cell axons associated with both the vestibulocerebellum and spinocerebellum project to the fastigial nucleus, while Purkinje cell axons associated with the cerebrocerebellum project to the interposed and dentate nuclei (Fig. 21-12). These relationships are central to our understanding of the functions of the cerebellum and disease states associated with different regions of the cerebellum.

EFFERENT CONNECTIONS OF THE VESTIBULOCEREBELLUM AND SPINOCEREBELLUM

The **fastigial nucleus**, which is related to functions of both the vestibulocerebellum and spinocerebellum, has two primary targets within the brainstem to which its axons project: the vestibular nuclei and reticular formation. The fibers project topographi-

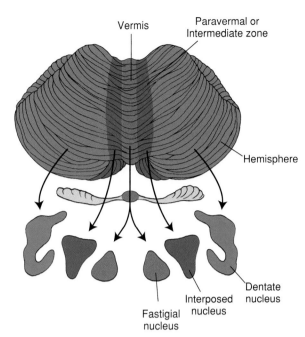

Figure 21-12 Medial to lateral zonal organization of the cerebellar cortex with respect to its outputs to the deep cerebellar nuclei. The vermal region and its projection target in the fastigial nuclei are shown in red; the paravermal region and its projection target in the interposed nuclei are shown in blue; and the region of the hemisphere and its projection target in the dentate nuclei are shown in green.

cally and bilaterally to vestibular nuclei and contralaterally to the parts of the reticular formation of the pons and medulla near the origins of the reticulospinal pathways (Fig. 21-13).

These connections thus establish two of the feedback circuits governing the axial musculature. One circuit involves the vestibular nuclei with the cerebellum, and the other involves the reticular formation with the cerebellum. The vestibular feedback circuit can be summarized as follows: vestibular input from the vestibular apparatus → vestibular nuclei (or primary vestibular fibers direct to) → flocculonodular lobe and posterior vermis → fastigial nucleus → vestibular nuclei → (to extensor motor neurons of spinal cord and cranial nerve nuclei III, IV, VI).

Thus, the vestibular-cerebellar feedback pathway enables the cerebellum to regulate the activity of neurons in the medial and lateral vestibular nucleus that control motor neuron activity within the spinal cord and brainstem. Concerning functions of the vestibulocerebellum and the medial vestibular nucleus, the feedback connections to the vestibular nuclei allow for cerebellar control over the position of the eyes via the vestibular inputs into the medial longitudinal fasciculus and over the position of the head via its connections with the medial vestibular nucleus and the medial vestibulospinal tract (which

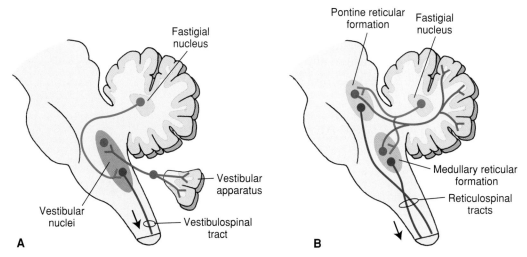

Figure 21–13 Diagrams illustrate the output relationships from the fastigial nucleus of cerebellum with (A) vestibular nuclei and spinal cord and (B) reticular nuclei and spinal cord. Inputs to the cerebellar cortex from the reticular formation and vestibular nuclei are shown in red; outputs of the fastigial nuclei of the cerebellum to the reticular formation and vestibular nuclei are shown in green; and the outputs of the reticular formation and vestibular nuclei (i.e., reticulospinal and vestibulospinal tracts) to the spinal cord are shown in blue.

influences the position of the head). In this manner, changes in postural position and head position result in activation of the vestibulocerebellum, which, in turn, transmits signals back to the vestibular nuclei that can modify the position of the head and eyes. Likewise, inputs into the lateral vestibular nucleus modulates the activity of the lateral vestibulospinal tract, which mediates control over limb extensor muscles and axial muscles, including motor tone of these muscles.

With respect to the spinocerebellum, the same general circuitry is involved through the feedback connection to the lateral vestibular nucleus. In particular, the inhibitory inputs to the lateral vestibular nucleus from Purkinje cell axons in the anterior lobe play an important role in extensor motor tone and general control over axial muscles and limb extensors. The control over muscle tone by the spinocerebellum is further mediated via the connections of the fastigial nucleus with the reticular formation of the pons and medulla. This circuitry, the reticular-cerebellar circuit, can be summarized as follows: nuclei of the reticular formation of the medulla and pons → anterior and posterior lobes (vermal and paravermal regions) → fastigial nucleus → nuclei of reticular formation of the pons and medulla (that project to extensor motor neurons of spinal cord).

This feedback circuit shares similarities with that of the vestibular-cerebellar feedback circuit in that both the reticular formation and lateral vestibular nucleus act on extensor motor neurons of the spinal cord and thus serve to regulate muscle tone and one's ability to stand erect. Thus, when taken collectively, the cerebellar cortical relation-

ships with these brainstem nuclei and ultimately with the spinal cord provide the feedback mechanisms by which the spinocerebellum can influence extensor motor processes within the spinal cord (Fig. 21-13).

EFFERENT CONNECTIONS OF THE CEREBELLAR HEMISPHERES

The cerebellar hemispheres are linked functionally to the cerebral cortex, which provides inputs to the hemispheres via the deep pontine nuclei or, more indirectly, through the red nucleus and inferior olivary nucleus. The Purkinje cell outputs from the intermediate zone of the hemisphere are directed onto the interposed nuclei, while the Purkinje cell axons of more lateral regions of the hemisphere project to the dentate nucleus (Fig. 21-12). The interposed nuclei project through the superior cerebellar peduncle to the contralateral red nucleus and thus complete a feedback circuit between the red nucleus and cerebellar cortex (Figs. 21-14 and 21-15). This feedback circuit can be summarized as follows: red nucleus → inferior olivary nucleus (crossed fibers that enter the inferior cerebellar peduncle) → contralateral intermediate zone of anterior and posterior lobes of cerebellar cortex → interposed nuclei → (superior cerebellar peduncle) → contralateral red nucleus → to excite flexor motor neurons of the side of spinal cord contralateral to the red nucleus (because the rubrospinal tract is crossed).

This feedback circuit to the red nucleus thus enables the intermediate zone of the cerebellar cortex to control neuronal activity within the red

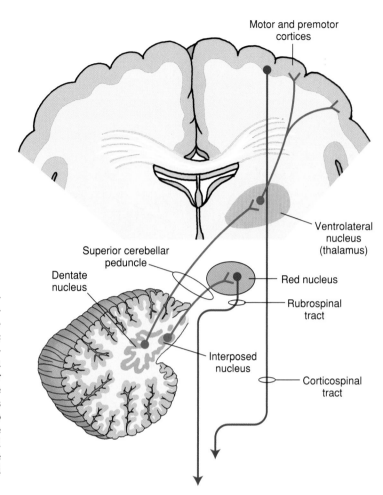

Figure 21–14 Diagram depicts the outflow pathways from the cerebellar cortex to the cerebral cortex and red nucleus. The linkage between the cerebellum and cerebral cortex involves a disynaptic pathway—an initial projection from the dentate nucleus to the ventrolateral thalamic nucleus and a second projection from the thalamus to the motor and premotor cortices (both shown in red). The pathway from the cerebellum to the red nucleus involves a projection from the interposed nuclei to the red nucleus (shown in green). Both of these outputs from the cerebellum to the contralateral thalamus and red nucleus are mediated through the superior cerebellar peduncle. The corticospinal and rubrospinal pathways are indicated in blue.

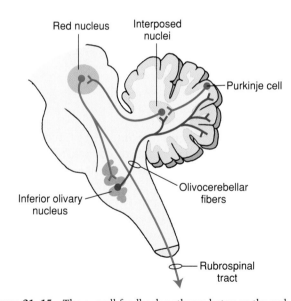

Figure 21–15 The overall feedback pathway between the red nucleus and cerebellum. The red nucleus projects to the cerebellum via a synapse in the inferior olivary nucleus (rubro-olivary projections shown in green and olivocerebellar fibers shown in blue). The cerebellum, in turn, projects back to the red nucleus from the interposed nucleus (shown in red, which includes a Purkinje cell axonal input to interposed nuclei). The relationship of this circuit with the spinal cord is indicated by the presence of the rubrospinal tract.

nucleus and ultimately of the flexor motor neurons of the cervical spinal cord. In effect, by controlling flexor motor neurons, it provides the cerebellar hemispheres with an additional mechanism by which it can control coordination and execution of movements associated mainly with muscles of the arm.

The most powerful means by which the cerebellar hemispheres can affect the planning, initiation, and coordination of motor responses is with its relationships with the cerebral cortex. As indicated previously, the primary region of cerebellum involved in these functions is the cerebellar hemisphere. It receives massive numbers of fibers from the cerebral cortex that are topographically relayed from the deep pontine nuclei via the middle cerebellar peduncle. In turn, the outflow from the cerebellar hemisphere is directed on the dentate nucleus. Fibers arising from the dentate nucleus enter the superior cerebellar peduncle and project beyond the red nucleus to the ventrolateral (VL) nucleus of the thalamus. Neurons arising from the ventrolateral nucleus project to the motor cortex (Fig. 21-16). This circuit thus comprises a feedback network linking the cerebral and cerebellar cortices

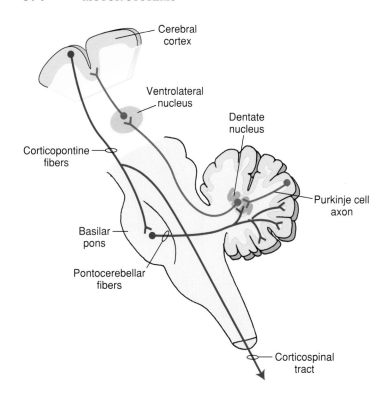

Figure 21-16 The overall feedback pathway between the cerebral cortex and cerebellar cortex. The cerebral cortex projects to the cerebellum via a synapse in the basilar pons (shown in blue); second-order neurons pass through the middle cerebellar peduncle as pontocerebellar fibers to the cerebellar cortex (shown in blue). The feedback to the cerebral cortex involves a projection from the dentate nucleus to the ventrolateral nucleus of the thalamus, which, in turn, projects to the motor and premotor cortices (both shown in red).

and is summarized as follows: cerebral cortex → deep pontine nuclei (middle cerebellar peduncle crossed to) → contralateral cerebellar hemispheres of the anterior and posterior lobes → dentate nucleus → (superior cerebellar peduncle crossed to) → contralateral ventrolateral thalamic nucleus → motor cortex (on side opposite the cerebellar hemisphere, which receives the cerebral cortical inputs and which gives rise to feedback pathway) (corticospinal tract) → contralateral spinal cord.

In this manner, feedback signals from the cerebellar cortex can assist in the planning, coordination, and execution of motor responses initiated from the cerebral cortex. Evidence that cerebellar neurons function in this manner was provided from experiments in which single unit recordings were taken from monkey motor and cerebellar cortices prior to and during motor activity. It was shown that cerebellar cortex neuronal discharges, as well as those discharges recorded from the motor cortex, preceded the movement. Experiments of this sort have clearly suggested that cerebellar cortical neurons likely help to organize and plan responses normally associated with the motor regions of the cerebral cortex.

When viewed as a whole, we can now see how the cerebellum powerfully regulates the activity of motor neurons of the spinal cord through each of these feedback circuits (Fig. 21-17). Postural mechanisms, balance, and muscle tone are regulated by the outputs of the fastigial nucleus to the

vestibular nuclei and reticular formation, whose axons innervate primarily extensor motor neurons. The outputs of the interposed and dentate nuclei to the red nucleus and motor regions of cerebral cortex (via the ventrolateral thalamic nucleus), respectively, can influence the distal musculature innervated by motor neurons of the spinal cord, which receive inputs from the red nucleus and motor cortex.

MOTOR LEARNING AND THE CEREBELLUM

Experimental evidence has suggested that the cerebellum is involved in motor learning. By this, it is meant that long-lasting changes in synaptic efficacy and modifications in synaptic connections take place after a response has taken place. Such changes can occur in any one of the synaptic connections that exist within the cerebellar cortex. However, it is more likely that the primary regions involved in motor learning include the mossy and climbing fiber connections that are made with the Purkinje cell. As indicated earlier, the Purkinje cell response to parallel fiber inputs is greatly modified following stimulation of climbing fibers. Therefore, it is reasonable to assume that repetition of a given response may quite easily lead to changes in synaptic plasticity involving Purkinje cells. Such changes would also likely produce changes in the patterns of coded neural signals

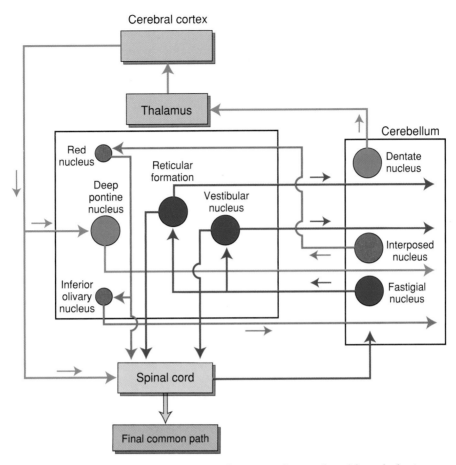

Figure 21–17 Feedback pathways. Diagram illustrates the overall inputs to the spinal cord from the brainstem and cerebral cortex. These inputs to the spinal cord are sculpted by the actions of the cerebellum via feedback pathways to key brainstem nuclei and cerebral cortex. Brainstem structures, which regulate spinal cord motor neurons and receive important feedback from the cerebellum, include the red nucleus, reticular formation, and vestibular nucleus. Likewise, the actions of the corticospinal tract on motor functions of the spinal cord are also powerfully regulated by the cerebellum. Reciprocal "feedback" relationships linking reticular formation and vestibular nuclei with the cerebellum and spinal cord are shown in blue; those linking the red nucleus, cerebellum, and spinal cord are shown in red; and those linking the cerebral cortex, deep pontine nuclei, cerebellum, and spinal cord are shown in green.

that are fed back to distal structures such as the cerebral cortex. The changes in the neural response pattern in the Purkinje cell as a function of movement would constitute a learned cerebellar response. The likelihood that learning takes place in the cerebellum is enhanced by the knowledge that the cerebellar cortex receives such a wide variety of sensory inputs, which include somatosensory, vestibular, visual, and auditory impulses. It is plausible to speculate that each of these sensory modalities may contribute to the learning process within the cerebellum.

There is much that we do not know about the role of learning in the cerebellum. We have little knowledge about the regions of cerebellum where learning takes place. We also have little understanding of the specific mechanisms involved in learning and what role specific sensory inputs play in the learning process. It is anticipated that future research will help to provide us with a better understanding of these mechanisms.

CEREBELLAR DISORDERS

The significance of the feedback pathways for motor functions is most appropriately understood when considered with respect to disorders of the cerebellum. When one or more of the feedback mechanisms are disrupted, a disorder of movement on the side of the body ipsilateral to the lesion emerges. The two types of such cerebellar disorders that have been described include **ataxia** (i.e., errors in the range, rate, force, and direction of movement resulting in loss of muscle coordination in producing smooth movements) and **hypotonia** (i.e., diminution of muscle tone).

ATAXIA

There are a number of disorders that include ataxic movements. In particular, loss of coordination (called **asynergy**) is quite frequent with patients who have incurred cerebellar lesions. The components of complex movements occur as a series of simple individual movements (called **decomposition of movement**). The patient may also not be able to accurately move his hand in space. For example, if the patient is asked to move his hand to touch his nose, he will either undershoot or overshoot the mark. This disorder is called **dysmetria**. Alternatively, the patient may be unable to make rapid alternating rotational movements of her hand. This disorder is called **dysdiadochokinesia**. As the patient voluntarily attempts to move her limb, she may display a tremor, which is called an **intention tremor**. All of these disorders most frequently involve the cerebellar hemispheres and presumably reflect a disruption of the feedback circuit between the cerebellar cortex and the cerebral cortex that governs movements of the distal musculature.

Ataxia may also result from damage to other regions of the cerebellum. If the lesion involves the flocculonodular lobe or the vermal region of the posterior or anterior lobes, patients will display a gait ataxia. They will walk with a very wide and slow gait (i.e., with legs widely separated), and they may also have a tendency to fall towards the side of the lesion. These symptoms have been shown to occur in cases of alcoholic cerebellar degeneration preferentially affecting the anterior lobe. Such lesions interfere with the feedback circuits involving either (or both) the vestibulocerebellum or spinocerebellum and their connections with the fastigial nucleus and its output pathways to the vestibular nuclei, reticular formation, and, ultimately, the spinal cord.

HYPOTONIA

Hypotonia has been associated with damage to parts of the cerebellar cortex, but the specific regions have not been clearly identified. It has been suggested that lesions, possibly of the paravermal region or hemisphere of the posterior lobe, are linked to this disorder. The precise mechanism underlying this disorder remains unknown. Because the outputs of the cerebellum to a brainstem structure, such as the lateral vestibular nucleus (which excites extensor motor neurons), are typically excitatory, such a lesion may cause loss of excitation to the lateral vestibular nucleus (from the fastigial nucleus), resulting in loss of excitatory input to the spinal cord motor neurons and subsequent hypotonia.

CEREBELLAR NYSTAGMUS AND GAIT ATAXIA

Lesions of the vermal region of the cerebellar cortex or fastigial nucleus can result in nystagmus. Presumably, the effect is due to a disruption of the inputs into the medial longitudinal fasciculus from vestibular nuclei. This is likely caused by the loss of or change in inputs into the vestibular nuclei from the fastigial nucleus because of the lesion in the fastigial nucleus or cerebellar cortical regions that project to the fastigial nucleus.

CLINICAL CASE

HISTORY

William is a 59-year-old man who has been drinking alcohol heavily since the age of 15. Sometimes, he would consume up to 2 pints of whiskey per day, although he would often drink cheap wine, cold syrup, or anything with alcohol in it that he could find in large amounts. He finally decided to seek medical attention when he began to have problems with an unsteady, "waddling" gait. He now needed to stand with his feet far apart in order to maintain his balance.

EXAMINATION

The physician who evaluated William tested his cognitive abilities and found some minor memory deficits. When asked to touch the doctor's finger, followed by touching his own nose, William's hand movements were somewhat unsteady and missed the target, which he then corrected. When asked to slide one heel down the contralateral shin, William's movements were clumsy and far worse than the arms. When asked to walk, his walk was slightly unsteady, with his feet placed wide apart. When attempting to walk in tandem fashion, with one foot in front of the other, he began to fall. The neurologist ordered a magnetic resonance imaging (MRI) scan of William's head.

EXPLANATION

William has alcoholic cerebellar degeneration. It is most likely caused by degeneration of neurons of the cerebellar cortex via nutritional deficiency. The cells of the cerebellum most affected are the Purkinje neurons, usually in the regions of the anterior aspects of the vermal and paravermal portions of the anterior lobe (see Fig. 21-7). Because of involvement of the midline of the cerebellum, structures such as the trunk are primarily affected, causing gait difficulties. Because the legs are represented in the anterior aspect of the paravermal portion of the anterior lobe in the cerebellar homunculus, the legs are affected more than the arms. The gait deficit described in William's legs is referred to as *ataxia*.

Imaging scans, such as an MRI scan, are able to demonstrate loss of volume in the vermis. This loss of volume is often indicative of a chronic, rather than an acute, problem and is irreversible. Therapies often used to minimize any further damage include vitamin replacement (i.e., nicotinic acid therapy plus other vitamins), discontinuation of alcohol, and physical therapy.

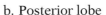

CHAPTER TEST

QUESTIONS

Choose the best answer for each question.

Questions 1 and 2. A middle-aged man was admitted to a local hospital with a cerebellar hemorrhage resulting from hypertension. Several days later, the patient displayed "past pointing" and "asynergia of movement."

1. The region of cerebellum that was most likely affected by the hemorrhage was:
   a. Fastigial nucleus
   b. Neocerebellar hemispheres
   c. Vermal region of the anterior lobe
   d. Vermal region of the posterior lobe
   e. Flocculonodular lobe

2. The region affected by the hemorrhage is one that shares direct or indirect connections with:
   a. Vestibular nuclei
   b. Reticular formation
   c. Fastigial nucleus
   d. Motor regions of cerebral cortex
   e. Sensory regions of spinal cord

Questions 3 and 4. An individual is diagnosed with a cerebellar tumor. As a result, the patient presents with nausea, vomiting, dizziness, nystagmus, and wide "ataxic" gait with disturbances of equilibrium.

3. The tumor is most likely located in the:
   a. Dentate nucleus
   b. Interposed nuclei
   c. Lateral aspect of neocerebellar hemispheres
   d. Anterior lobe
   e. Flocculonodular lobe

4. A primary source of input to the region where the tumor is located includes:
   a. Dentate nucleus
   b. Red nucleus
   c. Cerebral cortex
   d. Vestibular nuclei
   e. Ventral horn of spinal cord

5. There is a convergence of inputs from the dorsal spinocerebellar, ventral spinocerebellar, and cuneocerebellar tracts within the cerebellum. These major cerebellar afferent fibers terminate primarily in the:
   a. Anterior lobe

b. Posterior lobe
c. Flocculonodular lobe
d. Interposed nuclei
e. Dentate nucleus

ANSWERS AND EXPLANATIONS

1. Answer: b

A variety of the cerebellar ataxias are associated with lesions of the neocerebellar hemispheres, in particular, if the movement disorders involve the distal musculature. "Past pointing" involves the distal musculature, and asynergia of movement is associated with a failure of the planning mode of the cerebellar cortex, which is represented in the neocerebellar hemispheres. The axial musculature is represented in the vermal region.

2. Answer: d

The cerebellar hemisphere is linked anatomically and functionally (in a reciprocal manner) with motor regions of the cerebral cortex. The vestibular nuclei, reticular formation, and fastigial nucleus are all associated anatomically and functionally with more medial (vermal and paravermal) regions of the cerebellar cortex. Likewise, the relationship of the cerebellar hemisphere with sensory regions of the spinal cord is very indirect, if existent.

3 and 4. Answers: 3-e, 4-d

The flocculonodular lobe receives inputs from the vestibular system. Disruption of these inputs and the loss of ability to integrate such messages and provide the necessary feedback signals to the vestibular nuclei and reticular formation through the fastigial nuclei result in disturbances of gait and equilibrium as well as nystagmus. The cerebellar hemispheres are primarily concerned with movements associated with the distal musculature, as are the interposed and dentate nuclei, which are linked anatomically and functionally to the red nucleus and cerebral cortex. Axons of the ventral horn of the spinal cord project to skeletal muscle and not to the brainstem or cerebellum.

5. Answer: a

The anterior lobe receives major inputs from the spinal cord and is referred to as the spinocerebellum. These inputs contain fibers that convey signals associated with muscle spindle and Golgi tendon activity, as well as some tactile inputs that are transmitted through the dorsal spinocerebellar, ventral spinocerebellar, and cuneocerebellar tracts. The posterior lobe receives inputs mainly from the cerebral cortex, inferior olivary nucleus, red nucleus, and reticular formation. The flocculonodular lobe receives inputs from vestibular neurons. The dentate and interposed nuclei are anatomically and functionally related mainly to the posterior lobe and, in addition, receive only collateral inputs from fibers that are afferent to the cerebellum.

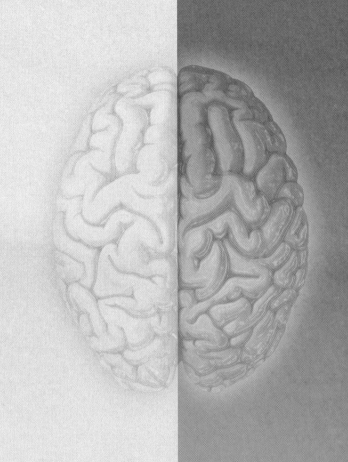

SECTION VI

Integrative Systems

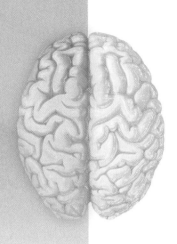

CHAPTER 22

THE AUTONOMIC NERVOUS SYSTEM

OBJECTIVES

After reading this chapter, the student should be able to:

1. Describe and diagram the three divisions (sympathetic, parasympathetic, and enteric) of the autonomic nervous system and list their functions

2. Describe and diagram the anatomy of the sympathetic pathways including the location of preganglionic and postganglionic neurons and the intervening ganglia

3. Describe and diagram the anatomy of the parasympathetic pathways including the location of preganglionic and postganglionic neurons and the intervening ganglia

4. Describe and diagram the autonomic innervation of some selected organs (e.g., the eye, salivary glands, heart, lungs, blood vessels, gastrointestinal tract, adrenal medulla, and urinary bladder)

5. Describe and diagram the cardiovascular and respiratory regulatory areas in the central nervous system

6. List and describe the major disorders of the autonomic nervous system

INTRODUCTION

The function of the autonomic nervous system is to maintain, *at a constant level*, the internal environment of the body (homeostasis). This system regulates involuntary functions such as blood pressure, heart rate, respiration, body temperature, glandular secretion, digestion, and reproduction. Based on the nature of its functions, the autonomic nervous system is also called the **involuntary or vegetative nervous system**. The system consists of both afferent and efferent components.

DIVISIONS OF THE AUTONOMIC NERVOUS SYSTEM

The autonomic nervous system is divided into three divisions: sympathetic, parasympathetic, and enteric.

SYMPATHETIC DIVISION

The neurons from which the outflow of the sympathetic division originates (sympathetic preganglionic neurons) are located in the **intermediolateral cell column** (IML) of the first thoracic to second lumbar (T1-L2) segments of the spinal cord. For this reason, the sympathetic nervous system is sometimes called the thoracolumbar division of the autonomic nervous system. An overview of the anatomical organization of the sympathetic and parasympathetic divisions of the autonomic nervous system is presented in the following sections (Figs. 22-1 and 22-2). A detailed description of autonomic innervation of important organs is provided later in this chapter.

Spinal Sympathetic Preganglionic Neurons

In the spinal cord, the distribution of sympathetic preganglionic neurons in the thoracolumbar cord

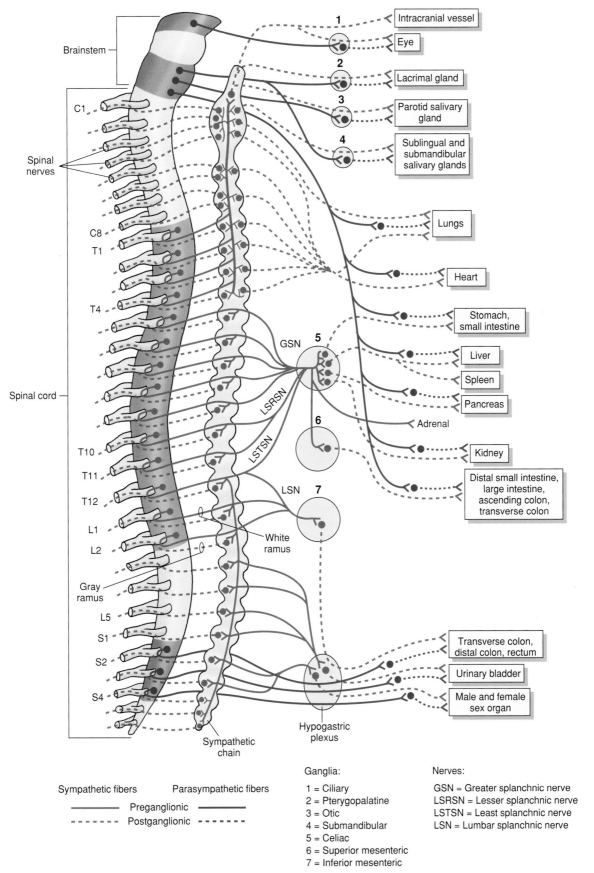

Figure 22–1 An overview of the sympathetic and parasympathetic components of the autonomic nervous system. Thoracolumbar division = red; craniosacral division = blue.
Abbreviations: C, cervical; T, thoracic; L, lumbar; S, sacral spinal segments (see text for details).

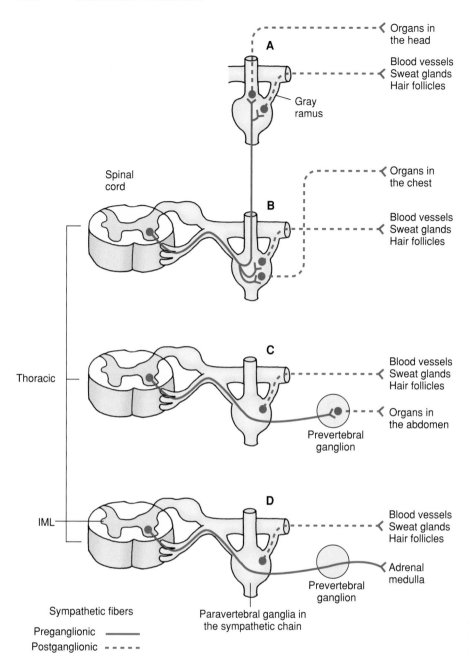

Figure 22–2 Examples of the course of preganglionic and postganglionic sympathetic fibers innervating different organs. (A) Organs in the head. (B) Organs in the chest. (C) Organs in the abdomen. (D) Adrenal gland. Also note that, at each level, the axons of the postganglionic neurons in the paravertebral ganglia re-enter the corresponding spinal nerves through gray rami, travel within or along the spinal nerve, and innervate the blood vessels, sweat glands, and erectile muscle of hair follicles.

exhibits rostral-to-caudal **viscerotopy**. Thus, the location of the sympathetic preganglionic neurons providing innervation to the eye is most rostral (T1-T2); the location of the neurons innervating the heart and lungs is more caudal; and the location of neurons innervating the gastrointestinal tract (GIT), bladder, and genitals is most caudal.

Paravertebral Ganglia and the Sympathetic Chains

There are two **sympathetic chains** (also called sympathetic trunks), one located on each side of the vertebral column. Each sympathetic chain consists of a ganglionated nerve trunk. These ganglia are called **paravertebral ganglia** (25 pairs) and represent one of the sites where the **sympathetic postganglionic neurons** are located. Axons of the sympathetic preganglionic neurons synapse on many **sympathetic postganglionic neurons** in the sympathetic chain; the ratio of preganglionic to postganglionic fibers is about 1:30. This divergence facilitates coordinated activity of sympathetic neurons at different levels of the spinal cord. In the autonomic nervous system, preganglionic axons are myelinated, whereas the postganglionic axons are unmyelinated.

The course of preganglionic and postganglionic sympathetic fibers at different levels of the spinal cord is shown in Figures 22-1 and 22-2. The axons of sympathetic preganglionic neurons located at T1-L2 exit the spinal cord via ventral roots, travel a short distance in the corresponding spinal nerves, and then enter the sympathetic chain via the **white rami** (they appear white because they contain myelinated axons). Some of these preganglionic axons synapse on postganglionic neurons located in the paravertebral ganglia, while others pass through the paravertebral ganglia without synapsing and finally synapse on postganglionic neurons located in the **prevertebral ganglia** (see next section). The axons of some of the postganglionic neurons located in the paravertebral ganglia exit the sympathetic chain via visceral branches and innervate different organs (Figs. 22-1 and 22-2). For example, sympathetic postganglionic fibers from the superior cervical ganglion exit the sympathetic chain and supply the organs located in the head and neck, including the blood vessels of the brain and cranial muscles, eyes, and lacrimal and salivary glands. Sympathetic postganglionic fibers from the middle and inferior cervical ganglia provide sympathetic innervation to the organs located in the chest cavity (e.g., the heart, lungs, and bronchi).

Some postganglionic fibers exit the sympathetic chain via the **gray rami** (they appear gray because the fibers passing through them are unmyelinated), re-enter the corresponding spinal nerve, course within or along the spinal nerve, and then innervate the blood vessels, sweat glands, and erectile muscles of some hair follicles in the tissues supplied by this spinal nerve (Fig. 22-2). It should be noted that gray rami are present at all levels of the sympathetic chain, whereas white rami are present only in the thoracolumbar region of the sympathetic chain (T1-L2 level).

Prevertebral Ganglia

As mentioned earlier, the sympathetic nervous system includes two types of ganglia: the paravertebral and the prevertebral ganglia. The sympathetic postganglionic neurons that innervate the abdominal viscera are located in the prevertebral ganglia. Unlike the paravertebral ganglia, the prevertebral ganglia are located distal to the sympathetic chain and closer to the organs that they innervate. The course of sympathetic fibers that innervate different abdominal organs is as follows. The axons of the sympathetic preganglionic neurons located in the IML at the T5-T9 spinal segments exit through the ventral roots, travel a short distance in the spinal nerve, enter the sympathetic chain via the white rami, exit the sympathetic chain without

synapsing, and form the **greater splanchnic nerve**. The axons of sympathetic preganglionic neurons located in the IML at T10-T12 follow a similar course and form the **lesser** and **least splanchnic nerves**. The axons of the greater, lesser, and least splanchnic nerves synapse on the postganglionic neurons located in the **celiac ganglion**.

The postganglionic fibers emerging from the celiac ganglion innervate the smooth muscle and glands in the stomach, small intestine, liver, spleen, pancreas, and kidney. Some sympathetic preganglionic fibers in the greater, lesser, and least splanchnic nerves pass through the celiac ganglion (without synapsing) and make a synapse on the cells in the **adrenal medulla** that secrete epinephrine and norepinephrine. It should be noted that the adrenal medulla is analogous to sympathetic ganglion, and the secretory cells present in it are functionally analogous to sympathetic postganglionic neurons.

Some sympathetic preganglionic fibers in the greater, lesser, and least splanchnic nerves pass through the celiac ganglion (without synapsing) and synapse on the postganglionic neurons located in the superior mesenteric ganglion. Postganglionic neurons located in this ganglion innervate the distal portions of the small intestine, large intestine, and ascending and transverse colon. Some sympathetic preganglionic fibers from L1-L2 spinal segments pass through the sympathetic chain without synapsing, travel in the lumbar splanchnic nerves, and synapse on the postganglionic neurons located in the inferior mesenteric ganglion. The postganglionic fibers from this ganglion then pass through inferior hypogastric (pelvic) plexus to innervate the transverse and distal colon and rectum. Some preganglionic fibers from L1-L2 spinal segments descend in the sympathetic chain, pass through the paravertebral ganglia, and synapse on postganglionic neurons in the inferior hypogastric plexus. The postganglionic fibers from these neurons then innervate the urinary bladder and male (penis) and female (clitoris) erectile tissue. Other preganglionic fibers from L1-L2 spinal segments descend in the sympathetic chain and synapse on postganglionic neurons in the paravertebral ganglia. Postganglionic fibers from these neurons then re-enter the spinal nerves via the gray rami and innervate the blood vessels, sweat glands, and erectile muscles of some hair follicles in the lower limb and lower part of the trunk.

Functions of the Sympathetic Nervous System

This division of the autonomic nervous system is activated in stressful situations. Thus, activation of the sympathetic nervous system results in an increase in blood flow in the skeletal muscles; an increase in heart rate, blood pressure, and blood sugar level; and pupillary dilation (mydriasis). These effects are widespread because one sympathetic preganglionic axon innervates several postganglionic neurons. All of these responses prepare the individual for "fight" or "flight." For example, in the need for "flight," an increase in blood flow in the skeletal muscles will help in running away from the site of danger. In the need for "fight," an increase in heart rate and blood pressure will help in better perfusion of different organs; an increase in blood sugar will provide energy; and pupillary dilation will provide better vision. The effects of simultaneous activation of the parasympathetic division of the autonomic nervous system (described later) complement the effects of sympathetic stimulation.

PARASYMPATHETIC DIVISION

The neurons from which the parasympathetic outflow arises (parasympathetic preganglionic neurons) are located in the brainstem (see Chapters 10 to 12; midbrain, pons, and medulla oblongata) and the sacral region of the spinal cord (second, third, and fourth sacral segments [S2-S4]). For this reason, this division is sometimes referred to as the **craniosacral division** (Fig. 22-1). A description of the parasympathetic preganglionic neurons, located in the brainstem and spinal cord, is provided in the following sections.

Brainstem Parasympathetic Preganglionic Neurons

The parasympathetic preganglionic neurons are located in the following nuclei of the brainstem.

The **Edinger-Westphal nucleus** of the oculomotor nerve (CN III), located in the midbrain, provides parasympathetic innervation to the constrictor muscles of the iris and circumferential muscles of the ciliary body. The **superior salivatory nucleus of the facial nerve** (CN VII), located in the lower pons, provides parasympathetic innervation to the lacrimal glands and sublingual and submandibular salivary glands. The **inferior salivatory nucleus of the glossopharyngeal nerve** (CN IX), located caudal to the superior salivatory nucleus in the upper medulla, provides parasympathetic innervation to the parotid salivary gland. Other nuclei where the parasympathetic preganglionic neurons are located include the **nucleus ambiguus** and the **dorsal motor nucleus of vagus.** The dorsal motor nucleus of vagus is located in the caudal aspect of the dorsal medulla, while the nucleus ambiguus is located more ventrally at approximately the same level of the medulla. The compact region of nucleus ambiguus provides innervation to the muscles of the larynx and pharynx. The region surrounding the compact zone of the nucleus ambiguus contains preganglionic neurons that provide parasympathetic innervation to the heart and mediate the decrease in heart rate following parasympathetic stimulation. The preganglionic neurons located in the dorsal motor nucleus of vagus provide primarily parasympathetic innervation to the lungs, pancreas, and gastrointestinal tract (GIT) and control secretions of the glands located in these organs. In addition, their activation elicits peristalsis in the GIT. These neurons may also play a role in eliciting cardiac inhibitory actions because they do provide parasympathetic innervation to the heart, although to a lesser extent than provided by the nucleus ambiguus.

Spinal Parasympathetic Preganglionic Neurons

As mentioned earlier, in the spinal cord, the parasympathetic preganglionic neurons are located in the IML of the sacral spinal cord at the S2-S4 level (Fig. 22-1). Their axons exit through the ventral roots, travel through pelvic nerves, and synapse on postganglionic neurons that are located close to or within the organs being innervated. It should be noted that, in the parasympathetic system, the terminal ganglia are located near or within the organs innervated. Thus, the parasympathetic postganglionic fibers are relatively short, while the sympathetic postganglionic fibers are relatively long.

Functions of the Parasympathetic Nervous System

Activation of the parasympathetic division of the autonomic nervous system results in conservation and restoration of body energy. For example, a decrease in heart rate brought about by the activation of the parasympathetic nervous system will also decrease the demand for energy, while the increased activity of the gastrointestinal system will promote restoration of body energy. The effects of parasympathetic activation are localized and last for a short time. Important differences between the sympathetic and parasympathetic nervous system are shown in Table 22-1.

ENTERIC DIVISION

The enteric division consists of neurons in the wall of the gut that regulate gastrointestinal motility and secretion. The enteric system consists of two layers of neurons that are present in the smooth muscle of the gut: the **myenteric (Auerbach's)** and

Table 22–1 A Comparison Between the Sympathetic and Parasympathetic Divisions of the Autonomic Nervous System

	Parasympathetic	Sympathetic
Preganglionic neurons: location	Nucleus of oculomotor nerve (pupil); superior salivatory nucleus of facial nerve, inferior salivatory nucleus of glossopharyngeal nerve (salivary glands); facial nerve (lacrimal glands); dorsal motor nucleus of vagus (GIT, kidney); nucleus ambiguus (heart); intermediolateral cell column of the sacral spinal cord at S2-S4 level. Target organ is shown in parentheses.	Intermediolateral cell column of the spinal cord (T1-L2)
Outflow	CN III, VII, IX, X; pelvic nerves	Ventral roots at T1-L2
Preganglionic fibers; transmitter at their terminals (within ganglia)	Myelinated; the preganglionic fibers are relatively long because the ganglia receiving them are located within the target organ or close to it; acetylcholine	Myelinated; the preganglionic fibers are relatively short because the ganglia receiving them are located at some distance from the target organ; acetylcholine
Ganglia	Ganglia located close to the organs (ciliary, otic); ganglia located within the organs (heart, bronchial tree, GIT)	Paravertebral ganglia in sympathetic chain (25 pairs); prevertebral ganglia (celiac, renal, superior, and inferior mesenteric)
Postganglionic fibers	Short, nonmyelinated	Long, nonmyelinated
Transmitter at the terminals of postganglionic fibers	Acetylcholine	Norepinephrine (acetylcholine in sweat glands)
Ratio of preganglionic to postganglionic neurons and extent of action	A single preganglionic fiber may connect with only one or two postganglionic neurons. This arrangement favors localized actions.	A single preganglionic fiber may connect with numerous postganglionic neurons; this arrangement results in widespread responses

submucosal (Meissner's) plexuses. The neurons of the myenteric (Auerbach's) plexus control gastrointestinal motility, while the neurons of the submucosal (Meissner's) plexus control water and ion movement across the intestinal epithelium. Excitatory transmitters of motor neurons and interneurons in the smooth muscle of the GIT are probably acetylcholine and substance P. Inhibitory transmitters are not yet known. The enteric nervous system is intrinsically active.

The enteric system is also controlled by sympathetic and parasympathetic innervation (extrinsic innervation). The sympathetic innervation is derived from branches of thoracic, lumbar, and sacral sympathetic chains. Most of the sympathetic fibers of the extrinsic innervation are postganglionic. The parasympathetic innervation is derived from the vagus and pelvic nerves. Most of the parasympathetic fibers of the extrinsic innervation are preganglionic. The extrinsic system can override the intrinsic system when the sympathetic or parasympathetic nervous system is activated.

AUTONOMIC INNERVATION OF SOME SELECTED ORGANS

Many organs receive dual innervation (i.e., from the sympathetic as well as the parasympathetic divisions of the autonomic nervous system). As a rule, in most of the organs with dual innervation, activation of the parasympathetic and sympathetic divisions has antagonistic actions. Exceptions to this rule are the salivary glands, where activation of either system results in increased secretion of saliva; sympathetic stimulation produces viscous saliva, whereas parasympathetic stimulation produces watery saliva. The autonomic innervation of some selected organs is discussed in the following sections.

UPPER EYELID

The **upper eyelid** is raised by the **levator palpebrae superioris** muscle. The bulk of levator palpebrae superioris is a skeletal muscle that is innervated by the caudal-central nucleus of the oculomotor nuclear complex. A small portion of this muscle, the tarsal muscle, consists of smooth muscle fibers that receive innervation from sympathetic postganglionic fibers arising from the superior cervical ganglion (Fig. 22-3A). The **orbital muscle of Müller** is also nonstriated and maintains the eyeball in a forward position in the orbit. This muscle is also innervated by sympathetic postganglionic fibers arising from the superior cervical ganglion. Sympathetic preganglionic fibers synapsing on the postganglionic neurons in the superior cervical ganglion arise from the

IML at the T1-T4 level. Interruption of the sympathetic innervation to the tarsal muscle results in **pseudoptosis** (partial drooping of the upper eyelid), and damage to the orbital muscle of Müller results in **enophthalmos** (sinking of the eyeball in the orbit). These symptoms are characteristic of Horner's syndrome (described later in this chapter). It should be noted that damage to the oculomotor nerve also causes paresis of the levator palpebrae superioris muscle, which results in **ptosis** (drooping of the upper eyelid).

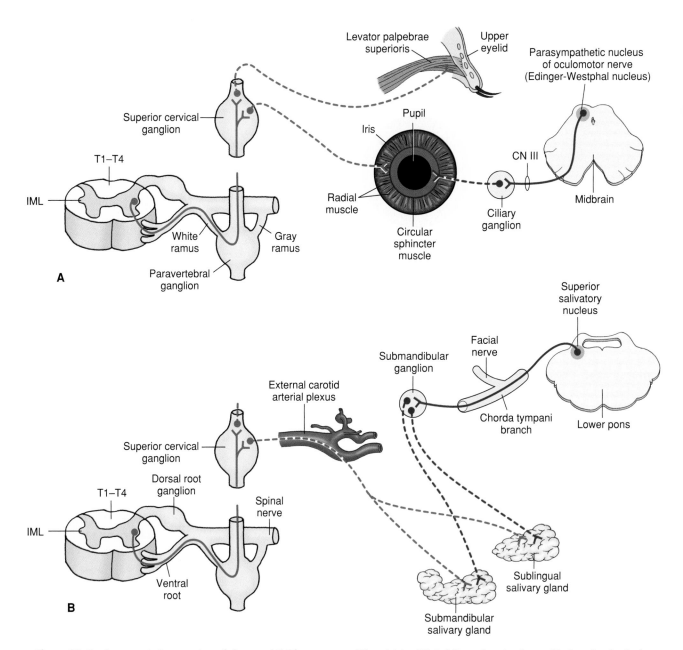

Figure 22–3 Autonomic innervation of the eye. (A) The upper eyelid and iris. (B) Sublingual and submandibular glands. Red = sympathetic nervous system, blue = parasympathetic nervous system. Solid lines = preganglionic fibers, dotted lines = postganglionic fibers.

IRIS AND THE CILIARY BODY OF THE EYE

Sympathetic Innervation

The axons of sympathetic preganglionic neurons, which are located in the IML at the T1 level, synapse on neurons in the superior cervical ganglia. The postganglionic sympathetic fibers arising from the latter innervate the radial smooth muscle fibers of the iris (Fig. 22-3A). Activation of the sympathetic nervous system results in contraction of the radial muscles of the iris, which causes **mydriasis** (pupillary dilation).

Parasympathetic Innervation

The axons of the parasympathetic preganglionic neurons located in the **Edinger-Westphal nucleus** (parasympathetic nucleus of the oculomotor nerve) leave the brainstem through the **oculomotor nerve (CN III)** and synapse on the parasympathetic postganglionic neurons in the ciliary ganglion that is located in the orbit. The postganglionic fibers from the ciliary ganglion enter the eyeball and innervate the circular (sphincter) smooth muscle fibers of the iris (Fig. 22-3A) and the circumferential muscles of the ciliary body. When the parasympathetic innervation to the eye is activated, the circular muscles of the pupil and the circumferential muscles of the ciliary body contract. Contraction of circular muscles of the iris causes **miosis** (constriction of the pupil). Contraction of circumferential muscles of the ciliary body results in the relaxation of the **suspensory ligaments of the lens**. The lens becomes more convex, thus allowing for greater refraction of the light rays, which is more suitable for near vision. These two responses (i.e., constriction of the pupil and making the lens more convex) are included in the **accommodation reflex** (see Chapter 16).

SUBLINGUAL AND SUBMANDIBULAR SALIVARY GLANDS

Sympathetic Innervation

The preganglionic neurons that provide sympathetic innervation to these glands are located in the T1-T4 level of the IML. The preganglionic fibers synapse on postganglionic neurons in the superior cervical ganglion. The postganglionic fibers pass through the external carotid arterial plexus and innervate these glands (Fig. 22-3B). Activation of the sympathetic innervation to these glands produces viscous salivary secretions.

Parasympathetic Innervation

The parasympathetic preganglionic fibers arising from the neurons located in the superior salivatory nucleus leave the lower pons through the facial nerve (CN VII). These fibers exit through the chorda tympani branch of the facial nerve and synapse on postganglionic neurons in the submandibular ganglion. The postganglionic parasympathetic fibers from the submandibular ganglion innervate sublingual and submandibular salivary glands (Fig. 22-3B). Activation of these parasympathetic fibers (secretomotor fibers) results in the secretion of watery saliva.

PAROTID SALIVARY GLANDS

Sympathetic Innervation

The preganglionic neurons that provide sympathetic innervation to the parotid salivary glands are located in the T1-T4 level of the IML. The preganglionic fibers synapse on postganglionic neurons in the superior cervical ganglion. The postganglionic fibers pass through the external carotid arterial plexus and innervate the parotid salivary gland (Fig. 22-4A). Activation of the sympathetic innervation to these glands produces viscous salivary secretions.

Parasympathetic Innervation

The axons of the neurons located in the **inferior salivatory nucleus**, which is located in the upper medulla, exit through the **glossopharyngeal nerve (CN IX)**. The parasympathetic preganglionic fibers pass through the tympanic plexus and synapse on postganglionic neurons located in the **otic ganglion**. The parasympathetic postganglionic fibers from the otic ganglion pass through the auriculotemporal nerve and innervate the parotid salivary gland (Fig. 22-4A). Activation of these fibers results in secretion of watery saliva from the parotid gland into the oral cavity.

LACRIMAL GLANDS

Sympathetic Innervation

The sympathetic fibers innervating the lacrimal gland follow the same course that was described for the sympathetic innervation of the sublingual and submandibular glands (Fig. 22-4B). The effects of activation of the sympathetic nervous system on secretion of the lacrimal glands are not clearly established.

Parasympathetic Innervation

The parasympathetic preganglionic fibers arising from the **superior salivatory nucleus** (located in the lower pons) exit through the greater petrosal

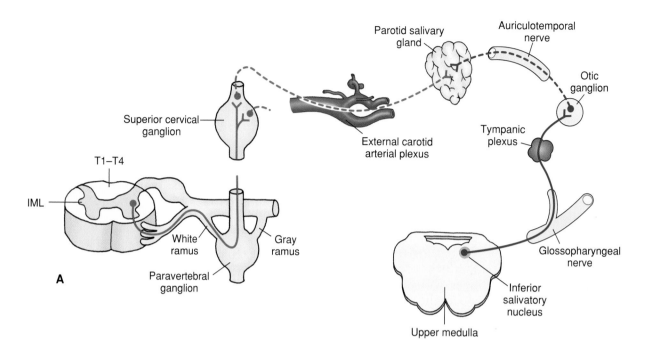

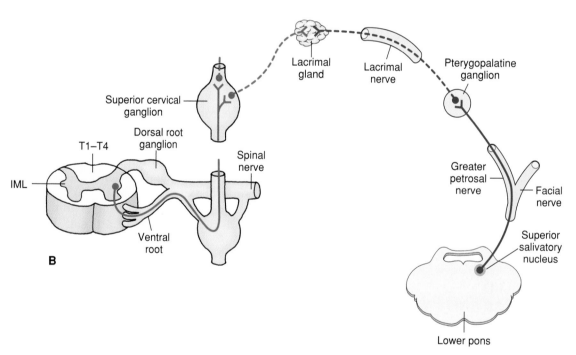

Figure 22–4 Autonomic innervation of (A) the parotid salivary gland and (B) the lacrimal gland (see text for details). Red = sympathetic nervous system, blue = parasympathetic nervous system. Solid lines = preganglionic fibers, dotted lines = postganglionic fibers.

branch of the facial nerve and synapse on the postganglionic neurons in the pterygopalatine ganglion. The postganglionic fibers from these neurons reach the lacrimal gland through the lacrimal nerve (Fig. 22-4B). Activation of these postganglionic parasympathetic fibers results in secretion of tears.

HEART

Sympathetic Innervation

The sympathetic preganglionic neurons innervating the heart are located in the T1-T4 spinal segments. The sympathetic preganglionic fibers enter the sympathetic chain via the ventral roots and synapse on postganglionic neurons located in the thoracic ganglia (1–4) and inferior, middle, and superior cervical ganglia. Sometimes, the last two cervical and first two thoracic ganglia are fused to form the star-shaped **stellate ganglion.** Sympathetic postganglionic innervation to the heart arises from thoracic ganglia (1–4) and inferior, middle, and superior cervical ganglia. Sympathetic postganglionic fibers innervating the heart also arise from the stel-

late ganglion when it is present. The sympathetic postganglionic fibers arising from these ganglia innervate all regions of the heart (**sinoatrial node, atria, atrioventricular node,** and **ventricles**) (Fig. 22-5). Activation of the sympathetic nervous system results in an increase in heart rate by increasing the pacemaker activity of the sinoatrial node cells. Impulse conduction at the atrioventricular node and the contractile force of atrial and ventricular muscle fibers are increased.

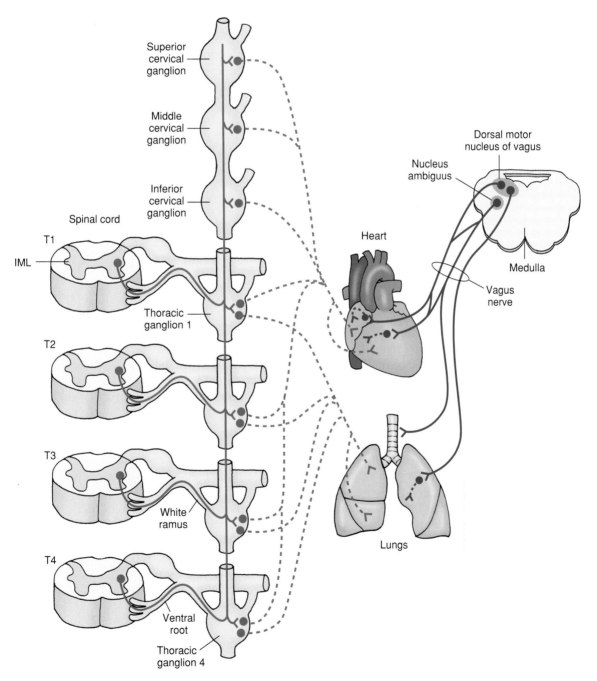

Figure 22–5 Autonomic innervation of the heart and lungs (see text for details). Red = sympathetic nervous system, blue = parasympathetic nervous system. Solid lines = preganglionic fibers, dotted lines = postganglionic fibers.

Parasympathetic Innervation

Animal experiments have shown that preganglionic neurons providing parasympathetic innervation to the heart are predominantly located in the region surrounding the compact zone of the **nucleus ambiguus** (Fig. 22-5). A component of the parasympathetic innervation to the heart arises also from the **dorsal motor nucleus of vagus**. These two nuclei are located in the medulla. The preganglionic fibers from parasympathetic preganglionic neurons located in the nucleus ambiguus and dorsal motor nucleus of vagus exit the ventrolateral medulla through the vagus and synapse on the postganglionic neurons located in the heart. The postganglionic parasympathetic fibers innervate the sinoatrial node, atria, and atrioventricular node. The ventricles of the heart receive relatively little postganglionic parasympathetic innervation. Activation of the parasympathetic division of the autonomic nervous system results in a decrease in heart rate by decreasing the pacemaker activity of the sinoatrial node cells. The impulse conduction through the atrioventricular node and the contractile force of the ventricular muscle are decreased.

LUNGS

Sympathetic Innervation

The sympathetic preganglionic neurons innervating the lungs are located in the IML at the T1-T4 spinal level. The sympathetic preganglionic fibers from these neurons synapse on T1-T4 ganglia in the sympathetic chain. Postganglionic fibers from these neurons innervate the smooth muscle of the bronchial tree (Fig. 22-5). Activation of the sympathetic nervous system results in bronchodilation.

Parasympathetic Innervation

The parasympathetic preganglionic fibers arise from neurons located in the dorsal motor nucleus of the vagus, travel to the thoracic cavity in the vagus nerves, and synapse on postganglionic neurons located in the lungs (Fig. 22-5). The postganglionic fibers then innervate the smooth muscles in the bronchial tree. Stimulation of the parasympathetic nervous system results in bronchoconstriction and an increase in the secretion of the bronchial glands.

GASTROINTESTINAL TRACT

Sympathetic Innervation

The axons from the sympathetic preganglionic neurons located in the IML at the T5-T9 level pass through the sympathetic chain without synapsing, travel through the greater splanchnic nerve, and synapse on neurons in the celiac ganglion. The preganglionic fibers arising from the IML at T10-T12 also pass through the sympathetic chain without synapsing and emerge as **lesser** and **least splanchnic nerves**. These fibers also synapse on postganglionic neurons in the celiac ganglion. The postganglionic fibers emerging from the celiac ganglion innervate the smooth muscle and glands of the stomach and small intestine. Some preganglionic fibers in the greater, lesser, and least splanchnic nerves pass through the celiac ganglion and synapse on postganglionic neurons located in the superior mesenteric ganglion. These postganglionic neurons then innervate the distal portions of the small intestine, large intestine, and ascending and transverse colon. The axons emerging from the sympathetic preganglionic neurons located in the IML at the T12-L2 pass through the sympathetic chain without synapsing and emerge as **lumbar splanchnic nerves**. These fibers then synapse on postganglionic neurons located in the inferior mesenteric ganglion. The postganglionic fibers emerging from the inferior mesenteric ganglion pass through the hypogastric plexus and innervate the transverse and distal colon and rectum (Fig. 22-6). Activation of the sympathetic nervous system, in different regions of the GIT, inhibits peristalsis and secretions of glands and contracts the sphincters.

Parasympathetic Innervation

The preganglionic neurons providing parasympathetic innervation to the stomach, small and large intestine, and colon are located in the dorsal motor nucleus of the vagus. These preganglionic fibers descend in the vagus nerves and synapse on postganglionic neurons located in the **myenteric (Auerbach's)** and **submucosal (Meissner's) plexuses** in these regions of the GIT. The postganglionic fibers from these plexuses then innervate the smooth muscle and glands of the stomach, small and large intestine, and ascending and transverse colon (Fig. 22-6). The parasympathetic preganglionic neurons innervating the transverse and distal colon and rectum are located in the IML of the sacral spinal cord at the S2-S4 level (Fig. 22-6). Their preganglionic fibers exit through the ventral roots, enter the pelvic nerves, and reach the myenteric (Auerbach's) and submucosal (Meissner's) plexuses. The postganglionic fibers arising from these plexuses innervate the smooth muscle and glands in these regions of the GIT. Stimulation of the parasympathetic nervous system, in this and other regions of the GIT, elicits peristalsis and secretion of glands and relaxes the sphincters.

As stated earlier, the enteric division of the autonomic nervous system, consisting of the myen-

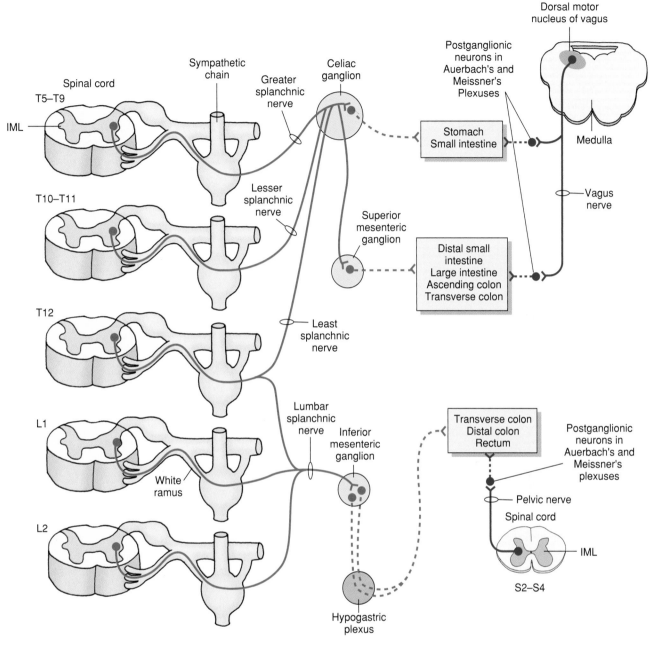

Figure 22–6 Autonomic innervation of the gastrointestinal tract (see text for details). Red = sympathetic nervous system, blue = parasympathetic nervous system. Solid lines = preganglionic fibers, dotted lines = postganglionic fibers.

teric (Auerbach's) and submucosal (Meissner's) plexuses, regulates gastrointestinal motility and secretion. This intrinsic system can be modulated by the extrinsic control of the GIT via sympathetic and parasympathetic innervation.

ADRENAL MEDULLA (SUPRARENAL GLAND)

The adrenal medulla is functionally analogous to a sympathetic ganglion; the adrenal medullary cells are directly innervated by the sympathetic pregan-

glionic neurons that are located in the IML at the T5-T9 level. The preganglionic fibers pass through the sympathetic chain, exit through the greater splanchnic nerve without synapsing on neurons in the celiac ganglion, and innervate the adrenal medulla. The preganglionic fibers arising from the neurons located in the IML at T10-T11 also contribute to the sympathetic innervation of the adrenal medulla. These preganglionic fibers pass through the sympathetic chain, exit through the lesser splanchnic nerve without synapsing in the celiac ganglion, and innervate the adrenal medulla

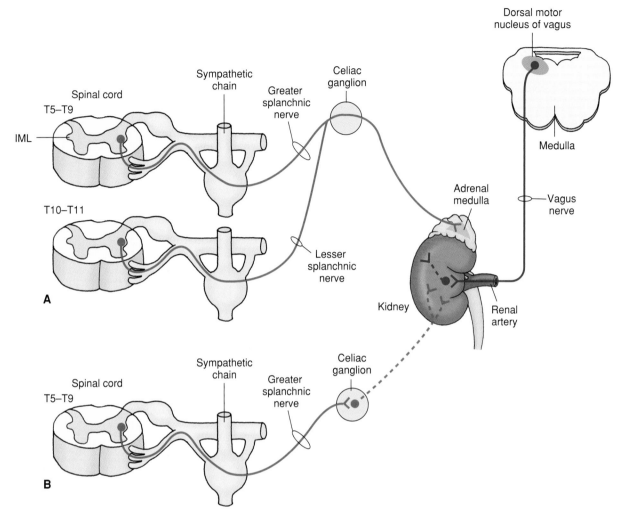

Figure 22–7 Autonomic innervation of the adrenal gland and kidney (see text for details). Red = sympathetic nervous system, blue = parasympathetic nervous system. Solid lines = preganglionic fibers, dotted lines = postganglionic fibers.

(Fig. 22-7). Acetylcholine is the transmitter released at the sympathetic preganglionic terminals innervating these cells. These cells secrete epinephrine (about 80%) and a small percentage (about 20%) of norepinephrine directly into the blood stream.

A rare catecholamine-secreting tumor of the neuroectodermal chromaffin cells is known as **pheochromocytoma.** These tumors occur in the adrenal medulla in a majority (85%) of these cases. Other major extra-adrenal sites where these tumors may be present include chromaffin cells associated with sympathetic nerves in the chest, abdomen, and pelvis. The tumors present in patients with pheochromocytoma contain secretory granules that release catecholamines, which elicit sustained or paroxysmal hypertension. Other disorders caused by excess circulating catecholamine concentrations include stroke, myocardial infarction, cardiac arrhythmias, and shock. Pheochromocytoma can be cured by surgical removal of the tumor. Phenoxybenzamine or

prazosin (alpha-adrenergic receptor blockers) or calcium channel blockers (e.g., verapamil) are used to control hypertension in these patients. Beta-adrenergic receptor blockers (e.g., propranolol) are used to prevent or treat supraventricular arrhythmias when present in these patients. For differential diagnosis of patients with primary hypertension and pheochromocytoma, an antihypertensive drug, clonidine, is administered orally. In patients with primary hypertension, plasma norepinephrine levels are decreased within 3 hours of the administration of clonidine, whereas this response is not observed in patients with pheochromocytoma.

KIDNEY

Sympathetic Innervation

The sympathetic preganglionic neurons are located in the IML at the T5-T9 level. The preganglionic fibers pass through the sympathetic chain, exit through the greater splanchnic nerve, and synapse on neurons in the celiac ganglia. The postganglionic fibers from the celiac ganglia innervate the kidney (Fig. 22-7). Sympathetic activation is believed to cause constriction of renal arteries.

Parasympathetic Innervation

The parasympathetic preganglionic fibers arising from the dorsal motor nucleus of vagus descend in the vagus nerves and enter the kidney along the renal artery (Fig. 22-7). It is believed that stimulation of these fibers causes vasodilation of the renal vascular bed.

URINARY BLADDER

Sympathetic Innervation

The sympathetic preganglionic neurons innervating the urinary bladder are located in the IML at the T12-L2 level. The sympathetic preganglionic fibers pass through the sympathetic chain and emerge in the lumbar splanchnic nerves. These fibers then synapse on the postganglionic neurons located in the inferior mesenteric ganglion. The postganglionic fibers from this ganglion reach the urinary bladder through the **hypogastric plexus** (Fig. 22-8). Traditionally, it was believed that activation of sympathetic fibers innervating the bladder results in relaxation of the detrusor muscle and contraction of the sphincter located at the neck of the bladder. However, it is now believed that sympathetic fibers innervating the bladder are primarily distributed to the blood vessels in this organ.

The sympathetic nerves innervating the sphincter located at the bladder neck (**sphincter vesicae**) play a minor role in maintaining urinary continence by contracting this sphincter. However, these nerves also play an important role during ejacula-

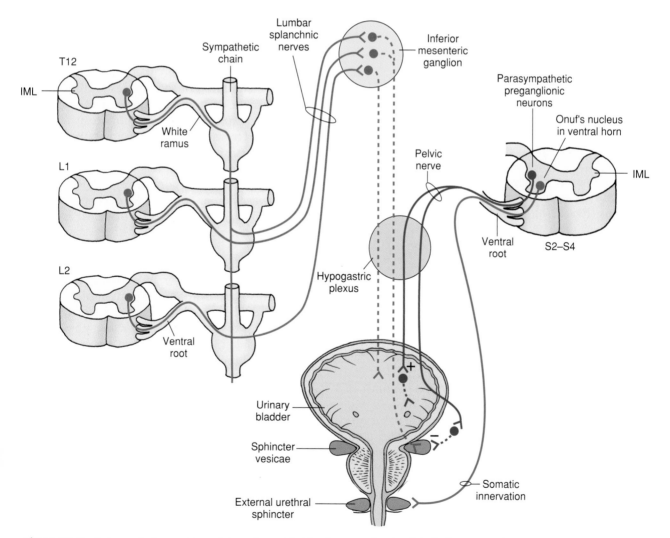

Figure 22–8 Autonomic innervation of the urinary bladder (see text for details). Red = sympathetic nervous system, blue = parasympathetic nervous system. Solid lines = preganglionic fibers, dotted lines = postganglionic fibers. The green line represents somatic innervation.

tion in the male. Ejaculation involves sympathetic activation. Sympathetic activation causes contraction of the sphincter vesicae during ejaculation and prevents seminal fluid from entering the bladder.

Parasympathetic Innervation

The parasympathetic preganglionic neurons innervating the bladder are located in the IML of the sacral spinal cord at the S2-S4 level. Their preganglionic axons exit from the ventral roots, travel in the pelvic nerves, pass through the hypogastric plexus, and synapse on postganglionic neurons located in the wall of the urinary bladder (Fig. 22-8). Activation of parasympathetic fibers results in contraction of the **detrusor muscle** of the bladder (smooth muscle of the bladder wall) and relaxation of the sphincter vesicae.

Afferent Innervation

Afferent impulses from the stretch receptors located in the bladder wall enter the spinal cord at T12-L2 levels via the hypogastric plexus. Such impulses also enter the spinal cord at S2-S4 levels via the pelvic nerve. Afferent information is transmitted to brainstem areas involved in coordination of bladder function.

Somatic Innervation

The **external urethral sphincter** consists of striated muscle that is innervated by alpha-motor neurons (somatic innervation) located in the ventral horn in the sacral segments S2-S4. This circumscribed region in the ventral horn is called **Onuf's nucleus** (Fig. 22-8).

Micturition

During bladder filling, alpha-motor neurons in Onuf's nucleus are active and keep the external urethral sphincter closed so that emptying of the bladder is prevented. During urination (voiding), the tonic activity of these alpha-motor neurons is temporarily inhibited, which results in relaxation of the external urethral sphincter. At the same time, parasympathetic neurons located in the IML at spinal sacral levels S2-S4, are activated to contract the detrusor muscle of the bladder wall. Thus, urination results from activation of sacral parasympathetic neurons innervating the bladder and temporary inhibition of alpha-motor neurons innervating the external urethral sphincter.

MALE REPRODUCTIVE SYSTEM

Sympathetic Innervation

The sympathetic preganglionic neurons innervating the male reproductive system (i.e., epididymis, vas deferens, seminal vesicles, and prostate glands) are located in the IML at the T12-L2 level. Their preganglionic fibers pass through the sympathetic chain, exit in the lumbar splanchnic nerves, and synapse on the neurons in the inferior mesenteric ganglion. The axons of these postganglionic neurons reach their target tissues in the male reproductive system via the hypogastric plexuses (Fig. 22-9). Activation of the sympathetic nervous system causes ejaculation of spermatozoa, along with secretions of the prostate and the seminal vesicles.

Parasympathetic Innervation

The parasympathetic preganglionic neurons innervating the erectile tissue (**corpora cavernosa**) in the male sexual organ are located in the IML of the sacral spinal cord at the S2-S4 level. The male erectile tissue is composed of many cavities. The parasympathetic preganglionic fibers exit from the ventral roots, travel in the pelvic nerves, pass through the hypogastric plexus, and are distributed to the erectile tissue (Fig. 22-9).

Male Erectile Dysfunction

Activation of the parasympathetic nervous system results in the dilation of the arteries and increased blood flow in the corpora cavernosa causing erection of the male sexual organ. In addition, nitric oxide (NO) released from nonadrenergic and noncholinergic nerve terminals increases cyclic guanosine monophosphate (cGMP) levels in the nonvascular smooth muscle of the corpora cavernosa. Relaxation of the nonvascular smooth muscle of corpora cavernosa caused by increased levels of cGMP permits inflow of blood into the sinuses of the cavernosa. This effect contributes to the erection of the male sexual organ (penis). Disruption of any of these mechanisms causes male erectile dysfunction.

In recent years, oral administration of sildenafil (Viagra) has been used to treat male erectile dysfunction. This drug inhibits an enzyme, phosphodiesterase-5, which is responsible for the breakdown of cGMP, and increases cGMP levels in the smooth muscle cells of corpora cavernosa. The blood flow in corpora cavernosa increases, causing it to swell up and produce an erection. The mechanism of action of vardenafil (Levitra) and tadalafil (Cialis), which have recently become available for oral treatment of male erectile dysfunction, is similar to that of sildenafil. It is important to note that currently available drugs used for the treatment of male erectile dysfunction should not be used by individuals who take nitrates and alpha-adrenergic receptor blockers for the treatment of other disorders because all of these drugs lower blood pressure and their combined use may reduce blood pressure to dangerous levels.

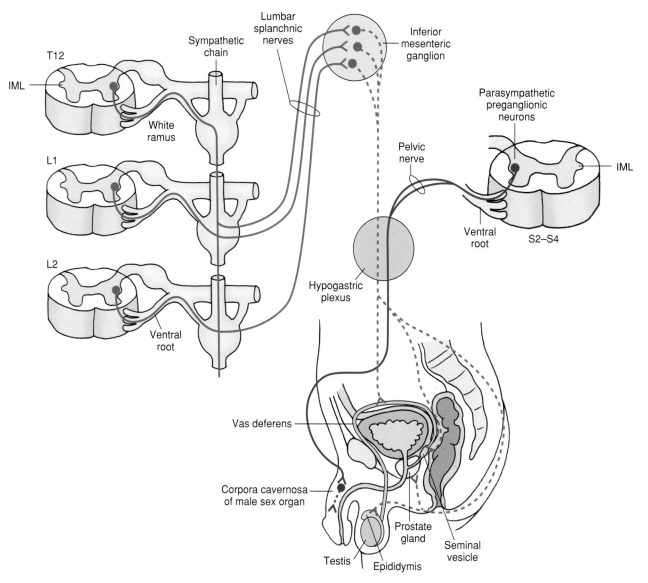

Figure 22–9 Autonomic innervation of the male reproductive system (see text for details). Red = sympathetic nervous system, blue = parasympathetic nervous system. Solid lines = preganglionic fibers, dotted lines = postganglionic fibers.

FEMALE REPRODUCTIVE SYSTEM

Sympathetic Innervation

The sympathetic preganglionic neurons innervating the smooth muscle of the uterine wall are located in the IML at the T12-L2 level. Their preganglionic fibers pass through the sympathetic chain, exit in the lumbar splanchnic nerves, and synapse on postganglionic neurons in the inferior mesenteric ganglion. The postganglionic fibers from these neurons pass through the hypogastric plexus and innervate the female sexual organ (vagina) and the uterus (Fig. 22-10). Activation of the sympathetic nervous system results in contraction of the uterus.

Parasympathetic Innervation

The location of the parasympathetic preganglionic neurons and the pathways they follow to innervate the uterus and female sexual organ are similar to those described for the male sexual organ (Fig. 22-10). The mechanism of vasodilation in the female erectile tissue (clitoris) is similar to that described for the male sexual organ. Parasympathetic stimulation causes stimulation of the female erectile tissue and relaxation of the uterine smooth muscle. The relaxation of the uterine smooth muscle may be variable due to hormonal influences on this muscle.

The pain-sensing neurons innervating the uterus are located in the dorsal root ganglia at T12-L2 and S2-S4. Their peripheral axons pass through

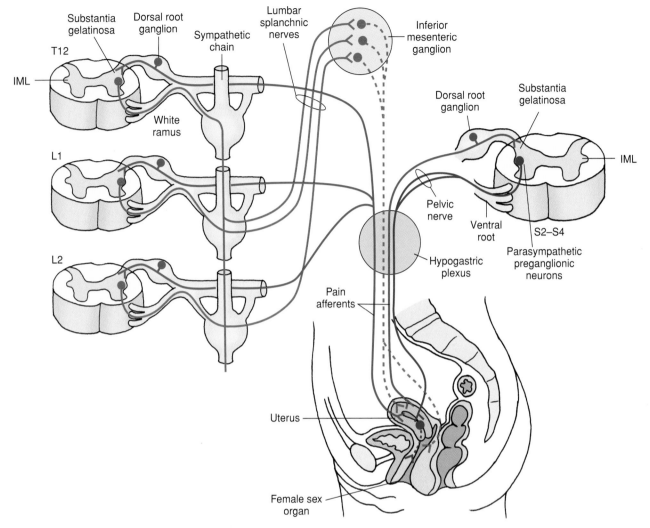

Figure 22–10 Autonomic innervation of the female reproductive system (see text for details). Red = sympathetic nervous system, blue = parasympathetic nervous system. Solid lines = preganglionic fibers, dotted lines = postganglionic fibers. The green lines indicate pain afferents.

the hypogastric plexus and terminate in the uterus, while their central terminals synapse in the substantia gelatinosa at the T12-L2 and S2-S4 levels. The secondary pain-sensing neurons then project to the cerebral cortex via the thalamus (see Chapter 15).

BLOOD VESSELS

Sympathetic Innervation

Sympathetic innervation to the blood vessels in most of the organs located in the head and chest cavity is provided by the postganglionic fibers emerging from the cervical ganglia (superior, middle, and inferior) and first four thoracic paravertebral ganglia. The blood vessels in most of the organs in the abdominal cavity are provided sympathetic innervation by postganglionic

fibers emerging from the prevertebral ganglia (e.g., celiac, superior mesenteric, and inferior mesenteric ganglia). As mentioned previously, sympathetic preganglionic fibers that synapse on the postganglionic neurons located in these prevertebral ganglia pass without synapsing in the paravertebral ganglia in the sympathetic chain.

The fibers providing sympathetic innervation of the blood vessels, sweat glands, and erectile muscles of hair follicles located in the upper and lower limbs and the trunk follow a different course. For example, the sympathetic preganglionic neurons innervating the upper limb are located in the IML at T1-T8. The axons of these preganglionic neurons enter the sympathetic chain via white rami, ascend through the sympathetic chain, and synapse on sympathetic postganglionic neurons located in the inferior and middle cervical paravertebral ganglia.

The axons of these postganglionic neurons re-enter the spinal nerves that form the brachial plexus via gray rami and are distributed to the arteries (**vasoconstrictor fibers**), sweat glands (**sudomotor fibers**), and erectile muscle of hairs (**pilomotor fibers**).

Sympathetic innervation to the lower limb is provided by sympathetic preganglionic neurons located in the IML at T10-L2. The axons of these neurons enter the sympathetic chain via white rami and synapse on postganglionic neurons in the lumbar and sacral ganglia. The axons of these postganglionic neurons join the branches of lumbar and sacral plexuses via the gray rami and innervate the blood vessels, sweat glands, and hair follicles located in the lower limb.

The postganglionic fibers that supply sympathetic innervation to the blood vessels, sweat glands, and hair follicles located in the trunk also re-enter the corresponding spinal nerves via the gray rami.

Parasympathetic Innervation

The parasympathetic nervous system does not innervate the arterioles in most of the organs. Some blood vessels that do receive parasympathetic innervation are located in the lacrimal and salivary glands and male erectile tissue.

Systemic Blood Pressure

An individual's blood pressure depends on the peripheral vascular resistance, which is determined primarily by the diameter of the systemic arterioles. The tone of the vascular smooth muscle is controlled by the activity of the noradrenergic postganglionic neurons that innervate the arterioles. Increased activity of the sympathetic nervous system results in the contraction of the arteriolar smooth muscle, thus causing an increase in peripheral vascular resistance and systemic blood pressure. A decrease in the activity of the sympathetic nervous system results in a decrease in systemic blood pressure due to a decrease in the peripheral vascular resistance, caused by relaxation of the arteriolar smooth muscle.

NEUROTRANSMITTERS IN THE AUTONOMIC NERVOUS SYSTEM

PREGANGLIONIC TERMINALS

Within the autonomic ganglia, **acetylcholine** is the transmitter released at the terminals of the sympathetic and parasympathetic preganglionic fibers. The terminal branches of the preganglionic fibers contain vesicles enclosing the neurotransmitter. The terminals make synaptic contacts with the postganglionic neurons located in the ganglia.

POSTGANGLIONIC TERMINALS

The terminals of the sympathetic and parasympathetic postganglionic neurons innervate the effector cells in the target organs. At the terminals of most sympathetic postganglionic neurons, **norepinephrine** is the transmitter, with the exception of those neurons innervating sweat glands and blood vessels of the skeletal muscles, where acetylcholine is the neurotransmitter. At the terminals of all the parasympathetic postganglionic neurons, acetylcholine is the neurotransmitter.

The synthesis, storage, release, and removal of acetylcholine and norepinephrine are described in detail in Chapter 8. To recapitulate, acetylcholine liberated in the synaptic cleft is removed by acetylcholinesterase that hydrolyzes the transmitter. Acetylcholinesterase inhibitors are used clinically in the treatment of many diseases. For example, donepezil (Aricept) is prescribed in Alzheimer's disease in an attempt to improve memory function (see Chapter 8). Pyridostigmine is used to improve muscle strength in myasthenia gravis (see Chapter 7). Abdominal cramps and diarrhea, due to increased levels of acetylcholine in the GIT, are the most common side effects of acetylcholinesterase inhibitors.

MAJOR RECEPTORS INVOLVED IN THE AUTONOMIC NERVOUS SYSTEM

The receptors (cholinergic and adrenergic) on which the two main transmitters of the autonomic nervous system act have been described in Chapter 8. A brief description of these receptors is given here.

CHOLINERGIC RECEPTORS

These receptors have been divided into two main classes: **cholinergic muscarinic** and **nicotinic receptors**. Cholinergic receptors located in the visceral effector organ cells (smooth and cardiac muscle and exocrine glands) are called cholinergic muscarinic receptors. Responses elicited by the stimulation of these receptors in the visceral effector organs, called muscarinic effects of acetylcholine, include decrease in heart rate, miosis, and secretions of different glands (lacrimal, salivary, and sweat glands and glands in the GIT). Cholinergic receptors located in the adrenal medulla and autonomic ganglia are called nicotinic receptors. Remember that acetylcholine is the transmitter at the preganglionic terminals synapsing on epinephrine- and norepinephrine-secreting cells of the adrenal medulla.

ADRENERGIC RECEPTORS

Adrenergic receptors are divided into two major classes: alpha- and beta-adrenergic receptors. These classes have been further subdivided into alpha$_1$- and alpha$_2$-adrenergic receptors and beta$_1$- and beta$_2$-adrenergic receptors. Alpha$_1$-adrenergic receptors are located on the membranes of postsynaptic cells. These receptors may be linked through a G-protein. G-proteins bind guanosine diphosphate (GDP) and guanosine triphosphate (GTP). When norepinephrine binds to an alpha$_1$-adrenergic receptor, the receptor is activated, and second messengers inositol 1,4,5-triphosphate (IP$_3$) and diacylglycerol (DAG) are liberated. IP$_3$ releases Ca^{2+} from its stores in the endoplasmic reticulum and is also phosphorylated to form inositol 1,3,4,5-tetraphosphate (IP$_4$), which opens calcium channels located in the cell membrane. Ca^{2+} then binds with calmodulin, and phosphorylation of a protein occurs to elicit a cellular response. DAG activates protein kinase C, which, in turn, promotes protein phosphorylation and subsequent cellular response.

Alpha$_2$-adrenergic receptors are present on the presynaptic membranes of adrenergic nerve terminals. Activation of alpha$_2$-adrenergic receptors at these endings by the released transmitter (norepinephrine) inhibits further release of the transmitter. This phenomenon is called autoinhibition (see Chapter 8). Stimulation of alpha$_2$-adrenergic receptors has been reported to inhibit adenylate cyclase and lower cyclic adenosine monophosphate (cAMP) levels in some effector cells. As mentioned previously (see Chapter 8), cAMP stimulates enzymes (e.g., protein kinase A), which then phosphorylate appropriate ion channels. Phosphorylation of ion channels by protein kinases results in the opening of these channels, ions flow across the cell membrane, and the cells are depolarized and rendered more excitable. Decrease in cAMP levels, therefore, elicits opposite responses.

Beta$_1$-adrenergic receptors are located in the heart; stimulation of these receptors results in an increase in heart rate and contractility. The biochemical mechanism responsible for the responses elicited by stimulation of beta-adrenergic receptors has been discussed in Chapter 8. Beta$_2$-adrenergic receptors are located in smooth muscles (e.g., bronchial smooth muscle); their activation results in the relaxation of these muscles.

BRAINSTEM AREAS REGULATING CARDIOVASCULAR FUNCTION

Regulation of the cardiovascular system is an autonomic function. Animal experiments have implicated several neuronal pools in this function. It is believed that the organization of these areas in humans is similar to that described for several animal species. The mechanisms that maintain cardiovascular function at an optimum level in healthy individuals are located in the brainstem (Fig. 22-11). However, higher integrative areas (e.g., hypothalamus and cortex) also have a profound influence on cardiovascular function. For example, specific stimulation of neurons located in different areas of the hypothalamus results in specific changes (either a decrease or increase) in blood pressure and heart rate.

THE SOLITARY NUCLEUS

This nucleus consists of a column of cells on each side of the fourth ventricle. At the rostral edge of the area postrema, the columns of the solitary nucleus (NTS) on the two sides merge in the midline to form the commissural subnucleus of the NTS (see Chapter 10). Recall that the area postrema is a circumventricular organ (i.e., it lacks a blood-brain barrier) that is located in the caudal region of the floor of the fourth ventricle (see Chapter 3). Medial and commissural subnuclei in the caudal regions of the NTS are the sites where the central terminals of baroreceptor, chemoreceptor, and cardiopulmonary sensory neurons make their first synapse. **Baroreceptor** neurons sense changes in blood pressure, **chemoreceptor** neurons sense changes in blood gases and pH, and **cardiopulmonary sensory neurons** are activated by noxious chemicals in the cardiopulmonary circulation. The role of the NTS in mediating the reflex cardiovascular responses to baroreceptor, chemoreceptor, and cardiopulmonary receptor activation is discussed in the following sections.

CAUDAL VENTROLATERAL MEDULLARY DEPRESSOR AREA

This region is located in the ventrolateral medulla, ventral to the NTS (Fig. 22-11). The caudal ventrolateral medullary depressor area (CVLM) is an important relay nucleus for mediating baroreflex and cardiopulmonary reflex, but not chemoreflex, responses. It contains a population of gamma-aminobutyric (GABA)-ergic neurons that projects to the rostral ventrolateral medullary pressor area (see next section). Activation of baroreceptors and

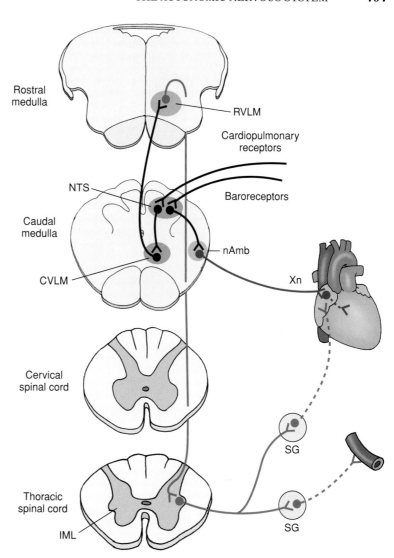

Figure 22-11 Cardiovascular neuronal pools involved in baroreflex (see text for details). Abbreviations: nAmb, nucleus ambiguus; Xn, vagus nerve; SG, sympathetic ganglion; IML, intermediolateral cell column of the spinal cord; CVLM, caudal ventrolateral medullary depressor area; NTS, solitary nucleus (also known as nucleus tractus solitarius); RVLM, rostral ventrolateral medullary pressor area. (Adapted with permission from Dun NJ, Machado BH, Pilowsky PM (eds.): Neural Mechanisms of Cardiovascular Regulation. Boston: Kluwer Academic Publishers, 2004, p. 87.)

cardiopulmonary receptors results in an activation of these GABAergic neurons. Release of GABA at their terminals causes an inhibition of rostral ventrolateral medullary neurons, which results in a decrease in blood pressure and heart rate (see the following sections, "Baroreceptor Reflex" and "Cardiopulmonary Reflex").

ROSTRAL VENTROLATERAL MEDULLARY PRESSOR AREA

This area is located in the ventrolateral medulla rostral to the CVLM and caudal to the facial nucleus (Fig. 22-11). The rostral ventrolateral medullary pressor area (RVLM) is believed to be one of the most important regions involved in the maintenance of sympathetic tone. The tonically active, barosensitive, sympathoexcitatory RVLM neurons send direct monosynaptic projections to the IML, where the sympathetic preganglionic neurons are located.

NUCLEUS AMBIGUUS

The role of nucleus ambiguus in regulating cardiac function has been discussed earlier in this chapter (see also Chapter 10). This nucleus receives direct or indirect excitatory projections from the NTS.

INTERMEDIOLATERAL CELL COLUMN

The location and function of the IML has been discussed earlier in this chapter (see also Chapter 9). As mentioned earlier, sympathetic preganglionic neurons are located in the IML of the thoracolumbar cord, and they receive monosynaptic projections from the RVLM neurons.

BARORECEPTOR REFLEX

The pathways and transmitters involved in the baroreceptor reflex can be summarized as follows (Fig. 22-11). Cardiovascular responses to the stimulation of baroreceptors are hypotension and bradycardia. Activation of baroreceptor afferents, in response to an elevation in systemic blood pressure, results in the release of an excitatory amino acid (most probably glutamate) in the dorsomedial NTS. Excitation of the second-order NTS neurons involved in the baroreflex results in the activation of an excitatory projection to the CVLM, and an excitatory amino acid is released in the CVLM. Activation of GABAergic neurons in the CVLM results in the release of GABA in the RVLM, causing inhibition of RVLM neurons. RVLM neurons normally provide a tonic excitatory input to the IML; glutamate is believed to be the transmitter released at the terminals of this projection. Therefore, inhibition of RVLM neurons results in a decrease in the excitatory input to the sympathetic preganglionic neurons in the IML. When this occurs, the activity of postganglionic sympathetic innervation to the arterioles and heart is decreased. Consequently, blood pressure and heart rate are decreased. However, activation of vagal innervation plays a major role in mediating reflex bradycardia. As mentioned earlier, vagal innervation to the heart is provided predominantly by the nucleus ambiguus. The presence of an excitatory projection from the NTS to the nucleus ambiguus has been reported; this projection is activated when the activity of baroreceptors increases in response to an increase in the systemic blood pressure.

ORTHOSTATIC HYPOTENSION

When an individual stands up suddenly from a recumbent position, the blood pressure in his or her upper body (including the brain) is temporarily reduced because relatively more blood is retained in the lower part of the body due to gravitational forces. The individual feels transient dizziness and dimness in vision and, sometimes, may even faint. The mechanism by which these symptoms are compensated in normal individuals is as follows. The baroreceptors located in the aortic arch and carotid sinus regions sense the fall in blood pressure induced by sudden standing and reflexly increase the activity of sympathetic nerves innervating the blood vessels, causing them to contract and increase blood pressure. Increase in the activity of sympathetic nerves innervating the blood vessels may result in an increase in the plasma norepinephrine levels. The organs in the upper part of the body (including the brain) then receive better blood perfusion, and the effects of postural hypotension are relieved. Sometimes, the symptoms of sudden standing (i.e., dizziness, dimness in vision, and feeling faint) are more severe and

prolonged. This is called **postural** or **orthostatic hypotension.** A decrease in systolic blood pressure greater than 20 mmHg and an increase in heart rate greater than 10 beats/min in response to sudden standing is considered to be orthostatic hypotension.

Patients suffering from diabetes and syphilis often experience postural hypotension because the sympathetic nerves are damaged in these conditions. Postural hypotension is also one of the side effects of **sympatholytic** drugs used in the treatment of systemic hypertension. Some individuals suffering from **autonomic insufficiency** also have postural hypotension. The plasma norepinephrine levels do not increase in response to standing up in these patients due to a defect in the central or peripheral nervous system. If the postural hypotension is caused by sympatholytic drugs, cessation of this treatment relieves this side effect. In other cases, mineralocorticoids (e.g., desoxicorticosterone) are used to relieve postural hypotension. These drugs increase blood volume by reabsorption of Na^+ from urine in the distal renal tubules.

CARDIOPULMONARY REFLEX

In experimental animals, injections of noxious chemicals (e.g., capsaicin, which is a pungent substance in hot chili peppers) via the right atrium elicit a triad of responses characterized by apnea, bradycardia, and hypotension. The receptors responding to these stimuli are located in the lungs and the heart, and the responses are mediated by vagal C-fiber afferents. The pathways involved in this reflex are identical to those described for baroreflex (Fig. 22-11). The exact physiological role of these receptors in humans has not been established. In experimental animals, injections of noxious chemicals in the right atrium are used to study the neural circuits involved in this reflex.

BRAINSTEM AREAS REGULATING RESPIRATORY FUNCTION

RESPIRATORY NEURONAL GROUPS

Regulation of respiration is an autonomic function. Based on animal experimentation, the following brainstem regions have been implicated in this function (Fig. 22-12). The medulla oblongata contains two main aggregates of respiration-related neurons. One aggregate, called the "**dorsal respiratory group (DRG)**," is located in the ventrolateral portion of the NTS. The DRG receives inputs from afferent fibers arising from the **pulmonary stretch receptors**. Periodic activation of pulmonary stretch receptors

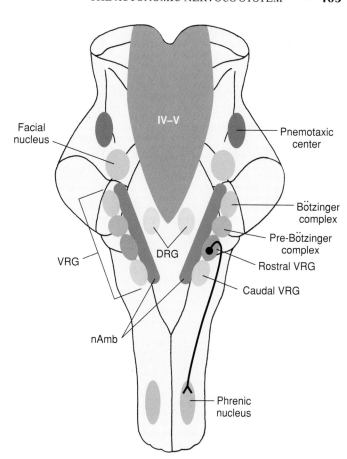

Figure 22–12 Brainstem respiratory neuronal pools (see text for details). Abbreviations: VRG, ventral respiratory group; nAmb, nucleus ambiguus; DRG, dorsal group of respiratory neurons; IV-V, fourth ventricle.

with each inspiration is believed to contribute to the rhythmic pattern of breathing. Another aggregate, called the "**ventral respiratory group (VRG),**" is located in the ventrolateral medulla. The VRG is divided into three functionally different parts: (1) the caudal part (called the **cVRG**) contains mostly expiratory neurons; (2) the part immediately rostral to the cVRG (called the **rVRG**) contains mostly inspiratory neurons; and (3) the neurons located rostral to the rVRG (called the **Bötzinger complex**) are mostly expiratory. Recently, an area just caudal to the Bötzinger complex, termed the **pre-Bötzinger complex**, has been implicated as the site of respiratory rhythm generation.

The axons of inspiratory neurons in the rVRG project to the **phrenic motor nucleus** (PMN) and other spinal neurons innervating respiratory muscles. The PMN is located in the ventral horn of the cervical spinal cord (C3-C5 level). The neurons in the PMN provide innervation to the diaphragm. The inspiratory neurons of the rVRG exhibit a burst pattern of activity. The phrenic motor neurons, which are driven predominantly by the inspiratory neurons located in the rVRG, also show similar bursts of activity. An excitatory amino acid is released as a transmitter at the terminals of the

rVRG neurons in the PMN. Each burst of phrenic motor neuron activity results in contraction of the diaphragm. Phrenic motor neurons are cholinergic, so acetylcholine is the transmitter released at the terminals of these neurons in the diaphragm.

Another group of respiratory neurons, named the **pneumotaxic center**, has been identified in the dorsolateral pontine tegmentum, just caudal to the **inferior colliculus** in most animal species. This neuronal pool is considered to be essential for maintaining a normal breathing pattern.

Interconnections between respiratory neuronal pools, transmitters involved in these circuits, and the mechanism of respiratory rhythm generation are not clearly known. Three models have been proposed for the generation of the respiratory rhythm: (1) in the network model, inhibitory and excitatory synaptic interactions are considered to be essential for the generation of respiratory rhythm; (2) in the pacemaker model, neurons with pacemaker properties, probably located in the pre-Bötzinger complex, generate respiratory rhythm; and (3) in the hybrid model, pacemaker neurons generate respiratory rhythm, while synaptic interactions between different respiratory neurons determine the pattern of respiration.

CHEMORECEPTOR REFLEX

Neural pathways involved in mediating the carotid chemoreflex can be summarized as follows (Fig. 22-13). Afferents from the carotid body terminate predominantly in the commissural subnucleus of the NTS. Activation of chemoreceptor afferents results in the release of an excitatory amino acid (EAA; probably glutamate) in the NTS. Secondary NTS neurons are believed to mediate the sympathoexcitatory responses to the carotid chemoreflex stimulation via a direct projection from the NTS to the RVLM, and EAA receptors in the RVLM mediate the sympathoexcitatory responses to chemoreceptor stimulation. Unlike in the baroreflex, the CVLM does not participate in mediating the cardiovascular responses to carotid chemoreceptor stimulation. As mentioned earlier, activation of RVLM neurons leads to excitation of sympathetic preganglionic neurons in the IML, and the activity of sympathetic nerves innervating the blood vessels increases. The net result of activation of these pathways is an increase in blood pressure. The predominant cardiac effect of chemoreflex stimulation is bradycardia, which may be mediated via a direct or indirect glutamatergic projection from the NTS to the nucleus ambiguus.

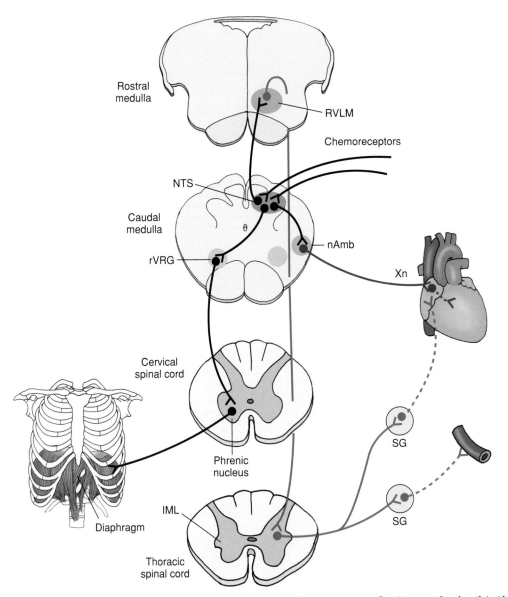

Figure 22–13 Cardiovascular and respiratory neuronal pools involved in chemoreceptor reflex (see text for details). Abbreviations: rVRG, rostral respiratory neuronal group; nAmb, nucleus ambiguus; Xn, vagus nerve; SG, sympathetic ganglion; IML, intermediolateral cell column of the spinal cord; NTS, solitary nucleus (also known as nucleus tractus solitarius); RVLM, rostral ventrolateral medullary pressor area. (Adapted with permission from Dun NJ, Machado BH, Pilowsky PM (eds.): Neural Mechanisms of Cardiovascular Regulation. Boston: Kluwer Academic Publishers, 2004, p. 87.)

Neural circuits mediating the respiratory responses to chemoreceptor stimulation have not been firmly established. It is known that EAA receptors in the ventrolateral medulla containing the rVRG are involved in these responses. Therefore, it is possible that activation of secondary NTS neurons results in the stimulation of rVRG neurons via EAA receptors. Activation of rVRG stimulates the PMN, and diaphragmatic movements are elicited via the activation of phrenic nerves. The role of other medullary respiratory areas in mediating responses to peripheral chemoreceptor stimulation has not been established.

SELECTED DISORDERS OF THE AUTONOMIC NERVOUS SYSTEM

HORNER'S SYNDROME

This syndrome is characterized by drooping of the upper eyelid (pseudoptosis), constriction of the pupil (miosis), enophthalmos (sinking of eyeball in the orbit), dilation of arterioles of the skin, and anhidrosis (loss of sweating) at the face. It is caused by lesions of the brainstem and upper cervical cord that interrupt the sympathetic fibers in the reticulospinal tract and fibers descending from the hypothalamus to the IML of the thoracolumbar cord. Such lesions are also encountered in multiple sclerosis. The interruption of the sympathetic innervation to the tarsal muscle of the eyelid (which is involved in the elevation of the upper eyelid) results in pseudoptosis. Disruption of similar inputs to the orbital muscle of Müller (which maintains the position of the eyeball forward in the orbit) results in **enophthalmos.** Decreased sympathetic activity and unopposed parasympathetic activity cause miosis; a decrease in the sympathetic activity of the facial skin arterioles and sweat glands also causes **vasodilation** and **anhidrosis** (decrease or lack of sweat), respectively (see also the Clinical Case in this chapter).

ARGYLL ROBERTSON PUPIL

As discussed in Chapter 16, this condition occurs in syphilitic patients with central nervous system complications. In brief, the chief symptom is that the pupils do not constrict in response to light, but they do constrict during the accommodation reflex.

HIRSCHSPRUNG'S DISEASE (MEGACOLON)

Patients with Hirschsprung's disease fail to develop the myenteric plexus in the distal colon. Therefore, peristalsis is absent in the distal colon and, consequently, the proximal part of the colon distends (megacolon), which is prone to impaction of feces. This disease usually develops in infancy.

FREY'S SYNDROME

In some patients with deep wounds in the parotid glands, the parasympathetic fibers eliciting secretory responses in these glands grow erroneously into the facial skin overlying these glands. In these patients, stimulation of the parasympathetic nervous system results in sweating of this facial region instead of producing saliva.

RAYNAUD'S DISEASE

The cause of this vascular disorder is unknown. Raynaud's disease is characterized by spasmodic vasoconstriction of arteries in the fingers and toes of upper and lower limbs, respectively. The vasoconstriction is often precipitated by the activation of the sympathetic nervous system in response to cold or emotional stress. The digits appear cyanosed periodically due to the deoxygenation of stagnant blood. Because the symptoms are precipitated by activation of the sympathetic nervous system, drugs that block sympathetically mediated vasoconstriction are useful in the treatment of this disease. These drugs include alpha-adrenergic receptor blockers (e.g., phenoxybenzamine and prazosin). Drugs that act directly on smooth muscle of the arteries to cause vasodilation (e.g., the calcium channel blocker nifedipine) are also useful in the treatment of this disease.

CLINICAL CASE

HISTORY

Harry is a 67-year-old man who has been a heavy smoker for 50 years and has suffered from a chronic cough that he attributed to smoking; however, he has never sought medical attention for it. Suddenly one day, Harry noticed that his left eyelid drooped slightly and that his left pupil was slightly smaller than the right. The inner side of his left hand was numb. When he attempted to shut off his alarm clock, he felt that his left hand was clumsy. He consulted his internist, who referred him to a neurologist.

EXAMINATION

The neurologist noted marked miosis (constriction) of the left pupil compared to the right, but the pupil remained reactive to light. Harry's left eyelid drooped slightly, but he was able to close his eye tightly. There was no sweat on the left side of his face. He was unable to feel a pin on the inner side of his left arm. His left triceps muscle and some of the muscles of the hand were weak.

EXPLANATION

Harry has Horner's syndrome, which is caused by the interruption of sympathetic fibers as they run their course from the hypothalamus through the brainstem to the IML of the upper thoracic spinal cord. Preganglionic neurons from this tract innervate the pupillary dilators and the levator palpebrae superioris muscle of the eyelid. They also supply the sweat glands of the face, and if these fibers are interrupted, the result is Horner's syndrome, as described.

Likewise, the symptoms that Harry had may be of peripheral origin, resulting from a different, but related, problem. Horner's syndrome here is caused by a compression of these sympathetic fibers by a tumor at the apex (most superior portion) of the lung, called a Pancoast tumor. The tumor compresses the sympathetic fibers as they run in close proximity to the spine and the apex of the lung. These tumors can also compress the exiting spinal nerves, especially at the level of C8, causing weakness of the triceps and hand muscles. Pancoast tumors often don't cause respiratory problems initially because they are located far from the main-stem bronchi, where most respiratory problems are first manifest. A computed tomography (CT) scan of the chest confirmed Harry's diagnosis.

CHAPTER TEST

QUESTIONS

Choose the best answer for each question.

1. Which of the following statements is correct regarding the location of the sympathetic preganglionic neurons?

   a. They are located in the intermediolateral cell column of the spinal cord at C2-C8.
   b. They are located in the intermediolateral cell column of the spinal cord at T1-L2.
   c. They are located in the intermediolateral cell column of the spinal cord at S2-S4.
   d. They are located in the prevertebral ganglia of the autonomic nervous system.
   e. They are located in the autonomic centers of the brainstem.

2. Which one of the following statements is correct regarding the autonomic innervation of the heart?

   a. Parasympathetic postganglionic fibers innervate primarily the ventricles.
   b. Sympathetic postganglionic fibers innervate all regions of the heart.
   c. Activation of postganglionic sympathetic fibers decreases conduction in the atrioventricular node.
   d. Activation of the postganglionic parasympathetic fibers increases sinoatrial node activity.
   e. The postganglionic neurons of the parasympathetic division are located in the sacral region of the spinal cord.

3. Which one of the following statements is correct concerning the autonomic innervation of different organs?

   a. Stimulation of the parasympathetic innervation of the circular muscles of the iris causes miosis.
   b. Activation of the sympathetic nervous system decreases myocardial contractility.
   c. Stimulation of the parasympathetic innervation of the gastrointestinal tract decreases its motility.
   d. Stimulation of the parasympathetic innervation of the systemic arterioles causes an increase in blood pressure.
   e. Activation of the parasympathetic nervous system inhibits secretion of saliva.

4. A 50-year-old woman was diagnosed as having Raynaud's disease. Which one of the following statements regarding this disease is correct?

   a. The disease is characterized by periodic cyanosis of digits.
   b. There is overactivation of the parasympathetic nervous system in this disorder.
   c. Alpha-adrenergic receptor blockers exaggerate the cyanosis of digits in this disorder.
   d. Acetylcholinesterase inhibitors are useful in the treatment of this disease.
   e. Beta-adrenergic receptor blockers are used to treat this disorder.

5. A 65-year-old man who has Alzheimer's disease was prescribed donepezil (Aricept) in an attempt to improve his memory. Which one of the following is the most likely side effect of the drug?

   a. Mydriasis
   b. Abdominal cramping and diarrhea
   c. Muscle weakness
   d. Hypertension
   e. Tachycardia

ANSWERS AND EXPLANATIONS

1. Answer: b

The sympathetic preganglionic neurons are located in the intermediolateral cell column (IML) of the thoracolumbar cord (T1-L2). The sympathetic division is also called the thoracolumbar division of the autonomic nervous system. The parasympathetic preganglionic neurons are located in the intermediolateral cell column at S2-S4. In addition, the parasympathetic preganglionic neurons, but not the sympathetic preganglionic neurons, are located in the brainstem (midbrain, pons, and medulla). The parasympathetic division is also called the craniosacral division of the autonomic nervous system.

2. Answer: b

Sympathetic postganglionic fibers innervate all regions of the heart. Parasympathetic innervation is provided by the vagus and is restricted to the sinoatrial (SA) node, atria, and atrioventricular (AV) node; the ventricles receive relatively sparse parasympathetic innervation. Activation of the parasympathetic nervous system decreases automaticity in the SA node cells and hence decreases heart rate. Activation of the sympathetic nervous system increases conduction through the AV node, while activation of the parasympathetic nervous system decreases conduction through the AV node. It should be noted that the postganglionic neurons of the parasympathetic nervous system are present either within the target organ or close to it.

3. Answer: a

Activation of the parasympathetic nervous system causes contraction of the circular muscles of the iris, which results in miosis. Sympathetic stimulation causes an increase in the heart rate and contractility. Stimulation of the parasympathetic nervous system causes an increase in the motility of the gastrointestinal tract. Blood vessels in most, but not all, organs are not innervated by the parasympathetic nervous system. Therefore, little or no change in systemic blood pressure results when the parasympathetic nervous system is stimulated. Activation of either the sympathetic or parasympathetic system results in an increase in the secretion of saliva; sympathetic stimulation produces viscous saliva, while parasympathetic stimulation produces watery saliva.

4. Answer: a

The cause of Raynaud's disease is not known. In this condition, cold or emotional stress precipitates vasoconstriction in the digits of the limbs; they appear cyanosed. The vasoconstriction is mediated by the sympathetic nervous system, which may be activated by stress. Alpha-adrenergic receptor blockers and calcium channel blockers are used to treat this vascular disorder. Therefore, treatment with alpha-adrenergic receptor blockers will relieve, not exaggerate, the symptoms. Since neurally released acetylcholine does not mediate vasodilation, drugs that increase acetylcholine levels (e.g., acetylcholinesterase inhibitors) are not used to treat this disease. Beta-adrenergic receptors do not play a role in vasoconstriction; therefore, blockers of these receptors are not used to treat this disease.

5. Answer: b

Donepezil, an acetylcholinesterase inhibitor that crosses the blood-brain barrier, is prescribed for the treatment of Alzheimer's disease. The drug increases acetylcholine levels in the brain, and patients show some improvement in their memory function. However, the drug increases acetylcholine levels in the gastrointestinal tract (GIT) in addition to other tissues. Increased levels of acetylcholine increase smooth muscle contractions in the GIT and peristalsis. These effects elicit abdominal cramps and diarrhea, respectively. Increased levels of acetylcholine are likely to cause miosis (not mydriasis), increased muscle strength (not muscle weakness), and bradycardia (not tachycardia). Although blood vessels in most organs do not receive innervation from the parasympathetic nervous system, noninnervated cholinergic muscarinic receptors are present in the blood vessels. Therefore, increased levels of acetylcholine may cause relaxation of these vessels, which may result in hypotension (not hypertension). In therapeutic doses, donepezil does not cause any change in systemic blood pressure.

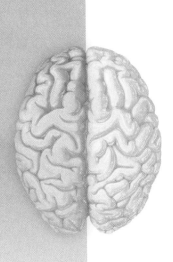

CHAPTER 23

THE RETICULAR FORMATION

OBJECTIVES

After reading this chapter, the student should be able to:

1. Describe and diagram (label) the general morphologic organization of the reticular formation and its overall boundaries

2. List, describe, and diagram the important sensory, motor, and visceral (autonomic) inputs to the reticular formation that relate to its basic functions

3. List, describe, and diagram the efferent projections of the reticular formation and the functions they mediate

4. Describe and diagram the basic input-output connections of the reticular formation and their relationship to functions of the reticular formation

5. Describe several of the key neurologic disorders resulting from damage to the reticular formation

Many of the structures discussed thus far appear to relate to unitary functions of the nervous system. For example, structures associated with either visual, auditory, vestibular, taste, or somatosensory information are dedicated to the transmission of a single sensory process. Likewise, other regions of the brain that we have just considered provide mechanisms related to motor processes but not to other functions. Additional structures and pathways considered in previous chapters are dedicated to autonomic functions.

In this chapter, we will examine the anatomical and functional organization of a region forming the core of the brainstem that is referred to as the **reticular formation**. The reticular formation of the brainstem differs from other regions of the brain in that it participates in a variety of processes. These functions include sensory, motor, and autonomic functions, sleep and wakefulness cycles, consciousness, and the regulation of emotional behavior. The questions that this chapter addresses are: (1) Which structures contribute to the processing of sensory information, and what are their contributions? (2) What are the regions of the reticular formation that contribute to motor functions, and what are their contributions? (3) How does the reticular formation contribute to autonomic functions? (4) How does the reticular formation help to regulate sleep and wakefulness cycles and states of consciousness? And, finally, (5) what is the role of the reticular formation in the regulation of emotional behavior? The remainder of this chapter attempts to answer these questions by analyzing the input-output relationships of the various regions of the reticular formation and their respective roles in mediating the different processes.

ANATOMICAL ORGANIZATION OF THE RETICULAR FORMATION

The reticular formation represents a phylogenetically older region of the brain because it is found in the core of the brainstem of lower forms of many species. Its appearance in lower forms is also similar to that found in humans. The reticular formation extends from the caudal medulla rostrally up to and including the midbrain (Fig. 23-1). At the upper end of the midbrain, the reticular formation becomes continuous with several nuclei of the thalamus, with which it is both anatomically and functionally related. These nuclei include the midline and intralaminar nuclei and are described later in this chapter. The reticular formation is surrounded laterally, dorsally, and ventrally by cranial nerve nuclei, which are the ascending and descending fiber pathways of the brainstem. The reticular formation, itself, consists of many cell groups situated among large numbers of fiber bundles. The name, reticular formation, was given to this region on the basis of its histological appearance, which can be described as a reticular network of fibers and cells.

GENERAL CHARACTERISTICS

As a general rule, the nuclei of the reticular formation are arranged in the following manner. The lateral third of the reticular formation contains small-sized cells (called **parvocellular** regions) whose function is to receive afferent fibers from both neighboring regions of the brainstem as well as from distant structures. The medial two thirds of the reticular formation contains different groups of large-sized cells (called **magnocellular** regions),

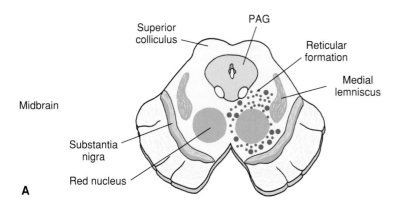

A Midbrain

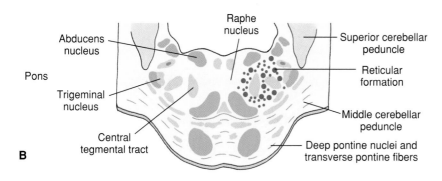

B Pons

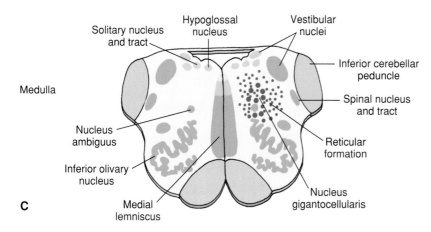

C Medulla

Figure 23–1 Position of the reticular formation in the brainstem. Diagrams illustrate the approximate positions of the reticular formation within the (A) midbrain, (B) pons, and (C) medulla as indicated by the dotted areas. Larger-sized dots represent magnocellular (large-celled regions), and smaller-sized dots represent parvocellular (small-celled regions).

which, in most instances, serve as the effector regions (i.e., the cell groups that give rise to the efferent projections of the reticular formation) (Fig. 23-2). At least two distinct magnocellular regions in the pons and one large region in the medulla have been identified. Additional groups of cells, which lie along or adjacent to the midline of the upper medulla, pons, and midbrain, are also included in the reticular formation. These cell groups comprise the **raphe** system of neurons. These cells are important because they produce serotonin that is distributed to wide regions of the brain and spinal cord. As will be discussed later in this chapter, the other types of monoamine neurons that supply the brain and spinal cord, namely, norepinephrine and

dopamine, are also located at different levels within the reticular formation.

AFFERENT CONNECTIONS

Cranial nerve nuclei and secondary sensory fibers form an outer shell that surrounds the reticular formation (and particularly the parvocellular region) on its dorsal, lateral, and ventral sides (Figs. 23-2 and 23-3). Because of this arrangement, the reticular formation is strategically positioned so that the various sensory systems can easily provide inputs into it. In this manner, the reticular formation is endowed with a capacity to modulate a wide variety of sensory processes.

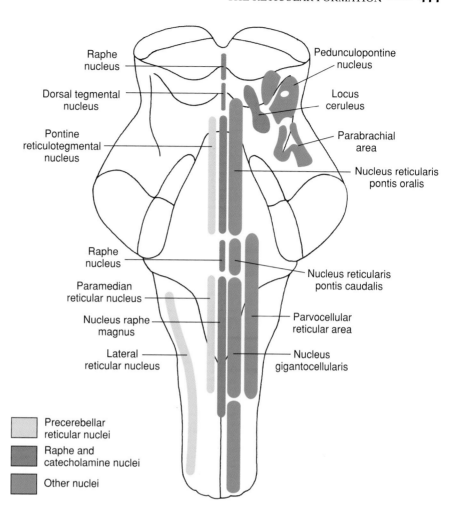

Figure 23–2 The positions of the magnocellular and parvocellular regions of the reticular formation. (Modified with permission from Barr ML, and Kiernan JA: The Human Nervous System, 6th ed. Philadelphia: Lippincott Williams & Wilkins, 1993, p. 150.)

The reticular formation receives inputs from brainstem and forebrain regions associated with sensory modalities, as well as from structures associated with motor functions, which include the cerebral cortex and cerebellum. Moreover, structures associated with autonomic and higher order visceral processes, such as the hypothalamus and limbic system, also contribute inputs to the reticular formation. The nature of these afferent sources to the reticular formation is considered in the following sections.

Sensory Systems

Somatosensory Signals from the Spinal Cord

As described in Chapter 9, pain and temperature signals are contained within the lateral spinothalamic tract, which passes directly from the spinal cord to the contralateral ventral posterolateral nucleus (VPL) of the thalamus. It is now well established that fibers arising from parts of the spinal cord gray matter (lamina VII) give off collaterals that terminate in specific parvocellular regions of the reticular formation, mainly adjacent to the magnocellular nuclei of the medulla (**nucleus gigantocellularis**) and pons (**nucleus reticularis pontis caudalis** and **nucleus reticularis pontis oralis**) (Figs. 23-3 and 23-4). In turn, these sensory signals are then transmitted from the parvocellular to the magnocellular nuclei. Neuronal groups with the reticular formation synapse with spinoreticular fibers and give rise to long ascending fibers Accordingly, the fibers projecting from spinal cord to the brainstem may be thought of as the first neurons in a chain of fibers that innervate the intralaminar nuclei of the thalamus, and these nuclei ultimately supply the cerebral cortex. It is believed that the information transmitted to the thalamus from the reticular formation mediates affective components of pain. We should also note that, as mentioned in Chapters 9 and 15, other fibers associated with pain modulation also supply the midbrain periaqueductal gray (PAG). Nociceptive inputs into the PAG represent part of a circuit whose descending component serves to inhibit ascending pain signals to the cerebral cortex.

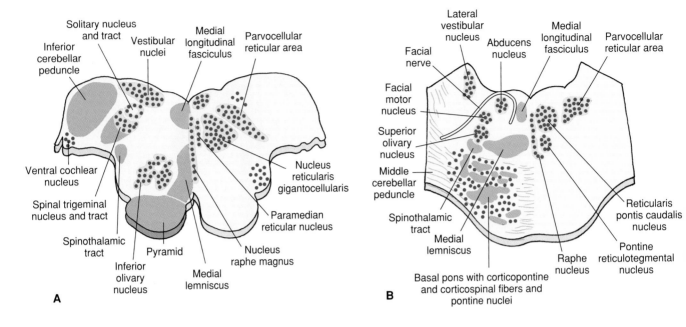

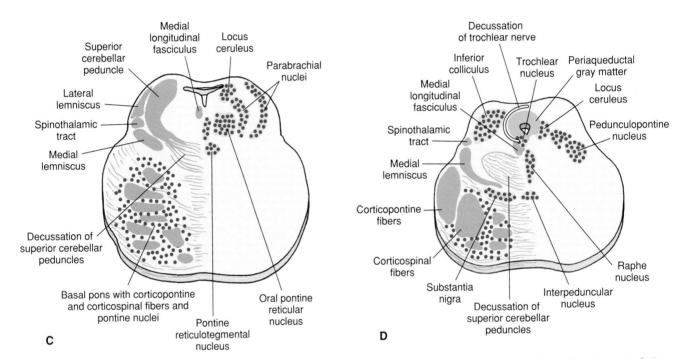

Figure 23–3 Cross sections of the brainstem. Note the principal nuclei of the reticular formation as well as other (nonreticular) nuclei situated adjacent to them. Many of these (other) nuclei make synaptic connections with nuclei of the reticular formation. (A) Medulla at level of rostral aspect of inferior olivary nucleus. (B) Level of caudal pons at the level of the abducens and facial nerves. (C) Rostral pons at level of the nucleus locus ceruleus and superior cerebellar peduncle. (D) Oblique section in which the dorsal aspect is at the level of the inferior colliculus of the caudal midbrain and the ventral aspect is at the level of the rostral aspect of the basilar pons. (Modified with permission from Barr ML, and Kiernan JA: The Human Nervous System, 6th ed. Philadelphia: Lippincott Williams & Wilkins, 1993, p. 153.)

The results of various studies have shown that other types of sensory signals can also produce cortical excitation by virtue of their connections with the brainstem reticular formation. On the basis of these studies dating back to the period of the 1940s and 1950s, the term **"reticular activating system"** was proposed as a mechanism by which sensory and other inputs to the reticular formation can modulate cortical neurons, cortical excitability, and states of consciousness. The importance of the

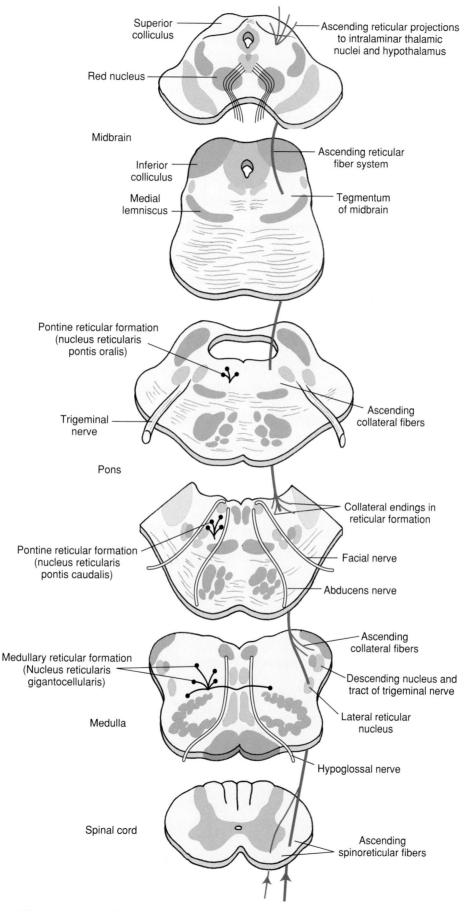

Figure 23–4 The connections of the lateral spinothalamic tract, including those made with the reticular formation.

reticular activating system is considered later in this chapter.

Other Secondary Sensory Systems

All sensory systems contribute fibers that ultimately make their way into the reticular formation. Trigeminal (for somatosensory information), solitary (for taste information), auditory, and vestibular nuclei lie adjacent to the reticular formation. Information is thus transmitted to the reticular formation from these structures, either as a result of the dendritic arborizations of neurons whose cell bodies lie in the lateral aspect of the reticular formation but which extend into these regions or by short axons that arise from these sensory regions that pass into the lateral aspects of the reticular formation.

In addition to these sensory inputs, impulses mediated from regions associated with olfactory and visual systems also contribute inputs to the reticular formation. Secondary olfactory signals are received by a number of limbic structures (amygdala, hippocampal formation, and septal area) that have known projections to the reticular formation (see page 415 and Chapters 24 and 25). Visual signals can reach the superior colliculus via optic tract fibers. From the superior colliculus, fibers project directly to the reticular formation of the midbrain and pons.

Thus, it is evident that the reticular formation receives multiple sensory inputs from all sensory systems. The reticular formation cannot maintain the specificity of the information that it receives from each of these sensory systems. Therefore, information of a nonspecific nature is transmitted via ascending fibers to the thalamus; this is in contrast to the specific transmission lines characteristic of other ascending sensory systems such as the dorsal column-medial lemniscus pathway. As indicated earlier, an important function of these signals that enter the reticular formation is to allow the reticular activating system to alter excitability levels of target neurons in the thalamus.

Motor Systems

It is clear that the reticular formation plays an important role in the processing of sensory information. The likely mechanisms are discussed in the following sections. As noted in previous chapters concerning motor systems, the reticular formation also plays an important role in the regulation of motor responses. The magnocellular nuclei of the reticular formation of the medulla and pons receive significant inputs from two key regions associated with motor functions: the cerebellum and sensorimotor cortex.

Cerebellum

The reticular formation and cerebellum share reciprocal connections, which complete a circuit comprising feedback pathways between these two regions for the regulation of motor functions associated with each of these two structures. Cerebellar fibers that project to the reticular formation of the medulla and pons arise from the **fastigial nucleus**. The fibers are both crossed and uncrossed and use the **uncinate fasciculus** (the pathway that passes just dorsal to the superior cerebellar peduncle).

Cerebral Cortex

Fibers from the same region of the sensorimotor cortex (areas 4, 3, 1, and 2) that give rise to much of the corticospinal tract also give rise to corticoreticular fibers. Corticoreticular fibers terminate in the pons and medulla near cell groups that give rise to the reticulospinal tracts (nucleus reticularis pontis oralis and nucleus reticularis pontis caudalis for the pons, and nucleus gigantocellularis for the medulla) (Fig. 23-5). In this way, corticoreticular fibers can influence both voluntary as well as reflex motor functions by acting on those neurons of the reticular formation that control extensor motoneuron activity.

Autonomic (and Higher Order Visceral Regulatory) Regions

The reticular formation receives autonomic inputs from different sources. One set of sources includes primary afferent fibers contained in cranial nerves (CN) IX and X. The other source includes fibers arising from higher order autonomic integrative regions, which include the hypothalamus, as well as parts of the limbic system.

Cranial Nerve (Autonomic) Nuclei

As indicated in Chapter 14, fibers of the glossopharyngeal and vagus nerves (CN IX and X) transmit both chemoreceptor and baroreceptor afferent signals to the brainstem. The signals arise from the aortic and carotid bodies (chemoreceptors) and the aortic arch and carotid sinus (baroreceptors) and terminate in the solitary nucleus. Secondary neurons located in the solitary nucleus then project to the nucleus ambiguus and the ventrolateral medullary depressor areas located in the medullary reticular formation. As noted earlier, this information is important for reflex regulation of blood pressure and respiration. Autonomic regions of the brainstem reticular formation that provide basic mechanisms for the control of blood pressure, heart rate, and respiration were considered in Chapter 22.

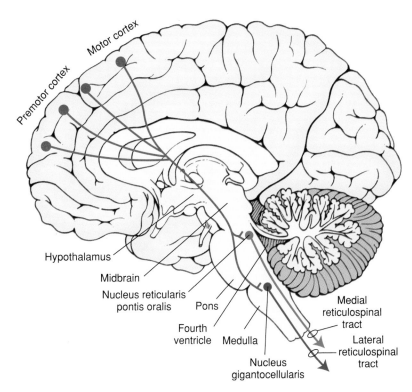

Figure 23–5 Corticoreticular projections. Sagittal view of the brain depicting the principal projections of fibers from the cerebral cortex to the reticular formation (shown in red). The largest majority of fibers arise from the motor and premotor cortices. The primary targets of these projections include the nucleus reticularis pontis oralis and nucleus reticularis gigantocellularis of the medulla, which give rise to the medial (green) and lateral (blue) reticulospinal tracts, respectively, and play important roles in regulating muscle tone.

Forebrain Regions (Hypothalamus and Limbic System)

Several different pathways that arise from both lateral and medial regions of the hypothalamus project downstream and make synaptic connections in different parts of the reticular formation, mainly the midbrain and pons. These regions of hypothalamus project most heavily to the midbrain PAG and neighboring regions of the dorsal and lateral tegmental fields of the reticular formation. Additional groups of fibers from the amygdala supply the PAG, tegmentum, and lower brainstem region (in and adjacent to the solitary nucleus). Other limbic structures also contribute fibers to the reticular formation. These include inputs from the prefrontal cortex and amygdala that are mainly directed to the midbrain PAG. These descending inputs provide a higher order control of central autonomic functions of the brainstem reticular formation.

EFFERENT PROJECTIONS

Organizational Considerations

As mentioned earlier, the reticular formation receives a variety of inputs from disparate regions of the central nervous system (CNS) that mediate different functions. The varied functions of the reticular formation are even more dramatically reflected by the nature of the outputs. Features concerning the basic organization of the neurons in the reticular formation should be pointed out before describing the output pathways of the reticular formation.

(1) The reticular formation contains cells whose axons travel long distances. Some ascend to the forebrain, and others descend to the spinal cord or project to the cerebellum. (2) The efferent fibers that travel long distances arise from the medial two thirds of the reticular formation, and those that travel only short distances as interneurons lie mainly in the lateral third of the reticular formation. (3) The main dendritic branches of the neurons are oriented in a plane perpendicular to the long axis of the brainstem (Fig. 23-6). This arrangement increases the probability that ascending and descending fibers of the reticular formation will make synaptic contact with other regions of the CNS. (4) Cells situated in the medial two thirds of the reticular formation of the medulla and pons give rise to bifurcating axons that travel for long distances in both directions (Fig. 23-7). By virtue of axon collaterals, each of these neurons can make synaptic contact with the other, thus providing an additional (sensorimotor) integrating mechanism by which signals transmitted downstream from the reticular formation can be synchronized with those projecting upstream.

Pathways to Regions Mediating Sensory Functions and Effects on Cortical Excitability Levels

There are at least three ways in which the reticular formation can modulate sensory functions and

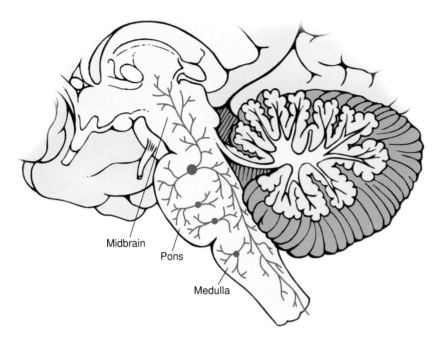

Figure 23–6 Ascending and descending axons in reticular formation. A sagittal section from the brainstem displays large cells in the magnocellular region of the reticular formation. Shown in this illustration is a neuron that bifurcates into an ascending and a descending branch. The branches give off collaterals to the structures adjacent to the reticular formation as well as to other nuclei of the reticular formation.

cortical excitability. The first two mechanisms involve projections from the reticular formation to the intralaminar nuclei of the thalamus, and the third mechanism involves direct projections from monoaminergic neurons of the reticular formation to the cerebral cortex.

Consider first the projections from the reticular formation to the thalamus. Fibers from nuclei within the reticular formation project to nonspecific thalamic nuclei, including the centromedian (CM) and parts of the ventral anterior (VA) nucleus, whose properties mimic those of a nonspecific thal-

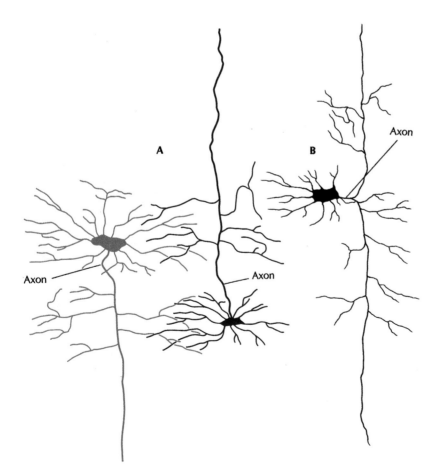

Figure 23–7 Different types of neurons in reticular formation can influence other regions along the neuraxis of the CNS. (A) The long descending neuron on the left (shown in red) gives off a collateral that makes synaptic contact with another neuron (shown in blue) that contains a long ascending axon. (B) Alternatively, a single neuron may bifurcate, giving rise to both long ascending and descending branches. (Used with permission from Barr ML, and Kiernan JA: The Human Nervous System, 6th ed. Philadelphia: Lippincott Williams & Wilkins, 1993, p. 156.)

THE RETICULAR FORMATION — **417**

amic nucleus (for further discussion, see Chapter 26). In turn, these nonspecific thalamic nuclei project to wide regions of cortex directly or indirectly through a synapse in the ventral anterior nucleus (Fig. 23-8). Although the projection from the ventral anterior nucleus to the cortex is extensive, its projection is directed principally to the frontal lobe. Because of the widespread projections, activation of the nonspecific thalamic nuclei by the reticular formation can lead to changes in cortical neuron excitability levels.

There is a second, alternative mechanism that could also be operative. Neurons in nonspecific thalamic nuclei are known to make synaptic contact with specific thalamic nuclei (Fig. 23-9). Here, nonspecific thalamic nuclei can modify sensory transmission at the level of the thalamus by interacting with specific thalamic nuclei before the signals can reach sensory regions of the cerebral cortex.

Evidence for a functional relationship between the reticular formation and cerebral cortex comes from electrical stimulation studies in which

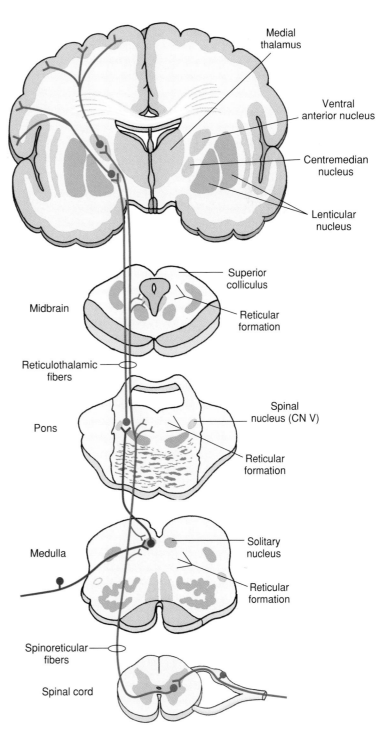

Figure 23–8 The ascending connections of the reticular formation and inputs into the reticular formation from lower levels of the CNS. The reticular formation receives spinoreticular fibers (shown in red). The ascending reticular fibers project either directly to the intralaminar nuclei (shown in red) or indirectly through an interneuron from the solitary nucleus to the dorsolateral pons first (shown in blue); neurons from intralaminar nuclei then project directly to the cortex (shown in red) or to specific thalamic nuclei, which then project to the cerebral cortex (not shown in this diagram). By either direct or indirect routes, inputs from the reticular formation can influence cortical activity and the transmission of sensory signals to the cortex.

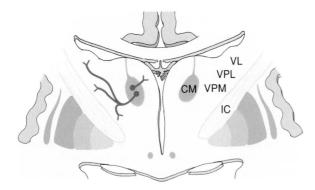

Figure 23–9 Cross section through the thalamus. Note the short efferent projections of a nonspecific thalamic nucleus, the center median nucleus (CM), to specific thalamic nuclei, such as the ventral posterior lateral (VPL), ventral posteromedial (VPM), and ventrolateral (VL) nuclei. IC, internal capsule.

low-frequency stimulation of nonspecific thalamic nuclei produces a distinctive cortical electrical pattern called a *recruiting response*. This response is characterized by a surface negative wave, which reaches a maximum amplitude rapidly and then slowly decreases in size. Additional stimulation results in a waxing and waning of the cortical wave. The behavioral response noted from such stimulation of the nonspecific thalamus is that the patient has a drowsy appearance. In contrast, electrical stimulation of the brainstem reticular formation suppresses the recruiting response as well as the electroencephalographic response that occurs during quiet, sometimes drowsy states referred to as the *alpha rhythm* (Fig. 23-10).[1] These findings provide evidence for the view that modulation of cortical excitability levels involves inputs to the nonspecific thalamus from the reticular formation that are ultimately relayed to the cortex (through the nonspecific thalamus).

Thus, one role of the reticular formation is to provide activation of the cerebral cortex (Fig. 23-11). The process of *arousal* is highly important because it serves to change excitability levels (i.e., prime the sensory [and other] neurons) of the cortex so that they will become more receptive to other sensory inputs that reach the cerebral cortex through the classical ascending sensory pathways. For example, upon awaking to the sound of fire

engines, there is activation of the reticular formation by descending cortical fibers and additional auditory signals (i.e., the continued sounding of the fire engines). This produces cortical desynchronization (*beta rhythm*) and enables the individual to respond in an appropriate way that generates conscious awareness of these stimuli.

It should further be pointed out that the reticular formation can also provide *inhibitory* modulation of sensory signals. In Chapter 15 (*Somatosensory System*), we indicated that the reticular formation comprises part of a descending pain-inhibitory pathway. This pathway originates in the midbrain PAG; it is enkephalinergic, and an enkephalinergic neuron synapses on serotonin neurons in the raphe magnus. This nucleus gives rise to a descending serotonin neuron that reaches the dorsal horn of the spinal cord and synapses on another enkephalin neuron, which ultimately modulates the primary afferent nociceptive pathway at this level of the spinal cord. It is possible that the reticular formation further modulates other sensory inputs, thus enabling us to "filter out" unwanted sensory information so that we can more clearly focus on more critical stimuli.

That cortical excitability is dependent on the capacity of the reticular formation to receive sensory information was demonstrated many years ago in experimental studies conducted in the cat. The studies showed that, if one produces a high spinal transection, called an **encephale isolé** preparation (Fig. 23-12), the cortical arousal pattern is retained. If, on the other hand, one produces a transection rostral to the trigeminal nerve (usually a mid-collicular cut), called a **cerveau isolé** preparation (Fig. 23-12), the electroencephalographic pattern that results is characteristic of a sleeping animal. After the spinal transection, sensory inputs to the reticular formation from cranial nerves remain largely intact. The only sensory loss is from secondary sensory fibers ascending from the spinal cord. However, following a mid-collicular cut, sensory inputs from both the spinal cord and most sensory cranial nerves are eliminated, especially those inputs from the trigeminal and auditory nerves.

These findings led to a passive theory concerning the basis for states of arousal and sleep. In this view, wakefulness results from activation of the reticular formation. Hence, the term "reticular activating system" was coined to describe this mechanism. Sleep was thought to be merely the absence of reticular activation or the shutting off of the reticular formation. But over the last several decades, this notion is no longer accepted. Instead, stages of sleep and wakefulness result from a dynamic interaction between different transmitter

---

[1]The electroencephalogram (EEG) samples the collective activity and summated charges of many neurons from given regions of the cortex (when measured with surface electrodes). The *alpha rhythm* contains waves of typical synchronization. They are slow (approximately 6 to 12/sec) and of relatively high amplitude. In contrast, states of heightened arousal are characterized by a desynchronized EEG pattern in which there is a much higher, irregular frequency and low voltage. This wave pattern is called the *beta rhythm*.

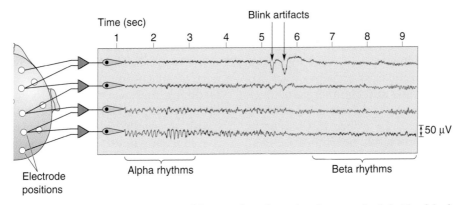

Figure 23–10 Tracings of a normal EEG. The locations of the recording electrodes, shown on the left side of the figure, are taken from an individual who is quiet but awake. Initially, the subject displays an alpha rhythm during the quiet period, but when he opens his eyes (shown by the blink artifacts), the alpha rhythm is replaced by a beta rhythm. (Used with permission from Bear MF, et al.: Neuroscience: Exploring the Brain, 2nd ed. Philadelphia: Lippincott Williams & Wilkins, 2001, p. 610.)

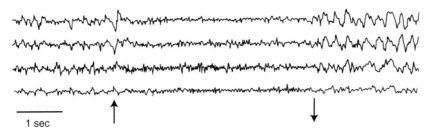

Figure 23–11 Electrical stimulation of the reticular formation. EEG recordings from the studies of Moruzzi and Magoun of the activating patterns of the brainstem reticular formation on the cortex. The four tracings are recorded over different parts of the cerebral cortex of the cat. The arrows pointing up and down indicate the onset and offset of electrical stimulation. Note the desynchronization of the EEG during stimulation followed by a return to a synchronized pattern after stimulation is terminated.

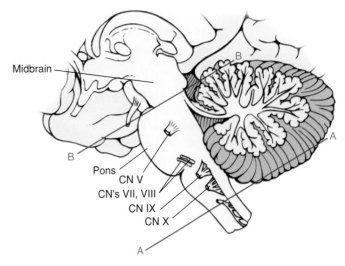

Figure 23–12 Experimental transection of the brainstem. Lateral view of the brainstem showing two levels of transection: (line A) near spinal cord-medulla juncture (encéphale isolé); and (line B) upper pons, rostral to the trigeminal nerve (cerveau isolé). An alert cortical EEG pattern characteristic of a beta rhythm can still be obtained after a cut shown in "A" but not in "B" because, after a transection of the spinal cord-medulla border, sensory information from cranial nerves is preserved, whereas this is not the case after a high pontine transection.

systems in the reticular formation as well as the activity of neuronal groups in other regions such as the hypothalamus.

The third way by which the reticular formation can influence sensory transmission is by direct projections from monoamine and cholinergic neurons of the brainstem to the cerebral cortex and other regions of the forebrain. As described in Chapters 8, 10, 11, and 12, monoaminergic neurons arise from different regions of the brainstem to supply the entire CNS, including the cerebral cortex, hypothalamus, and limbic system. In brief, the key neuronal groups include: (1) the raphe neurons, which give rise to serotonergic projections; (2) the nucleus locus ceruleus, which gives rise to noradrenergic projections; (3) cholinergic neurons from the region of the pedunculopontine nucleus, which project to the forebrain, and (4) the ventral tegmental area, which contains dopaminergic neurons that project to the entire forebrain with the exception of the neostriatum (which is supplied by the *pars compacta* of the substantia nigra).

Pathways to Regions Mediating Motor Functions

We have previously established that the reticular formation receives inputs from two regions that mediate motor functions: the sensorimotor cortex and cerebellum. Inputs from both of these regions modulate the activity of neurons in the reticular formation that project to the spinal cord. Recall that the afferents from both of these regions and, in particular, corticoreticular fibers terminate near the origins of these descending reticulospinal fibers.

The primary motor outputs of the reticular formation are directed on the spinal cord as reticulospinal fibers. As indicated in Chapters 9, 19, and 21, these fibers arise from the pons and medulla. The fibers arising from the pons form the medial reticulospinal tract and issue from the nucleus reticularis pontis oralis and nucleus reticularis pontis caudalis. They pass in the ventral funiculus of the spinal cord and facilitate both alpha and gamma motor neurons of extensors. In contrast, fibers from the medulla arise from the magnocellular nuclei, such as the nucleus gigantocellularis, and descend in the ventral funiculus as the lateral reticulospinal tract, where they also terminate on alpha and gamma motor neurons of extensors. However, their action on these neurons is inhibitory. Collectively, the actions of the reticulospinal fibers serve to modulate muscle tone, regulate posture, and participate in automatic reflex mechanisms involving the extensor musculature (Figs. 23-13 and 23-14) (see also Chapter 19).

Alterations in posture and muscle tone can be mediated by the corticoreticular pathways as part of the overall voluntary motor control system (see Chapter 19). The actions of the cerebellum are somewhat different. The reticular formation receives feedback signals from the fastigial nucleus as part of an automatic regulatory mechanism. The feedback message to the reticular formation is produced in response to signals that the cerebellar cortex receives from the reticular formation. Thus, the efferent connections of the reticular formation to the cerebellar cortex complete a feedback circuit linking these two important structures for the regulation of posture and muscle tone. The efferent pathways to the cerebellar cortex from the reticular formation arise from two nuclei of the medulla (the lateral and paramedian reticular nuclei) and one nucleus from the pons (reticulotegmental nucleus).

The closely integrated response network between the cerebellum, cerebral cortex, and reticular formation is extremely important for the proper maintenance of postural mechanisms and standing erect, especially since there is a delicate balance between the excitatory and inhibitory actions of different regions of the reticular formation on extensor motor neurons. Disruption of any component of this network can lead to significant motor deficits. These deficits include *spasticity* if the inhibitory components of the reticulospinal pathways are disrupted by loss of corticoreticular inputs, *rigidity* if the inputs from the cerebellum to the inhibitory zones of the reticular formation are disrupted, and *hypertonicity* if cerebellar inputs on the excitatory components are disrupted.

Other motor functions that involve the reticular formation include the control of horizontal eye movements. As described in Chapter 14, the **horizontal gaze center** is located in the reticular formation and adjacent to the abducens nucleus and is chiefly responsible for the organization of horizontal eye movements. This region integrates signals from the cerebral cortex (frontal eye fields) and vestibular nuclei. As a result, the horizontal gaze center enables conjugate horizontal movements of the eyes to occur, especially in response to changes in body posture and position of the head in space.

Pathways Mediating Autonomic Functions

Earlier in this chapter, we noted that parts of the reticular formation receive autonomic-related inputs from first-order signals associated with changes in levels of blood oxygen and carbon dioxide levels and changes in blood pressure and inputs from higher order regions of the brain that function to regulate blood pressure and heart rate. As documented in Chapters 10, 14, and 22, the

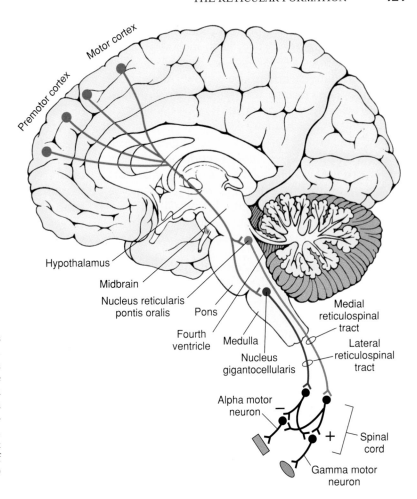

Figure 23–13 Descending motor pathways to the spinal cord from the pons and medulla. Note also that corticoreticular fibers from motor and premotor cortices modulate the activity neurons of the reticular formation that give rise to the reticulospinal tracts. In turn, reticulospinal tracts modulate the activity of alpha and gamma motor neurons. Activation of the lateral reticulospinal tract inhibits spinal reflexes (−), and activation of the medial reticulospinal tract facilitates (+) spinal reflexes.

reticular formation is well equipped with mechanisms that can respond to these autonomic changes. In brief, the reticular formation of the lower brainstem possesses both excitatory and inhibitory regions that provide neural control over cardiovascular functions. The most important controlling regions include the solitary nucleus and the caudal and rostral ventrolateral medulla for blood pressure because they receive inputs from primary and secondary autonomic afferents as well as from higher regulatory centers of the brain such as the hypothalamus, midbrain PAG, and amygdala.

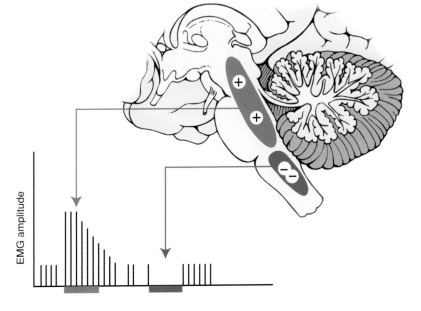

Figure 23–14 Effects of stimulation of reticular formation on spinal reflexes. Stimulation of the facilitory zone (+) (shown in green) of the reticular formation causes a dramatic increase in the patellar reflex as determined by EMG measurements, whereas marked suppression of this reflex follows stimulation of the inhibitory zone (−) (shown in red) of the reticular formation.

Recall that the solitary nucleus and ventrolateral medulla share reciprocal connections and that the ventrolateral medulla can influence cardiovascular functions relatively directly because its descending axons reach the intermediolateral cell column of the thoracic and lumbar cord.

Respiratory mechanisms involve nuclear groups located in both the dorsal and ventrolateral medulla and pons. Descending reticulospinal projections to the cervical cord make synaptic contact with somatic motor neurons of the phrenic nerve that innervate the diaphragm. This provides the efferent pathway by which the reticular formation can modify respiratory responses.

Pathways Modulating Functions of the Hypothalamus and Limbic System

Projections from different regions of the reticular formation (but most notably, the midbrain PAG) and neuronal groups containing monoamine neurons to the hypothalamus and limbic structures are now well established. These efferent projections probably play significant roles in the regulation of higher order autonomic, endocrine, and behavioral functions associated with these structures.

The importance of these ascending fibers is demonstrated by two types of experiments. The first is that lesions of the reticular formation disrupt functions associated with the hypothalamus and limbic system. The second is that administration of drugs that block one or more of the monoamine systems can affect mood changes that are normally associated with the hypothalamus and limbic system.

SLEEP AND WAKEFULNESS

Many regions of the CNS mediate sleep and wakefulness. These regions include specific nuclei of the reticular formation, thalamus, hypothalamus, and basal forebrain. In this section, we will concentrate on the involvement of the reticular formation in sleep and wakefulness.

STAGES OF SLEEP

Most of nighttime sleep (approximately 75%) is not associated with rapid eye movements (REM) (Fig. 23-15). This activity is mediated mainly by thalamo-cortical circuits. These circuits are ultimately activated by the brainstem. There is an increase in gamma-aminobutyric acid (GABA)-ergic neuronal activity in the anterior hypothalamus and a decrease in noradrenergic, serotonergic, and cholinergic activity. The neuronal activity affected by these neuro-

transmitters is likely mediated on the thalamus and cortex and is linked to non-REM sleep.

The initiation of non-REM sleep begins with brain wave (EEG) slowing and vertex waves or high-voltage slow waves recorded from the vertex of the head, called drowsiness or *stage 1* sleep. As sleep deepens, *stage 2* evolves from *stage 1* and is characterized by slowing of the EEG and clusters of 12 to 14 Hz rhythmic waves recorded in the central head region called sleep spindles. A combination of sleep spindles and K-complexes are high-voltage, irregular, slow waves also seen during stage 2 sleep. *Stage 3* is characterized by high-voltage (75 μV) slow waves of frequencies in the range of 2 Hz. Sleep is moderate to deep and spindle activity declines. *Stage 4* sleep is characterized by more than 50% slow wave activity. The circuitry of lighter non-REM sleep consists of rhythmic activity generated by thalamic and cortical neurons. As sleep deepens, cortical neurons generate slow (delta frequency) waves. *Stage 4* sleep is the most difficult stage in which to wake someone from, although sleep walking and talking are recorded from stage 3 or 4 sleep.

RAPID EYE MOVEMENT OR PARADOXICAL SLEEP AND ITS ANATOMICAL LOCI

Studies have demonstrated that the pontine reticular formation is necessary for rapid eye movement (REM) or "dreaming" sleep. These studies also demonstrated that the pons was also instrumental in the inhibition of muscle tone during REM sleep. Projections from the pontine reticular formation to the spinal cord are essential to prevent the "acting out" of dreams. Ponto-geniculo-occipital (PGO) waves, as measured in electrical recordings, occur in bursts during REM sleep and originate in the nucleus pontis oralis and project to the forebrain. These waves serve as a marker for REM sleep in the cat but have never been demonstrated in humans.

Two pontine reticular nuclei initiate REM sleep. Because of their functional similarity, the **pedunculopontine nucleus** and the **lateral dorsal nucleus** are often considered to be one region. These neurons contain cholinergic nuclei that project to other regions of the reticular formation, hypothalamus, basal forebrain, and thalamus. When the cholinergic regions become activated, there is a change in the activity within the thalamus and cortex. Moreover, as indicated earlier, REM sleep is associated with activation of these cholinergic neurons and a reduction of catecholaminergic activity.

Multiple regions modulate REM sleep. The **locus ceruleus**, a major norepinephrine cell group of

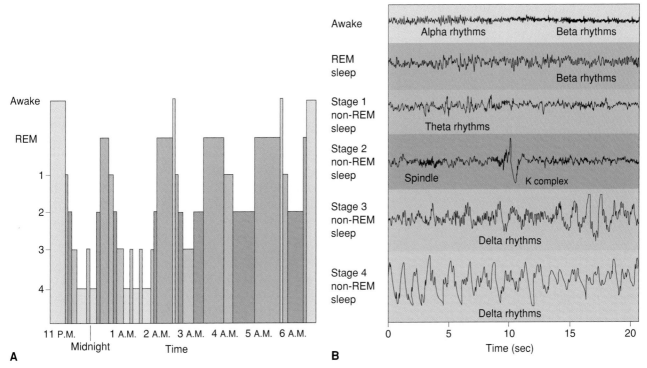

Figure 23–15 EEG rhythms during different stages of sleep. (A) Graph depicts the extent to which different stages of sleep are present throughout the night, beginning at 11:00 PM when sleep began. Initially, there were deeper periods of non-REM sleep, which were eventually replaced by longer periods of REM sleep. The sleep cycles tended to be repeated, with the REM sleep becoming more prominent. (B) The four stages of sleep are characterized by the presence of different EEG rhythms. For example, theta rhythms are present during stage 1, sleep spindles are present in stage 2, and delta rhythms are present in stages 3 and 4. Note that, during REM sleep, the EEG displays a beta rhythm, which is characteristic of the waking state. (From Bear MF, et al.: Neuroscience: Exploring the Brain, 2nd ed. Philadelphia: Lippincott Williams & Wilkins, 2001, p. 616.)

the rostral pontine reticular formation, projects to the thalamus and cerebral and cerebellar cortices. These connections provide the anatomical bases for the regulation of sensory functions of the cerebral cortex as well as cortical activation itself, which can affect REM sleep. The serotonergic region of the reticular formation, the raphe nuclei, innervates much of the forebrain. It has been hypothesized that serotonin contributes to the process of REM sleep. Consistent with this hypothesis is the observation that destruction or pharmacological depletion of serotonin levels in the brain results in long periods of wakefulness (insomnia). Replacement therapy with 5-hydroxytryptophan (the serotonin precursor) can restore normal states of slow-wave sleep.

Wakefulness, as well as REM sleep, is modulated by the reticular formation. The direct connections of the monoaminergic fibers to the cerebral cortex endow this region with a simple mechanism by which the reticular formation can regulate levels of cortical excitability. In particular, the noradrenergic neurons located in the nucleus locus ceruleus seem to play an important role in cortical excitabil-

ity and wakefulness. Sleep onset occurs when circadian rhythms, any sleep deprivations, and environmental stimulation (such as a dark room) are optimal. Removal of the cortical-activating influence occurs, and non-REM sleep is initiated.

In experimental studies, the nucleus locus ceruleus has also been linked to the regulation of **REM** or **paradoxical sleep**. Lesions placed in the locus ceruleus or administration of the drug alpha methyldopa (from which the false neurotransmitter alpha methylnorepinephrine is synthesized) can suppress paradoxical sleep. Moreover, long-lasting states of wakefulness are produced after cerebral catecholamine levels are elevated.

ROLE OF OTHER REGIONS IN SLEEP AND WAKEFULNESS

Although not part of the reticular formation, neurons in the suprachiasmatic nucleus of the hypothalamus also appear to play an important role in the sleep-wakefulness cycle. These neurons show a clear-cut diurnal rhythm for light and darkness. They receive direct retinal inputs, and if the nucleus is destroyed, other rhythms, such as those for endocrine function and sleep-wakefulness cycles, are disrupted. What remains unknown is the specific triggering mechanism for sleep. It had previously been thought that it was located in the raphe complex, but as indicated earlier, more recent studies suggest involvement of the cholinergic neurons in the pedunculopontine region. Other investigators further suggest that the suprachiasmatic nucleus serves this function. Whatever mechanism(s) regulate sleep and wakefulness, it is clear that it is an active, not a passive, process that is present, and one that involves the reticular formation and other nuclei in the brainstem and forebrain.

SLEEP DISORDERS

A number of common types of sleep disorders have been identified and are summarized here.

Narcolepsy

Narcolepsy is frequently a disabling form of somnolence. The individual experiences attacks of sleep at times and places where sleep does not normally occur. For example, the individual may fall asleep in the car while driving or while giving a lecture. Such individuals may also be subject to a condition called **cataplexy,** which is a loss of muscle tone. Narcoleptic individuals may also display a sleep paralysis in which they remain awake at night, begin to hallucinate, and are unable to move. This disorder may be associated with abnormal functions of cholinergic neurons.

Sleep Apnea

Sleep apnea is a condition characterized by an interruption of breathing. In individuals with this condition, there is a decline in the oxygen content of the blood. The interruption of breathing leads to arousal from sleep or results in lighter stages of non-REM sleep in order for breathing to be maintained. Muscle tone in individuals suffering from sleep apnea is further compromised by REM sleep, which, by itself, results in reduced muscle tone. The net effect in such individuals is that excessive reduction in muscle tone of the airway muscles leads to a further narrowing of the airway passages. In addition, patients with sleep apnea may show impaired performance in work-related functions and reduced intellectual capacity as well as excessive daytime sleepiness. This condition could be dangerous to the afflicted individual in such circumstances as driving a car or operating machines that may be lethal if misused. Sleep apnea is exacerbated in individuals who are obese because the added fatty tissue may further reduce the air passages.

Sleep Disorders in Psychiatric Patients

In certain psychiatric conditions, there is a marked reduction in the amount of sleep that an individual may receive. These disorders include **depression**, in which the individual awakens very early or during the nighttime (in addition to the characteristic conditions of excessive guilt, depressed mood and appetite, and difficulties in concentrating on one's work and remembering), and **posttraumatic stress disorder**, in which a life-threatening event in the distant past of the individual reappears in her memory during the daytime or in the evening in dreams. It is possible that this disorder may relate to the disruption of mechanisms that control REM sleep.

COMA

What are the consequences of lesions of the reticular formation? From the earlier discussion, it is not surprising that lesions of the brainstem reticular formation are associated with disturbances of consciousness. Damage (typically associated with a cerebrovascular accident) to the reticular formation of the pons or midbrain will produce **coma** in most instances. The electroencephalographic patterns resulting from lesions of different regions of the reticular formation may vary significantly. For example, lesions of the midbrain reticular formation result in the appearance of slow waves of large amplitude. In contrast, lesions of the pons are frequently characterized by an alpha rhythm typically seen in a normal drowsy person. With other lesions, the patient may display an EEG pattern characteristic of slow-wave sleep. In the case of a pontine lesion, the patient lies quietly and displays a variety of autonomic and somatomotor reflexes as well as normal eye movements. This constellation of responses is referred to as **coma vigil** or **akinetic mutism**. Lesions involving the lower brainstem also produce a loss of consciousness. However, lesions involving the lower brainstem are frequently fatal because of the severity of the accompanying cardiovascular respiratory disturbances.

CLINICAL CASE

HISTORY

Bill is a 23-year-old man who has had bouts of difficulty remaining awake for several years. Throughout high school, he was unable to remain awake during class and while taking tests. He would fall asleep while on the telephone, watching television, playing video games, and during driving instruction to such an extent that he was not permitted to obtain a driver's license. If he heard a joke or reacted to another emotional stimulus, he would often have a loss of muscle tone in his head and jaw and, in severe cases, would fall to the floor. He required at least one nap during the day, which refreshed him even if it lasted only 15 or 20 minutes. He felt as though he had dreamed during these naps, although they were short. Although he had no trouble falling asleep at night, his nighttime sleep was fragmented, with frequent kicking and awakening. Upon falling asleep or awaking, he often felt paralyzed or had hallucinations similar to dreaming. He sought medical attention when it took him 6 years to complete college, despite having a superior intellectual ability.

EXAMINATION

A neurologist saw Bill and completed a history and physical examination. The neurologic examination was normal, except that when the lights were lowered to perform a fundoscopic examination, the neurologist observed the **Bell effect**, which involves the rolling back of the eyes, which is a normal response upon closing one's eyes. A nighttime sleep study was ordered, followed by a test consisting of a series of naps called **multiple sleep latency tests**, where Bill was asked to take a 20-minute nap every 2

hours. A magnetic resonance imaging (MRI) scan of Bill's head was ordered.

EXPLANATION

Bill has **narcolepsy**, a neurologic disorder characterized by excessive daytime somnolence with frequent, uncontrollable napping, cataplexy (drop attacks, or loss of tone in the antigravity muscles), sleep paralysis (feeling paralyzed while falling asleep or awaking), and hypnagogic hallucinations (hallucinations upon falling asleep and awaking). One neurophysiological characteristic of narcolepsy is called **sleep-onset REM** (or REM sleep), which occurs in the first hour of nighttime sleep or anytime during daytime multiple sleep latency tests. This provides evidence that narcolepsy is a disorder of the intrusion of REM sleep during inappropriate times, even wakefulness in response to an emotional stimulus (cataplexy—muscle tone is normally lost during REM sleep). Experimental evidence has been unable to pinpoint a precise lesion causing narcolepsy. Moreover, hypothalamic and brainstem tumors involving the reticular formation have been rarely found in new cases of narcolepsy. Most cases of narcolepsy are idiopathic and begin during the teenage years or even earlier.

CHAPTER TEST

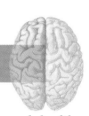

QUESTIONS

Choose the best answer for each question.

1. Central control of cardiovascular function is mediated primarily from the:
   a. Prefrontal cortex
   b. Dorsomedial pons
   c. Ventromedial medulla
   d. Ventrolateral medulla
   e. Midbrain tectum

2. Rapid eye movement (REM) sleep is believed to originate in the:
   a. Caudal medulla
   b. Pons
   c. Midbrain
   d. Lateral hypothalamus
   e. Medial thalamus

3. A 72-year-old man was found unconscious in his home and was taken to the emergency room of the local hospital. After a few days, the patient remained in a coma, and the pattern on his EEG

revealed mainly the presence of an alpha-like rhythm. In addition, the patient presented with normal eye movements and a variety of autonomic and somatomotor reflexes. On the basis of these observations as well as an MRI, the neurologist concluded that the lesion was localized to the:
   a. Medulla
   b. Pons
   c. Midbrain
   d. Diencephalon
   e. Cerebral cortex

4. A middle-aged, male professor of neuroscience at a Northeastern medical school began to experience intermittent episodes of uncontrollable sleep, even while giving lectures to the first-year medical class. At the request of colleagues and students, it was suggested that he see a neurologist in the university hospital. The neurologic examination revealed temporary loss of muscle tone in the trunk and extremities, and in the sleep clinic, he experienced some hallucinations and

tended to remain awake at night. The neurologist concluded that the patient was suffering from:

a. A brainstem stroke
b. A cortical stroke
c. Narcolepsy
d. Depression
e. Sleep apnea

5. A 67-year-old woman complained to her ophthalmologist that she was experiencing double vision. After a thorough examination, the patient was given a neurologic examination. An MRI revealed the presence of a small stroke. The most likely locus of the lesion was:

a. Ventrolateral medulla
b. Dorsomedial medulla
c. Dorsolateral pons
d. Dorsomedial pons
e. Dorsolateral midbrain

ANSWERS AND EXPLANATIONS

1. Answer: d

The ventrolateral medulla gives rise to neurons that project to the intermediolateral cell column of the thoracolumbar spinal cord. In this manner, this region of the medulla regulates sympathetic activity. The prefrontal cortex may exert some influence on autonomic functions; the primary properties of this region are associated with intellectual and affective functions. The dorsomedial pons, ventromedial medulla, and tectum are not known to contain fiber systems that directly affect autonomic functions.

2. Answer: b

Electrophysiological studies have indicated that REM sleep originates in the pontine reticular formation. Activation of this pathway modulates cortical activity in association with REM sleep. Other choices include regions that have never been associated with induction of REM sleep. The caudal medulla contains few reticular formation neurons, and the general region of the caudal medulla contains cell bodies and axons associated with transmission of sensory information to higher regions, cranial nerve function, and descending fibers to the spinal cord. The midbrain contains neurons comprising part of the reticular formation but lacks the cholinergic cell groups essential for generation of REM sleep, which is characteristic of those pre-

sent in the pontine reticular formation. The lateral hypothalamus is associated with visceral processes, such as feeding, and contains ascending and descending fibers associated with limbic structures and monoaminergic systems that are unrelated to REM sleep. The medial thalamus is concerned with the transmission of impulses mainly to the frontal lobe and has no known relationship to REM sleep.

3. Answer: b

The disorder described in this case is referred to as "coma vigil." It is characteristic of a pontine lesion, which includes parts of the tegmentum but spares the dorsomedial region, which is associated with the control of horizontal eye movements. Although the patient is comatose, his EEG response is characteristic of an alpha rhythm, and horizontal eye movements are clearly present. Lesions of that medulla usually are fatal; lesions involving the other choices do not produce the symptoms described in this case, such as the alpha-like rhythms and eye movements.

4. Answer: c

The constellation of symptoms described in this case is characteristic of narcolepsy. In narcolepsy, the patient has frequent bouts of sleep during the day, an inability to sleep at night, and loss of muscle tone. Sleep apnea is characterized by an interruption of breathing during sleep, with considerable snoring. A cortical or brainstem stroke would significantly disable the patient, and the symptoms associated with these lesions are totally distinct from those described in this case and would likely involve paralysis and perhaps coma. Although depression oftentimes is associated with problems in sleeping, it does not involve either loss of muscle tone or frequent bouts of sleep during the day as described in this case.

5. Answer: d

The paramedian reticular formation of the caudal pons in the region of the abducens nucleus contains the horizontal gaze center. It serves to integrate cortical and vestibular inputs for the control of conjugate horizontal gaze. Damage to this region would result in loss of coordination of the eyes, causing double vision. The other choices involve regions that are not associated with the regulation of eye movements. Damage to these regions would cause significantly different neurologic deficits that are unrelated to double vision.

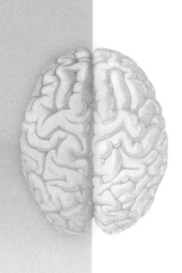

CHAPTER 24

THE HYPOTHALAMUS

OBJECTIVES

After reading this chapter, the student should be able to:

1. Describe and diagram the morphological organization of the hypothalamus

2. List and diagram the primary afferent fiber connections of the hypothalamus

3. List and diagram the primary efferent fiber connections of the hypothalamus

4. Describe the basic functional properties of the hypothalamus regarding:
   a. Control of endocrine functions
   b. Role in temperature regulation
   c. Regulation of cardiovascular function
   d. Regulation of feeding and drinking behavior
   e. Role in sexual behavior
   f. Regulation of aggression, rage, and related forms of emotional behavior
   g. Role in sleep

5. List and describe some of the basic disorders associated with hypothalamic dysfunctions

As described in Chapter 13, the hypothalamus occupies only a very small part of the tissue of the forebrain. Yet, it plays a vital role in the organization of a number of autonomic functions and in the expression of related visceral behavioral processes. For example, endocrine function is controlled by the activity of different neurons of the hypothalamus. Likewise, temperature regulation is governed by the actions of different regions of the hypothalamus. The control of water balance, drinking, feeding, and sexual behaviors are also governed by distinct neuronal mechanisms within the hypothalamus, as are the mechanisms regulating aggression, rage, and flight behaviors. This chapter focuses on the anatomical and functional relationships of the hypothalamus with other regions of the brain and pituitary gland.

HYPOTHALAMIC ANATOMY

HYPOTHALAMIC NUCLEI

Details concerning the anatomical organization of the nuclei of the hypothalamus can be found in Chapter 13. The relative positions of the major nuclei are outlined in Figure 24-1. The key nuclei include the **preoptic, supraoptic, paraventricular, ventromedial, suprachiasmatic, dorsomedial, arcuate, tuberal,** and **mammillary bodies**. Additionally, there are four other regional areas, which are designated as the **anterior, lateral, dorsal,** and **posterior hypothalamic areas.**

CONNECTIONS OF THE HYPOTHALAMUS

Afferent Connections

Significant modulation of hypothalamic processes is mediated by different groups of afferent fibers that originate primarily from the limbic system and reticular formation. The specific pathways over which such modulation occurs are described in the following sections.

Fornix

The origin, course, and distribution of the fibers that make up the fornix are described in detail in Chapter 25. Briefly, the postcommissural fornix projects to the hypothalamus and anterior nucleus of the thalamus. This branch of the fornix arises from the subicular cortex of the hippocampal formation, and the hypothalamic component terminates largely in the medial hypothalamus and mammillary bodies (Figs. 24-1 and 24-2).

Stria Terminalis

A description of the position and course of these fibers was presented in Chapter 13. In brief, this important pathway arises from the medial amygdala, and the periamygdalar cortex projects to the bed nucleus of the stria terminalis and much of the rostro-caudal extent of the medial hypothalamus (Fig. 24-2).

Ventral Amygdalofugal Pathway

This fiber bundle arises chiefly from the basolateral amygdala and parts of the adjoining pyriform cortex. Fibers of this bundle course medially from the amygdala into the lateral hypothalamus, where many terminate. Other axons of this bundle continue to pass in a caudal direction, where most synapse in the midbrain periaqueductal gray (PAG) (see Chapter 25).

Medial Forebrain Bundle

The medial forebrain bundle is the principal pathway that traverses the rostro-caudal extent of the lateral hypothalamus. Many of the fibers constitute hypothalamic efferent projections to the brainstem.

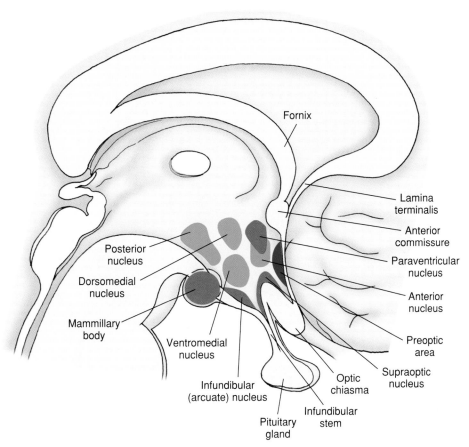

Figure 24–1 A schematic three-dimensional reconstruction of the loci of the nuclei of the hypothalamus. (From Barr ML, and Kiernan JA: The Human Nervous System, 6th ed. Philadelphia: Lippincott Williams & Wilkins, 1993.)

Other fibers represent ascending monoaminergic projections from the brainstem that supply much of the forebrain, including the cerebral cortex. Still other fibers arise from the septal area and diagonal band of Broca and project directly to the lateral and medial regions of hypothalamus, including the mammillary bodies (Fig. 24-2).

Thalamohypothalamic Fibers

The mediodorsal thalamic nucleus receives major inputs from the prefrontal cortex and adjoining portions of the anterior cingulate gyrus. Fibers that issue from the mediodorsal nucleus project to posterior midline thalamic nuclei. From the posterior midline thalamus, a chain of neurons then pass rostrally through midline nuclei. Neurons that arise from the rostral aspect of the midline thalamus (nucleus reuniens) project to the anterior lateral hypothalamus (Fig. 24-3). This circuitry provides an important anatomical substrate by which the prefrontal cortex and anterior cingulate gyrus can regulate functions associated with the lateral hypothalamus. Recent findings have provided evidence that the prefrontal cortex can influence hypothalamic functions via a monosynaptic projection to the hypothalamus.

Retinohypothalamic Fibers

An overwhelming number of retinal fibers terminate in the lateral geniculate nucleus, pretectal region, and superior colliculus. Nevertheless, it has been shown that some optic fibers terminate in the region of the suprachiasmatic nucleus. Such inputs are important in regulating the sleep-wakefulness cycle (pages 423–424) and circadian rhythms that govern endocrine functions (see pages 209–210).

Mammillary Peduncle

This tract arises mainly from the ventral and dorsal tegmental nuclei of the midbrain and presumably serves as a relay for ascending impulses to the hypothalamus from lower regions of the brainstem tegmentum. Ascending fibers from the dorsal tegmental nuclei terminate principally in the mammillary bodies, while those in the ventral tegmentum pass through the medial forebrain bundle to more rostral levels of the hypothalamus and limbic structures.

Midbrain Periaqueductal Gray (PAG)

The midbrain PAG matter is functionally related to the medial hypothalamus. Consequently, it shares reciprocal connections with parts of the medial

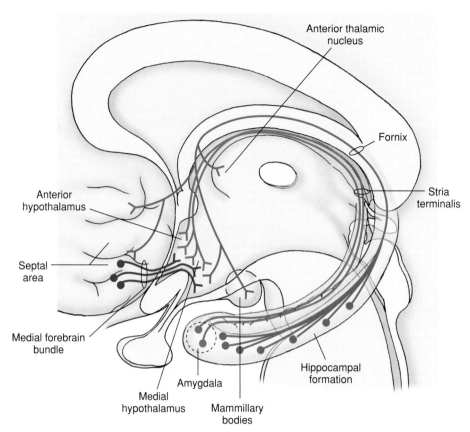

Figure 24–2 Inputs from limbic structures. Projections from hippocampal formation through the fornix (shown in red), amygdala through the stria terminalis (shown in green), and septal area through the medial forebrain bundle (shown in blue) to the hypothalamus. Other inputs, such as those from the brainstem, are omitted from this diagram.

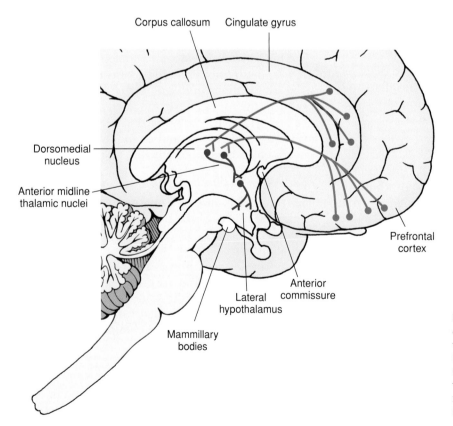

Figure 24–3 Inputs from cerebral cortex. Diagrams illustrate the pathways by which the prefrontal cortex (green) and anterior cingulate gyrus (red) supply the hypothalamus by virtue of relays in the mediodorsal and midline thalamic nuclear groups (blue).

hypothalamus. The dorsal part of the midbrain PAG contains both ascending and descending projections. Its ascending projections reach the posterior half of the medial hypothalamus and thus serve as a feedback mechanism with respect to several of the functions of the medial hypothalamus, which are mediated via their descending projections to the midbrain PAG.

Monoaminergic Pathways

As noted in Chapter 23, the hypothalamus and other forebrain regions receive monoaminergic projections from the raphe complex (containing serotonin), locus ceruleus (containing norepinephrine), and ventral tegmental area (containing dopamine). These inputs from the brainstem tegmentum, together with the inputs from limbic structures, provide significant modulation of hypothalamic processes.

Efferent Projections

Projections from the Mammillary Bodies

The mammillary bodies give rise to at least two groups of fiber projections. One ascends to the thalamus, and the other descends to the brainstem (Fig. 24-4). The ascending pathway is called the **mammillothalamic tract**. It projects to the anterior thalamic nucleus and comprises a component of the **Papez Circuit**, which is a circular series of

pathways linking the cingulate gyrus to the hippocampal formation to the mammillary bodies to the anterior thalamic nucleus, with a return flow back to the cingulate gyrus. This circuit, which is discussed in more detail in Chapter 25, was originally believed to be associated with the regulation of emotional behavior, but more recent evidence suggests that it may be more closely linked with short-term memory functions.

A second pathway arising from the mammillary bodies is called the **mammillotegmental tract**, which projects to the midbrain tegmentum (Fig. 24-4). Other fibers forming a multisynaptic chain descend in the mammillary peduncle from the mammillary bodies to the reticular formation. Projections from the midbrain tegmentum to autonomic nuclei of the lower brainstem and spinal cord may provide an anatomical substrate for hypothalamic control of autonomic functions. However, as described on page 432, other descending pathways from the hypothalamus are equally (if not more) tenable.

Projections from the Medial Hypothalamus

Fibers originating from the medial hypothalamus have both ascending and descending projections. The ascending projections reach the medial nucleus of the amygdala (Fig. 24-5). This projection could be viewed as a feedback pathway to the amygdala associated with a major descending

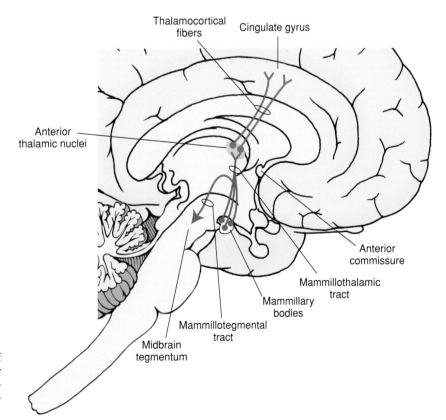

Figure 24–4 Efferent projections of the mammillary bodies to the anterior thalamic nucleus via the mammillothalamic tract and to the midbrain tegmentum via the mammillotegmental tract.

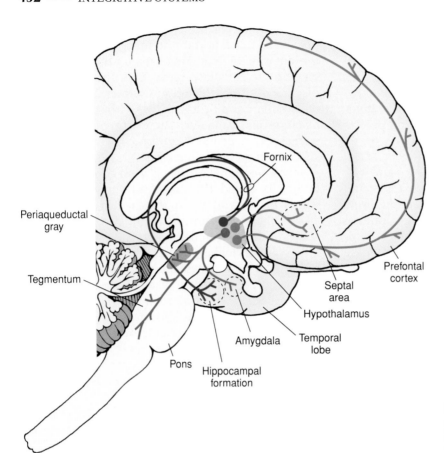

Figure 24–5 Major efferent projections of the hypothalamus. Not shown in this illustration are connections from the hypothalamus to the pituitary gland.

projection from the medial amygdala to the medial hypothalamus that regulates emotional behavior and related hypothalamic processes.

Descending fibers project principally to the dorsal half of the midbrain PAG. This pathway enables emotional (i.e., aggression, rage, and flight) and autonomic (i.e., marked changes in heart rate and blood pressure) responses integrated within the medial hypothalamus to be transmitted downstream to the midbrain PAG. For this reason, the midbrain PAG can be viewed functionally as a caudal extension of the medial hypothalamus. Moreover, the midbrain PAG then transmits this information to the lower sympathetic, parasympathetic (i.e., pontine tegmentum, solitary nucleus, ventrolateral medulla, dorsal motor nucleus of CN X, and intermediolateral cell column of the spinal cord), and somatic motor regions of the lower brainstem and spinal cord; from here, ultimate expression of these responses is achieved.

Projections from the Medial Forebrain Bundle (Lateral Hypothalamus)

Cells situated at all levels of the lateral hypothalamus give rise to axons that pass both rostrally and caudally within the medial forebrain bundle. Ascending fibers within the medial forebrain bundle supply the septal area, preoptic region, and nuclei of the diagonal band of Broca. In addition, some fibers of the far rostral lateral hypothalamus have been shown to have long axons that project as far as the hippocampal formation, prefrontal cortex, and other parts of the frontal and parietal lobes (Fig. 24–5). Such a pathway could provide the cerebral cortex with direct information concerning the internal milieu of the organism as well as synchronize cortical activity with hypothalamic functions. Other fibers ascending in the medial forebrain bundle enter the **stria medullaris** and pass caudally to the habenular complex, where they terminate in the lateral habenular nucleus.

Descending fibers of the lateral hypothalamus pass through the medial forebrain bundle to ventral regions of the midbrain PAG and other regions of the midbrain and pontine tegmentum. This pathway could also serve as an anatomical substrate by which the lateral regions of the hypothalamus could regulate autonomic and somatomotor components of emotional responses normally associated with this region.

Hypothalamic Efferents to the Pituitary

Effects on Neuroendocrine Functions to the Posterior Pituitary from the Paraventricular and Supraoptic Nuclei. The paraventricular and supraoptic nuclei share a number of similarities.

Both have large cells, both have axonal projections that reach rich vascular beds in the posterior pituitary, and both synthesize the same peptides: antidiuretic hormone (ADH, vasopressin) and oxytocin.

These peptides, which are synthesized in the cell bodies, are then transported down the hypothalamohypophyseal tract and are released into the portal circulation (Fig. 24-6). These neurons are accordingly referred to as **neurosecretory**. Fibers from these hypothalamic nuclei also reach the median eminence, where the hormones are released into the vascular beds. From the vascular beds, the hormones can be transported elsewhere, including the anterior pituitary. The triggers that release the hormones from the nerve endings in the posterior pituitary are action potentials that are conducted down the neurons in response to different types of stimuli (see, for example, the following paragraphs and *Drinking Behavior* on page 439).

Functionally, **ADH** produces its major effects by increasing water absorption in the kidneys. ADH release is triggered by two factors: (1) neuronal impulses from afferent sources of the supraoptic nucleus (frequently occurring in response to sudden increases in emotional states); and (2) the sensory properties of supraoptic nuclei that enable them to sense changes in blood osmolarity. In this sense, the supraoptic and paraventricular nuclei serve as osmoreceptors. Under conditions in which there is an increase in osmotic pressure resulting from such factors as reduced fluid intake, increased amount of salt intake, or fluid loss due to diarrhea or sweating, supraoptic neurons discharge more rapidly and release increased amounts of ADH into the vascular system. The primary target of ADH is the distal convoluted tubules of the kidney. The mechanism of action of ADH hormone is as follows: when the plasma concentration of salt increases, the osmotic pressure increases within the arterial blood vessels that supply the hypothalamus. This results in an increase in production and release of ADH, which acts on its target organ, the distal convoluted tubule, causing reabsorption of excess water, thus allowing the blood to re-establish osmolality. Damage to the posterior pituitary or the pituitary stalk produces a condition in which there is an excess of excretion of low-gravity urine. This condition is referred to as **diabetes insipidus** and results from loss of secretion of ADH.

The mechanism of action of **oxytocin** and the stimuli affecting its release are somewhat different. The main actions of oxytocin are: (1) to produce the contractions of the myoepithelial cells around the nipple of the mammary gland for the ejection of milk (called the **milk ejection reflex**), and (2) to aid in producing contractions of the smooth muscles of the uterus during birth. The trigger for production and release of oxytocin involves a neural mechanism. Sensory stimuli associated with

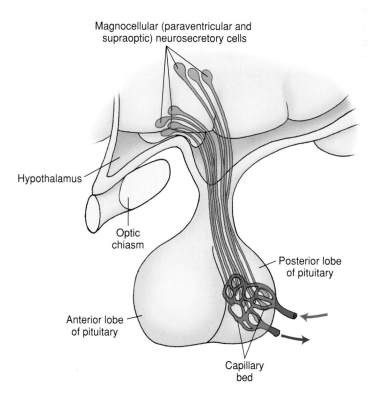

Magnocellular (paraventricular and supraoptic) neurosecretory cells

Hypothalamus

Optic chiasm

Posterior lobe of pituitary

Anterior lobe of pituitary

Capillary bed

Figure 24–6 Hypothalamoneurohypophyseal tracts are used by the paraventricular and supraoptic nuclei as projection pathways to the posterior pituitary.

suckling produce sensory impulses that ascend to the forebrain through multisynaptic pathways, ultimately causing increased neuronal discharges within the paraventricular nucleus. Increased firing of these neurons results in increased secretion of oxytocin into the circulatory system, where it acts on the mammary gland soon afterwards.

Effects on Neuroendocrine Functions to the Anterior Pituitary from the Hypophysiotropic Zone. The anterior pituitary differs from the posterior pituitary in that it does not contain any nerve fiber terminals from the hypothalamus. Instead, communication between the hypothalamus and anterior pituitary is achieved through a portal system of blood vessels called the **hypothalamohypophyseal portal vascular system**. The hypothalamohypophyseal portal system arises from a capillary bed in the median eminence and the pituitary stalk that is drained by other portal vessels. This system thus transports releasing hormones through the blood to the sinuses of the anterior lobe of the pituitary (Fig. 24-7).

NATURE AND FUNCTIONS OF HYPOTHALAMIC PEPTIDES

HORMONES THAT TARGET THE ANTERIOR PITUITARY

It should be pointed out that the primary capillary plexus is situated in the infundibular stalk and lies proximal to the region of convergence of nerve terminals. Because of this anatomical arrangement, the peptides, which are synthesized in the cell bodies of hypothalamic neurons, can easily be released into the hypophyseal portal system. The cell bodies that synthesize these peptides are found over wide regions of the hypothalamus. Some of these cell bodies extend rostrally as far as the ventral aspect of the septal area. For the most part, however, the cells are present in greatest quantities within the medial hypothalamus in proximity to the third ventricle.

Each of the hormones in the anterior pituitary is produced by a specific epithelial cell type (called **gonadotropes, thyrotropes, corticotropes,** and

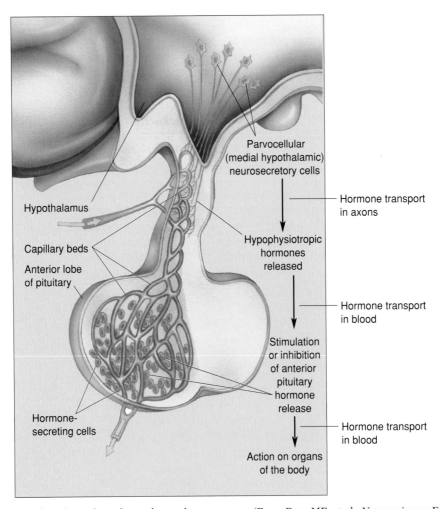

Figure 24–7 The hypothalamohypophyseal portal vasculature system. (From Bear MF, et al.: Neuroscience: Exploring the Brain, 2nd ed. Philadelphia: Lippincott Williams & Wilkins, 2001, p. 504.)

somatotropes for the respective cell types). In turn, these hormones are controlled by hypothalamic peptides called **releasing hormones**. Each releasing hormone acts on one cell type within the anterior pituitary. In addition to releasing hormones, some of the peptides that are produced have inhibitory effects on secretion and release of anterior pituitary hormones. These are called **inhibiting hormones**. The hormones of the anterior pituitary, their functions, and their hypothalamic releasing and/or inhibiting hormones are summarized in the following sections.

Growth Hormone (GH)

Growth hormone (GH) stimulates growth of the body and, particularly, the long bones. Its release is controlled by **growth hormone-releasing hormone (GHrH)**, which is present in greatest quantities within the arcuate nucleus of the hypothalamus. GH can also be inhibited by **growth hormone-inhibiting hormone (somatostatin)**. Somatostatin is widely distributed throughout the central nervous system but is present in dense quantities in the preoptic region and anterior hypothalamus. Many of these neurons project directly to the capillary beds of the median eminence where somatostatin is released into the portal system. On reaching the anterior pituitary, the neurons directly inhibit the release of GH. The effects of somatostatin on the anterior pituitary are not entirely specific because this peptide also inhibits thyrotropin and prolactin.

Thyroid-Stimulating Hormone (TSH)

Thyroid-stimulating hormone (TSH) is controlled by **thyrotropin-releasing hormone (TRH)**. TRH cells are located principally in the periventricular region and adjoining areas of the hypothalamus. The peptide is released from axon terminals located in the median eminence into the portal system.

Adrenocorticotropic Hormone (ACTH)

Adrenocorticotropic hormone (ACTH) controls the release of steroid hormones, such as cortisol, in the adrenal cortex. In turn, it is controlled by **corticotropin-releasing hormone (CRH)**. CRH, synthesized in the paraventricular, supraoptic, and arcuate nuclei, as well as outside the hypothalamus, enters the portal system from axon terminals in the median eminence. CRH also stimulates the release of **β-endorphin** from the anterior pituitary. CRH is activated by conditions of stress, which increase the release of ACTH from the anterior pituitary. This, in turn, causes the release of corticosteroids from the adrenal glands. Increased levels of circulating corticosteroids within the brain provide a negative feedback mechanism to the CRH-containing hypothalamic neurons, which, ultimately, inhibit the further release of CRH.

Gonadotropic Hormones

Gonadotropic hormones include **follicle-stimulating hormone (FSH)**, which facilitates growth of follicles and oocytes, and **luteinizing hormone (LH)**, which is critical for induction of ovulation and formulation of the corpus luteum. These hormones are controlled by **gonadotropin-releasing hormone (GnRH)**. The cells that synthesize GnRH are distributed widely over a region extending from the septal area to the posterior hypothalamus. But the cells modulating and controlling the release of LH are found in most abundant quantities in the arcuate region and area surrounding the median eminence. An example is **neuropeptide Y**, which is synthesized in the arcuate nucleus of the hypothalamus and acts as a neuromodulator of GnRH-containing neurons. Neuropeptide Y also stimulates feeding behavior.

Prolactin

Prolactin is released from the anterior pituitary by prolactin-releasing factor and causes growth of the mammary glands in women prior to and following birth. It is believed to be inhibited by several substances, including somatostatin, endothelins, and dopamine. In fact, dopamine may even constitute the prolactin release-inhibiting hormone.

OTHER PEPTIDES FOUND IN THE HYPOTHALAMUS

Other peptides have been discovered in the hypothalamus and likely serve as neuromodulators or neurotransmitters that specifically act on one or more of the releasing hormones. For the most part, they constitute brain-gut peptides because they have been identified immunocytochemically in the gut and in the brain. These peptides provide a variety of functions within the gut. In the brain, these peptides have recently been discovered, and attempts to identify their functions are currently under investigation.

Vasoactive Intestinal Polypeptide (VIP)

VIP is present in very high concentrations in the cerebral cortex and is also present within the suprachiasmatic nucleus of the hypothalamus. It appears to modulate functions associated with this nucleus. VIP is also present in the anterior pituitary, where it may act to modulate the release of anterior pituitary hormones.

Cholecystokinin (CCK)

The biologically active form of CCK (CCK-8, the carboxyl-terminal octapeptide) is found widely throughout the nervous system. It is also present in the supraoptic and paraventricular nuclei as well as in the posterior lobe of the pituitary. It likely modulates the release of oxytocin and vasopressin from these hypothalamic nuclei. Recent studies have shown that activation of CCK receptors in the PAG can also facilitate rage behavior in the cat. Peripherally, CCK plays an important role in evacuation of the gallbladder by causing contraction of this organ, resulting in increased secretion of bile and increased flow of biliary contents into the duodenum. Likewise, it also induces secretion from the pancreas.

Neurotensin

Neurotensin neurons have been identified in the preoptic area and adjoining regions of the anterior hypothalamus, including the paraventricular, arcuate, and dorsomedial nuclei. The presence of neurotensin within the dorsomedial hypothalamus suggests that it may modulate the release of anterior pituitary hormones. Neurotensin is also co-localized within dopamine neurons in the tuberoinfundibular region, further suggesting that it may also modulate the release of dopamine into the portal system.

Substance P

Substance P-immunopositive cell bodies and axon terminals are found in the anterior and medial hypothalamus. Substance P-positive cell bodies are also present in the medial nucleus of the amygdala, the axons of which project to the medial hypothalamus. It is likely that substance P acts as a neurotransmitter or neuromodulator of neuronal functions associated with the medial hypothalamus. Like CCK, activation of substance P (neurokinin-1) receptors in the hypothalamus potentiates emotional forms of behavior such as flight and rage.

Pro-Opiomelanocortin Peptides

A large protein (pro-opiomelanocortin) serves as a precursor for a number of peptides that have been identified within the hypothalamus. These include β-lipotropin, melanocyte-stimulating hormones, and β-endorphin. Although the functions of β-lipotropin have not been identified, enkephalins generally have inhibitory effects on neuronal functions.

Angiotensin II

Another peptide, **angiotensin II**, has cell bodies localized within the supraoptic and paraventricular region. Receptors for angiotensin II are found in a variety of areas but are highly prominent in the anterior hypothalamus and preoptic region. Angiotensin II plays an important role in the regulation of blood pressure and in drinking behavior. In the periphery, angiotensin II is formed in the following manner. The enzyme, renin (formed and stored in the kidney), acts on the liver peptide, angiotensinogen, to produce angiotensin I. Angiotensin I is converted to the biologically active peptide, angiotensin II, by a converting enzyme (localized on the surface of endothelial cells mainly in the lung). Administration of angiotensin II to the subfornical organ (a circumventricular organ that lies outside the blood-brain barrier adjacent to the fornix and that contains dense quantities of angiotensin II receptors) results in an increase in blood pressure and also induces drinking behavior. A similar mechanism is believed to be responsible for the synthesis of angiotensin II in the brain. A number of drugs, such as clonidine, reserpine, beta-blockers, and methyldopa, can block renin secretion. In addition, there is another class of drugs that inhibit the angiotensin-converting enzyme (see earlier discussion), called ACE inhibitors. Collectively, these drugs are effective in treating hypertension.

The likely basis for angiotensin II-induced drinking is that it causes the release of aldosterone from the adrenal cortex, leading to sodium retention in the kidneys. Increases in blood osmolarity are sensed by receptors located in the anterior hypothalamus and preoptic region. Although the specific neural mechanism has not been elaborated, it is reasonable to assume that the neural circuits organizing drinking behavior emanate from these regions of the hypothalamus in the form of a series of downstream pathways. This mechanism illustrates the presence of a hormonal-neural reflex mechanism.

In general, increased sodium retention activates a related kind of homeostatic hormonal-neural-(hormonal) mechanism. This involves axons from the subfornical organ (activated by angiotensin II) that project to the supraoptic and paraventricular nuclei and that activate a mechanism that promotes water retention from the kidneys and induces drinking behavior.

OVERVIEW OF THE INTEGRATIVE FUNCTIONS OF THE HYPOTHALAMUS

The integrative functions of the hypothalamus include cardiovascular regulation, temperature regulation, sexual behavior, feeding behavior, and drinking, aggression, rage, and flight behaviors.

The specific nature of each of these response patterns is highly complex, and our present understanding of the precise role of the underlying mechanisms remains incomplete. Our current knowledge of these functions is briefly reviewed here.

REGULATION OF CARDIOVASCULAR PROCESSES

In chapters 22 and 23, we discussed central regulation of blood pressure and heart rate. It was pointed out that the basic cardiovascular mechanisms present at the level of the intermediolateral cell columns of the thoracic and lumbar levels of the spinal cord are controlled extensively by other mechanisms residing in the ventrolateral medulla and solitary nucleus of the lower brainstem. Superimposed on these brainstem mechanisms are other mechanisms residing in the hypothalamus and limbic system. The most important region mediating sympathetic responses includes the posterior two thirds of the medial aspect of the hypothalamus. Sympathetic responses are also mediated by the lateral hypothalamus but are less intense than those mediated from the medial hypothalamus. Parasympathetic responses have been reported after stimulation of parts of the anterior hypothalamus and preoptic region. These autonomic responses are presumably mediated through descending pathways that reach the lower brainstem. Some investigators have even suggested that descending hypothalamic fibers may reach as far as the intermediolateral cell column of the thoracic cord, thus providing the basis for direct hypothalamic mediation of sympathetic functions.

TEMPERATURE REGULATION

Temperature regulation requires the integration of a number of processes associated with hypothalamic functions. These include: (1) activation of temperature-sensitive neurons (thermoreceptors) that can respond to increases or decreases in blood temperature; (2) the capacity of the hypothalamus to activate thyroid-releasing hormone, which leads to secretion of TSH, with subsequent secretion of thyroid hormone for increases in metabolic rates; (3) activation of autonomic mechanisms, which, in turn, *dilate or constrict* peripheral blood vessels that serve to cause loss or conservation of body temperature, respectively; and (4) activation of behavioral responses such as panting (to generate heat loss) and shivering (to conserve heat).

That body temperature normally remains relatively constant is the result of a balance between neuronal mechanisms subserving heat loss and heat conservation. A group of neurons situated in the anterior hypothalamus-preoptic region responds to changes in blood temperature. These neurons are specifically designed to prevent body temperature from rising above set values. When body temperature does increase, anterior hypothalamic neurons discharge, and efferent volleys are conducted down their axons to respiratory and cardiovascular neuronal groups of the lower brainstem and spinal cord. The net effect of such activation is initiation of vasodilation and perspiration, leading to heat loss. Therefore, this region of the hypothalamus is often referred to as a **heat loss center** (Fig. 24-8). Moreover, neurons in this region respond to substances called **pyrogens** (which cause marked increases in body temperature) by discharging in an attempt to re-establish normal body temperature. In addition, certain neurons in this region, as well as in adjoining regions of the septal area that contain **vasopressin**, are capable of counteracting the actions of pyrogens. Accordingly, this group of neurons is referred to as an **antipyrogenic region**.

Other neurons located in the posterior lateral hypothalamus appear to be more closely linked with **heat conservation**. These neurons discharge when body temperature declines, and impulses are conducted down similar pathways to lower autonomic regions of the brainstem and spinal cord. The net effects include vasoconstriction, increases in cardiac rate, elevation of the basal metabolic rate, piloerection, and shivering. Shivering contributes to heat conservation because the rapid, involuntary contractions of the somatic musculature (through a multisynaptic descending pathway to ventral horn cells of the spinal cord) produce heat.

FEEDING BEHAVIOR

Extensive research conducted in animals has demonstrated that feeding and ingestive behaviors are clearly regulated by the hypothalamus. Such studies have pointed out that two regions of the hypothalamus, the medial and lateral hypothalamus, play key roles in the regulation of feeding responses. Stimulation of the lateral hypothalamus has been shown to induce feeding behavior, while stimulation of the medial hypothalamus suppresses this behavior. Moreover, lesions of the lateral hypothalamus induce **aphagia**, while lesions of the medial hypothalamus result in **hyperphagia**. Based on such evidence, the lateral hypothalamus has often been referred to as a **feeding center**, while the ventromedial hypothalamus has been called a **satiety center**.

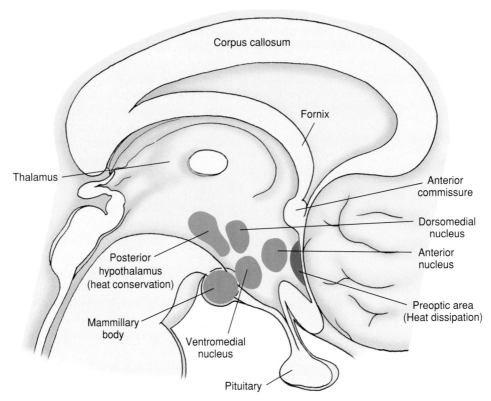

Figure 24–8 Sagittal view of the brain indicating the relationship of the regions of the hypothalamus associated with heat conservation and heat loss.

The data in support of two opposing regions that regulate feeding is significant, although interpretation of the data may be somewhat oversimplified. It appears that a number of different mechanisms may be operative within these hypothalamic nuclei. The ventromedial nucleus appears to play a critical role here. For example, it has recently been shown that the ventromedial nucleus responds to changes in caloric intake. There is believed to be a **set-point** governing hypothalamic regulation of food intake. The set-point is governed by such factors as metabolic rate of the organism, immediate past history of food intake, and present level of food intake. Lesions of the medial hypothalamus disrupt this set-point, leading to large increases in food intake and weight gain. The ventromedial hypothalamus and adjoining nuclei have been linked to several neurotransmitter and hormonal systems. For example, inhibition of feeding behavior occurs after administration of CCK to the paraventricular region. This finding suggests that part of the satiety mechanism involves a release of CCK from the medial hypothalamus following food intake. Other compounds associated with the medial hypothalamus, such as glucagon and neurotensin, appear to have similar functions. Thus, lesions of the medial hypothalamus may result in hyperphagia because of disruption of these compounds and may affect the release of other hormones, such as ACTH and insulin, that normally regulate metabolic rates.

Several mechanisms may also be operative with respect to food intake functions involving several nuclei of the hypothalamus. Sensory processes play an important role in feeding behavior. Of particular significance are the learned sensory cues associated with olfaction and taste. These signals, which intensify the drive for food, involve signals that reach the amygdala, which, in turn, are relayed to the lateral hypothalamus via the ventral amygdalofugal pathway. The loss of motivation for food following lesions of the lateral hypothalamus may be related, in part, to the disruption of inputs to the lateral hypothalamus from the amygdala triggered by sensory signals associated with food.

In addition to the lateral hypothalamus, the paraventricular nucleus also appears to contribute to feeding behavior. Recent studies have shown that several different peptides (galanin, neuropeptide Y, and opioids) and norepinephrine can induce feeding responses in rats when microinjected into the paraventricular nucleus. The precise mechanisms governing how these compounds affect feeding responses remain unknown.

DRINKING BEHAVIOR

The basic mechanisms governing drinking behavior were described previously in this chapter. They include the role of the paraventricular nucleus in releasing ADH in response to increases in tissue osmolarity and the role of the subfornical organ in responding to the presence of angiotensin II by exciting neurons in the anterior hypothalamus and preoptic region. As noted earlier, stimulation of the paraventricular nucleus activates a mechanism that induces water retention from the kidneys. A separate mechanism has also been described: activation of the tissue surrounding the anteroventral aspect of the third ventricle, which includes the preoptic region, is believed to excite a process that induces the behavioral process of drinking. However, the specific neural circuits underlying how drinking behavior occurs remain obscure.

SEXUAL BEHAVIOR

Female sexual behavior is directly dependent on the relationship between endocrine function, the presence of hormonal-neural interactions, and activation of neural circuits that govern the elicitation of species-specific sexual responses. One of the key structures controlling sexual behavior is the ventromedial hypothalamus. It contains estrogen and progesterone receptors. In fact, experimental studies in rats have shown that stimulation of the ventromedial nucleus by chemicals (i.e., cholinergic stimulation) induces a sexual response referred to as **lordosis**. This response is characterized by arching of the back (by the female) coupled with a rigid posture and a deflection of the tail, all of which allows intromission by the male. In contrast, lesions of the ventromedial nucleus significantly reduce sexual behavior.

The correlation between sexual behavior and estrogen levels is quite high. Therefore, it is reasonable to conclude that increased levels of estrogen act on estrogen receptors within the ventromedial hypothalamus to trigger a neural mechanism that excites other neurons in lower regions of the central nervous system, such as the midbrain PAG and spinal cord, which serve to induce the expression of sexual behavior. Progesterone also likely acts on ventromedial neurons, the net effect of which is to intensify the sexual response to estrogen. Experimental studies have also shown that the lordosis reaction is also modulated by monoaminergic inputs and acetylcholine. In particular, lordosis behavior is enhanced by norepinephrine, suppressed by serotonin, and induced by acetylcholine when each of the agonists for these transmitters is microinjected directly into the rat ventromedial hypothalamus.

Part of the overall hypothalamic mechanism underlying sexual behavior may involve the release of GnRH from the anterior hypothalamus (preoptic region). These neurons project to the median eminence, where the peptide is released into the portal circulation. The peptide is then transported to the anterior pituitary, resulting in increases in estrogen levels. In addition, the gonadotropin pathway from the anterior hypothalamus also reaches the midbrain PAG, where the release of gonadotropin-releasing hormone can induce lordosis. It is reasonable to conclude that all of these mechanisms come into play when sexual behavior occurs normally in humans.

Male sexual behavior is induced or augmented by the presence of testosterone. Testosterone appears to act on the preoptic region to produce the various behavioral characteristics of sexual behavior. This suggests that the preoptic region plays an important role in sexual behavior in both males and females. It is of interest to note that the morphological appearance of the preoptic region differs between males and females (at least in rodents), and the appearance is dependent on the extent of release of LH from the anterior pituitary. For this reason, the preoptic region contains the **sexually dimorphic nucleus**, which is a somewhat rounded, compact structure that is larger in males than females. It may be that the kind of morphology present in the preoptic region may provide the neural substrate for the kind of sexual behavior that is expressed by a given organism. Like the female, male sexual responses are modulated by various neurotransmitters, such as dopamine, and by neuropeptides (gonadotropin-releasing hormone, substance P, and neuropeptide Y).

AGGRESSION AND RAGE

We have previously pointed out the role of the hypothalamus in regulating cardiovascular and related autonomic functions of the nervous system. These functions comprise components of the various forms of emotional behavior that are integrated within different regions of the hypothalamus.

Several forms of emotional behavior have been identified, mainly from feline models of aggression and rage. Stimulation of the medial hypothalamus produces a rage-like response called **defensive rage behavior**. In cats, for example, the response includes piloerection, marked vocalization, such as hissing and growling, retraction of the claws, significant pupillary dilatation and other forms of sympathetic reactions, arching of the paws,

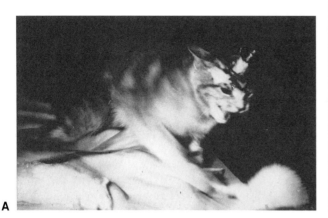
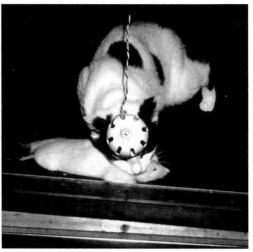

A   B

Figure 24–9 Defensive rage and predatory behavior. (A) Defensive rage behavior elicited by electrical stimulation of the medial hypothalamus. (B) Predatory attack behavior elicited by electrical stimulation of the lateral hypothalamus of the cat. (Courtesy of Allan Siegel, Ph.D.)

and striking out at a moving object within its visual field (Fig. 24-9). The response is essentially defensive in nature and occurs naturally when the cat perceives itself as being threatened by another animal.

The pathways and putative neurotransmitters that regulate defensive rage behavior have recently been described. The primary pathway mediating defensive rage behavior from the medial hypothalamus projects to the dorsal aspect of the midbrain PAG from which this response can also be elicited. Excitatory amino acids that act on N-methyl-D-asparate (NMDA) receptors have been identified as the neurotransmitters associated with this pathway. Because the most caudal level of the brainstem at which this response is integrated is the PAG, the autonomic and somatomotor components that comprise the defensive rage response are activated by descending fibers from the PAG that reach autonomic regions of the lower brainstem and somatomotor regions of the brainstem (e.g., trigeminal and facial motor nuclei for vocalization) and spinal cord (for paw striking).

Other regions of the brain play important roles in modulating defensive rage behavior. Perhaps the most significant group of structures includes the limbic system (see Chapter 25). Structures, such as the amygdala, hippocampal formation, septal area, and prefrontal cortex, powerfully control this response through direct or indirect connections with the hypothalamus or midbrain PAG. For example, the medial amygdala generates a very powerful excitatory effect on defensive rage behavior by virtue of a direct excitatory pathway to the medial hypothalamus, which uses substance P as a neurotransmitter. Inhibitory effects on defensive rage

behavior become manifest when the central nucleus is stimulated. This structure provides a direct, inhibitory pathway to the midbrain periaqueductal gray, which is mediated by opioid peptides acting through receptors. Monoamine neurotransmitters have also been studied, and the results indicate that dopamine and norepinephrine facilitate defensive rage, whereas serotonin is inhibitory.

Stimulation of the lateral hypothalamus in the cat produces a different form of aggressive behavior. It is called **quiet biting (predatory) attack** behavior. In this form of attack behavior, cats, which do not normally attack rats, will stalk and then bite the back of the neck of the rat and/or strike it with its forepaw (Fig. 24-9). This form of aggressive behavior resembles the natural predatory response of a cat on a prey object. This response is accompanied by few overt autonomic signs other than some pupillary dilation and increases in heart rate and blood pressure.

The pathways mediating this response descend through the medial forebrain bundle from the lateral hypothalamus and synapse in several areas of the brainstem, including the ventral aspect of the midbrain PAG, tegmental fields, and motor nucleus of the trigeminal nerve. Secondary fibers from the brainstem descend to lower levels of the brainstem and spinal cord, where they synapse with somatomotor and autonomic nuclei, which must be activated for this response to occur. In addition, because of the complexity of the response, it is also likely that the sensorimotor cortex also becomes activated following stimulation of the lateral hypothalamus, which may account for the precise character of the behavioral response. The anatomical pathway by which the cerebral cortex becomes activated following stimulation of the lateral hypothalamus remains obscure.

Predatory attack behavior is also powerfully modulated by different regions of the limbic system that project directly or indirectly to the lateral hypothalamus. Monoamine neurotransmitters appear to have effects on predatory attack behavior that are similar to those mediated on defensive rage behavior.

The relationship between the medial and lateral hypothalamus with respect to these two forms of aggression is mutual inhibition. When the predatory attack mechanism is activated in the lateral hypothalamus, neurons in the medial hypothalamus subserving defensive rage are suppressed, and likewise, when the defensive rage mechanism is activated, neurons mediating predatory attack are suppressed. These opposing effects likely involve inhibitory connections between the medial and lateral hypothalamus. Such an interactive mechanism would be of obvious survival value to an organism: an animal about to display predatory attack on a prey object would not find it useful to elicit vocalization associated with defensive rage behavior. Similarly, predatory attack-like responses would be of little survival value when an animal's life space is threatened by another organism of the same or different species.

A third type of emotional response elicited by electrical stimulation of wide regions of the hypothalamus and dorsal aspect of the midbrain PAG gray is **flight behavior**. It is characterized by an attempt of the cat to escape from its cage after electrical stimulation is applied to either of these brain regions. The pathways mediating flight behavior have been described and indicate that direct descending fibers to the midbrain PAG most likely mediate this response. The neurotransmitters associated with elicitation or modulation of this response have yet to be identified.

BIOLOGICAL RHYTHMS

As indicated earlier, specific regions of the hypothalamus play an important role in pacemaker activities (i.e., setting and maintaining biological rhythms) for different endocrine and behaviorally related functions. Of particular importance are the suprachiasmatic nucleus and the preoptic area. The suprachiasmatic nucleus receives retinal inputs that appear to be critical for triggering circadian rhythms for a number of sex hormones, corticosterone, and the pineal hormone melatonin. The multisynaptic pathway connecting the suprachiasmatic nucleus with the pineal gland was described in Chapter 13. Associated with these hormonal rhythms are circadian rhythms for body temperature and sexual behavior. It is possible and even likely that the preoptic area also plays an important role in governing the circadian rhythm for the release of LH from the anterior pituitary because GnRH neurons are located within the preoptic region.

SLEEP

We have previously considered in detail the process of sleep in Chapter 23. The hypothalamus and the reticular formation have been associated with the regulation of sleep. Thus, a brief summary of the role of the hypothalamus in sleep is considered here.

Early experiments conducted in rats demonstrated that lesions of the posterior hypothalamus produced prolonged periods of sleep. This led to the view that mechanisms regulating sleep involve the hypothalamus. Subsequent experiments have revealed that such lesions may have produced sleep because of the disruption of ascending fibers from the reticular formation rather than because of the cell damage within the hypothalamus. However, more recent studies have suggested that portions of the cholinergic basal forebrain region, such as the preoptic area and substantia innominata, are likely involved and function in concert with other cholinergic and monoaminergic mechanisms within the reticular formation of the brainstem to regulate sleep and wakefulness cycles.

DYSFUNCTIONS OF THE HYPOTHALAMUS

Destruction of hypothalamic tissue can result in a number of different disorders related to the processes considered earlier in this chapter. These include: obesity, diabetes insipidus, hyperaggressivity and violent behavior, disruption of thermal regulation, emaciation, alterations in sexual development, sleep disorders, and hypertension.

Disorders of the hypothalamus may result from specific lesions caused by vascular disturbances, inflammation of hypothalamic tissue, or by tumors that usually emanate from the floor of the third ventricle or pituitary gland.

HYPERTHERMIA

Hyperthermia is characterized by high temperature that could be fatal. It is sometimes associated with surgery involving the region adjacent to the pituitary and is believed to involve the anterior hypothalamus that controls the *heat-loss* mechanism.

GENITAL DYSTROPHY AND ABNORMALITIES IN SEXUAL DEVELOPMENT

Genital dystrophy can occur following lesions believed to be located in or around the tuberal region of the hypothalamus but that may extend to the ventromedial nucleus as well. This type of dystrophy is characterized by loss of sexual activity and genital atrophy. Other forms of alterations in sexual development may also occur from lesions, tumors, encephalitis, or even hematomas of the hypothalamus. In children, the disorder may result in retardation of sexual organs and sexual function. It is also possible for the disorder to lead to an opposite effect, resulting in premature sexual development of the genitalia.

FEEDING, OBESITY, AND EMACIATION

Marked increases in appetite occur as a result of lesions of the ventromedial hypothalamus. This is associated with significant weight gain and striking changes in emotional behavior (usually characterized by expressions of rage). Lesions of the lateral hypothalamus, on the other hand, result in loss of appetite and emaciation.

HYPERTENSION

Excessive release of corticotropin-releasing factor causes oversecretion of adrenocorticotropins. This, in turn, results in hypertension because of several factors, such as changes in sodium and water metabolism, and a release of renin from the kidney, which leads to increased synthesis of angiotensin II.

SLEEP DISORDERS

Sleep disorders may result from damage (such as encephalitis) to the posterior region of the hypothalamus (i.e., the diencephalic-midbrain juncture). The result is prolonged periods of sleep. As noted earlier, the effects may be due to damage to ascending fibers from the reticular formation to the thalamus and cortex rather than damage to neurons situated within the hypothalamus.

AGGRESSION AND RAGE

Tumors located near the base of the brain but that impinge on the ventromedial hypothalamus have been known to produce marked expressions of violent behavior. The tumors likely have a stimulation-like effect in causing aberrant expressions of emotional behavior. Such effects may also be due to vascular disturbances and inflammatory disorders. Sometimes, such disturbances were treated two to three decades ago by placing surgical lesions in the posteromedial region of the hypothalamus (sometimes called the ergotropic triangle). Surgical lesions placed in schizophrenic patients generally reduced sympathetic activity and aggressive responses. It is likely that such lesions disrupt the major descending outputs of the medial hypothalamus to the midbrain PAG and other regions of the tegmentum. In recent times, surgical approaches have generally been replaced by noninvasive methods emphasizing drug therapy.

CLINICAL CASE

HISTORY

Iris is a 29-year-old woman who stopped taking birth control pills 6 months ago to try to become pregnant. However, her menstrual periods failed to resume. Her cycles had been normal prior to starting the pills 4 years ago, and she'd taken them steadily during that period. She also noted that she had been having dull headaches, which were worsening over the past few months, as well as some problems with her peripheral vision, but didn't pay much attention to either symptom. She thought that she already might be pregnant, so she went to see her gynecologist.

EXAMINATION

A pregnancy test was negative at her doctor's office, and there was no evidence of any pregnancy from her physical examination. As a result, her gynecologist sent Iris's blood for blood hormone levels. On returning for her test results, Iris learned that her prolactin level (a hormone that mediates lactation and inhibits menstruation) was high. She was also surprised that her gynecologist referred her to a neurologist but agreed to go because of her headaches and vision problems.

The neurologist found that Iris was unable to see objects in the lateral half of each visual field (heteronymous hemianopsia), but the remainder of her examination was normal. A magnetic resonance imaging (MRI) scan of Iris's head was ordered.

EXPLANATION

The MRI scan revealed a mass in the pituitary gland called a microadenoma (a benign tumor arising from the anterior pituitary gland). Most microadenomas secrete the hormone prolactin, as this one did (as evidenced by the high serum level). The pituitary gland is in close proximity to the optic chiasm, so it is common for pituitary tumors to put pressure on it. The pituitary sits near the medial aspect of the optic chiasm where the fibers associated with the temporal visual fields run. Recall that the temporal visual fields are linked with the nasal retina and that the fibers from the nasal retina cross in the optic chiasm. Thus, the vision lost is from the lateral temporal visual fields.

Prolactin-releasing factor is manufactured in the arcuate nucleus of the hypothalamus, activating the lactotropic cells of the anterior pituitary gland. Several substances, including dopamine, are able to raise serum prolactin levels. Therefore, dopamine agonists are given to treat these tumors because, by raising serum prolactin, the tumor cells producing prolactin are inhibited, resulting in a shrinking of the tumor.

CHAPTER TEST

QUESTIONS

Choose the best answer for each question.

1. Oxytocin is:
   a. Synthesized in the medial hypothalamus and released in the posterior pituitary
   b. Synthesized in the medial hypothalamus and released in the anterior pituitary
   c. Synthesized in the paraventricular nucleus and released in the anterior pituitary
   d. Synthesized in the paraventricular nucleus and released in the posterior pituitary
   e. Synthesized in the lateral hypothalamus and released in the median eminence

2. An experiment was conducted in cats to determine the effects of stimulation of the medial amygdala on the activity of medial hypothalamic neurons. After determining that stimulation of the medial amygdala powerfully excited medial amygdaloid neurons, the investigator sought to further test the relationship between these regions by destroying the major pathway that links these two regions and then testing to see whether stimulation of the medial amygdala no longer affected medial hypothalamic neuronal activity. The most likely pathway that was destroyed by the investigator was the:
   a. Mammillothalamic tract
   b. Medial forebrain bundle
   c. Stria terminalis
   d. Stria medullaris
   e. Ventral amygdalofugal fibers

3. Lesions of the medial hypothalamus will result in:
   a. Aphagia
   b. Diabetes insipidus
   c. Hyperphagia
   d. Increased sexual behavior
   e. Failure to regulate body temperature

4. A lesion of the lateral hypothalamus is discovered after an examination in which a magnetic resonance imaging (MRI) scan was done. Which of the following disorders would likely be present, and which pathway would most likely be damaged?
   a. Hyperphagia – stria terminalis
   b. Aphagia – medial forebrain bundle
   c. Dysphagia – stria medullaris
   d. Hypertension – mammillotegmental fibers
   e. Fever – corticohypothalamic fibers

5. Surgical lesions designed to reduce blood pressure and manifestations of violent and related emotional responses in schizophrenic patients have been made in the:
   a. Medial preoptic region
   b. Lateral preoptic region
   c. Posterior lateral hypothalamus
   d. Posterior medial hypothalamus
   e. Supraoptic nucleus

ANSWERS AND EXPLANATIONS

1. **Answer: d**

   Oxytocin is synthesized in the paraventricular nucleus and is transported down the axons to their terminals in the posterior pituitary. Oxytocin is then distributed through the blood stream to its target organ in and around the epithelial cells of the mammary gland, where it helps to trigger the milk ejection reflex upon sensory stimulation.

2. **Answer: c**

   The investigator experimentally cut the stria terminalis because it arises from the medial amygdala and projects directly to the rostrocaudal extent of the medial hypothalamus. It serves as a very important source of excitatory input to this region of the hypothalamus. The mammillothalamic tract projects from the mammillary bodies to the anterior thalamic nucleus. The medial forebrain bundle contains ascending and descending fibers that pass through the lateral hypothalamus and do not directly link the amygdala with the medial hypothalamus. The stria medullaris contains fibers that pass mainly from the habenular nuclei to the ventral aspect of the rostral forebrain and has no direct relationship to either the medial hypothalamus or medial amygdala. Ventral amygdalofugal fibers connect mainly the lateral aspects of the amygdala with the lateral hypothalamus and parts of the brainstem. Again, this pathway does not mediate direct inputs from the medial amygdala to the medial hypothalamus.

3. Answer: c

Lesions of the medial hypothalamus result in a disorder called hypothalamic hyperphagia, which is characterized by marked increases in food intake and obesity. Aphagia is produced by lesions of the lateral hypothalamus. Diabetes insipidus is associated with lesions of the supraoptic region. Destruction of the medial hypothalamus blocks sexual behavior. Thermal regulation is governed by the anterior (for heat loss) and posterior (for heat conservation) regions of the hypothalamus.

4. Answer: b

Lesions of the lateral hypothalamus have been associated with aphagia. The major pathway passing through the lateral hypothalamus is the medial forebrain bundle. It contains descending fibers, which arise from different groups of neurons in the lateral hypothalamus and septal area, and ascending fibers that pass to different regions of the forebrain, which also arise from the lateral hypothalamus as well as from the brainstem, including monoaminergic cell groups. The medial hypothalamus is the region that most directly is associated with hyperphagia. Dysphagia is associated with lesions of the lower brainstem and, in particular, neurons associated with cranial nerves (CN) IX and X. Hypertension is most closely associated with the posterior hypothalamus and the region of the medial hypothalamus. Lesions of the lateral hypothalamus are not known to result in hypertension. Fever is associated with excitation of the preoptic region and septal area. Lesions of the lateral hypothalamus would most likely not cause major increases in body temperature.

5. Answer: d

The posterior medial hypothalamus is referred to as the *ergotropic triangle* of the hypothalamus and is the region where surgical lesions have been placed to cause reductions in blood pressure. Lesions of this region also reduce aggressive and related forms of emotional responses. Presumably, the sites of the lesions serve to disrupt many of the descending fibers from the medial hypothalamus to the midbrain PAG and lower regions of the brainstem that integrate forebrain control of sympathetic activity as well as rage and violent forms of behavior. The preoptic region, lateral hypothalamus, and supraoptic nucleus have not been known to cause increases in blood pressure and are not associated specifically with the control of rage behavior. The preoptic region is closely associated with temperature regulation; the lateral hypothalamus is associated with feeding and predatory behavior, and the supraoptic nucleus is associated with control of functions of the posterior pituitary.

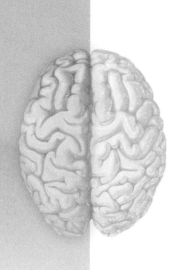

CHAPTER 25

THE LIMBIC SYSTEM

OBJECTIVES

After reading this chapter, the student should be able to:

1. Describe and diagram the basic morphology of the structures comprising the limbic system

2. Describe and diagram the input-output relationships of limbic nuclei

3. Characterize the functions of limbic brain structures and their underlying mechanisms (where known)

4. Develop an understanding of the structural and functional bases for clinical and behavioral disorders associated with dysfunctions of the limbic system

As stated in Chapter 13, the limbic system links a group of functionally related structures that are interposed between the cerebral cortex and the underlying diencephalon. The limbic system includes the phylogenetically older regions of the brain and consists of the **hippocampal formation**, **septal area**, and **amygdala**. In discussing the limbic system, most authors also include the **prefrontal cortex** and **cingulate gyrus** as components within this system. Some authors also include the hypothalamus as part of the limbic system, but in the present context, we have limited our analysis of these structures based on criteria described in the following paragraph. It should also be pointed out that the expression "limbic system" implies that the component structures making up this system have similar or identical functions. However, this is not the case. The structures that are discussed in this chapter are not uniform in their functions and differ with respect to physiological, pharmacological, and behavioral properties. Nevertheless, we use the term "limbic system" because of the overriding common features of the different structures and because of historical reasons where this term has been in use for over 40 years.

As an overall defining property, limbic structures either directly or indirectly communicate with the hypothalamus or midbrain periaqueductal gray (PAG). Thus, a critical property of limbic structures is to modulate the functions normally attributed to the hypothalamus and/or midbrain PAG. Accordingly, one of the primary objectives of this chapter is to examine how each of the limbic structures can regulate processes associated with the hypothalamus and PAG. It should also be pointed out that limbic structures also serve other functions, such as short-term memory and epileptogenic activity, that do not relate to functions of the hypothalamus. These functions are also considered separately in this chapter.

One of the major themes regarding functions of the limbic system relates to its role in modulating processes normally associated with the hypothalamus. To gain a better understanding of the functional properties of the various limbic structures, it is important to consider their input-output relationships. These relationships are depicted in Figure 25-1. As a general rule, limbic structures receive inputs from at least two sources: (1) from one or more sensory systems, either directly or indirectly through interneurons in the cerebral cortex; and (2) from brainstem monoaminergic fiber systems. Limbic neurons then project directly or indirectly to the hypothalamus (and/or midbrain PAG). These projections enable the

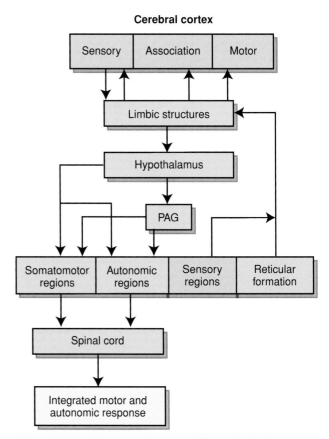

Figure 25–1 Information flow to and from the limbic system. Note that the limbic system receives inputs from sensory systems, including the cerebral cortex, and monoamine neuronal groups of the brainstem reticular formation. Primary outputs of the limbic system are directed to the hypothalamus. This arrangement allows the limbic system to alter the activity of the hypothalamus in response to sensory input. Because the hypothalamus provides the integrating mechanism for different forms of emotional behaviors as well as for other visceral and autonomic responses, the limbic system serves as a key modulating region of these processes by virtue of its inputs into the hypothalamus. Inputs to the limbic system from monoamine pathways can provide the substrates underlying mood changes.

limbic structures to modulate the outputs of the hypothalamus and PAG that are directed on somatic motor and autonomic neurons of the lower brainstem and spinal cord for the integration of specific forms of visceral responses. Feedback signals can also reach the limbic system from the hypothalamus. Similarly, limbic structures can also send feedback signals to the cerebral cortex, which provide the cortex with visceral signals that are contiguous with other sensory signals that initially caused excitation of limbic nuclei. It is likely that the contiguity of these signals helps to provide the emotional quality to sensory signals.

HIPPOCAMPAL FORMATION

HISTOLOGY AND LOCAL ANATOMICAL CONNECTIONS

The hippocampal formation consists of the **hippocampus**, **dentate gyrus**, and **subicular cortex** (Fig. 25-2A). The primary cell type within the hippocampus is the pyramidal cell, which has both basal and apical dendrites. The basal dendrites extend laterally and slightly in the direction of the ventricular surface. The apical dendrites extend away from the ventricular surface towards the dentate gyrus. The axon of the pyramidal cell, which constitutes the primary efferent process of the hippocampal formation, passes into the superficial layer of the hippocampus, called the **alveus** (a fiber layer adjacent to the inferior horn of the lateral ventricle), and ultimately into either the fimbria-fornix or entorhinal cortex (Fig. 25-2B).

The **hippocampus** can be viewed as a primitive form of three-layered cortical tissue. Accordingly, it has the following layers extending from the ventricular surface to the dentate gyrus: (1) an **external plexiform layer**, situated adjacent to the inferior horn of the lateral ventricle, which contains axons of pyramidal cells that project outside the hippocampus as well as hippocampal afferent fibers from the entorhinal cortex (i.e., the alvear pathway); (2) **stratum oriens**, which contains basal dendrites and basket cells; (3) a **pyramidal cell layer**, which contains the pyramidal cells of the hippocampus; and (4) the **stratum radiatum** and **stratum lacunosum-moleculare**, which are two layers that contain the apical dendrites of the pyramidal cells and hippocampal afferents from the entorhinal cortex (i.e., perforant pathway) (Fig. 25-2, A and B).

As shown in Figure 25-2A, the pyramidal cells of the hippocampus are arranged in a C-shaped fashion, which is interlocked with another C-shaped arrangement of the dentate gyrus. The hippocampus is divided into a number of distinct fields. The fields, according to one classification, include four sectors (i.e., CA1, CA2, CA3, and CA4). The pyramidal cells situated closest to the subiculum are referred to as the CA1 field, whereas the CA4 field is located within the hilus of the dentate gyrus. The CA2 and CA3 fields are located between the CA1 and CA4 fields. Collaterals of axons arising from CA3 pyramidal cells (called **recurrent** or **Schaffer collaterals**) project back to the CA1 field. The CA1 field is of particular interest because the pyramidal cells are highly susceptible to anoxia, especially during periods of temporal lobe epilepsy. This region is referred to as **Sommer's sector**.

The **dentate gyrus** can also be thought of as a primitive three-layered cortical structure. It is multilayered, and the principal cell type is the **granule cell**. The axon of the granule cell, called a **mossy fiber**, makes synaptic contact with pyramidal cells

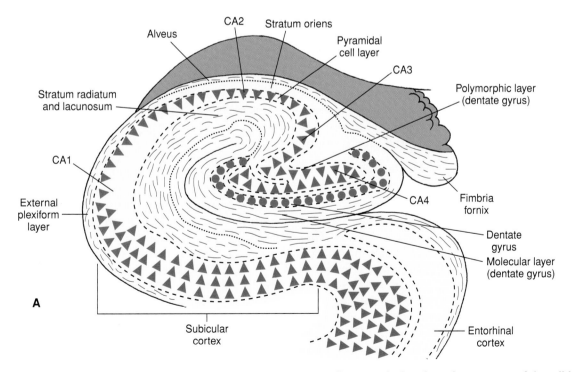

Figure 25–2 Hippocampal anatomy and internal circuitry. (A) Diagram illustrates the histological appearance of the cell layers within the hippocampus and loci of the hippocampal fields, dentate gyrus, and subicular cortex.

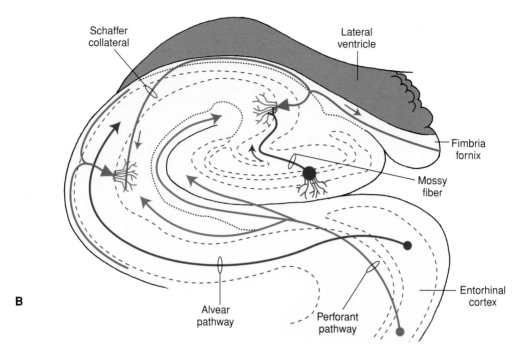

Figure 25–2 (*continued*) (B) Semischematic diagram illustrates: (1) inputs from the entorhinal region, which include the perforant and alvear pathways; (2) internal circuitry, which includes the connections of the mossy fibers and Schaffer collaterals; and (3) efferent projections of the hippocampal formation through the fimbria-fornix system of fibers. CA1-CA4 denote the four sectors of the hippocampus.

in the CA3 region. A **polymorphic cell layer**, composed of modified pyramidal cells, lies deep to the granule cell layer. External to the granule cell layer lies the **molecular cell layer**, which is apposed to the molecular layer of the hippocampus. The molecular layer mainly contains axons of hippocampal afferent fibers.

The last component of the hippocampal formation is the **subicular cortex**. It constitutes a transitional region between the entorhinal cortex and hippocampus. The primary histological distinction between the hippocampus and subicular cortex is that the pyramidal cell layer is considerably thicker in the subicular cortex than in the hippocampus (Fig. 25-2A).

AFFERENT CONNECTIONS

There are a variety of sources that contribute afferent fibers to the hippocampal formation. One major source of inputs includes the entorhinal cortex. Separate groups of fibers arising from the lateral and medial parts of the entorhinal cortex pass through the alveus and molecular layers of the hippocampus and dentate gyrus, respectively, to supply much of the hippocampus. The lateral pathway is called the "**lateral perforant pathway**" and passes from the lateral entorhinal cortex into the molecular layer of the hippocampus. The medial pathway is called the "**medial perforant path-**

way" and enters the alveus of the hippocampus after passing through the white matter adjoining the subiculum (Fig. 25-2B). Many of these inputs represent tertiary olfactory, visual, and auditory fibers that reach the hippocampus after making synaptic connections within the entorhinal region. A second group of fibers arises from the diagonal band of Broca (of the septal area) and supplies much of the hippocampal formation (see discussion in the section on efferent connections of the septal area, page 454). These fibers may be viewed as a feedback circuit to the hippocampal formation from the septal area, which, in turn, receives inputs from the hippocampal formation via the precommissural fornix (see discussion on page 449). Other sources of hippocampal afferent fibers include the prefrontal cortex, anterior cingulate gyrus, and premammillary region. A final source of hippocampal afferent fibers includes monoamine neuronal projections from the brainstem reticular formation (i.e., locus ceruleus, ventral tegmental area, and pontine and midbrain raphe neurons). These projections of the brainstem, which also supply other parts of the limbic system, provide the anatomical and physiological substrates that regulate mood changes. Thus, by receiving inputs from these varied sources, the hippocampal formation can respond to sudden changes in brainstem and cortical events and relay such changes to the hypothalamus (see page 450), which then provides a visceral (and/or emotional) quality to these events.

EFFERENT CONNECTIONS

The efferent connections of the hippocampal formation arise from pyramidal cells located in both the hippocampus and subicular cortex. The axons of these cells contribute the largest component to the fornix system of fibers. With respect to efferent connections of the hippocampal formation, there are three components of the fornix system. One component, called the **precommissural fornix** (Fig. 25-3), passes rostral to the anterior commissure and supplies the septal area. The precommissural fornix projection is topographically organized in that fibers situated near the anterior pole of the hippocampal formation project to the lateral aspect of the lateral septal nucleus, while neurons situated more posteriorly in the hippocampal formation project to progressively more medial aspects of this nucleus.

A second component, called the **postcommissural fornix**, innervates the diencephalon. The postcommissural fornix innervates the anterior thalamic nucleus, mammillary bodies, and adjoining regions of the medial hypothalamus (Fig. 25-3). While the precommissural fornix arises from the hippocampus and subicular cortex, the postcommissural fornix arises solely from the subicular cortex. Neurons located in the subiculum also project to the entorhinal cortex, cingulate cortex, and various parts of the prefrontal cortex. The entorhinal cortex, in turn, projects to the amygdala and adjoining regions of temporal neocortex. Taken collectively, the significance of the projections of the subicular and entorhinal cortex is that they enable the hippocampal formation to communicate with widespread regions of neocortex, including areas that receive different modalities of sensory information. Such projections may constitute the substrate by which signals from limbic regions of the brain serve to provide affective properties to various modalities of sensory signals.

The third component of the fornix system is its **commissural component**, which provides connections between the hippocampus on each side of the brain. In general, the hippocampal fibers that provide commissural connections arise mainly from the CA3–CA4 region and terminate in the homotypical region of the contralateral hippocampus. The presence of a commissural connection has

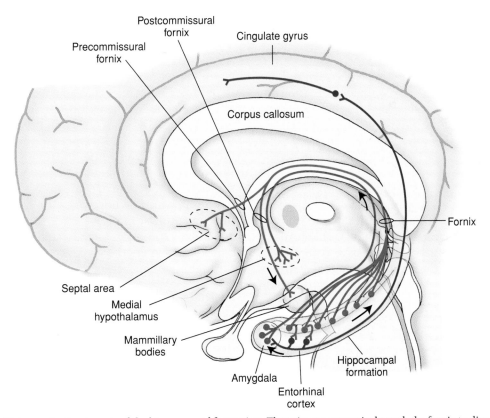

Figure 25–3 Major projection targets of the hippocampal formation. The primary output is through the fornix to diencephalon (i.e., medial hypothalamus, mammillary bodies, and anterior thalamic nucleus) via the postcommissural fornix and to the septal area via the precommissural fornix. Other connections shown include efferent fibers that synapse in entorhinal cortex, which, in turn, project to amygdala and cingulate gyrus.

important clinical significance. It may provide the structural basis by which seizures spread from the hippocampus on one side of the brain to the hippocampus on the other side, allowing for the formation of secondary epileptogenic foci on the side of the temporal lobe contralateral to the site where the primary focus is present.

FUNCTIONS OF THE HIPPOCAMPAL FORMATION

The hippocampal formation has been linked to a number of different functions. These include modulation of aggressive behavior, autonomic and endocrine functions, and certain forms of learning and memory. Modulation of aggression and autonomic and endocrine functions likely results from direct or indirect hippocampal inputs to different regions of the hypothalamus. The underlying anatomical substrates and functional mechanisms for learning and memory remain largely unknown.

Aggression and Rage

Experimental studies in animals and human clinical reports have indicated that the hippocampal formation plays an important role in the control of aggression and rage behavior. Electrical stimulation of the hippocampal formation of the cat at current levels below threshold for elicitation of seizure activity significantly alters the propensity for elicitation of aggressive responses elicited from the hypothalamus (see Chapter 24). As is true with several other regions of the limbic system, the hippocampal formation differentially modulates aggressive reactions. For example, activation of the part of the hippocampal formation closest to the amygdala (i.e., temporal pole) facilitates predatory attack behavior, while activation of the portion closest to the septal pole suppresses this form of aggression. It is important to note that the fibers arising from each of these regions of the hippocampal formation project to different regions of the septal area. That such fibers likely mediate hippocampal control of aggressive responses is further suggested by the fact that the septal area projects extensively to the hypothalamus (see discussion on pages 454–455). In this manner, the septal area may be viewed, in part, as a relay nucleus of the hippocampal formation of signals that are ultimately transmitted to the hypothalamus.

In humans, there have been a number of published reports linking lesions, tumors, and epileptogenic activity of the hippocampal formation with aggressive reactions. These responses vary in content but include reactions such as hostility and explosive acts of physical violence. It is difficult to know whether tumors have stimulation-like or lesion-like properties and whether the effects of

such trauma originate directly from the hippocampal formation or are a result of secondary effects generated elsewhere in the limbic system. Nevertheless, these clinical findings provide support for the view that, in humans, the hippocampal formation contributes to the regulation of aggressive forms of behavior. It is likely that such effects are mediated on the hypothalamus via interneurons in the septal area.

Endocrine Functions

The hippocampal formation (like other regions of the limbic system) has significant inputs to different parts of the hypothalamus, so it is not surprising that this region can also modulate endocrine functions normally associated with the hypothalamus. The supporting evidence is as follows: (1) estradiol-concentrating neurons are densely packed in the ventral regions of the hippocampal formation; (2) corticosterone is also localized in heavy concentrations in the hippocampal formation and has inhibitory effects on these neurons; (3) stimulation of the hippocampal formation inhibits ovulation in spontaneously ovulating rats; and (4) lesions of the hippocampus or section of the fornix disrupt the diurnal rhythm for adrenocorticotropic hormone (ACTH) release.

One possible mechanism guiding these effects is that the hippocampal formation may be selectively sensitive to various hormone levels and, therefore, serve as part of a feedback pathway to the pituitary via its direct and indirect projections to the hypothalamus. Such effects may be mediated by a direct pathway called the **medial corticohypothalamic tract**. This pathway arises from the subiculum near the temporal pole of hippocampus and projects directly to the ventromedial region of the hypothalamus. It terminates in the region between suprachiasmatic and arcuate nuclei, which contain hypophysiotrophic hormones that control anterior pituitary function. As we have indicated, the hippocampal formation can also indirectly communicate with the medial hypothalamus. It does so through a synaptic relay in the septal area.

Learning and Memory Functions of the Hippocampal Formation

There is abundant literature concerning both animal and human studies that indicates that the hippocampal formation plays a significant role in learning processes. In animals, a number of different types of studies have been carried out that link the hippocampus with learning and memory functions. One of the earliest studies demonstrated that a hippocampal **theta rhythm** (a slow wave of 4 to 7 Hz) appears as an animal is approaching a goal and during different phases of classical or operant conditioning. Other studies showed that animals with hippocampal lesions persevere by responding in the same way in a learning situation even if the responses are incorrect. If animals are required to delay their responses for a fixed period of time, animals with hippocampal lesions fail to do so and respond during the period when no responses should be made.

The phenomenon of **spatial learning (spatial memory)** has also been associated with the hippocampal formation. Normally, a rat can learn to enter the correct arm of a Y-maze or the correct series of arms in a more complicated maze such as an eight-armed radial maze. Animals sustaining hippocampal lesions consistently fail to approach the correct arm of the maze and consistently make the same or similar kinds of errors. Other related studies have suggested that a *cognitive map* exists within the hippocampal formation. The researchers have based their conclusion on the fact that individual hippocampal cells change their discharge patterns as the animal moves to different parts of the cage or when it is placed in different arms of a radial maze.

The human literature is equally extensive with respect to learning and memory functions. One of the earliest reported disorders, called **Korsakoff's syndrome**, is a memory disorder in which the patient displays amnesia (memory loss) of both anterograde

and retrograde memory. Anterograde memory consists of memory loss that occurs after hippocampal damage, while retrograde memory loss refers to loss of memory that occurs before damage to the hippocampus. In Korsakoff's syndrome, the patient experiences a great deal of difficulty in recalling events in the recent past and handling and retaining new information, as well as remembering those events that took place in the distant past. Korsakoff's syndrome is typically associated with the toxic effects of alcohol or from a vitamin B deficiency. Neurons in the hippocampal formation and other parts of the Papez circuit (i.e., the pathway linking the hippocampal formation, especially the mammillary bodies, anterior thalamic nucleus, and cingulate gyrus; Fig. 25-4) seem to be particularly affected.

Patients sustaining hippocampal lobectomies display perseveration of response tendencies and further display a **short-term memory disorder**. In such instances, the patient displays anterograde amnesia, but retrograde amnesia is less severe, with little diminution of intellectual abilities. The patient can remember events that took place in the distant past but cannot remember events that occurred recently. For example, if a patient is required to select a geometric form from another series of objects that he was shown 1 minute earlier, he is unable to perform that task. Such a patient

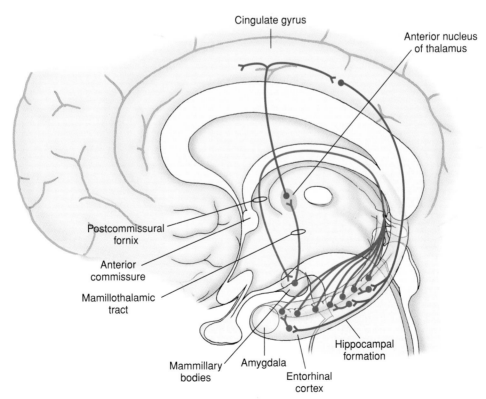

Figure 25–4 Papez circuit. In the Papez circuit, hippocampal fibers project to the mammillary bodies, which, in turn, project through the mammillothalamic tract to the anterior nucleus. The anterior thalamic nucleus then projects to the cingulate gyrus, and the axons of the cingulate gyrus then project back to the hippocampal formation.

may also have difficulty in reading, in that he is unable to remember a previously read line. In contrast, a normal population has little difficulty in successfully completing these tasks.

The following is an example of a memory disorder associated with hippocampal ablation. A patient received a bilateral temporal lobectomy (involving much of the hippocampal formation on each side of the brain) to eliminate the spread of severe seizure activity. He was able to remember such facts as the place where he lived years earlier, but he could not remember where he recently moved after the surgery. Similarly, he was able to recall other facts in his distant past, such as people and songs that he had known from years past, but he was unable to remember the people who he met or music that he heard after the surgery. Surprisingly, other forms of intellectual abilities remained intact. He was able to show normal levels of abstract reasoning and perform equally well on related forms of intelligence tests.

These results suggest that one of the functions of the hippocampal formation is to contribute to the consolidation of memory functions by transferring short-term memories to long-term memories. Adequate explanations of the mechanisms underlying the role of the hippocampal formation in memory functions are still lacking in the literature. It is reasonable, however, to suggest that the hippocampal formation normally receives, processes, and

categorizes sensory information during learning. Thus, lesions of the hippocampal formation would likely disrupt these events and further interfere with related attentional mechanisms required for the processing and storage of sensory events (in different regions of the cerebral cortex) that are critical for conditioned learning to take place. This kind of loss may be reflected in patients with hippocampal lesions by their inability to encode, categorize, and abstract relevant information necessary for the learning process and, thus, prevents new long-term memories from becoming established.

One hippocampal mechanism that has been proposed as a model for memory consolidation is called **long-term potentiation** (LTP). It represents a change in synaptic strength as a manifestation of synaptic plasticity. LTP can be produced by stimulating fibers that make excitatory connections with hippocampal pyramidal cells. For example, short bursts of high-frequency stimulation of the entorhinal afferents or Schaffer collaterals to hippocampal pyramidal cells over a period of time result in an increased efficiency of the CA1 pyramidal cell response. The increase in excitatory response potency in pyramidal cells that lasts over a period of many minutes and even weeks may constitute a cellular mechanism by which learning takes place (Fig. 25-5, A-C). The suspected synaptic mechanism is believed to involve the release of glutamate that binds to N-methyl-D-aspartate

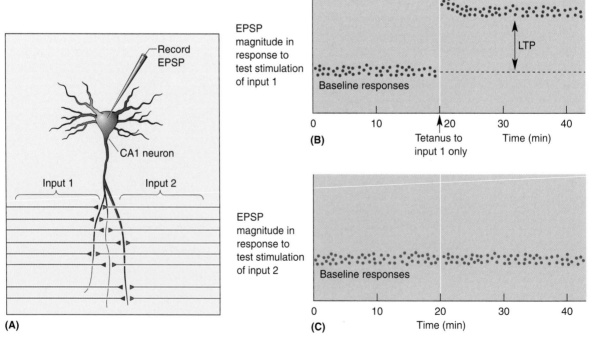

Figure 25–5 Long-term potentiation (LTP). (A) Activity within the CA1 field of hippocampus is recorded with a microelectrode following alternate stimulation of inputs 1 and 2. (B) In this experiment, high-frequency (tetanus) stimulation applied in input 1 at the time indicated by the arrow potentiated the response as shown in the time period to the right of the arrow. (C) This graph shows the specificity of the response because there was no change in response following stimulation of input 2.

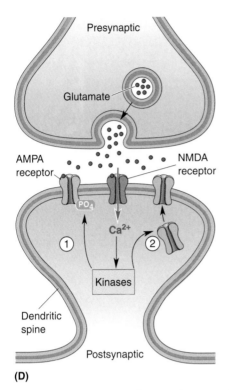

(D)

Figure 25–5 *(continued)* (D) Ca^{2+}, which enters through NMDA receptors and activates protein kinases, can induce LTP by either altering the efficiency of AMPA receptors or inducing new AMPA receptors. (From Bear MF, et al.: Neuroscience: Exploring the Brain, 2nd ed. Philadelphia: Lippincott, Williams & Wilkins, 2001, p. 793.)

(NMDA) receptors (Fig. 25-5D). This conclusion is based on the fact that NMDA receptor blockade in the hippocampus eliminates LTP. The suggested basis for these events may be as follows. During low-frequency stimulation of the hippocampus, glutamate is released from the Schaffer collaterals and binds to both NMDA and non-NMDA receptors. However, the presence of magnesium blocks the NMDA channels. During high-frequency stimu-

lation, magnesium is released from NMDA channels, and current then flows through both NMDA and non-NMDA channels. Apparently, the essential feature here is that NMDA channels are highly permeable to calcium. Therefore, when these events open calcium channels, there is a likely increase in synaptic efficiency as well as the number of terminals present at that synapse, reflecting a functional change at the synapse during LTP.

SEPTAL AREA

HISTOLOGY

As noted in Chapter 13, the histological appearance of the septal area differs between humans and other animals. In animals, there exists a dorsal septal area, which includes the lateral septal nucleus and medial septal nucleus. The medial septal nucleus becomes continuous with the vertical limb of the diagonal band of Broca, which lies ventral to the dorsal septal area and is referred to as the ventral septal area (Fig. 25-6A). In humans, a dorsal septal area is not present, and the corresponding area is relegated to the region of the ventral septal area. Two cell groups are sometimes associated with the septal area. These include: (1) the bed nucleus of the stria terminalis, which lies adjacent to the ventrolateral aspect of the lateral septal nucleus; and (2) the nucleus accumbens, which lies just lateral to the vertical limb of the diagonal band of Broca (Fig. 25-6A).

AFFERENT CONNECTIONS

The septal area receives sensory afferent fibers from the medial olfactory stria, monoaminergic systems of the brainstem, hippocampal formation, amygdala, and feedback signals from the lateral

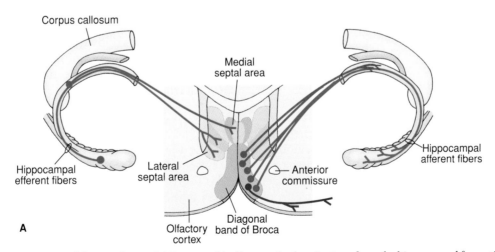

Figure 25–6 Connections of the septal area. (A) Topographically organized projections from the hippocampal formation to the septal area (*left side*) and topographically arranged efferent projections from the diagonal band of Broca to the hippocampal formation (*right side*).

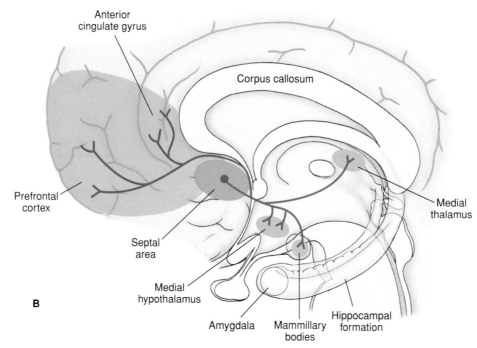

Figure 25–6 (*continued*) (B) Diagram illustrates other projections from the septal area to the medial hypothalamus, mammillary bodies, medial thalamus, prefrontal cortex, and anterior cingulate gyrus.

hypothalamus. The monoaminergic inputs presumably serve to modulate septal neuronal activity, as do the olfactory inputs. As previously pointed out, the septal area serves principally as a relay of the hippocampal formation to the hypothalamus. Thus, the topographically organized inputs from the hippocampal formation (Fig. 25-6A) are considered to be highly significant.

EFFERENT CONNECTIONS

The primary efferent projections of the septal area are directed on the hypothalamus and hippocampal formation (Fig. 25-6B). The projections to the hypothalamus arise primarily from the lateral septal nucleus and contribute significant quantities of fibers to the descending component of the medial forebrain bundle. These fibers terminate mainly in the medial hypothalamus. In this manner, the hippocampal formation uses the septal area as a relay nucleus to modulate functions of the hypothalamus.

The hippocampal formation and septal nuclei are reciprocally connected. We have previously pointed out that the hippocampal formation projects topographically to the septal area. The nuclei of the diagonal band, which receive inputs from the lateral septal nucleus, also project topographically back to the hippocampal formation in such a manner that neurons situated most medially project to that part of the hippocampal formation that

is located near the septal pole, while neurons situated progressively more laterally within the diagonal band project to progressively more ventral and anterior regions that approach the temporal pole of the hippocampal formation (Fig. 25-6B).

The nuclei of the diagonal band of Broca actually have widespread projections that make synaptic connections with other parts of the limbic system (Fig. 25-6B). They project to olfactory, prefrontal, and anterior cingulate cortices, as well as to the amygdala, mammillary bodies, habenular complex, and mediodorsal thalamic nucleus. Accordingly, the nuclei of the diagonal band parallel the projection patterns of the subicular cortex in that both regions are able to communicate with much of the limbic system, thus allowing neurons of the septal-hippocampal axis to communicate and synchronize their activity with much of the limbic system and related nuclei.

FUNCTIONS OF THE SEPTAL AREA

Because the septal area is reciprocally related to the hippocampal formation, it serves not only as a relay for the transmission of hippocampal impulses to the hypothalamus, but also as a feedback system to the hippocampal formation. Therefore, it is understandable that the functions of the septal area are highly similar to those of the hippocampal formation. Like the hippocampal formation, the septal area has been implicated in the control of functions normally attributable to the hypothalamus, such as aggression, rage, autonomic functions, self-stimulation, and drinking behavior. For example, lesions of the septal area in rats cause them to be highly irritable, aggressive, easily startled, and very difficult to handle. This syndrome is referred to as **septal rage**. Electrical stimulation of the septal area of the cat modulates aggressive behavior, cardiovascular responses, and single-cell activity in the hypothalamus. Electrical stimulation of the septal area also modulates self-stimulation and drinking behavior elicited from the lateral hypothalamus.

The neuroanatomical basis for these functions of the septal area can be attributed to the septal area's direct projections to the hypothalamus. Along these lines, direct septal-hypothalamic projections can also account for the modulatory effects that the septal area exerts on the endocrine system via the hypothalamic-pituitary axis. For example, stimulation of the septal area suppresses ACTH secretion and adrenal activity in the rat. Conversely, lesions of the septal area facilitate ACTH release.

The pathway from the septal area to the hippocampal formation may function in ways other than as a feedback mechanism. It has been shown that the nuclei of the diagonal band likely serve as the origin of the hippocampal theta rhythm. Moreover, the septal-hippocampal pathway may also contribute inputs that significantly contribute to some of the learning functions normally associated with the hippocampal formation. That such a mechanism may exist is suggested from behavioral studies in which lesions of the septal area impair passive avoidance learning (which also occurs with damage to the hippocampal formation).

RELATED BASAL FOREBRAIN NUCLEI

The adjoining nuclei of the bed nucleus of the stria terminalis, nucleus accumbens, and substantia innominata also link these regions of the limbic forebrain with the hypothalamus and midbrain tegmentum (Fig. 25-7, see also Fig. 13-15). The bed nucleus of the stria terminalis receives significant inputs from various nuclei of the amygdala and projects its axons to both the hypothalamus and midbrain PAG. Thus, it serves as a parallel pathway by which the amygdala can modulate visceral functions of the hypothalamus and PAG. Some authors view the nucleus accumbens as a region that integrates motor and motivational processes associated with the basal ganglia and limbic system, respectively. Projections from this region include

short axons to the substantia innominata, whose axons are then directed onto the hypothalamus and amygdala (as well as to wide regions of cortex). Other projections of the nucleus accumbens descend to the ventral tegmentum. The ventral tegmentum is a major source of dopaminergic fibers to the limbic system and neocortex. Thus, inputs into the ventral tegmentum from the nucleus accumbens can serve to regulate neuronal activity within much of the limbic system. Monoaminergic inputs into the limbic system are believed to provide a basis for the regulation of mood states. Accordingly, the inputs from the nucleus accumbens may play an important role in controlling this process.

A region of the substantia innominata, called the **basal nucleus of Meynert** (see Fig. 13-15), is of particular interest with respect to the development of **Alzheimer's disease.** The basal nucleus of Meynert lies immediately lateral to the horizontal limb of the diagonal band. Like the diagonal band nuclei, the neurons of the basal nucleus are cholinergic and project to wide regions of the cerebral cortex and limbic system. Alzheimer's disease, which is associated with severe loss of memory functions, is correlated with: (1) the presence of neurofibrillary tangles; (2) extracellular deposition of the abnormal amyloid protein β-amyloid cortex plaques in the cerebral cortex; and (3) cell loss in the basal nucleus and reduced cholinergic content of cortical tissue. Because of the widespread projections of the basal nucleus to limbic structures, it is possible that disruption of these connections may contribute to the affective changes seen in these Alzheimer's patients. Moreover, evidence further suggests that neuronal cell damage may not be limited to the basal nucleus but may also include limbic nuclei as well. Limbic structures believed to contain cell loss in Alzheimer's patients include the diagonal band of Broca and the subicular cortex. Recent studies have suggested that the amyloid deposits result from a mutation of the gene that encodes the amyloid precursor protein. Moreover, the ε4 allele of the apolipoprotein E situated on chromosome 19 has been shown to be a risk factor for onset of Alzheimer's disease. One approach to combating this disorder involves drug therapy. One drug, called Alzhemed (still in clinical trials at the time of publication), has been reported to function as an anti-amyloid compound and may be effective in reducing the effects of amyloid fibers in the cerebral cortex. Another drug that has been used for the treatment of Alzheimer's disease is Aricept, a reversible acetylcholinesterase inhibitor (see Chapter 8). It has met with some success with patients in nursing homes.

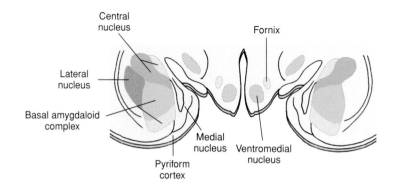

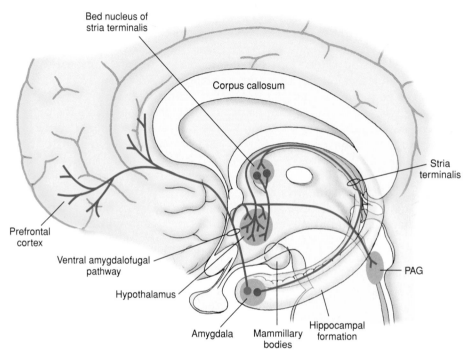

Figure 25–7   Efferent projections of the amygdala. The diagram in the upper panel indicates the organization of the nuclei of the amygdala. Schematic diagram in the lower panel identifies the major efferent projections of the amygdala. One principal output includes the stria terminalis, which projects to the bed nucleus of the stria terminalis and to the rostro-caudal extent of the medial hypothalamus. Fibers from the bed nucleus also supply similar regions of the hypothalamus. Another important output to the hypothalamus and midbrain PAG uses the ventral amygdalofugal pathway. Other fibers pass rostrally from the amygdala to the prefrontal cortex.

AMYGDALA

HISTOLOGY

The amygdala is located deep to the uncus in humans and is comprised of different nuclei, which differ in their anatomical connections and neurochemical and physiological properties. The amygdala contains a cortical mantle called the **pyriform lobe** that provides significant input to the amygdala and is, thus, functionally associated with it. The major groups of nuclei include the **lateral, basal, medial, anterior, central,** and **cortical nuclei**. However, from a functional point of view, it is convenient to divide the amygdaloid complex into two components: (1) a **corticomedial group**, which includes mainly the cortical, medial, and medial aspect of the basal nuclei that lie within its dorsal and medial aspects; and (2) a **basolateral group**, which includes the lateral, central, and lateral aspects of the basal nuclei (see Fig. 1-4). As indicated earlier, the amygdala is intimately related to the pyriform lobe. The cortex immediately adjacent to the amygdala at rostral levels of this structure is referred to as the **prepyriform area**, and more posterior regions of the pyriform lobe are referred to as the **periamygdaloid cortex**.

AFFERENT CONNECTIONS

Like the hippocampal formation, the amygdala receives inputs from sensory and monoaminergic systems. Afferent fibers to the amygdala arise from structures linked with transmission of both olfactory and taste signals. These include direct inputs from the olfactory bulb, indirect inputs from the pyriform lobe (which also receives afferents from the olfactory bulb), and direct and indirect inputs from the solitary nucleus. The amygdala also receives inputs from the neocortex. These include auditory signals from the temporal neocortex and integrative signals from the prefrontal cortex. Additional regions of the forebrain projecting (nonsensory) information to the amygdala include the ventromedial hypothalamus, substantia innominata, nuclei of the diagonal band of Broca, and medial thalamus.

EFFERENT CONNECTIONS

The most significant projections of the amygdala are those that innervate the hypothalamus, bed nucleus of the stria terminalis, and midbrain PAG. These projections are deemed to be highly significant because they provide the anatomical substrate by which the amygdala regulates visceral processes normally associated with these structures.

Consider first the amygdaloid projections to the hypothalamus. Communication from the amygdala to the hypothalamus can be achieved by direct or indirect pathways. Direct routes involve the **stria terminalis** and **ventral amygdalofugal pathway**. The stria terminalis arises mainly from the corticomedial group of nuclei, and a primary projection of these fibers is directed to the rostrocaudal extent of the preopticomedial hypothalamus. The ventral amygdalofugal pathway arises mainly from the basolateral complex of amygdala, passes deep to the pyriform cortex, and supplies primarily the lateral hypothalamus and midbrain PAG (Fig. 25-7). These two groups of fibers enable the corticomedial amygdala to directly control the medial hypothalamus and enable the basolateral amygdala to directly control the lateral hypothalamus and PAG. The amygdala can also modulate activity of the hypothalamus and PAG indirectly. It does so by virtue of its connections with the bed nucleus of the stria terminalis, which, in turn, project directly to these structures. The amygdala also maintains a significant anatomical relationship with the prefrontal cortex with which it shares reciprocal connections.

FUNCTIONS OF THE AMYGDALA

Perhaps of all the limbic structures, it is the amygdala that exerts the most potent control over visceral processes of the hypothalamus. Many studies have been conducted that involved ablations, lesions, and electrical stimulation to identify the role of the amygdala in aggression and rage, feeding, and cardiovascular and endocrine functions.

One of the classic studies depicting the behavioral effects of amygdaloid ablations was carried out in 1937 by Klüver and Bucy. They described a constellation of behavioral response changes as a result of amygdaloid lesions in the monkey, which consisted of hypersexuality, a change in dietary habits, a decrease in anxiety toward fear-producing objects, a tendency to orally explore and contact inedible objects, and visual agnosia. These response tendencies are referred to as the **Klüver-Bucy syndrome**. However, in humans, only some of these symptoms are typically seen in a given patient.

Other studies, however, have demonstrated that the modulating properties of the amygdala on aggressive behavior are not uniform. Different regions of amygdala exert differential effects on different forms of aggressive behavior. For example, stimulation of the corticomedial amygdala has a powerful, facilitating effect on defensive rage behavior but has an equally potent suppression on predatory attack behavior. In contrast, stimulation of the basolateral region of amygdala has just the opposite effects on these forms of aggressive behavior. Some of the underlying mechanisms have also been discovered. Medial amygdaloid potentiation of defensive rage behavior is mediated by fibers of the stria terminalis that excite medial hypothalamic neurons and that use substance P as a neurotransmitter, whereas central and lateral amygdaloid suppression of this form of aggression is mediated through an inhibitory enkephalinergic projection to the midbrain PAG.

Studies concerning the relationship of the amygdala to aggression and rage have also been reported in humans. In such studies, which are usually carried out in cases with intractable epilepsy, lesions have been reported to produce a general taming effect, with decreases in aggressive and explosive behaviors and decreases in hyperactivity. The loci of the lesions (presumably involving mainly the amygdala) have not been clearly identified. However, studies involving tumors of this region have often been associated with increases in rage behavior, impulsivity, and loss of emotional control in response to an event that normally would be perceived as a minor annoyance to most people.

Electrical stimulation of the amygdala in both animals and humans does not produce aggressive responses. In humans, it has been reported that stimulation can evoke different types of emotional feelings such as relief, relaxation, detachment, and a general pleasant sensation.

Stimulation of the amygdala has likewise produced different effects on the cardiovascular system. Generally, pressor responses appear to be dominant, such as increases in blood pressure, heart rate, and pupillary dilation, especially in regions that facilitate defensive rage behavior (i.e., corticomedial amygdala). Stimulation of the amygdala has also been reported to produce micturition and occasional depressor responses.

The amygdala has also been shown to play a role in other functions. This area of the limbic system modulates feeding and drinking functions associated with the hypothalamus. Stimulation and lesion studies suggest that the basolateral amygdala has a facilitative effect, while the corticomedial region is inhibitory. The amygdala also affects endocrine function. Stimulation of the corticomedial amygdala can induce ovulation, while transection of the stria terminalis abolishes this response. Moreover, activation of the basolateral amygdala facilitates growth hormone release, while the corticomedial amygdala inhibits growth hormone release. Basolateral amygdaloid stimulation and lesions of the corticomedial region also facilitate the release of ACTH. Collectively, it appears that the pathways arising from basolateral and corticomedial amygdala that target the lateral and medial regions of hypothalamus (and midbrain PAG) serve to differentially modulate the various visceral functions normally associated with the hypothalamus.

LIMBIC COMPONENTS OF THE CEREBRAL CORTEX

ANATOMICAL CONNECTIONS

The prefrontal cortex and the anterior cingulate gyrus are included as parts of the limbic system principally because they send indirect projections to the hypothalamus and have been shown to modulate functions normally associated with the hypothalamus. It should be noted, however, that some of the functions of both the prefrontal cortex and anterior cingulate gyrus are likely mediated through projections to other parts of the brain as well. These include the basal ganglia, other regions of cerebral cortex, brainstem nuclei, and thalamic structures.

As a cortical structure, the prefrontal cortex is unique in that it receives afferent fibers from all re-

gions of the cerebral cortex. It also receives inputs from all brainstem monoaminergic systems and limbic-related structures. These structures include the mediodorsal thalamic nucleus (with which it shares reciprocal connections), lateral hypothalamus, nuclei of the diagonal band of Broca, basolateral amygdala, and subicular cortex. Fibers arising from the prefrontal cortex project to the temporal neocortex and to deep temporal lobe structures, which include the amygdala and subicular cortex. The influence of the prefrontal cortex on hypothalamic functions is mediated via both direct and indirect routes. The direct route has recently been discovered and involves a monosynaptic projection from the prefrontal cortex to the hypothalamus. The indirect route involves an initial projection to the mediodorsal nucleus, and through a series of interneurons directed rostrally from the mediodorsal nucleus and midline thalamus, impulses from the prefrontal cortex can also reach the anterior lateral hypothalamus (see Fig. 24-3).

The anterior cingulate gyrus receives inputs from the following areas: (1) the anterior thalamic nucleus; (2) dopaminergic fibers that arise in the ventral tegmental area; and (3) the diagonal band of Broca. Efferent fibers of the anterior cingulate gyrus project to the mediodorsal thalamic nucleus and to the subicular cortex. In this manner, the anterior cingulate gyrus can also modulate visceral processes by using the same circuitry to the hypothalamus as is used by the prefrontal cortex (i.e., mediodorsal thalamic nucleus → midline thalamic nuclei → anterior lateral hypothalamus). Other parts of the cingulate gyrus project through the cingulum bundle to the hippocampal formation, forming a component of the Papez circuit (Fig. 25-4), and may function to modulate memory functions.

FUNCTIONS OF THE CEREBRAL CORTEX

Prefrontal Cortex

The prefrontal cortex experiences significant evolutionary changes. It is rudimentary in rodents, is more clearly identifiable in the cat, and becomes considerably larger in primates, reaching its largest relative size in humans, which suggests an increasingly important role for this region.

The prefrontal cortex is associated with both emotional and intellectual processes. Concerning emotional behavior, stimulation of either the orbital frontal region or the medial aspect of the prefrontal cortex powerfully suppresses predatory attack and defensive rage responses elicited from the hypothalamus, as well as spontaneously elicited aggressive behavior. The inhibitory effects of the prefrontal cortex on the attack response are dependent on an intact pathway from the prefrontal cortex to the mediodorsal nucleus. When this pathway is severed or when a lesion is placed in the mediodorsal nucleus, the inhibitory effects of prefrontal cortex stimulation are blocked.

The importance of the human prefrontal cortex in the control of human aggression has also been recognized for many years. The first reported case of prefrontal damage was reported in the middle of the 19th century as a result of an industrial accident in Vermont of a railroad worker named Phineas Gage. Gage was wounded by a spike that pierced through his skull, severing the prefrontal region of his brain. Amazingly, he was able to recover from the incident without significant motor damage. However, soon afterwards, he began to experience significant emotional and personality changes, characterized principally by irritable, irrational, and hostile behavior, all of which were absent prior to the accident. Therefore, these observations would suggest that the prefrontal cortex normally inhibits aggression and rage behavior.

Therefore, it was surprising that a technique called **prefrontal lobotomy** was developed in 1936 by Egaz Moniz for controlling human violence and manifestations of psychotic behavior that involved the undercutting of the afferent and efferent connections of the prefrontal cortex. For developing this procedure, Moniz received a Nobel prize. The procedure had met with some minor success, and some mild personality changes were reported on varying occasions. However, consistent effects in reducing aggressive tendencies were never reported over extended periods of time. The use of prefrontal lobotomies has been replaced by other (noninvasive) therapeutic measures such as antipsychotic drugs. Accordingly, such surgical procedures are rarely performed at the present time.

The prefrontal cortex also exerts a powerful modulatory effect on other processes associated with the hypothalamus. For example, lesions of the prefrontal cortex lead to an increase in feeding behavior, while stimulation of this region inhibits feeding. Electrical stimulation also inhibits respiratory movements, changes blood pressure, inhibits gastric motility, and raises the temperature of the extremities.

With respect to intellectual functions, lesions of the prefrontal cortex also have profound effects. Perhaps one of the clear-cut demonstrations of loss of function following prefrontal lesions involves experiments conducted on animals in which delayed alternation tests were used. In this type of experiment, the animal is shown which of two places

food has been placed. However, the animal must learn to postpone its response for a specific length of time. Normally, an intact animal will master this task within a short period of time. However, animals sustaining lesions of the prefrontal cortex commit many errors, mostly relating to failure to wait the requisite amount of time before eliciting the response. In addition, if the prefrontal damaged animal has to discriminate between two sounds or between two visual signals, many more errors are committed than by intact animals.

In humans, patients sustaining damage to the prefrontal cortex also display a number of characteristic intellectual and perceptual deficits. The patients experience difficulty in accurately identifying the perceived vertical when the body is placed in a tilted position. If these patients are given a card-sorting task in which they are asked to sort the cards on the basis of color, shape, or number of figures on the card, they can easily master this task until they are requested to shift their criteria for categorization (i.e., change from shape to numbers). Under these circumstances, these patients tend to persevere with their original strategies and appear to lose sight of the original purpose of their goals and objectives. These behavioral dysfunctions can be characterized as a "derangement in behavioral programming," which likely involves a disruption of the connections between the frontal lobe and parietal and temporal cortices.

Anterior Cingulate Gyrus

Experimental evidence suggests that the anterior cingulate gyrus also plays an important role in the regulation of visceral processes, which are, in part, associated with the hypothalamus. For example, electrical stimulation of this region of cortex suppresses predatory attack behavior elicited from the lateral hypothalamus in the cat, whereas lesions facilitate the occurrence of this response in several species. Case history studies have revealed that, in humans, tumors of this region have been associated with aggressive responses, while electrical stimulation produces respiratory arrest, a fall in blood pressure, and cardiac slowing. Thus, it would appear that the anterior cingulate gyrus functions similarly to the prefrontal cortex in that it exerts a general suppressive effect on a variety of visceral processes associated with the hypothalamic functions in addition to its reported effects on aggressive behavior. However, as noted earlier, it is quite possible that the modulating effects of the prefrontal cortex and cingulate gyrus with respect to these functions are also mediated through different circuits on other groups of neurons in the forebrain and brainstem.

PATHOLOGICAL ACTIVITY WITHIN LIMBIC CIRCUITS

Because epilepsy is a major disorder associated with the limbic system and, in particular, with temporal lobe structures, we include the following discussions of epilepsy and the application of the electroencephalogram (EEG).

MEASUREMENT OF BRAIN ACTIVITY: THE ELECTROENCEPHALOGRAM

The **EEG** is recorded at the scalp and sometimes from the surface of the brain during epilepsy surgery. It measures potential differences between two active electrodes on the scalp or between a scalp electrode and an inactive electrode, which is usually placed behind the ear. The EEG measures the summation of excitatory postsynaptic potentials (EPSPs) and inhibitory postsynaptic potentials (IPSPs) from the scalp. Because these signals are low in amplitude, a differential amplifier is used to make the waves more visible. Gold or platinum electrodes are placed on the scalp after thorough cleaning with an abrasive agent. The pins from the wire attached to the electrodes are plugged into a jackbox that is attached by cable to the amplifier.

There are many characteristic waveforms seen on both normal and abnormal EEGs. For instance, when a normal subject lies quietly, an **alpha rhythm** is found in the occipital leads. This disappears with eye opening. If this rhythm is slow or absent, then there may be a neurologic problem. States of alertness are characterized by waves of lower amplitude and higher frequency (see Fig. 23-10). Similarly, epileptiform spikes are sharp waves followed by a slow wave, and the presence of these entities is abnormal. If the patient has had seizures or questionable seizures in the past, then the presence of epileptiform spikes will assist in making the diagnosis. Additionally, certain patterns, such as a 3-per-second spike and wave when the patient has had a history of staring spells, will assist in making the diagnosis of an absence seizure. Likewise, waves of 4 to 7 Hz recorded over the temporal lobes or within the hippocampal formation, called a **theta rhythm**, reflect a dysfunction of hippocampal tissue in humans. In lower forms of animals, theta rhythms may appear normal when recorded from hippocampal tissue, especially during conditions reflecting altered motivational states, such as when an animal is approaching a goal. **Delta rhythms** are defined as very slow, 1- to 3-Hz, synchronous waves that occur under conditions of severe trauma to the brain (e.g., such as brain tumors). They also occur normally for short periods during sleep. EEG is also useful in other disorders, such as coma.

EPILEPSY

Seizures can be defined as paroxysmal events in which there is a significant change in the EEG that correlates with a change in behavior and/or consciousness. Seizures may also include generalized "convulsions," sensory experiences (either prior to or during the seizure), and a variety of motor activities. Seizures are usually stereotyped for each patient, and some patients with severe epilepsy may have multiple seizure types.

Epilepsy can be defined as a condition in which seizures are recurrent. Seizures may develop as a result of the spreading of excitatory postsynaptic potentials, which discharge synchronously from either abnormal neurons or metabolic problems that lower seizure potential. Seizure disorders may be idiopathic, but they also may occur as a result of a mass lesion, such as brain tumors and vascular malformations, infections, drugs and drug withdrawal, and metabolic problems. The time of the occurrence of the seizure is called the **ictal period**; the time following the seizure is called the **postictal period**; and the time between seizures is called the **interictal period**.

Seizures can be classified into two basic types: (1) partial or focal, meaning that the seizure arises from specific regions of the brain and is limited to one hemisphere; or (2) generalized, meaning seizures arise diffusely throughout the brain, causing a loss of consciousness. The EEG also classifies seizure types. The EEG helps to define whether seizures arise from one or more specific areas or whether they develop diffusely.

Partial seizures can be classified as either simple partial or complex partial (sometimes called psychomotor) seizures. Simple partial seizures do not cause a change in consciousness, but the patient experiences various sensory and motor symptoms, usually not lasting more than 1 to 2 minutes. Motor signs described in simple partial seizures include focal motor clonic activity and a focal **Jacksonian March**, where seizure activity begins locally over the cortex, causing either sensory or motor activity directly corresponding to the **homunculus** of either the sensory or motor cortex. The patient experiences a "march" of sensory or motor activity from muscle to muscle in the same order as the homunculus. Other types of simple partial seizures include those that generate sensory phenomena such as somatosensory, visual, olfactory, gustatory, and vestibular sensations. These seizures may also contain autonomic symptoms including a rising epigastric sensation, pallor, sweating, and pupillary dilation. Psychic symptoms may also be found in simple partial seizures, but when these are present, the patient will also progress to a complex partial seizure with impairment of consciousness. Examples of psychic phenomena include **dysphasia**, which is a speech difficulty that is a less severe form of aphasia. The patient may also experience déjà vu, fear, anger, macropsia (i.e., things appearing larger than they are), or micropsia (i.e., things appearing smaller than they are). Often, simple partial seizures are called an **aura**, meaning that they provide a warning of the spread of the seizure, causing a complex partial seizure.

The most common type of seizure is the **complex partial seizure**. These seizures are characterized by an impairment of consciousness, although not usually a loss of consciousness. They may begin with an aura (simple partial seizure), but this is not necessary for the diagnosis of this seizure type. During the seizure, the patient may stare and not respond to commands. The patient may exhibit automatisms, which are automatic, stereotypic, and nonpurposeful behaviors such as chewing, lip smacking, or grabbing objects. Complex partial seizures may spread from a single focus to the entire cortex, resulting in secondary generalization. The patient initially has complex partial seizures that evolve into generalized tonic-clonic seizures as a result of the diffuse spread of the seizure. Postictal periods of sleepiness are common in this seizure type.

Generalized seizures arise diffusely from the cerebral cortex. All generalized seizures reveal epileptic activity diffusely. One common type of generalized seizure is the generalized **tonic-clonic seizure** (Fig. 25-8). These seizures, often called convulsions, involve a tonic phase or stiffening, followed by a clonic phase in which the extremities contract the agonistic and antagonistic

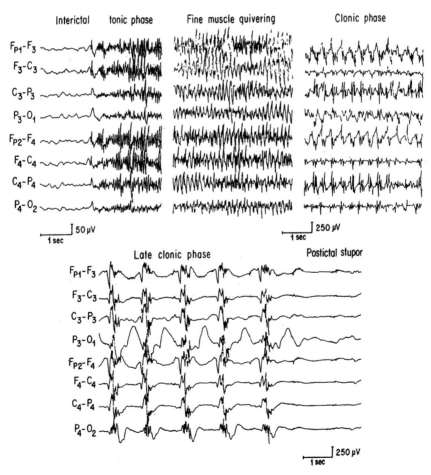

Figure 25–8 EEG records showing a generalized tonic-clonic seizure. The various segments illustrate the interictal phase (prior to the seizure); the tonic phase (where the body is stiff) with repetitive spiking; a clonic phase (where body is jerking), which shows spike and waves; and a postictal phase (where no seizure activity is present). (From Westmoreland BF, et al.: Medical Neurosciences, 3rd ed. Boston: Little, Brown & Co., 1994, p. 484.)

muscles. The clonic phase begins with rapid movements, which then slow until they stop, and the patient remains unconscious. Often at the beginning of these seizures, the patient will attempt to force air through a tonic airway, causing an "epileptic cry." Most of these seizures are not dangerous and last only a minute or two. Prolonged seizure activity or the generation of two or more of these seizures in a row without regaining consciousness is called **status epilepticus**. This condition is a neurologic emergency with a high morbidity and mortality.

Other types of generalized seizures include **absence**, **myoclonic**, and **atonic** seizures. Absence seizures are very brief (approximately 3 to 10 seconds long), and the patient is unresponsive and is often seen as "daydreaming" (Fig. 25-9). When the patient is tested during the seizure, all behavioral functions cease but begin again after the seizure, indicating that there is no effective postictal period. The classic finding on the EEG is a **3-per-second spike** and **wave complex**. Myoclonic seizures are very brief and characterized by a rapid muscle jerk accompanied by polyspike and wave complexes, which are also brief. Atonic seizures, which are found mainly in children with neurologic disorders, consist of a very brief complete loss of muscle tone. These seizures are further characterized by a brief burst of polyspike and slow wave complexes.

One of the unique features of temporal lobe neurons, which include those cells that lie in the pyriform cortex, hippocampal formation, and parts of the amygdala, is their low threshold for seizure discharges. In particular, one region of the hippocampus, called Sommer's sector, consists of CA1 neurons that are highly susceptible to anoxia at

birth and that are also damaged in patients who have epilepsy with a primary focus in the hippocampus. Seizure discharges associated with hippocampal epilepsy are frequently characterized by high-frequency, high-amplitude synchronous discharges of large groups of cells that become self-sustaining. Frequently, partial seizures are limited to the region of the hippocampus that has no behavioral concomitant. The patient sits quietly and appears unaware of his surroundings during the time of the seizure (i.e., ictal period). The patient may appear confused and experience auditory, olfactory, vertiginous, or even gustatory hallucinations. Such seizures are often identified by EEG recordings. As indicated earlier in this chapter, such emotional responses as aggressive behavior may be associated with seizures of the temporal lobe, occurring in the postictal or interictal periods. Such responses occur frequently when attempting to look toward the patient or give the patient directions. Seizures may evolve from multiple sources. Typically, they result from anoxia at birth or from head injuries or tumors in adults. Such damage may involve vascularization, glial formation, or fibrosis, which serve as irritative foci for seizure development.

Seizures are mainly treated with anticonvulsant medications. However, patients with seizures that are intractable to multiple medications may be candidates for other options, such as the surgical removal of the epileptic focus (if there is one clear focus); vagus nerve stimulation, which has been used successfully for the treatment of seizures when drug therapy is unsuccessful; and in young children suffering from an inborn error of metabolism (phenylketonuria), a restricted protein diet, which gives rise to ketones.

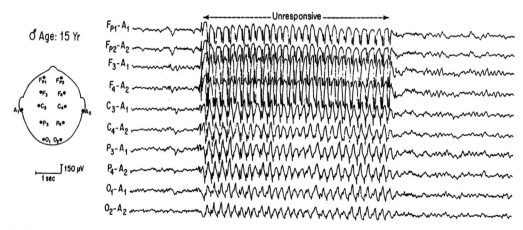

Figure 25–9 Absence seizure. EEG records illustrating an absence seizure consisting of a 3-Hz spike and wave pattern, at which time the patient was unresponsive. (From Westmoreland BF, et al.: Medical Neurosciences, 3rd ed. Boston: Little, Brown & Co., 1994, p. 485.)

CLINICAL CASE

HISTORY

Chuck is a 58-year-old chairman of a neurology department, who has always performed well professionally and never had any significant health problems. In the past year or two, both his colleagues and family have noticed that his behavior has changed. Although he was mildly impulsive and prone to rage attacks at home in the past, recently, Chuck has begun to have more violent, inappropriate rage attacks at work, as well. When a nurse was slow in passing him a reflex hammer while examining a patient in his office, he threw it at her. When he believed that a colleague did not produce a result quickly enough, he accused her of not trying hard enough, threw a floppy disc at her, and ordered her out of the hospital. Additionally, he was pursuing women inappropriately, even at work, despite having a relatively stable marriage. One of his colleagues found him taking liberties with his secretary, despite obvious protests on her part. He propositioned women in front of his wife, who became so upset that she demanded that she either see a psychiatrist or she would divorce him. However, 2 days prior to his appointment, Chuck had an episode characterized by a "funny smell" and then stared motionless for approximately 2 minutes. While he was staring into space, his secretary observed him chewing and smacking his lips. When she asked him if he was all right, he did not answer. When he began to speak again, he simply said that he was tired and went to lie down. At this point, his secretary became concerned, and she called a fellow neurologist, who examined him the same day.

EXAMINATION

On examination, there were no obvious abnormalities, with the exception of a visual field deficit in the right upper quadrant of each eye. Smell and hearing were intact. All motor functions and language function were also normal. The neurologist ordered a magnetic resonance imaging (MRI) scan and an EEG. The MRI of Chuck's head revealed a left side anterior temporal mass, which, upon further investigation, was identified as a glioma. The tumor was apparently growing slowly because of the lack of significant swelling surrounding the tumor.

EXPLANATION

The staring episode is called a complex partial seizure or paroxysmal storm of initially localized activity, which appears on an EEG to be rhythmic, excitatory activity. Clinically, these seizures are manifested as stereotypic staring spells, sometimes involving various automatic behaviors. Since stimulation of certain regions of the limbic system, including the corticomedial amygdaloid nuclei, can induce anger and rage, a tumor in this region can produce behavioral changes of this sort. Hypersexuality and indiscriminate sexual behavior can also be found with lesions of this region, even unilaterally. Bilateral lesions of the amygdala frequently cause hypersexuality as part of the Klüver-Bucy syndrome. The superior quadrantanopsia or "pie-in-the-sky" visual field defect occurs as a result of interruption of fibers from the upper visual field as they travel through the temporal lobe. It may go unnoticed initially because the patient is easily able to compensate for small visual field defects.

CHAPTER TEST

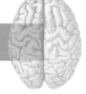

QUESTIONS

Choose the best answer for each question.

1. The postcommissural fornix arises from the:
   a. Hippocampus
   b. Subicular cortex
   c. Dentate gyrus
   d. Entorhinal cortex
   e. Medial septal nucleus

2. After a neurological examination, a 34-year-old man was diagnosed with temporal lobe epilepsy, the focus of which was estimated to be Sommer's sector. This region is associated with the:
   a. CA1 hippocampal field
   b. CA3 hippocampal field
   c. Dentate gyrus
   d. Central nucleus of amygdala
   e. Nuclei of the diagonal band of Broca

3. A 63-year-old man was transferred from a psychiatric clinic to the local hospital for a neurological examination because he showed signs of a Klüver-Bucy syndrome.

INTEGRATIVE SYSTEMS

An MRI revealed the presence of a small tumor in the brain. The locus of this tumor likely included the:

a. Hippocampal formation
b. Septal area
c. Amygdala
d. Prefrontal cortex
e. Anterior cingulate gyrus

4. A 63-year-old woman was experiencing difficulties in a card-sorting test (as a measure of cognitive function), and failed to accurately perceive the vertical when seated in a tilted chair. An MRI revealed the presence of a lesion in the:

a. Hippocampal formation
b. Septal area
c. Amygdala
d. Prefrontal cortex
e. Cingulate gyrus

5. A 78-year-old man was admitted to a neurological clinic because he was having memory difficulties. The diagnosis was that the patient was experiencing the early stages of Alzheimer's disease. His disorder most likely involved loss of or damage to neurons in the:

a. Reticular formation
b. Hypothalamus
c. Central nucleus of amygdala
d. Dentate gyrus
e. Basal nucleus of Meynert

ANSWERS AND EXPLANATIONS

1. Answer: **b**

The postcommissural fornix refers to those hippocampal fibers that arise from the subicular cortex and innervate several regions of the diencephalon. These regions include the anterior thalamic nucleus, mammillary bodies, and the ventromedial region of the hypothalamus (medial corticothalamic tract in rodents). The cornu ammonis does not contribute to the postcommissural fornix, but only to the precommissural fornix and to commissural fibers of the fornix. The dentate gyrus does not project outside of the hippocampal formation. The sep-

tal area and entorhinal cortex do not contribute any fibers to the postcommissural fornix.

2. Answer: **a**

Sommer's sector refers to the CA1 field of the hippocampus. This region of the hippocampus is particularly susceptible to anoxia at birth and to seizure discharges. Accordingly, neuropathology of this region can be noted under conditions where anoxia is likely to occur.

3. Answer: **c**

Lesions of the amygdala or adjoining pyriform cortex produce a disorder referred to as the Klüver-Bucy syndrome. It is characterized by placidity, hypersexuality, visual agnosia, oral tendencies, and loss of fear of objects that previously produced fear. Damage to the septal area, parts of the hippocampal formation, cingulate gyrus, and prefrontal cortex are typically associated with increases in aggression, which is opposite of what occurs in the Klüver-Bucy syndrome.

4. Answer: **d**

Lesions of the prefrontal cortex produce unique intellectual and perceptual deficits, which are not generally associated with the other choices provided (hippocampus, amygdala, septal area, and cingulate gyrus). In a card-sorting task, the patient will not vary her strategy for sorting cards even when asked to do so. In a perceptual task, when the patient is placed in a tilted chair in the dark and asked to identify the true vertical, she is unable to do so, although normal individuals have little difficulty in doing so.

5. Answer: **e**

Alzheimer's disease has been correlated with cell loss in the basal nucleus of Meynert, which is a group of large cells located in the ventral aspect of the basal forebrain adjacent to the horizontal limb of the diagonal band and substantia innominata. These cells are cholinergic and project to wide areas of the cerebral cortex. In Alzheimer's disease, there is a sharp reduction in the cholinergic content of cortical tissue. The regions shown as other choices do not contain cholinergic neurons that are known to project to the cerebral cortex.

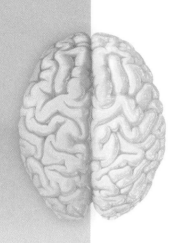

CHAPTER 26

THE THALAMUS AND CEREBRAL CORTEX

465

OBJECTIVES

After reading this chapter, the student should be able to:

1. Describe and diagram the histological arrangement of the cerebral cortex and its columnar organization

2. Identify the major afferent sources of the cerebral cortex

3. Review the organization and functional properties of thalamic nuclei considered in Chapter 13 and analysis of the projections from thalamic nuclei to the cerebral cortex and related regions of the forebrain

4. Identify the afferent fibers that arise from the basal forebrain and monoaminergic afferent fibers that arise from the brainstem

5. Review the motor functions of the cerebral cortex, including the descending motor projections

6. Review the somatosensory, visual, auditory, and taste functions of the cerebral cortex

7. Describe the functions of the prefrontal cortex and other regions of the cortex, including the process of cerebral dominance

8. List and describe several of the key disorders of the cerebral cortex

9. List and characterize disorders of language, learning, and memory

The cerebral cortex in humans reflects the pinnacle of phylogenetic development with respect to cortical size and complexity. It is estimated that the human cerebral cortex contains 15 billion neurons, encompassing an area of approximately 220 cm^2. Much of the cortex is out of view because of the convexities of the sulci. Different parts of the cerebral cortex receive many afferent fibers. The largest source of fibers is from the thalamus, but other regions, such as the brainstem monoaminergic systems and parts of the basal forebrain, contribute fibers as well. Cortical afferent fibers also arise from other regions of the cortex (called association fibers) and from the contralateral cerebral cortex (via the corpus callosum). The complexities of the functions attributable to the cerebral cortex derive, in part, from the nature of the histological organization of the cortex, which differs from one cortical region to another. The histological arrangement of a given region of cortex can be subdivided into basic functional units called **cortical columns**. Collectively, the integrated actions of groups of cortical columns serve to mediate voluntary motor activity, sensory perception, learning, memory, language functions, and affective processes.

The varied processes associated with the cerebral cortex can be better understood by examining the nature of the organization of different regions of cortex, including the functional properties of cortical columns, followed by an analysis of the afferent and efferent connections of this region of the brain. Accordingly, this chapter begins with an ex-amination of the histology of the cerebral cortex followed by a review and discussion of the input-output relationships of the cerebral cortex.

ANATOMICAL AND FUNCTIONAL CHARACTERISTICS OF THE GRAY MATTER OF THE CEREBRAL CORTEX

We begin this chapter by considering the organization of the basic functional units of the cerebral cortex. The functional units are composed of narrow bands of gray matter of cortex arranged vertically through all cell layers called cortical columns. To understand how a cortical column functions, as well as its relationship to the overall functions of the region of cortex of which it is a part, it is first necessary to consider the histological arrangement of the gray matter of the cerebral cortex, which differs somewhat from region to region.

MORPHOLOGICAL FEATURES

Typically, the cerebral cortex contains six layers arranged parallel to the cortical surface (Fig. 26-1). The layers are generally classified according to the cell type that is most prominent for a given layer (Fig. 26-2). The most superficial layer, layer I, is called the **molecular layer**. It contains mainly axons, dendrites whose cell bodies are located in deeper layers, and axon terminals of neurons whose cell bodies are also located in deeper layers. The only cell type found in this layer is a *horizontal*

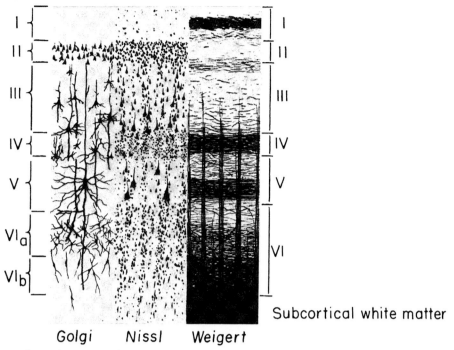

Figure 26–1 Six-layered structure of the cerebral cortex. The sections are arranged perpendicular to the cortical surface so that the top layer is the one closest to the cortical surface. The illustration on the left depicts the cells as they appear in a Golgi stained section (for identification of neuronal and glial cells and their processes); the illustration in the middle shows the cortical appearance when it is stained for cells; and the illustration on the right depicts the cortex when stained for fibers. (From Parent A: Carpenter's Human Neuroanatomy, 9th ed. Baltimore: Williams & Wilkins, 1996, p. 866.)

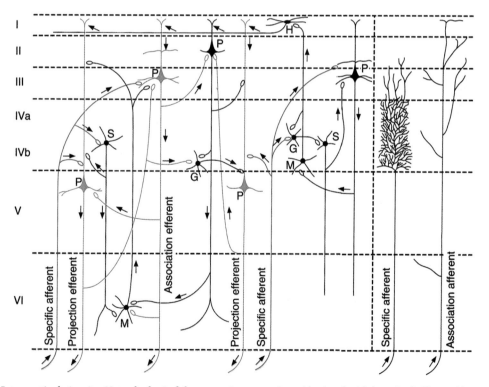

Figure 26–2 Intracortical circuits. Note the loci of the synaptic connections (depicted with loops) of afferent fiber projections, the origins of the efferent projections, and the origins of intracortical connections within a given column. The specific region of cortex is not defined in this illustration. Abbreviations: G, granule cell; H, horizontal cell; M, Martinotti cell; P, pyramidal cell; S, stellate cell. Arrows indicate direction of information flow. (From Parent A: Carpenter's Human Neuroanatomy, 9th ed. Baltimore: Williams & Wilkins, 1996, p. 868.)

cell, the axon of which passes laterally in this layer parallel to the surface of the cortex.

Layers II and IV are similar in that they both contain densely packed **granule cells**. Thus, layer II is called the external granule cell layer, and layer IV is called the internal granule cell layer. The granule cell may be one of several types. It may contain a very short axon that ramifies close to the cell body (called a Golgi type II cell) or a longer axon that extends beyond the dendritic tree (called a Golgi type I cell, which ascends toward the cortical surface where it may make contact with the cell body of a pyramidal cell or contact the dendrites of other cells). The most important feature of the granule cell layers (layer II and especially layer IV) is that they are basically receiving areas for inputs from the thalamus and other regions of cortex. Likewise, layers III and V contain mainly pyramidal cells and are thus referred to as **pyramidal cell layers**. Layer III is called an external pyramidal cell layer, and layer V is called an internal pyramidal cell layer. The pyramidal cell, which is largest in layer V, contains an apical dendrite that extends toward the surface of the cortex and basal dendrites that extend outward from the cell body. The primary efferents of the cortex include axons of pyramidal cells that project throughout the central nervous system. Layer VI (multiform layer) contains several different types of neurons (spindle-shaped cells with long ascending dendrites, Martinotti cells with long ascending axons, variations of Golgi cells, and some pyramidal cells) (Fig 26-2). Because of this anatomical arrangement, afferent signals received at almost any layer of cortex can result in excitation of cells located in other cell layers. It is this synchronized form of activation of cells located within a given vertical plane of the cortex that defines the **cortical column** and thus provides the cortex with its basic functional properties (Fig. 26-2). The concept of a cortical column is discussed again later in this chapter in reference to functions of the visual cortex.

CYTOARCHITECTONIC DIVISION OF THE CEREBRAL CORTEX

The histological appearance of the cerebral cortex varies from region to region. These variations are frequently associated with functional differences as well. The histological variations were first recognized by Brodmann at the beginning of the 20th century. Consequently, he assigned numbers and symbols to each cortical area to define and characterize the different regions of the cortex (Fig. 26-3). This numbering system has remained in the literature for almost a century and is commonly used to define a given functional region. More recently, specific regions of the brain have been defined in terms of other characteristics, such as their afferent and efferent connections, physiological and receptor characteristics, and relationships to behavioral functions.

As a general rule, histological differences in the appearance of cortical tissue are most apparent when comparing sensory and motor regions of the brain. One of the clearest examples is the difference between the histological appearance of the primary motor (area 4) and primary somatosensory (areas 3, 1, and 2) cortices (Fig 26-3). These differences indicate that, with respect to area 4, the granule cell layers (layers II and IV) are quite small, whereas pyramidal cell layers III and V are rather extensive. In contrast, in a portion of the primary somatosensory cortex (area 3), the granule cell lay-

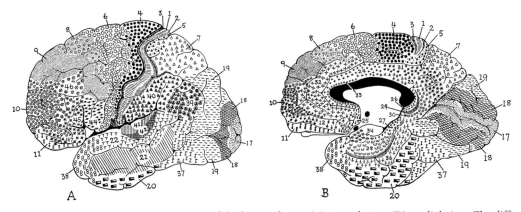

Figure 26–3 Brodmann's cytoarchitectonic mapping of the human brain. (A) Lateral view; (B) medial view. The different regions are labeled with different symbols and numbers. Note the key regions that have been identified using Brodmann's numbering scheme. Several of these regions include: area 4: primary motor cortex; area 6: premotor area; areas 3, 1, and 2: primary somatosensory receiving areas; areas 5 and 7: posterior parietal cortex; area 17: primary visual cortex; and area 41: primary auditory receiving area. See text for further discussion of Brodmann's areas. (From Parent A: Carpenter's Human Neuroanatomy, 9th ed. Baltimore: Williams & Wilkins, 1996, p. 882.)

ers are more extensive, and the pyramidal cell layers are reduced in size.

Other examples of cortical regions that contain an abundance of pyramidal cells relative to populations of granule cells include the medial aspect of the prefrontal cortex and anterior cingulate gyrus. The regions that contain an abundance of granule cells relative to pyramidal cell populations include the primary auditory and visual cortices.

NEUROTRANSMITTERS

Both excitatory and inhibitory neurons are present within the cortex. Excitatory effects may be generated from cortical interneurons that have short projections within a given column or between adjacent columns as well as by thalamocortical and other cortical afferent fibers. Inhibitory interneurons within the cortex are extensive, including those acting within the same column from where they originate or between adjacent columns. Excitatory interneurons are mediated mainly by excitatory amino acids (aspartate and glutamate) that act on glutamate receptors (kainate, quisqualate, and N-methyl-D-aspartate [NMDA]). Other neurotransmitters associated with intrinsic cortical neurons include a variety of neuropeptides. The neuropeptides include somatostatin, substance P, enkephalin, cholecystokinin, and vasoactive intestinal peptide and presumably serve a modulating function on cortical neurons. With regard to extrinsic neurons, monoamine neurons arising from different regions of the brainstem act on many cell groups within the cerebral cortex, releasing dopamine, norepinephrine, and serotonin from their nerve terminals. These monoaminergic neurons also modulate neuronal excitability levels and play an important role in the processes of sleep and wakefulness and in the regulation of emotional states. In addition, acetylcholine originating from neurons in the basal forebrain supplies wide regions of cerebral cortex. This excitatory transmitter has been linked to functions of learning and memory, and loss of such inputs to the cortex has been reported to occur in disorders such as Alzheimer's disease.

CORTICAL LAYERS ASSOCIATED WITH INPUTS AND OUTPUTS

Different layers of the cortex serve different functions with respect to its afferent and efferent connections. Layer I is primarily a receiving area for nonspecific afferent fibers from the intralaminar thalamus and brainstem monoaminergic neurons. Layers II and IV are primarily receiving areas: layer II is a receiving area for cortical (callosal and asso-

ciation) afferents, and layer IV is a receiving area for afferents from the thalamus. Layers III and V primarily contain efferents: layer III contains callosal and cortical association fibers, and layer V contains efferents that project to the neostriatum, brainstem, and spinal cord (Fig. 26-4). Concerning layer VI, some of these neurons project to the thalamus, whereas others contain short projections that ramify within the same cortical columns from which they arise.

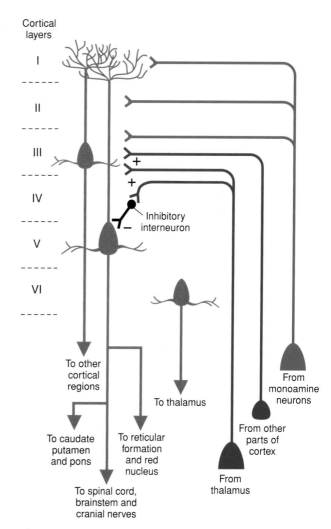

Figure 26–4 Input-output relationships of cortex. Schematic diagram depicts the intrinsic organization and input-output relationships of the cerebral cortex. Excitatory connections are indicated by (+), and inhibitory synapse is indicated by (−). Note that thalamocortical and intracortical projections terminate mainly in layer IV, and monoaminergic projections are distributed mainly to more superficial layers. Cortical afferents terminating in layer IV can either excite or inhibit pyramidal cells in layer V, which contribute significantly to the outputs of the cerebral cortex. The major outputs to the spinal cord, cranial nerve motor nuclei, other brainstem structures, thalamus, and neostriatum arise in layers V-VI, whereas projections to other regions of cortex either on the ipsilateral or contralateral side arise from layer III. (Adapted from Conn PM: Neuroscience in Medicine. Philadelphia: J.B. Lippincott, 1995, p. 316.)

EXCITABILITY CHARACTERISTICS OF NEURONS WITHIN A CORTICAL COLUMN

Two factors that regulate cortical excitability should be noted. The first is that large cortical cells, such as pyramidal cells, integrate the activity of many neurons that impinge on these cells. Pyramidal cells also transmit signals to other layers of the cortex by virtue of their axon collaterals. Some connections are excitatory, whereby other neurons within a given cortical column are then excited. Other connections are inhibitory, especially with neurons in an adjacent column. The inhibitory neurons may then make synapse with additional neurons that are either inhibitory (producing cortical disinhibition) or excitatory. Thus, excitation of the pyramidal cell can lead to wide variations in the patterns of cortical excitability. For this reason, the nature of the functional patterns governing excitation within a cortical column still remains poorly understood.

The second factor is that cortical afferents, such as those arising from the thalamus or from other regions of the cortex, have the capacity to activate large numbers of cortical neurons at any one given moment. These sources typically have fast excitatory synaptic actions. Other inputs that are mediated by acetylcholine, monoamines, or peptides appear to have a slow, modulatory-like action on these cells.

AFFERENT CONNECTIONS OF THE CEREBRAL CORTEX

THE THALAMUS

Defining Characteristics of Thalamic Nuclei

The gross anatomical organization of the thalamus and the respective nuclei are described in detail in Chapter 13. In brief, the major thalamic nuclei can be divided into the following groups: anterior, medial, lateral, midline, and intralaminar nuclei. In addition, the terms specific, association, and nonspecific nuclei have also been used to functionally define and characterize the thalamic nuclei. These terms are defined in the following sections.

Specific Thalamic Nuclei

The characteristics of this group of thalamic nuclei include the following: (1) they receive specific signals from sensory pathways such as the inferior colliculus (auditory), retina (visual), medial lemniscus, and spinothalamic and trigeminothalamic tracts (somatosensory); and (2) they project topographically to specific regions of the cerebral cortex (e.g., temporal neocortex, visual cortex, and primary somatosensory cortex). Thus, the function of these nuclei is to relay specific sensory information originating in the periphery to a specific region of the neocortex.

Association Nuclei

These nuclei receive few, if any, afferents from ascending sensory pathways. They do, however, receive inputs from regions such as the cerebral cortex, limbic nuclei, basal ganglia, and nonspecific thalamic nuclei. Association nuclei also project to specific regions of the cerebral cortex. Their functions appear to be complex and integrative in nature and, in many cases, are not entirely understood. Figure 26-5 depicts the anatomical arrangement of the thalamic nuclei and their output relationships with the cerebral cortex.

Nonspecific Thalamic Nuclei

The unique feature of nonspecific thalamic nuclei is that they appear to project to wide regions of cerebral cortex rather than to localized areas like the specific and association nuclei. Specific and association nuclei generally project topographically to specific regions of the cerebral cortex. The projections from nonspecific nuclei to the cortex are not topographically organized. Nonspecific thalamic nuclei also possess another feature: they project to specific thalamic nuclei. In this manner, they are capable of modulating the activity of wide numbers of cortical neurons either from direct projections to various regions of cortex or, indirectly, through their actions on different specific and association nuclei of the thalamus, which then project to their respective target regions of cortex. Inasmuch as monoaminergic (and other) axons of the reticular formation project to nonspecific thalamic nuclei, these direct and indirect connections between nonspecific thalamic nuclei and cortex provide important substrates by which the reticular formation can significantly alter cortical excitability levels (see Chapter 23).

Two other general features concerning thalamocortical relationships are to be noted. The first is that, since the nonspecific thalamus projects to wide areas of cortex, most regions of cortex thus receive converging inputs from both specific (or association) nuclei and nonspecific thalamic nuclei. Specific and association thalamic nuclei project most commonly to layers III and IV of the neocortex, whereas the projections of nonspecific thalamic nuclei may reach more superficial layers, including layer I (Fig. 26-4). Because such an arrangement makes it possible for regions such as the reticular formation to alter cortical excitability

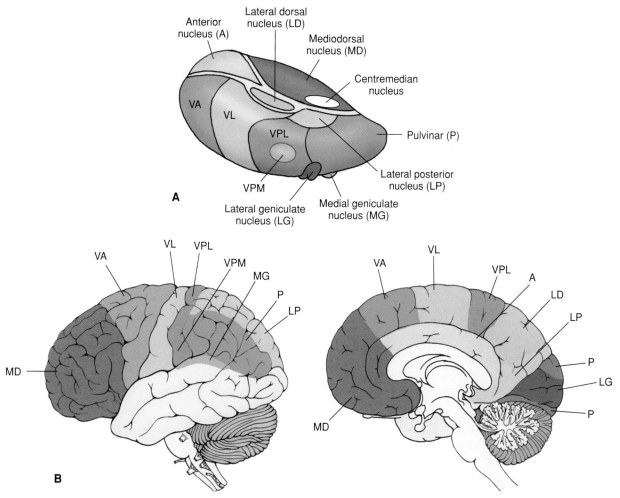

Figure 26–5 Thalamocortical relationships. (A) The relative positions of thalamic nuclei. (B) Lateral (left) and medial (right) views of the cerebral cortex that demonstrate the projection targets of thalamic nuclei. Color coding is to facilitate visualization of the projection targets of thalamic nuclei on the cerebral cortex. Abbreviations: VPM, ventral posteromedial nucleus; VPL, ventral posterolateral nucleus; VA, ventral anterior nucleus; VL, ventrolateral nucleus.

levels, they further serve to increase (or decrease) the likelihood that cortical neurons will respond more effectively to other inputs from specific or association thalamic nuclei.

The second feature is that specific, association, and nonspecific thalamic nuclei share reciprocal connections with the cerebral cortex. The apparent significance of such reciprocal connections is that they provide the basis for a feedback mechanism from the cortex to the thalamus, which ultimately serves to control the amount of information that reaches a specific region of cortex at any given moment.

Functional Organization of the Thalamus
Specific Thalamic Nuclei

Somatosensory Relays. The primary receiving areas for inputs from the body associated with touch, pressure, and movement at the joints (i.e., conscious proprioception) is the ventral posterolateral nucleus

(VPL). The VPL receives afferents fibers from the medial lemniscus and spinothalamic tracts. As noted in Chapter 9, these fiber tracts are **somatotopically** organized; and, likewise, their relay projections from the VPL to the postcentral gyrus are also somatotopically arranged. Fibers arising from the medial aspect of the VPL project to the arm region (lateral aspect) of the postcentral gyrus, while the lateral aspect of the VPL projects to the leg region of the postcentral gyrus (midline region) (Figs. 9-7 and 26-6).

The ventral posteromedial nucleus (VPM) receives similar somesthetic kinds of inputs from the trigeminothalamic tract. The VPM, in turn, projects its axons to the head region (far lateral aspect) of the postcentral gyrus. Collectively, the VPL and VPM are referred to as the ventral basal complex and contain all the ascending somatosensory inputs from the whole body (including the head region).

Pain Relays. The lateral spinothalamic and ventral trigeminothalamic tracts mediate ascending

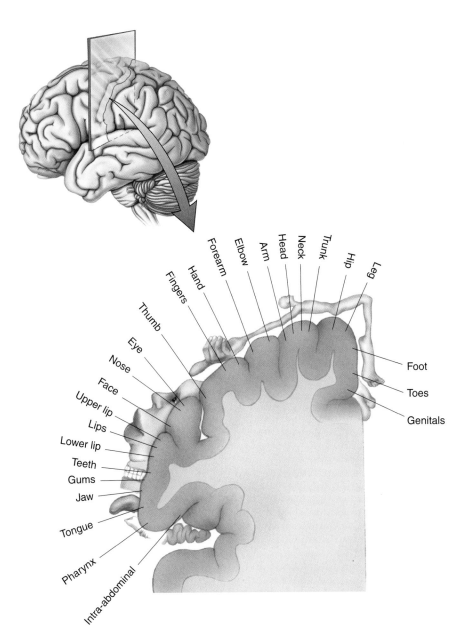

Figure 26–6 Cortical homunculus. Somatotopic organization of the body surface as represented on the postcentral gyrus of the cerebral cortex. Neurons situated along the medial-to-lateral surface of the postcentral gyrus are responsive to stimulation of a specific aspect of the body region as indicated in this illustration. (From Bear MF, et al.: Neuroscience: Exploring the Brain, 2nd ed. Philadelphia: Lippincott Williams & Wilkins, 2001, p. 415.)

pain signals to the thalamus from the body (cell bodies for tract fibers lie in the contralateral proper sensory nucleus [lamina IV] of the spinal cord) and head (contralateral spinal trigeminal nucleus of the lower brainstem), respectively. The primary targets of these signals are the posterior thalamic complex (which is composed of several different nuclear groups) and the intralaminar nuclei (such as the centromedian and parafascicular nuclei), although some fibers also terminate in the VPL and VPM of the thalamus. It could be that the more affective components of pain are directed to the posterior thalamic complex and intralaminar nuclei. Our understanding of the functional organization of the posterior thalamic complex is made more complex by the fact that this nucleus also integrates other so-matosensory and auditory signals as well. The precise locations of pain inputs within the cerebral cortex have not been clearly localized. However, studies conducted in cat and monkey suggest that cortical neurons that respond most clearly to nociceptive stimuli lie in a region called the second somatic area and the area immediately caudal to it. In humans, these regions would approximately correspond to the supramarginal gyrus and insular region.

Thermal Relays. The lateral spinothalamic tract mediates thermal signals from the spinal cord to VPL. Thermal signals are then transmitted to the postcentral gyrus, but the sites where these fibers are distributed do not appear to be localized to any one area of the postcentral gyrus.

Auditory Relays. The medial geniculate nucleus is the thalamic relay nucleus that receives inputs from the inferior colliculus via the brachium of the inferior colliculus. The pathway is tonotopically organized (i.e., different groups of neurons respond to different sound frequencies) at both brainstem levels as well as in the medial geniculate nucleus. The medial geniculate nucleus projects mainly to the transverse temporal gyri of Heschl (called Brodmann's area 41), which is the primary auditory receiving area. Additional auditory fibers project to the surrounding auditory association area (called Brodmann's area 42) (Fig 26-3).

Visual Relays. The primary visual relay nucleus in the thalamus is the lateral geniculate nucleus. As pointed out in Chapter 16, the lateral geniculate nucleus contains six layers and receives retinal inputs from both eyes. The retinal inputs to the lateral geniculate nucleus on the left side of the brain represent the right hemifield, and the left hemifield is represented on the right lateral geniculate nucleus. Neurons located in both magnocellular (layers 1 and 2) and parvocellular (layers 3 through 6) regions of the lateral geniculate nucleus project to the primary visual cortex (area 17).

Taste Relays. As indicated earlier, parts of the VPM receive somatosensory inputs from the trigeminal system. Other groups of neurons within this nucleus, however, receive inputs from the solitary nucleus (which includes a relay in the pontine taste [parabrachial] nucleus). These inputs mediate taste signals from the periphery. The region of VPM receiving taste inputs projects to the far lateral aspect of the postcentral gyrus bordering on the Sylvian fissure.

Vestibular Relays. The vestibular nuclei project their axons either to the cerebellum or into the medial longitudinal fasciculus. While most fibers contained within the medial longitudinal fasciculus terminate on the motor nuclei of cranial nerves (CN) III, IV, and VI, some axons are believed to bypass these nuclei and reach parts of the VPL nucleus. In turn, these vestibular inputs are then relayed to the postcentral gyrus. Although the validity of these connections has been suggested, it is questionable whether the conscious awareness of vestibular sensations is specifically associated with this pathway. Instead, it may be that such inputs may relate more closely to the regulation of motor functions and that the conscious awareness of vestibular signals may reside elsewhere in the cortex.

Olfactory Relays. Of all the sensory relay systems, the olfactory pathway is the only one that can reach the cerebral cortex without having to synapse in the thalamus. As described in Chapter 18, this pathway involves initial olfactory bulb projections (i.e., mitral cell axons) to the prepyriform area, periamygdalar cortex, and the corticomedial amygdala and secondary projections from these regions to the prefrontal cortex and septal area. However, a parallel pathway by which olfactory signals can reach the cerebral cortex via the thalamus also exists. This pathway involves amygdaloid and prepyriform cortex projections to the mediodorsal thalamic nucleus, which, in turn, project to wide areas of the anterior aspect of the frontal lobe, including the prefrontal cortex.

Association Nuclei

Nuclei Mediating Motor Functions. Different portions of the ventral anterior (VA) and ventrolateral (VL) receive inputs from structures associated with motor functions. These projections arise from the cerebellum and basal ganglia. Specifically, fibers arising from the **dentate nucleus** of the contralateral cerebellum project to the posterior part of the VL. The anterior part of the VL receives inputs from the medial pallidal segment and substantia nigra. These two components of the basal ganglia also project to the VA as well. The projections to motor regions of the cortex from these regions are as follows: the VL projects to the primary motor cortex (area 4) and to the premotor cortex (parts of area 6), and the VA projects more diffusely to the supplementary and premotor areas (area 6). Thus, the VA and VL provide the substrate by which different components of the motor systems can provide feedback signals back to the motor regions of the cerebral cortex that are essential for normal motor functions to take place. When such feedback is lost, significant motor dysfunctions ensue (see Chapters 19 and 20 for details). Also note that parts of the VA also function as a nonspecific nucleus and produce widespread excitability changes of cortical neurons.

Nuclei Mediating Functions Associated with the Limbic System. The connections of the **anterior nucleus** contribute to part of the Papez circuit (see Fig. 25-4). The anterior nucleus receives inputs from the subicular cortex of the hippocampal formation and from the mammillary bodies via the mammillothalamic tract. The anterior nucleus, in turn, projects its axons to the cingulate cortex. The cingulate cortex projects to the hippocampal formation, thus completing the circuit referred to as the Papez circuit. As pointed out in Chapter 25, this circuit was originally thought to be associated with the regulation of emotional behavior. However, more recent studies have suggested that the Papez circuit may also be associated with memory functions.

Aside from inputs from the posterior parietal cortex, known inputs to the **lateral dorsal nucleus** have not been clearly defined but are thought to arise from several limbic nuclei (i.e., septal area and hippocampal formation). The outputs of the lateral dorsal nucleus have been shown to project to several regions of the limbic system, including the cingulate cortex, and to the medial wall of the posterior parietal cortex. Its functions remain obscure.

The **mediodorsal thalamic nucleus** receives converging inputs from a number of limbic structures (Fig. 26-7). These include the amygdala, prepyriform area, septal area, anterior cingulate gyrus, and prefrontal cortex. The mediodorsal thalamic nucleus has two important projections. The first is a massive distribution of fibers to the prefrontal cortex and to adjoining regions of the frontal lobe. The second is a projection (described in Chapter 25) to the midline thalamus that forms the first limb of a polysynaptic pathway to the anterior lateral hypothalamus. The likely function of these converging inputs to the mediodorsal nucleus is that it provides an additional substrate by which limbic structures can modulate hypothalamic processes. Evidence that this nucleus also mediates affective components of pain comes from clinical reports that revealed that surgical lesions of the mediodorsal nucleus have sometimes been carried out to alleviate the severity of certain forms of pain. Patients subjected to these surgical procedures report that they still physically experience pain but show little of the distress that is normally associated with severe pain.

Nuclei Associated with Complex Integrative Functions. The **lateral posterior nucleus** receives inputs mainly from the parietal lobe. Subcortical projections to this nucleus have not been clearly identified. The major cortical projection target of the lateral posterior nucleus is the superior parietal lobule (areas 5 and 7). Recall that these regions are associated with complex sensorimotor integration. They receive polysensory inputs from other sensory regions of cortex, and their fibers project to the premotor and supplementary motor areas (area 6). These regions are believed to help program the sequences of motor responses involved in complex motor processes. Accordingly, by providing significant inputs to the posterior parietal cortex, it is likely that the lateral posterior nucleus also contributes to the functions of areas 5 and 7.

The **pulvinar** primarily receives inputs from visual (from the superior colliculus and visual cortex) and auditory (from the temporal neocortex) regions of the brain. Its projections are directed to a wide expanse of the inferior parietal lobule and to adjoining regions of the temporal lobe. It appears that the pulvinar integrates auditory and visual inputs and perhaps some somesthetic impulses as well. It is thought to mediate complex sensory discrimination learning and cognitive functions.

Intralaminar and Midline Thalamic Nuclei

Centromedian Nucleus. Some of the anatomical and functional properties of the intralaminar and midline thalamic nuclei were described earlier in this chapter and were also discussed in Chapters 13 and 23. These nuclei comprise the nonspecific thalamus. The largest of the nonspecific intralaminar thalamic nuclei is the **centromedian nucleus**. It receives inputs from the cerebral cortex and reticular formation, nociceptive stimuli from the spinal cord, and some fibers from the medial pallidal segment. The centromedian is the only thalamic nucleus that projects to the basal ganglia (i.e., the thalamostriate projection to the putamen). Moreover, the centromedian nucleus, like other nonspecific thalamic nuclei, projects to specific thalamic nuclei and can thus influence the transmission of sensory information to the cortex.

The Thalamic Reticular Nucleus. The **reticular nucleus** differs from other thalamic nuclei and does not readily fit the classification scheme of thalamic nuclei mainly because it does not project to the cortex. It is located on the lateral margin

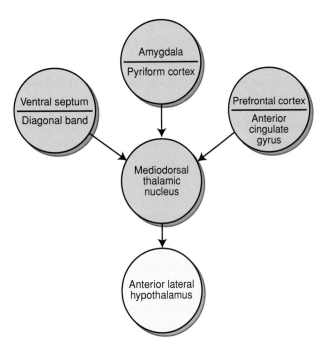

Figure 26–7 The mediodorsal thalamic nucleus. Schematic diagram illustrating the converging limbic inputs on the mediodorsal thalamic nucleus and its output onto the hypothalamus.

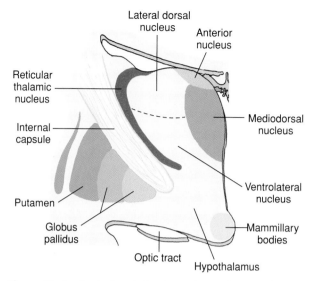

Figure 26–8. Reticular thalamic nucleus. The reticular nucleus of the thalamus lies just medial to the internal capsule. It differs from other thalamic nuclei in that it does not project to the cerebral cortex. Instead, it contains inhibitory neurons, which modulate thalamic neurons that project to the cortex.

and dorsal aspect (within the external medullary lamina) of the thalamus (Fig. 26-8). As a result of its location, most, if not all, corticothalamic fibers pass through this nucleus and provide collateral connections with it. Thalamocortical relay neurons also provide collaterals that synapse with neurons of the reticular nucleus. Moreover, both thalamocortical and corticothalamic fibers that provide inputs to the reticular nucleus are reciprocally connected. Such an arrangement permits the reticular nucleus to evaluate the amount of information that is descending from the cortex as well as the amount that is ascending to the cortex. Adjustments to marked changes in descending or ascending inputs can be made by the reticular nucleus because its output neurons, which are γ-aminobutyric acid (GABA)-ergic, inhibit the specific thalamic nuclei with which they make synaptic contact. The interrelationships among these nuclei may be associated with states of sleep and wakefulness. Here, activation of the reticular nucleus may serve to functionally disconnect the cerebral cortex from the thalamus for periods of time when reticular neurons display bursting or tonic discharges during sleep.

OTHER (NONTHALAMIC) REGIONS THAT PROJECT TO THE CEREBRAL CORTEX

Brainstem Reticular Formation

Monoaminergic fibers arising mainly from the pons and midbrain project to wide areas of the cerebral cortex (see Chapters 8 and 23 for details) and serve as significant modulators of cortical neurons. Serotonergic fibers from the raphe neurons (mainly of the pons) project to most, if not all, regions of the cerebral cortex and reach all cell layers. Dopaminergic fibers (see Fig. 8-8) and noradrenergic fibers also project to wide areas of the cerebral cortex but in less abundant quantities than serotonin fibers (Figs. 26-9 and 26-10). The dopaminergic fibers arise from the ventral tegmental area of the midbrain. The densest quantities of fibers appear to supply motor regions and the prefrontal cortex.

Noradrenergic fibers arising from the nucleus locus ceruleus of the pons also project to wide areas of the cerebral cortex similar to the distributions for dopamine and serotonin.

Forebrain

The cerebral cortex also receives a significant contribution of cholinergic fibers from the basal nucleus of Meynert (see Chapter 25). These fibers supply cholinergic fibers to most regions of the cerebral cortex (see Fig. 8-3). Damage to these cholinergic neurons has been associated with **Alzheimer's disease** (see Chapter 25 for discussion). The etiology of this disease remains unknown.

LOCALIZATION OF FUNCTION WITHIN THE CEREBRAL CORTEX

Our understanding of cortical localization is derived from two main sources: basic laboratory investigations and clinical studies. For each of the functional regions that will be considered in the following sections, the discussion begins with a brief analysis of the basic functional properties of that region and then uses information derived from clinical studies to evaluate the region's overall functions.

THE PARIETAL LOBE

The principal unit of organization is the cortical column (Fig. 26-11). Within each column, neurons located in each of the layers within a given column respond best to a single class of receptors, and all of the neurons respond to stimulation applied to the same local region of the body surface (Fig. 26-11). Adjoining columns representing the same body surface have different physiological properties, such as being rapidly adapting or slowly adapting to sensory stimulation.

Other characteristics concerning somatosensory neurons should also be noted. For example,

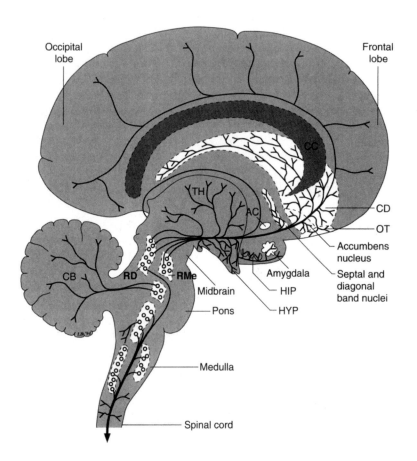

Figure 26–9 Serotonergic projections. Diagram illustrates the projection pathways of the serotonergic fiber systems from the raphe complex of the pons and midbrain to the cerebral cortex. Other serotonergic projections to the cerebellum, diencephalon, and spinal cord are presented for purposes of completion. Abbreviations: AC, anterior commissure; CB, cerebellum; CC, corpus callosum; CD, caudate nucleus; HIP, hippocampal formation; HYP, hypothalamus; OT, olfactory tubercle; RD, dorsal raphe nucleus; RMe, median raphe nucleus. (From Parent A: Carpenter's Human Neuroanatomy, 9th ed. Baltimore: Williams & Wilkins, 1996, p. 518.)

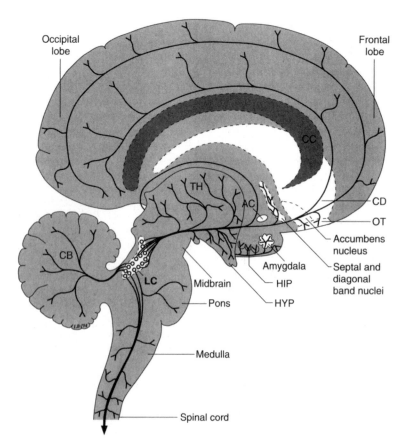

Figure 26–10 Noradrenergic projections. Diagram illustrates the projection pathways from the locus ceruleus (LC) to the hypothalamus (HYP), thalamus (TH), limbic regions including the amygdala and hippocampus (HIP), and the wide regions of the cerebral cortex. Other projections are presented for purposes of completion, including the spinal cord, medulla, and cerebellum (CB). Abbreviations: AC, anterior commissure; CD, caudate nucleus; OT, olfactory tubercle. (From Parent A: Carpenter's Human Neuroanatomy, 9th ed. Baltimore: Williams & Wilkins, 1996, p. 514.)

direction of stimulation. Such response properties suggest that these neurons have larger receptor fields and are capable of integrating the activities of other more basic neurons located in a slightly different region of somatosensory cortex. In fact, it is suggested that the neurons that respond to the more simple aspects of stimulation lie in the region of area 3 and the neurons that respond to the more complex properties of stimulation lie in area 2. It is the increased complexity of the response properties of these neurons that likely provides the neuronal basis for spatial perception that is essential for recognition of three-dimensional objects (i.e., stereognosis). It is important to note that such perceptual discriminations are essential for complex skilled movements to be made.

Effects of Lesions

Complex sensory discriminations require the presence of an intact somatosensory cortex of the parietal lobe, which is organized along lines of complexities of hierarchies of neurons that integrate different kinds of sensory stimuli. Thus, it is not difficult to appreciate how damage to different cell groups in the somatosensory cortex can produce different types of disorders. Lesions of the primary somatosensory cortex produce paresthesias consisting of abnormal tingling sensations and numbness on the side of the body opposite to the lesion. In addition, there is loss of ability to characterize the specific types of stimuli impinging on the individual as well as an inability to localize or evaluate the intensity of the stimulus.

Other parts of the parietal and frontal lobes, which receive inputs from sensory regions of the cortex, require the engagement of neuronal networks processing the appropriate memories to function properly. The arousal of such memories represents the basis of understanding for carrying out specific tasks and is referred to as "gnosis." When this process is disrupted, several different kinds of disorders occur, including agnosia, apraxia, and aphasia.

Agnosia

A separate class of disorders usually involving a part of the parietal lobe called the posterior parietal cortex (which receives inputs from sensory regions of the cortex) is referred to as **agnosia**. Agnosia is defined as a difficulty or inability to recognize objects. Different types of agnosias have been identified and characterized.

In one type, called **astereognosia**, the patient cannot recognize an object felt with the hand of the side contralateral to the parietal lobe lesion. Another parietal lobe lesion of much interest is

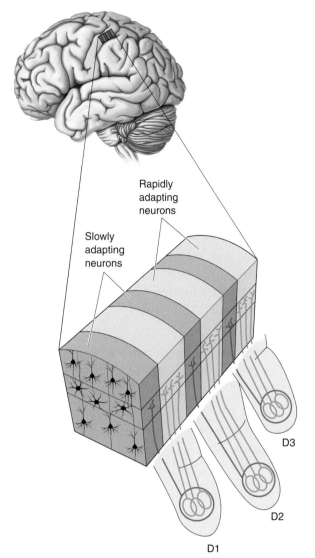

Figure 26–11. Columnar organization of somatosensory cortex. Diagram illustrates that different fingers (D1-D3) are represented on adjoining regions of somatosensory cortex. Within the area represented by each finger, there are alternating columns of neurons that are rapidly adapting (green) and slowly adapting (red). The inputs for each type of receptor for each digit are organized into separate columns. (From Bear MF, et al.: Neuroscience: Exploring the Brain, 2nd ed. Philadelphia: Lippincott Williams & Wilkins, 2001, p. 414.)

as indicated earlier, different regions of the somatosensory cortex may respond to different modalities of stimulation, but they also have a preference for responding to a single type of stimulus. Like other sensory modalities, certain classes of somatosensory neurons appear to respond to complex aspects of a given form of stimulation. For example, although one class of neurons may respond to any form of tactile stimulation applied to a certain region of the body surface, other more complex neurons may respond to the orientation and anosognosia. In this disorder, the patient either denies having an illness or lacks awareness of it. This occurs with a left hemiparesis in which the patient will deny the presence of limbs that are paralyzed or deny their presence on his body. In a related syndrome, called **sensory neglect** (described in Chapter 19), on the side contralateral to the lesion of the posterior parietal cortex, the patient fails to respond to half of his visual field and may also ignore tactile and auditory stimuli. Moreover, the patient may fail to shave or dress that side of the body. An additional syndrome that results from damage to the parietal lobes is called the **Gerstmann syndrome**. The symptoms include: (1) a **finger agnosia** (the patient is unable to recognize the different fingers on his or someone else's hands); (2) **agraphia** (the patient is unable to write); (3) inability to distinguish left from right; (4) **alexia** (the patient is deficient in being able to read); and (5) acalculia (inability to perform calculations).

Apraxia

We initially described this disorder in Chapter 19. Apraxia is basically the inability to carry out motor functions properly, and depending on the form of apraxia considered, it could involve the parietal or frontal lobes. In one type of apraxia, called **ideational apraxia**, the patient experiences difficulty in conceptualizing how to sequence and perform the required task, even though the separate movements comprising the sequence can be performed adequately. This disorder typically involves the posterior parietal lobe with some possible involvement of the adjoining regions of the temporal and occipital lobes. Recall that the posterior parietal cortex receives and integrates many kinds of sensory signals; it further contributes to the programming mechanism of the premotor and supplementary motor areas for the execution of complex motor tasks by virtue of its projections to these motor regions of cortex. Therefore, it is understandable why damage to the posterior parietal cortex is associated with ideational apraxia.

A variation of this disorder is called *ideomotor apraxia*. In this disorder, the patient apparently knows what she wants to do but is unable to execute the acts. This disorder may involve motor areas of the cortex as well as the association (probably from sensory regions) fibers that project to the motor areas.

REGIONS ASSOCIATED WITH VISUAL FUNCTIONS

We have noted in Chapter 16 that, like the other sensory systems, the visual cortex consists of a primary visual receiving area and secondary and tertiary visual processing areas. In fact, some processing of visual information actually involves adjoining regions of the temporal lobe as well (see discussion on pages 479–480 and 482–485). As we pointed out for the somatosensory systems, the cortical column plays a very important role in the processing of sensory information and in providing the basis for the perception of somatosensory signals. Likewise, for the visual system, the cortical column is also critical for the processing of visual signals and for the establishment of form perception.

Projection Patterns from the Lateral Geniculate Nucleus

Both the retina and lateral geniculate nucleus contain neurons that have concentric receptor fields with surround inhibition. Some of the cells are "on-center" and "off-surround," whereas others are "off-center" and "on-surround." Each of these cell groups gives rise to distinct pathways that reach the primary visual cortex (referred to as v1; the secondary visual area is called v2). Several of the pathways are associated with **magnocellular** neurons, and other pathways are associated with **parvocellular** neurons of the lateral geniculate nucleus. The pathways arising from magnocellular neurons are associated with identifying the location of the visual image, whereas the parvocellular pathway is associated with form and color.

When a special stain for identifying mitochondrial enzymes (called cytochrome oxidase) is applied to this region of cortex, the visual cortex reveals two types of staining patterns. One pattern includes intense staining of small, ovoid areas called **blob** areas. The surrounding areas stain less intensely and are called **interblob** areas (Fig. 26-12). The important point to note is that color processing takes place in the blob areas, while the interblob areas contain **orientation columns** (i.e., vertically oriented columns that include neurons that respond to bars of lines having a specific spatial orientation). Thus, one pathway arising from the parvocellular portions of the lateral geniculate nucleus projects to blob regions of v1 and terminates in specific parts of layer IV (Fig. 26-13).[1] This pathway is associated

---

[1] These groups of fibers project to different parts (sublayers) of layer IV of the primary visual cortex (v1). These layers are referred to as 4A, 4B, 4Cα, and 4Cβ (Fig. 26-13). Most magnocellular cells from the lateral geniculate nucleus (which detect movement) terminate in the upper part of layer 4C (sublayer 4Cα). The parvocellular interblob pathway (concerned with shapes and spatial orientation) terminates in the lower half of layer IV (sublayer 4Cβ). Another group of parvocellular neurons projects to blob areas in other parts of layers IV and II and is concerned with color analysis.

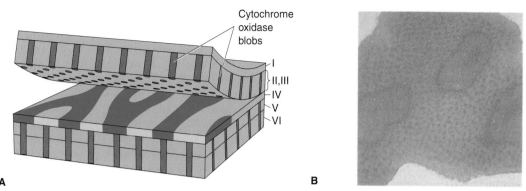

Figure 26–12 Blobs shown with cytochrome oxidase staining. (A) Diagram illustrates the distribution of the enzyme cytochrome oxidase in blob areas of the visual (also called "striate") cortex of a monkey. (B) Photomicrograph taken from the blob area in layer III (as shown in A) revealing intense positive staining for cytochrome oxidase. (From Bear MF, et al.: Neuroscience: Exploring the Brain, 2nd ed. Philadelphia: Lippincott Williams & Wilkins, 2001, p. 330.)

with the processing of color vision. But completion of the process for color vision and form requires the activation of additional pathways and regions of the visual cortex. These include a pathway with connections from v1 to v2 (area 18), then to v4 (area 19), and ultimately to the inferotemporal cortex (Fig. 26-14). This pathway is specifically concerned with color perception and is sometimes called the **parvocellular blob stream pathway**. A second pathway originating from the parvocellular region of the lateral geniculate also projects to v1, which in turn,

projects to v2, then to v4, and finally to the inferotemporal cortex. This pathway, however, is concerned with the processing of form perception (i.e., the outline and orientation of images critical to form perception) and is sometimes referred to as the **parvocellular interblob pathway**. A third pathway originates from the magnocellular region of the lateral geniculate nucleus and projects through the interblob region, terminating, in part, within layer IV of v1. From this region, fibers project to v2, v3, and the middle temporal gyrus (MT or v5; Fig. 26-

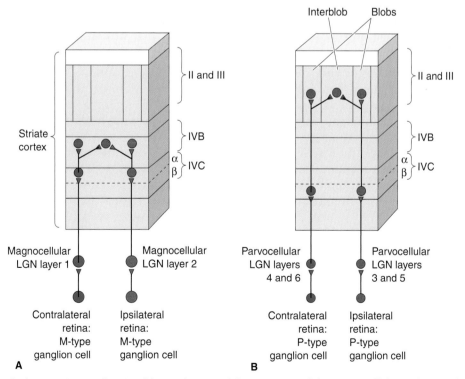

Figure 26–13 Retinal projections to the visual (striate) cortex. (A) Projections of the magnocellular pathway, which is associated with identification of the visual image, to upper parts of layer IV. (B) Parvocellular pathway, which is associated with form and color, to lower parts of layer IV. Abbreviations: LGN, lateral geniculate nucleus; IVB, layer IVB of visual cortex; IVC, layer IVC of visual cortex. (From Bear MF, et al.: Neuroscience: Exploring the Brain, 2nd ed. Philadelphia: Lippincott Williams & Wilkins, 2001, p. 331.)

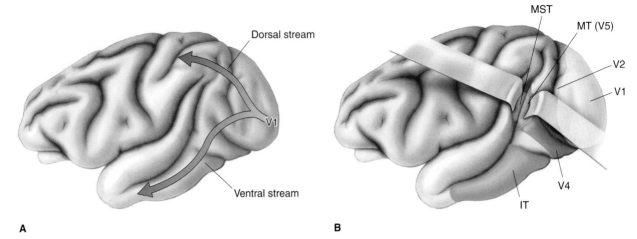

A   **B**

Figure 26–14. Processing of visual information outside the visual cortex. (A) Fibers mediating visual information pass both dorsally and ventrally from the primary visual cortex to both the parietal and temporal lobes. (B) The dorsal pathway also supplies neurons of the temporal and neighboring parietal cortices (labeled as MT [middle temporal gyrus] and MST [medial superior temporal gyrus]) that respond to specific directional properties of movement of objects. The ventral pathway supplies neurons of the inferotemporal (IT) aspect of the temporal lobe, which respond to faces. (From Bear MF, et al.: Neuroscience: Exploring the Brain, 2nd ed. Philadelphia: Lippincott Williams & Wilkins, 2001, p. 338.)

14). This pathway is associated with neurons that detect directional movement of objects. In addition, this pathway also projects to an adjoining region of the parietal lobe, called the medial superior temporal gyrus (MST). Neurons in this region respond to a wider variety of motion, which is linear, circular, or spatial in direction (Fig. 26-14). Overall, this pathway is referred to as the **magnocellular stream pathway**. It is not known to what extent each of these systems may interact with each other in producing visual perception of objects. It has been suggested that the processing of color information may be independent of the systems mediating depth, form, and general figure-ground relationships. On the other hand, one parvocellular pathway (the parvocellular interblob pathway) may use such stimuli as orientation cues to produce fine visual discriminations, whereas the magnocellular stream pathway may use the same information for generating an impression of the location of the object in space.

Analysis of Form Perception

Several of the basic questions that have confronted investigators are: (1) how do neurons in the visual cortex respond to visual stimuli, and (2) how do such changes relate to our capacity to recognize objects? Answers to these basic questions were provided following the discovery of different classes of neurons in the visual cortex that respond, not to a point of light (as do geniculate and retinal ganglion cells), but to bars (linear properties) of light and their orientations.

One class of cell is called a **simple cell**. It is located near the region of sublayer 4Cβ. Within this sublayer, stellate cells, which have circular receptive fields, receive inputs from the lateral geniculate nucleus. The simple cells receive converging inputs from groups of stellate cells. Thus, the receptive fields of the simple cells are considerably larger than stellate cells. Because the inputs to the simple cell from the stellate cells are arranged at slightly different retinal positions, the integrated response of the simple cell is to a group of points of light (i.e., a beam of light). The key feature here is that the simple cells are rectangular in form and have specific excitatory foci and inhibitory surrounds. For example, in the illustration shown in Figure 26-15, a simple cell responds most effectively to a bar of light that is presented in a vertical position. This occurs because the neuron from which the recording was taken has a receptive field whose excitatory zone is oriented vertically, with parallel inhibitory zones located on either side of the excitatory zone. Thus, when the bar of light is reoriented from a vertical to a horizontal position, the neuron ceases to discharge. Note that the cell could also respond to a variety of changes in the vertical position of the bar of light (Fig. 26-15). In this manner, different groups of cells can respond to various orientations of light. Ultimately, any possible orientation of light will excite some neurons in the visual cortex.

Another class of cells has been identified that responds to somewhat different characteristics of light beams. **Complex cells** differ from simple cells in that complex cells have larger receptive fields. In addition, the "on" and "off" zones are not clearly defined. The complex cell responds to a specific

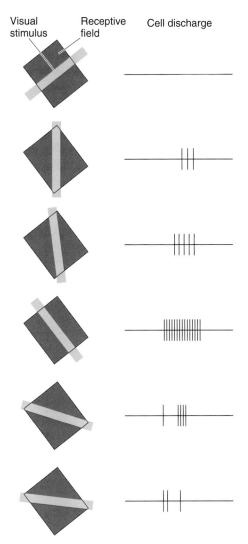

Visual stimulus   Receptive field   Cell discharge

Figure 26–15 Orientation-sensitive simple cell. Illustration demonstrates that a simple cell in the primary visual cortex responds maximally to a bar of light oriented approximately 45° to the vertical. Bars of light oriented differently evoke a much weaker neuronal response, especially if the orientation is opposite of that which evokes a maximal response. When spots of light are presented, the response of the cortical neuron is much weaker and diffuses light. The basic concept involves the notion of a convergence of similar center-surround organizations that are simultaneously excited when light falls along a straight line in the retina and thus strikes the receptive fields of these cells. These cells then converge upon a single cell in the visual cortex, thus establishing an excitatory region that is elongated. (From Bear MF, et al.: Neuroscience: Exploring the Brain, 2nd ed. Philadelphia: Lippincott Williams & Wilkins, 2001, p. 332.)

orientation of the beam of light, but the precise position of the image within the receptive field is not critical (Fig. 26-16). In addition, movement of the image across the receptive field is also an effective stimulus for exciting this (complex) cell. Complex cells, which receive inputs from simple cells, are located in other layers of the primary visual cortex than are simple cells (mainly in layers II, III, V, and VI).

The perception of edges, which provides the basis for form perception, is achieved by the combined actions of the simple and complex cells. Recall that the simple cell will respond to a beam of light within a specific receptive field, while the complex cell will respond to the same orientation of the beam but will extend to different receptive fields. If one's eye is focused on an edge of a line or figure, then certain simple and complex cells will respond to that edge. If the eye then shifts to a different aspect of the figure, another group of simple cells associated with the new receptive field will discharge, but the complex cells that responded to the first aspect of the figure may continue to discharge even though the focus is shifted slightly to another aspect of the figure. In this manner, the complex cell is capable of recognizing a certain aspect of the image at any point within its receptive field. Therefore, the combined actions of the various simple cells coupled with those of the complex cells likely provide the neuronal basis for perceiving edges, borders, boundaries, and contrasts.

Other evidence suggests that there is even a third type of cell, which is a cell that responds like a complex cell in that the cell increases its firing frequency as the bar (held in a certain orientation) is extended. However, these cells differ from other complex cells because, as the beam of light is extended beyond a certain length, the neuron ceases to discharge. This type of variant of a complex cell is referred to as **end-stopped**. End-stopped cells are believed to receive inputs from groups of complex cells and possibly signal the length of a line of an object as well as its borders and curvatures. Thus, when viewed in its totality, a general principle appears to emerge from our analysis of the visual system. This principle is that, as the visual signals pass to higher levels within the visual pathway, the level of complexity governing the discharge patterns of the neurons increases. The levels of complexity are heavily dependent on the converging inputs from different groups of neurons located at lower levels within the visual pathway.

Features of Cortical Columns Within the Occipital Cortex

Like the somatosensory systems, cortical columns within the visual cortex are also arranged in terms of the similarities of the receptive properties of the neurons located in each of the columns. As shown in Figure 26-13, area 17 of the visual cortex is organized into separate vertical columns that receive magnocellular and parvocellular pathways. This means that a given interblob pathway will terminate in a column that will activate cells that will

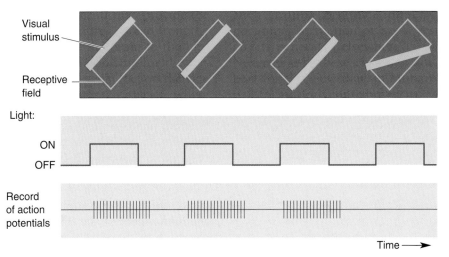

Figure 26–16 Complex cells. These neurons respond best to a bar oriented in a specific direction, but they also respond to different positions of the bar within the visual field. (From Bear MF, et al.: Neuroscience: Exploring the Brain, 2nd ed. Philadelphia: Lippincott Williams & Wilkins, 2001, p. 333.)

respond to a single orientation of an object in space. The orientation column contains complex and simple cells, providing the basis for higher levels of integration and abstraction to take place within the column. Orientation columns are oriented in a radial fashion, much like the spokes of a wheel. The cortex contains many orientation columns arranged in this fashion with different axes of orientation radiating outward from different columns. The center of this array is called an orientation center, and a given axis of orientation is represented only once within a given array.

As described earlier, cortical columns are concerned with color perception (blob areas) and orientation of objects (interblob areas). The cortical column can also be defined in terms of the inputs it receives from each eye. An ocular dominance column receives inputs from one eye (Fig. 26-17), and the inputs are arranged in patterns of alternate columns for each eye. Collectively, sets of orientation columns coupled with blob areas (for color vision) and sets of ocular dominance columns form a unit referred to as a *hypercolumn*. The hypercolumn is responsible for analyzing a single point on the retina. Thus, the primary visual cortex consists of large numbers of hypercolumns, which provide the overall basis for form perception. Moreover, adjoining hypercolumns are capable of communicating with each other by virtue of short, horizontally arranged axons. Typically, an orientation from one hypercolumn associated with a specific spatial orientation can communicate with a counterpart of a neighboring hypercolumn that is associated with the same spatial orientation. Likewise, blob areas within neighboring hypercolumns asso-

ciated with the same color can also communicate with each other. Such arrangements allow for higher levels of integration of visual signals.

FUNCTIONS OF THE TEMPORAL NEOCORTEX

Inferotemporal Cortex (Inferior Temporal and Occipitotemporal [Fusiform] Gyri)

We have seen that the primary visual cortex deals with the initial analysis of visual information in terms of lines and primitive aspects of form perception. Clearly, visual perception requires higher complexities of analysis for images such as faces and forms (shapes) to have clear-cut recognition value. Specifically, the mechanism for face and shape recognition is represented in the **inferior temporal cortex** (see Fig. 1-4). This region receives inputs from tertiary (v4) parts of the visual cortex (which, in turn, receive inputs from the primary [v1] and secondary [v2] visual areas). Neurons in this region specifically respond to faces and shapes, such as the position of a hand in the visual field.

Middle Temporal Cortex

Other parts of the temporal neocortex also contribute to a different aspect of vision—the detection of motion. Recall that certain retinal ganglion cells (type M cells) initially respond to circular fields with changing levels of contrast over time. These neurons project to the magnocellular regions of the lateral geniculate nucleus, which, in turn, project to those regions of the primary visual cortex in which the neurons respond to specific changes in the

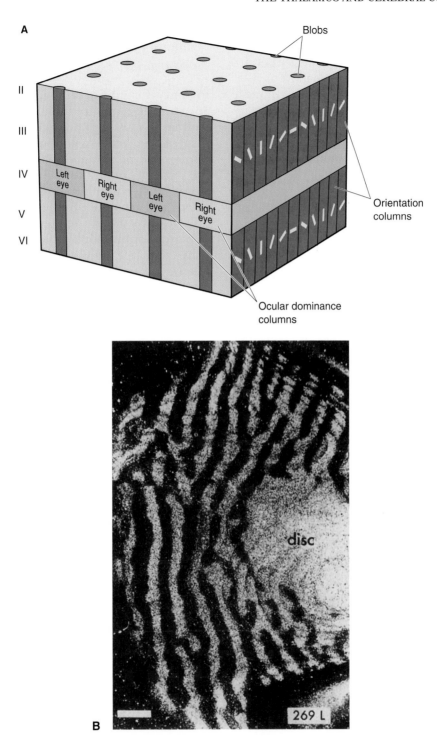

Figure 26–17 Hypercolumn and ocular dominance. (A) Model displaying sets of orientation and ocular dominance columns together with blob areas (for color vision), which, collectively, is referred to as a hypercolumn. (B) Autoradiograph of area 17 of the visual cortex of a monkey whose right eye was removed as an adult. The left eye was injected with the tracer, ^{3}H-proline, which was then transported through the visual pathways to area 17. The autoradiograph reveals alternating patterns of uniformly labeled ocular dominance columns with unlabeled bands. The uniformly labeled region is the optic disc (of the monocular area) covering the blind spot of the right eye that was enucleated. (Reproduced with permission from Parent A: Carpenter's Human Neuroanatomy, 9th ed. Baltimore: Williams & Wilkins, 1996, pp. 337 [panel A] and 900 [panel B].)

movement of objects. Neurons located in the middle temporal gyrus receive such information from parts of the primary visual cortex (i.e., layer IV) and are thus capable of responding to the movement of the object within the visual field. Neurons in these regions of the temporal neocortex then relay signals concerning movement of the object to parts of the parietal lobe that further process the direction and speed of the object's movement.

Superior Temporal Gyrus

On the dorsal aspect of the superior temporal gyrus lie the transverse gyri of Heschl, which face the lateral sulcus. The primary auditory receiving area for auditory signals transmitted to the cerebral cortex from the medial geniculate nucleus is located in the middle part of the anterior transverse gyrus and corresponds to Brodmann's area 41. Adjacent regions of the posterior transverse gyrus include area 42 and largely represent an auditory association area. While characteristics of neural processing of auditory signals within the auditory cortex are not as well delineated as those for vision, a number of similar characteristics to other sensory systems have been described. The auditory cortex, similar to other sensory regions, contains primary, secondary, and tertiary auditory receiving areas that play roles in auditory perception. The cortical neurons in the auditory cortex also respond to a higher level of complexity to auditory signals. For example, neurons located in lower regions of the auditory relay system respond to specific frequencies of stimulation and are thus tonotopically organized. While different regions of the auditory cortex, including the primary receiving areas, may display a tonotopic organization, other neurons located in the auditory cortex respond effectively when the frequency is either increasing or decreasing, reflecting a higher level of integration of the auditory signals.

One additional feature of the primary auditory cortex should be noted. This region of cortex may be divided into two alternating zones or bands that are arranged at right angles to the axis of tonotopic organization. One zone contains neurons that respond to stimuli from either ear, although the effects of stimulation of the contralateral side are more prominent. The second type of zone contains neurons that are excited by stimuli from one side and inhibited by stimuli from the other side. Because of this arrangement, the primary auditory receiving area can respond to all frequencies and to different forms of binaural interaction. This kind of functional organization thus resembles the functional arrangement of the visual cortex with respect to ocular dominance columns.

Effects of Lesions of the Occipital and Temporal Regions of the Cortex
Visual Deficits

Primary Visual Cortex. As described in Chapter 16, a total lesion of the visual cortex (or a lesion affecting all of the geniculocortical fibers) on one side of the brain will produce a contralateral **homonymous hemianopsia** (i.e., loss of vision of the same half of the visual fields of both eyes). A lesion restricted to the inferior bank of the calcarine sulcus will cause an **upper quadrantanopia**. If the lesion affects the left side of the brain, then a **right upper quadrantanopia** will result. If the lesion involves the upper bank of the calcarine sulcus, then a **lower quadrantanopia** (i.e., loss of vision of one quarter of the visual field of both eyes) will result.

Secondary Visual Areas (in Occipital Cortex). Lesions in the secondary visual areas can produce a variety of deficits, including **visual agnosia** (i.e., failure to understand the meaning or use of an object) and **color agnosia** (i.e., inability to associate colors with objects and inability to name or distinguish colors).

Inferotemporal Cortex. Another disorder involves the loss of the ability to recognize familiar faces even though the patient is able to describe the physical features of such individuals. This disorder is called **prosopagnosia** and appears to be associated with lesions of the inferotemporal cortex. It is likely that such lesions disrupt the neurons that receive inputs from interblob regions of the visual cortex that mediate shapes, contours, and edges of figures.

Middle Temporal Cortex. As noted earlier, neurons in the middle temporal cortex respond to the movement of objects. Lesions of this region can produce a disorder called **movement agnosia** in which the patient cannot distinguish between objects that are stationary and those that are moving. A person with this disorder will recognize another individual at both a far distance and then at a closer distance but is incapable of recognizing the movement of that individual.

Auditory Deficits: Superior Temporal Cortex

Bilateral lesions of the auditory cortex do not significantly alter the capacity to discriminate tones or hear sounds. Such lesions, however, appear to interfere with the ability to interpret patterns of sounds. This deficit may extend to the inability to recognize the sounds of animals, speech of individuals, and mechanical sounds such as horns and bells. This disorder is sometimes referred to as an **acoustic agnosia**.

REGIONS ASSOCIATED WITH SPEECH DEFICITS

Temporal-Parietal Region (Wernicke's Area)

Lesions involving the superior temporal gyrus and adjoining parts of the parietal cortex (angular and supramarginal gyri) (Fig. 26-18) produce a disorder referred to as **receptive, sensory,** or **fluent aphasia**. In this disorder, patients are unable to understand either written or spoken language. They may be able to speak, but they do not make sense.

Frontal Lobe (Broca's Area)

A different form of aphasia called **motor** or **nonfluent aphasia** results from a lesion of the posterior aspect of the inferior frontal gyrus (called **Broca's area**). In motor aphasia, the patient is unable to express ideas in spoken words. With respect to both receptive and motor forms of aphasia, two points should be noted. The first is that it is likely that Broca's area and Wernicke's area are functionally interrelated because they can communicate with each other through a pathway referred to as the **arcuate fasciculus** (Fig. 26-18). The second point is that both forms of aphasia occur only when the dominant hemisphere is affected (see discussion on pages 487–490 concerning cerebral dominance).

FUNCTIONS OF THE FRONTAL LOBE

Motor Regions of the Cortex

Details concerning the anatomical and functional properties of motor regions of the frontal lobe have been presented in Chapter 19 and are briefly summarized here.

Three motor regions of the cortex have been identified: a primary motor cortex (area 4), and area 6, which contains both a supplemental motor area and a premotor area. The precentral gyrus gives rise to a component of the corticospinal tract that is critical for generating voluntary control over precise movements that affect primarily the distal musculature. The precentral gyrus is somatotopically organized, and the motor homunculus is depicted in Figure 19-3. As shown in Figure 19-3, motor functions of the head region (corticobulbar tract) are represented in the ventrolateral aspect of the precentral gyrus. The hand and fingers are represented on the dorsal aspect of the cortex, and the lower limb extends onto the medial aspect of the hemisphere. Fibers arising from the precentral gyrus make synaptic contact with ventral horn cells via short interneurons within the spinal cord. Descending cortical neurons are continually modulated by other inputs. These inputs include sensory (conscious proprioceptive) signals from the region of the limb associated with the movement as well as inputs from other motor regions. The motor regions in question include the cerebellum, basal ganglia, and supplemental motor cortex.

Other components of the corticospinal tract include fibers that arise from area 6 and the postcentral gyrus. The fibers arising from the postcentral gyrus make synaptic contact with ascending sensory neurons at the levels of the dorsal column nuclei and dorsal horn of the spinal cord. The function of this descending component is to filter extraneous sensory signals that otherwise might reach the motor cortex, the net effect of which is to enhance the excitatory focus and inhibitory

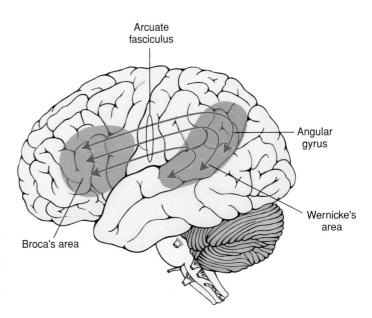

Figure 26–18 Relationship of Wernicke's and Broca's areas. Diagram is of the left cerebral hemisphere indicating the loci of Broca's motor speech area and Wernicke's area. There are reciprocal connections between the two regions, which pass in a bundle called the arcuate fasciculus.

surround with respect to the appropriate sensory signals that affect motor neurons of the precentral gyrus. The supplementary and premotor cortices (area 6) serve to provide the programming mechanisms for the sequencing of response patterns that are critical for complex motor events such as walking, writing, and lacing one's shoes. The outputs of these regions are directed to both the spinal cord and precentral gyrus. The actions of the neurons in area 6 are dependent upon the integrated output of the posterior parietal cortex, which receives both somatosensory and visual signals (see Figs. 19-7 and 26-19).

Two additional motor regions should also be noted. One is located in the posterior aspect of the inferior frontal gyrus and is called **Broca's area**. This region, the functions of which have been described earlier, is associated with the motor expression of speech. The second region lies rostral to area 6 in the middle frontal gyrus and is called the **frontal eye fields (area 8)**. The frontal eye fields coordinate voluntary control of eye movements. Because there are no known projections from the frontal eye fields to cranial nerve nuclei whose axons innervate extraocular eye muscles, area 8 likely controls eye movements by projecting its axons to the horizontal gaze center located in the pontine reticular formation indirectly through projections to the superior

colliculus. Specifically, area 8 projects to the ipsilateral superior colliculus, which, in turn, projects to the contralateral paramedian pontine nucleus (horizontal gaze center). Thus, stimulation of the right area 8 causes conjugate movement of the eyes to the left. If area 8 is damaged, the eyes will look towards the side of the lesion.

It should be noted that there exists an **occipital eye field**. Stimulation of parts of the occipital cortex similarly produces conjugate deviation of the eyes to the contralateral side, and lesions of this region produce conjugate deviation to the side of the lesion. It is believed that occipital control of eye movements is reflexive in nature and serves as a tracking center. These functions are mediated through descending fibers to the superior colliculus.

Summary and Review of Descending Cortical Pathways

The primary descending motor pathways include the following.

1. **Corticospinal tract**: arises from areas 4, 6, 3, 1, and 2 and passes to all levels of the contralateral spinal cord. Its basic function is to produce voluntary control of movement.

2. **Corticobulbar tract**: arises from the head regions of the precentral and postcentral gyri and projects mainly bilaterally to the motor nuclei of the cranial nerves. Its primary function is to produce voluntary movement of the region of the head (i.e., facial expression, movements of the tongue, phonation, jaw opening and closing, eye blinking and squinting).

3. **Corticostriate fibers**: arise from wide regions of the cerebral cortex, although the large majority originates from the frontal lobe. They provide the primary inputs into the neostriatum and use glutamate as a neurotransmitter. This pathway forms an afferent limb (to the basal ganglia) of an overall feedback circuit relating the motor regions of cortex with the basal ganglia.

4. **Corticoreticular fibers**: arise mainly from sensorimotor regions of cortex and project to magnocellular neurons of the pons and medulla (i.e., brainstem motor regions), which, in turn, give rise to the reticulospinal tracts. In this manner, the cerebral cortex can exert control over extensor motor functions normally attributed to the reticular formation.

5. **Corticorubral fibers**: arise mainly from sensorimotor cortex. Because the rubrospinal tract normally controls the activity of flexor motor neurons of the upper limbs (in humans), corticorubral fibers represent a means by which the sensorimotor cortex can influence the

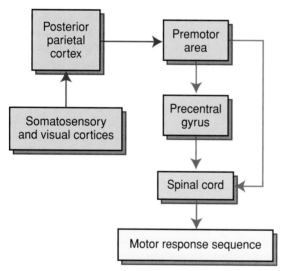

Figure 26–19 Cortical inputs to motor regions. Diagram illustrates the inputs into the posterior parietal cortex from somatosensory and visual cortices as well as the relationship of the posterior parietal cortex with the premotor area, precentral gyrus, and spinal cord. The significance of this relationship is that: (1) the posterior parietal cortex integrates different kinds of sensory information; and (2) these signals are then integrated and transmitted to the premotor area. In this manner, the posterior parietal area contributes to the programming of the sequences of movement with respect to any given motor task. When this mechanism is disrupted, motor functions are impaired, resulting in apraxia.

flexor motor system as well. The cortico-rubrospinal tract can be viewed as a parallel circuit to that of the corticospinal tract for control of the flexor motor system to the neck and upper extremities.

6. **Corticopontine fibers**: arise from all regions of the cerebral cortex, but the largest contribution is from the frontal lobe. This pathway represents a way by which the cerebral cortex can provide important inputs (related to planned movements) to the contralateral cerebellar cortex since these fibers terminate in the deep pontine nuclei (which, in turn, project to the contralateral cortex of the anterior and posterior lobes).

7. **Corticothalamic fibers**: arise from all regions of cortex that receive inputs from specific thalamic nuclei. These fibers project back to the nuclei from which they receive projections. Thus, structures such as the lateral geniculate nucleus and visual cortex are reciprocally connected, as are other regions such as the ventrolateral nucleus and precentral gyrus and the prefrontal cortex and mediodorsal thalamic nucleus. These descending corticothalamic fibers presumably provide feedback functions with respect to the inputs that they receive from the respective thalamic nuclei.

8. **Corticocollicular projections**: these projections were described earlier; in brief, they arise from the frontal and occipital eye fields, project to the superior colliculus and to the horizontal gaze center, and coordinate voluntary and involuntary movements of the eyes from the frontal and occipital eye fields, respectively.

Lesions of the Motor Regions of the Frontal Lobe

The effects of lesions of motor regions of the cerebral cortex have been described previously (see Chapter 19). In brief, a moderate to large lesion of the motor cortex will produce an **upper motor neuron paralysis** (as opposed to a discrete lesion of motor cortex, which has been reported to produce a flaccid paralysis). The upper motor neuron paralysis is characterized by a paralysis of the contralateral limb(s), hyperreflexia, hypertonia, and a Babinski sign. A lesion of parts of area 6 will produce **apraxia**, which is the inability to carry out certain types of complex learned movements (see discussion in Chapter 19). It is presumably due to the loss of the programming mechanism for the execution of movements. A lesion of the posterior aspect of the inferior frontal cortex (Broca's area) will produce **expressive** or **motor (nonfluent) aphasia**. As noted previously, this disorder is characterized by difficulty in expressing ideas in a meaningful manner.

FUNCTIONS OF THE PREFRONTAL CORTEX

The functions of the prefrontal cortex, which are described in detail in Chapter 25, are briefly summarized here. The prefrontal cortex receives inputs from all regions of the cerebral cortex, including sensory regions of the parietal, temporal, and occipital cortices. The prefrontal cortex also receives inputs from the limbic system and monaminergic nuclei of the brainstem. The prefrontal cortex also projects widely to different regions of the brain, including the neostriatum, hypothalamus (directly and indirectly), mediodorsal thalamic nucleus, and brainstem nuclei mediating sensory, motor, and autonomic functions. These connections provide the anatomical bases by which the prefrontal cortex can play important roles in the regulation of visceral, emotional, and cognitive processes.

Animal studies have demonstrated that stimulation of the prefrontal cortex powerfully suppresses predatory attack and defensive rage behavior in the cat. This phenomenon is mediated through a multisynaptic pathway passing through the mediodorsal nucleus and midline thalamic nuclei to the hypothalamus. In humans, destruction of the prefrontal cortex produces variable symptoms. On one hand, there is a general loss or reduction in affect, especially following prefrontal lobotomy; on the other hand, prefrontal lesions have also been associated with increased or heightened emotionality, as originally described in the case of Phineas Gage (see Chapter 25). Lesions of the prefrontal cortex also produce significant intellectual changes. Examples of such changes include: (1) the failure of animals to perform delayed alternation tasks accurately; (2) perceptual deficits, such as the failure to accurately perceive the vertical when the body is placed in a tilted position; and (3) perseveration with original, incorrect strategies in attempting to solve problems. These deficits likely result from the disconnection of the fiber connections between the prefrontal cortex and other regions of the cerebral cortex.

GENERAL FUNCTIONS OF THE CEREBRAL CORTEX: CEREBRAL DOMINANCE, CORTICAL EXCITABILITY, AND LEARNING AND MEMORY

CEREBRAL DOMINANCE

As we have described throughout this chapter, the cerebral cortex participates in a wide range of functions. Although these functions are represented on both sides of the brain, they are *not* represented equally on both sides of the brain. By this, it is meant that, for a given function, one side of the brain plays a more active role and has more neurons dedicated to that function than the other side. We say that there is *cerebral dominance* on that side of the brain for the function in question. Yet, to a lesser extent, that function is also represented on the nondominant side of the brain.

Role of the Corpus Callosum in Hemispheric Transfer of Information

Information acquired on one side of the brain can be typically transferred to the homotypical region (i.e., the corresponding region) on the contralateral cortex. Almost all of the fibers that transfer such information from one side of the cortex to the other involve the corpus callosum. Callosal fibers arise from pyramidal cells of layers II and III of a given region of cortex and terminate in the more superficial layers of the homotypical cortex.

Most regions of cortex share connections with homotypical regions of the contralateral side. However, there are several regions where such connections appear to be limited or even absent. These include parts of the visual cortex and the primary sensory and motor regions of the cortex that are associated with the distal parts of the upper and lower limbs. The apparent reason for this is that, although each hemisphere does receive information concerning the status of the limbs on each side of the body, certain parts of the body, like the distal musculature, function somewhat independently (on each side). In comparison, proximal regions of the body on each side, such as the back, neck, and stomach, function in concert with their opposite counterpart. Consequently, relatively greater quantities of callosal fibers arising from cortical regions associated with these parts of the body connect the sensory and motor cortices on each side.

Illustrations of the significance of the transfer of information from one hemisphere to the other through the corpus callosum were demonstrated from a series of studies by Roger Sperry, for which he received the Nobel Prize in 1981. In one of the studies, a monkey was trained in a visual discrimination task in which the animal was required to distinguish between two types of objects that enabled it to receive a food reward. In the experimental animals, the optic chiasm was severed, as was the anterior commissure and corpus callosum (called a **split-brain** preparation). Because the optic chiasm was cut, each eye then projected only to the ipsilateral hemisphere with the uncrossed temporal retinal fibers. Then, a patch was placed over one eye, and a training task was then given to the animal. For example, if the patch was placed over the left eye, information could only be provided through the right eye and then to the right hemisphere. Both the experimental and control animals (those whose corpus callosum were intact) clearly learned such a task when the patch was placed over the left eye. When experimental animals were then tested with the patch over the right eye, no evidence of learning was present. In contrast, control animals similarly tested demonstrated clear-cut learning after the patch was placed over the right eye, indicating that there is, indeed, transfer of information from one hemisphere to the other.

Similar kinds of demonstrations of transfer of information from one hemisphere to the other were provided by Sperry with respect to discrimination tasks requiring the using of other sensory modalities such as somatosensory (i.e., tactile, kinesthetic) sensations. These studies also revealed that the region of the corpus callosum proximal to the splenium (i.e., fibers connecting parts of the occipital cortices) was critical for the transfer of information concerning visual discriminations, whereas the body of the corpus callosum connecting the parietal and adjoining parts of the frontal lobes was essential for the tasks involving discriminations of somatosensory sensations.

Examples of Cerebral Dominance

The phenomenon of cerebral dominance exists for both animals and humans. Much of our knowledge of cerebral dominance in humans is derived from studies involving patients suffering from severe cases of epilepsy in which the corpus callosum was surgically cut in order to limit the spread of seizure activity throughout the cerebral cortex.

From these studies, it is most likely that, although lateralization of specific brain functions is present for a variety of cortical functions (Fig. 26-20), normally, both cortices work in concert with respect to the successful execution of different functions. However, one side of the brain is very highly dominant with respect to certain functions. The classic example is that of *speech*, which is basically represented in the left hemisphere. For example, individuals who have suffered strokes involving the left hemisphere have a much greater likelihood of suffering from speech deficits than individuals sustaining strokes of the right hemisphere. In fact, the various forms of aphasia (described earlier) typically result from strokes sustained in the left cerebral hemisphere. Other illustrations of cerebral dominance with respect to speech have been demonstrated with split-brain patients. For example, when the patient is handed an object in his right hand and asked to name the

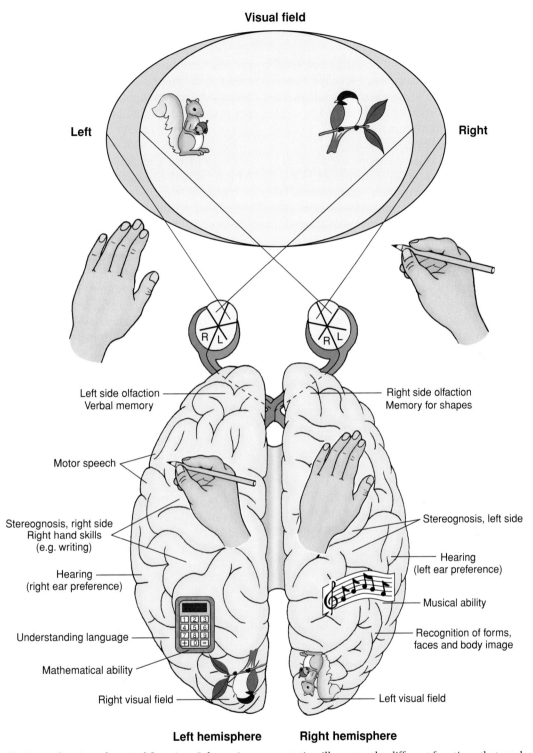

Figure 26–20 Lateralization of cortical function. Schematic representation illustrates the different functions that are localized in each of the hemispheres. These findings were determined from clinical cases involving patients with a sectioned corpus callosum.

object without having seen it, he has little difficulty in doing so. However, when given the same task with the object placed in his left hand, he is unable to name it. The likely explanation for this finding is that the sensation from the right hand reaches the left cerebral cortex, which is the dominant hemi-

sphere for speech. Since the right hemisphere plays little role in speech, the patient has great difficulty in naming the object when it is placed in his left hand. Nevertheless, he does show some signs of understanding the nature of the object even though the language function is absent. For example, if the patient were specifically asked to pick out a pencil from several other objects, he would have little difficulty in doing so.

In addition to language and speech, cerebral dominance is present for a variety of other functions. A most commonly observed function is **handedness**. Most people are right-handed and are, therefore, left-hemisphere dominant. It has been suggested that the handedness may be due, in part, to the anatomical differences in the shape of the dominant hemisphere relative to the nondominant one. The significance of the differences in shape remains unclear. Handedness is also affected by such factors as learning and social conditions. In fact, people quite frequently learn how to use the hand associated with the nondominant hemisphere as effectively as the other hand, indicating the presence of significant cross talk between the two hemispheres. Handedness is also highly correlated with the dominant hemisphere for speech. Almost all right-handed individuals contain left hemispheres that are dominant for both speech and handedness. On the other hand, most left-handed individuals contain right hemispheres that are dominant for handedness and left hemispheres that are dominant for speech.

It has been suggested that the left hemisphere also appears to be dominant for understanding arithmetic and the visual appearance of written words and letters (i.e., right visual field). The right hemisphere is believed to be dominant for spatial design, emotional expression, understanding of music, complex visual patterns, and also the affective part of speech.

CORTICAL EXCITABILITY: A SUMMARY

Excitation of a region (or regions) of the cerebral cortex is governed by a number of factors, including the types of inputs that the cortical region receives from other regions of the central nervous system. One type of input that significantly affects cortical excitability is from specific thalamic afferent fibers. They directly excite cortical cells initially in layer IV and, ultimately, cells in most, if not all, layers of a given cortical column associated with the region receiving the initial input. A second source of excitation includes nonspecific afferent fibers from the thalamus and brainstem. Thalamic afferents arise from such nonspecific nuclei as the centromedian and parts of the ventral anterior nucleus. Brainstem afferents arise from monoaminergic cell groups (i.e., cell groups containing serotonin, dopamine, and norepinephrine). Both of these types of inputs serve to modulate the activity

of cortical neurons and significantly alter cortical excitability levels. A fourth source of cortical inputs includes cholinergic afferent fibers that arise from the **nucleus basalis of Meynert** of the basal forebrain. Cholinergic fibers are generally excitatory. Thus, their inputs to wide areas of the cerebral cortex presumably serve to significantly enhance cortical excitability levels.

Finally, excitation of cortical neurons is also dependent on the actions of local interneurons, which may be excitatory or inhibitory. Many cortical interneurons are excitatory and likely use excitatory amino acids as their neurotransmitters. The inhibitory interneurons appear to be mainly GABAergic but may also be co-localized with a neuropeptide (e.g., somatostatin, cholecystokinin). In fact, a major question central to present theories concerning the development of epilepsy is whether epileptogenic events reflect an *increase* in glutamatergic activity or a *decrease* in GABAergic activity or a combination of the two types of activity.

LEARNING AND MEMORY

Learning may be defined as the acquisition of new information. *Memory* may be defined as the process by which information is retrieved or stored, and forgetting reflects a process by which information is lost.

Definitions of memory may be made along several different dimensions. One dimension involves temporal parameters, and the second dimension deals with the qualitative characteristics of conscious awareness. With respect to the temporal dimension, the following definitions have evolved. **Immediate memory** refers to recalling an event a few seconds after it occurs. **Short-term memory** is the retention of an event for several minutes after it has occurred. **Working memory** is a form of short-term memory and requires recall of a sequence of events for a few minutes to complete a task. An example would be an individual who makes a series of successive approximations that are required for the completion of a task. Here, successful completion of the task necessitates knowledge and recall of the previous response patterns, including those that are correct as well as those that are erratic. **Long-term memory** refers to events that are remembered weeks, months, or years after they have occurred. It is a generally accepted view that long-term memory involves a change in synaptic organization or an increase in the efficiency of the synapse. It is apparent that, at some point in time, short-term memory is converted into long-term memory. The mechanism by which this transformation takes place is still poorly understood.

The second dimension, qualitative characteristics of *conscious awareness*, can be divided into two categories. The first category, called **declarative memory**, represents the memory for such facts as an address, directions to get to a specific place, or a string of numbers such as a telephone number or a personal bank card pin number. The principal feature of this form of memory is that the individual is conscious of the information that is remembered. The second category is called **procedural memory**. This form of memory differs from declarative memory in that the individual may not be consciously aware of the procedures involved in carrying out a task (e.g., shooting a basketball, skiing, or hitting a baseball).

The process by which information had been retained but then is lost is called **forgetting**. Forgetting is a normal and useful process that enables new information to be learned, especially if the information forgotten is of little or no consequence. A special, pathological form of forgetting is called **amnesia**. Amnesia can occur most often as a result of head injury or a cerebrovascular accident, most typically involving the temporal lobe, particularly the hippocampus, or medial aspects of the thalamus. Difficulty in retrieving old memories is called **retrograde amnesia**. Difficulty in generating new memories is called **anterograde amnesia**. Alzheimer's patients typically suffer from these forms of amnesia. Individuals with hippocampal damage or damage to other parts of the Papez circuit have great difficulty in establishing new anterograde memories because they suffer from anterograde amnesia.

There are other general functions that clearly involve the cerebral cortex. Several of these functions include the topics of sleep and wakefulness, electroencephalogram (EEG) activity, and epilepsy. Because these topics were covered extensively in Chapters 23 and 25, they are omitted here. However, it is recommended that one review these sections to gain a more complete understanding of the varied functions of the cerebral cortex.

CLINICAL CASES

THALAMUS
HISTORY

Norma is a 75-year-old woman who had a stroke several months ago, which resulted in numbness (i.e., inability to feel sensory stimulation) on her right side, including her arm, face, trunk, and leg. The numbness had improved somewhat over time but did not completely disappear. One day, she noticed that brushing her right arm against a door was very painful. Thinking that perhaps this was "in her mind," she tried touching the right arm with her left hand, and this, too, was painful. Fearful that she may be having another stroke, she went immediately to see her neurologist at her local hospital.

EXAMINATION

Norma's neurologist examined her and found that sensation for pain, temperature, and vibration were diminished on the entire right side of her body. The degree of sensory loss was unchanged from an examination several months before. However, she had a large amount of discomfort with any type of stimulus, accompanied by some emotional disturbance. The discomfort was far out of proportion to the degree of the stimulus; for instance, a light touch to her right arm would engender a scream similar to that elicited by a knife. The remainder of her examination was normal.

The neurologist told Norma that he didn't think that she had another stroke but would order a head computed tomography (CT) scan to be sure that there was no tumor or bleeding. In addition, he told her that if the head CT showed nothing new, that she could begin a new medication that would help with the pain.

EXPLANATION

Norma's head CT showed an old stroke in her left ventral thalamus and no new lesions. A stroke involving the ventral posterolateral nucleus of the thalamus can produce a disorder called the syndrome of Dejerine-Roussy, or thalamic pain syndrome, which usually occurs several months after the stroke. Although there is sensory loss on the contralateral side, there is pain or discomfort out of proportion to the stimulus on the affected side of the body. Emotional disturbance aggravates the response. Some patients describe the sensation as "knife-like" or "hot." As the deficit (numbness) resolves, the pain may lessen. This syndrome may also occur in lesions of the parietal white matter and is thought to occur as a result of an imbalance of afferent sensory impulses.

In the past, neurosurgery has been used for the ablation of the ventral posterolateral nucleus of the thalamus to relieve the pain in extreme cases. In more recent years, with the advent of a class of drugs called tricyclic antidepressants, these patients can be treated medically. The methylated forms of these medications are useful blockers of serotonin re-uptake. Because serotonin is a pain modulator, it is believed that blocking the re-uptake of serotonin enhances its action and facilitates the action of intrinsic opiates to relieve pain.

CEREBRAL CORTEX
HISTORY

June is a 65-year-old woman who was previously healthy. One day, while taking a walk in the park, she noticed her right fingers twitching, then her right hand, then her arm and shoulder, followed by a march of twitches down her leg. She did not remember any more than this because she lost consciousness. An onlooker saw her drop to the ground and deviate her neck backwards, while making a high-pitched noise. Then, both of her arms and legs began to jerk for approximately 1 to 2 minutes and then stopped abruptly. She had lost control of her bladder during this event. When the onlooker attempted to speak to June to ask her if she was okay, she opened her eyes but mumbled and closed them again. The onlooker called an ambulance, which brought June to the nearest hospital.

EXAMINATION

A doctor met June at the emergency room entrance and asked her what had happened. By this time, June was slightly drowsy but able to answer questions appropriately. Her speech was fluent and grammatically correct. She knew the month but not the day of the week or where she was. The remainder of her examination was normal. The doctor ordered a CT of June's head and drew some blood.

EXPLANATION

June had a seizure, which began focally on the left motor strip (the left precentral gyrus), moved up the motor strip, and then secondarily generalized, or spread throughout the cortex. The phenomenon whereby there is twitching of an extremity that spreads to other areas on that extremity or other areas of the body is called a Jacksonian march. This phenomenon is named for Hughlings Jackson, a neurosurgeon who was instrumental in mapping out the cerebral cortex and describing the somatotopic organization of the neocortex called a homunculus (meaning "little man"). Observing patients with a Jacksonian march helped him to identify which areas are represented on each location of the motor strip.

Sometimes, epileptic discharges spread to other areas of the cortex, recruiting contiguous areas of cortex through callosal, commissural, and sometimes thalamic circuits to eventually involve a large area of the cortex, causing the movements of the entire body. This occurs with a generalized seizure. The cells (often pyramidal cells) in the cortex can generate a seizure through high-frequency, synchronous discharges in large groups. These cells can be epileptogenic for several reasons: (1) intrinsic membrane properties that allow the cells to generate pacemaker-like slow depolarization, (2) a large degree of excitatory coupling among the neurons, and (3) the loss of inhibitory control mechanisms. Cells may become epileptogenic for many reasons, including irritative lesions on or near the cortex, metabolic abnormalities, drug withdrawal, strokes, and infections of the CNS. Very often, there is inhibition after a seizure, which accounts for drowsiness in a "post-ictal state" after the seizure has finished.

June had a CT of her head, which revealed a meningioma (a benign tumor originating in the meninges) over the precentral gyrus. She was given a medication called phenytoin, which helps to prevent seizures by blocking Na^+ channels and also by facilitating the movement of K^+ to the extracellular space, thereby decreasing neuronal excitability. June was admitted to the hospital to have surgery to remove the tumor.

CHAPTER TEST

QUESTIONS

Choose the best answer for each question.

1. A patient exhibits a variety of behavioral and language problems such as a failure to inhibit responses that are socially inappropriate. Such an individual is most likely to suffer from dementia involving the:

   a. Parieto-occipital region
   b. Frontal cortex
   c. Inferior temporal cortex
   d. Corpus callosum
   e. Caudate nucleus

2. The corpus callosum of each of 20 patients was severed in order to reduce the spread of seizure activity. The patients were then asked to participate in a research study to identify specific features of brain function. The most likely purpose of this study was to:

   a. Identify the different areas of the cortex that mediate speech functions
   b. Identify how the corpus callosum mediates visual functions
   c. Identify the various properties of cerebral dominance
   d. Identify the cortical sites mediating movement of the fingers
   e. Characterize thalamocortical relationships

3. A patient exhibits clumsiness, weakness, and somatosensory loss of the right leg. The most likely cause of these symptoms is a:

   a. Seizure of the left frontal lobe
   b. Tumor of the left prefrontal cortex
   c. Tumor of the right cerebellar hemisphere

d. Hemorrhagic stroke of the left anterior cerebral artery

e. Left frontal lobe concussion resulting from an automobile accident

Questions 4 and 5. A 68-year-old man is admitted to the emergency room after initially complaining of dizziness. In the emergency room, the patient indicated that he could not move his right arm or leg, and his speech were slurred. The tongue was directed to the right side when the patient was asked to protrude it, and the patient's jaw drooped to the right side as well. Sensory functions on each side of the body appeared normal as well as motor functions on the left side.

4. The patient suffered a stroke involving the:

a. Anterior cerebral artery

b. Middle cerebral artery

c. Posterior cerebral artery

d. Anterior spinal artery

e. Vertebral artery

5. The stroke involved the:

a. Right precentral gyrus

b. Left postcentral gyrus

c. Left internal capsule

d. Right internal capsule

e. Left medullary pyramids

ANSWERS AND EXPLANATIONS

1. Answer: b

The frontal cortex, particularly the prefrontal region, plays an important role in cognitive functions and in the regulation of emotional behavior. Parts of the frontal lobe (i.e., Broca's area) and superior aspect of the temporal lobe (Wernicke's area) mediate the motor and receptive components of speech. Neither the parieto-occipital region nor inferior temporal cortex is directly involved in these functions. The corpus callosum mediates the transmission of information from one side of the cortex to the other, and the caudate nucleus is associated with the cognitive aspects of motor functions.

2. Answer: c

Much of the knowledge we have recently obtained concerning cerebral dominance has come from studies of patients whose corpus callosum has been cut in order to reduce the spread of seizure activity. These patients have been ideal subjects for determining which side of the cerebral cortex is dominant with respect to a variety of functions such as music, language, mathematics, and spatial percep-

tion. The corpus callosum plays a minimal role in transferring visual information and information concerning movements of the fingers. Removal of the corpus callosum is not necessary to characterize the different areas of the cortex that mediate speech functions. Also, sectioning of the corpus callosum would not serve any purpose in examining thalamocortical connections, which typically involve relationships on the same side of the brain.

3. Answer: d

The anterior cerebral artery supplies, in part, the motor and somatosensory neurons associated with the leg region of the cerebral cortex. A stroke involving the left anterior cerebral artery will damage neurons in the left medial sensorimotor region, thus causing weakness and loss of sensation in the right leg. The other choices are incorrect because they involve different regions of the cerebral cortex that are not involved in sensorimotor regulation of the leg region.

4 and 5. Answers: 4-b, 5-c

The lenticulostriate branches of the middle cerebral artery supply the internal capsule, including the region of the posterior limb and genu. The key point here is that these regions of the internal capsule contain corticobulbar and corticospinal fibers that mediate functions of the head and body that were affected in the patient, likely producing a right central palsy. Thus, of the choices given in this question, only the middle cerebral artery is correct because its branches supply these regions and none of the other arteries supply fibers that mediate these functions. Note that both the anterior spinal and vertebral arteries are present at medullary levels, while the corticobulbar fibers mediating motor control of the jaw exit at the level of the pons. The anterior cerebral artery, which passes on the medial aspect of the cortex, does not supply neurons that mediate speech (located laterally on the cortex).

As indicated in the explanation to question 4, branches of the middle cerebral artery supply descending fibers in the internal capsule, which are associated with the motor functions disrupted in this patient. Other choices involving fiber bundles on the right side of the brain are wrong because the right side of the body was affected in this case, requiring an answer that included damage to the left corticospinal tract. The left postcentral gyrus is not directly involved in motor functions, and the left medullary pyramids lie below the level where corticobulbar fibers exit to innervate motor neurons of the facial nerve.

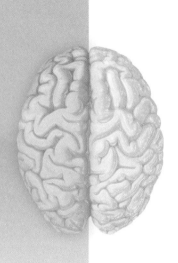

CHAPTER 27

VASCULAR SYNDROMES

OBJECTIVES

After reading this chapter, the student should be able to:

1. List the common neuroimaging techniques and describe the principles on which they are based

2. Describe the deficits and symptoms caused by the occlusion of different arteries

3. Describe the salient characteristics of stroke

Blood flow in the cerebral vasculature serves the critical function of supplying oxygen, glucose, and other nutrients to the central nervous system (CNS). In addition, removal of carbon dioxide, lactic acid, and other metabolic products is also dependent on the blood circulating in the CNS. As mentioned in Chapter 4, the blood flow to the brain is about 700 to 750 mL/min. A major fraction of this blood flow (about 350 mL/min) is provided by the internal carotid arteries, while the remaining blood supply comes via the vertebral arteries. Serious neurologic disorders occur when there is a complete or partial occlusion of one or more arteries supplying the CNS. The nature of deficits varies according to the arterial system that is occluded and the region of the CNS affected.

Reliable techniques have recently been developed to identify the areas of the CNS in which the blood supply is compromised due to vascular disease. This chapter begins with a brief description of these techniques, after which follows a discussion of the neurologic deficits that may occur after the occlusion of the most frequently affected arteries.

NEUROIMAGING

In recent years, several neuroimaging techniques have been used to identify defects or alterations in blood flow in different regions of the brain. Many modalities exist to visualize the human nervous system, both noninvasively and invasively. In the early evaluation of patients with neurologic problems, noninvasive imaging is usually used first. The most common noninvasive neuroimaging modalities are **computed tomography (CT) scanning** and **magnetic resonance imaging (MRI)**. Other modalities used less commonly include **magnetic resonance angiography (MRA)**, **magnetic resonance spectroscopy (MRS)**, **positron emission tomography (PET)**, and **single-photon emission computed tomography (SPECT)**.

COMPUTED TOMOGRAPHY

Conventional x-ray radiography suffers from several limitations. First, the x-ray attenuation information regarding the three-dimensional anatomy of the patient is projected on the radiograph in only two dimensions. Second, x-rays provide poor soft-tissue contrast. Third, x-rays involve relatively high radiation exposure. Because of these limitations, other techniques, such as CT scanning, have been developed for neuroimaging.

CT scanning uses basic x-ray principles. An x-ray assembly (Fig. 27-1A) consists of a negatively charged electrode (the cathode), which is the source of electrons, and a positively charged electrode (the anode), which serves as a target for the electrons. A large potential difference is applied between the two electrodes in an evacuated envelope. Electrons are released from the cathode and are accelerated as they travel towards the anode; the electrons acquire kinetic energy as they travel across the potential difference. When these electrons come close to the large electric field generated by the positive charge of the anode, they are decelerated and lose their kinetic energy, which results in the production of high-energy x-rays. The x-rays emitted by the x-ray tube are uniformly distributed on one side of the patient. Inside the patient's body, the x-rays are attenuated by absorption and scattering, and the x-ray distribution is altered. The transmitted x-ray pattern is then imaged by the detector (a conventional x-ray film or comparable device) placed on the other side of the patient. A thicker structure in the patient's

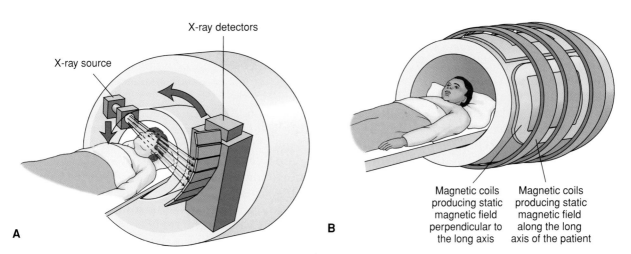

Figure 27–1 Assemblies for commonly used neuroimaging techniques. (A) An assembly for computed tomography (CT) scanning. (B) An assembly for magnetic resonance imaging (MRI). See text for details.

body produces a greater attenuation of x-rays. Consequently, fewer x-rays reach the detector, which results in a lower optical density at the corresponding site on the radiograph. Thus, lower and higher optical densities appear white and dark, respectively, on the radiograph.

In CT scanning of the head, a movable x-ray tube is rotated around the patient's head. Very sensitive x-ray detectors are placed opposite to the x-ray tube on the other side of the patient's head. Because of high sensitivity of the detectors, shorter exposure times are needed, and therefore, there is a less risk due to the radiation damage. The CT scanner acquires a large number (100 to 1200) of projections around the desired region of the patient's head. The detectors obtain data around the tissue along a thin line. A tomographic image is a representation of a slice of the patient's body where the x-rays penetrated. The table on which the patient is laying is then moved slightly so that a different axial slice of the tissue is placed in the path of the x-ray beam. Thus, a series of x-rays representing different slices of the tissue is obtained. These data are converted into CT images by a computer. If the patient's head is scanned in this manner, it is possible to acquire tomograms (slices) of different planes through the brain. Thus, internal structures at any desired plane can be visualized.

An example of a CT scan is presented in Figure 27-2, which was taken in the transaxial plane. The figure shows an acute cerebral infarction. The CT scan was taken 6 hours after the acute onset of a right hemianopsia. A subtle loss of gray-white contrast in the infarcted left visual cortex due to the embolization of the left posterior cerebral artery is observed (Fig. 27-2A). A marked hypodensity of gray and white matter is visible 48 hours after the onset of the infarct (Fig. 27-2B).

MAGNETIC RESONANCE IMAGING

MRI is based on the principles of nuclear magnetic resonance (NMR), which is a technique used to acquire chemical, physical, and microscopic information about molecules. Water in the human body consists of many hydrogen atoms. The nucleus of a hydrogen atom consists of a single proton. The proton possesses a property called "spin," which is a small magnetic field causing the nucleus to produce an NMR signal. The NMR signal produced by the nuclei of hydrogen atoms is used for imaging in MRI. In an MRI assembly (Fig. 27-1B), graded spatial variations in the magnetic field are generated by different sets of gradient magnets oriented along different axes. When all the atomic nuclei are aligned by the magnetic field, a brief radiofrequency pulse is applied. The atomic nuclei emit energy in an oscillatory pattern as they return to the alignment imposed by the magnetic field. The radiofrequencies emitted by the oscillating nuclei are detected by sensitive detectors, and a computer attached to the MRI assembly converts signal intensities and magnetic gradient parameters into spatial locations. Detailed images of the tissue under examination are then constructed based on this information. The brain and spinal cord can thus be imaged in three dimensions to reproduce the locations of specific structures. A few examples follow.

Figure 27-3 shows an MRI axial section through the isthmus of the pons. A hypointensity within the aqueduct consistent with a venous angioma of the subependymal venous system is observed (Fig. 27-3A). A section at the level of the inferior cerebellar peduncle demonstrates the tributaries of the - venous angioma and an associated cavernous angioma in the left cerebellar hemisphere (Fig. 27-3B).

An MRI of a patient with congenital optic atrophy, taken in the coronal plane, is shown in Figure 27-4. The cisternal segment of the left optic nerve is small and has abnormal hyperintensity. The visual abnormality in this patient was monocular.

A sagittal MRI image taken from a patient suffering from an ectopic neurohypophysis is shown in Figure 27-5. When the pituitary stalk is unable to transmit releasing factors to the anterior pituitary, panhypopituitarism develops. A hyperintense signal arising from the secretary granules is visible in the MRI. Detailed anatomy of the suprasellar region, including the optic chiasm, lamina terminalis, anterior commissure, and mammillary body, is shown in Figure 27-6.

MAGNETIC RESONANCE ANGIOGRAPHY

Magnetic resonance angiography (MRA) is a noninvasive method for visualizing the cerebral vasculature. The basic principle behind MRA is that there are macroscopic changes in spins within the nuclei in the blood that are detectable in a similar fashion to MRI. This technique uses the fact that blood flows and provides a signal that is different from that of the surrounding tissue. This procedure is often used in stroke patients before conventional angiography because it is far less invasive. MRA is useful in visualizing arteries in which blood flow is relatively fast (e.g., carotid arteries and proximal intracranial vessels). Screening for large vascular atherosclerotic plaques, stenosis, or occlusion of arteries and venous sinuses can be done using this procedure. Computer processing

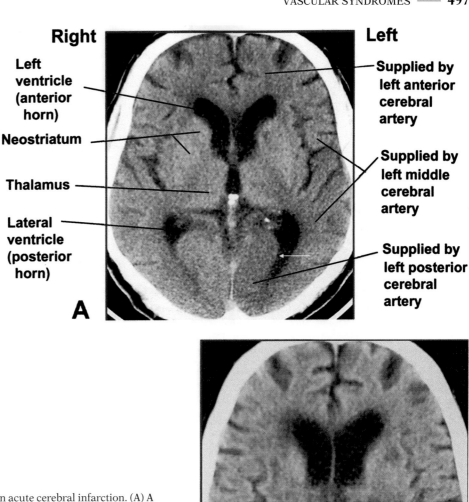

Right　　　　　　　　　**Left**

Left ventricle (anterior horn)

Neostriatum

Thalamus

Lateral ventricle (posterior horn)

A

Supplied by left anterior cerebral artery

Supplied by left middle cerebral artery

Supplied by left posterior cerebral artery

B

Figure 27–2 CT scan showing an acute cerebral infarction. (A) A CT scan taken in the transaxial plane 6 hours after acute onset of right homonymous hemianopsia (hyperacute infarct). Subtle loss of gray-white tissue contrast in the infarcted left visual cortex (*arrow*) due to embolization of the left posterior cerebral artery is visible. (B) A CT scan taken in transaxial plane 48 hours after the initial symptoms shows marked hypodensity of gray and white matter in the infarcted left visual cortex (*arrow*). Rapid evolution of these changes is the hallmark of infarction. Labeling of regions supplied by different arteries is identical in A and B. (Courtesy of Dr. Leo J. Wolansky, Department of Radiology, New Jersey Medical School.)

allows three-dimensional reconstruction of MRAs. However, in vessels where blood flow is slow, the resolution of MRA images is inferior to that of conventional angiography.

MAGNETIC RESONANCE SPECTROSCOPY

Magnetic resonance spectroscopy (MRS), also known as NMR spectroscopy, has been used in chemistry laboratories as a method for distinguishing different chemical species. Different materials have slightly different magnetic shielding that changes the net magnetic field. This tech-

nique is now being used in neuroscience research to identify specific neurotransmitters and other substances in specific regions of the brain. The presence or absence of certain substances may someday serve as markers for specific neurologic diseases.

POSITRON EMISSION TOMOGRAPHY

Positron emission tomography (PET) scanning involves injecting a solution containing molecules labeled with an unstable radionuclide into the blood circulation. The excess protons in the unstable radionuclide are converted into neutrons by

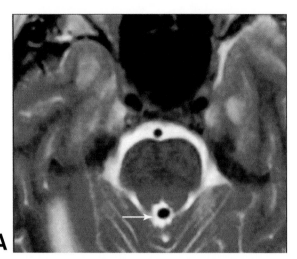

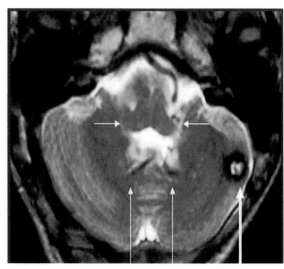

Figure 27–3 An MRI of a patient with intra-aqueductal venous angioma. (A) An axial section through the isthmus of the pons demonstrates a hypointensity within the aqueduct (arrow) consistent with a venous angioma of the subependymal venous system. (B) An axial section at the level of the inferior cerebellar peduncles (*short arrows*) demonstrates the tributaries of the venous angioma (*long arrows*) and an associated cavernous angioma (*thick arrow*) in the left cerebellar hemisphere. (Courtesy of Dr. Leo J. Wolansky, Department of Radiology, New Jersey Medical School.)

radioactive decay. During this conversion, a positron (a positively charged electron) is emitted. The positron collides with an electron, releasing two photons that are sensed by detectors placed around the head. Usually blood flow in the brain is monitored by injecting oxygen 15 (^{15}O)-labeled water, and glucose utilization is assessed by injecting fluorine-18–labeled 2-deoxyglucose. When

a particular brain region is activated by a given task (e.g., visual stimulation), neuronal activity, blood flow, and glucose utilization are increased in that region. A common radionuclide used for localization of a seizure focus in patients with epilepsy is ^{18}F-deoxyglucose. This radiolabeled substance displaces glucose. As the unstable isotope decays, a positron is generated that collides

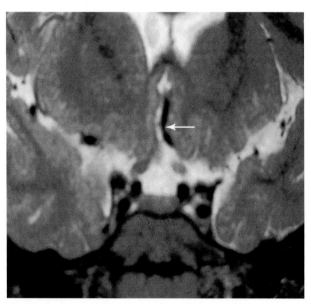

Figure 27–4 An MRI of a patient with congenital optic atrophy. The MRI was taken in a coronal plane. The cisternal segment of the left optic nerve (arrow) is small and has abnormal hyperintensity. The visual abnormality in this patient was monocular. (Courtesy of Dr. Leo J. Wolansky, Department of Radiology, New Jersey Medical School.)

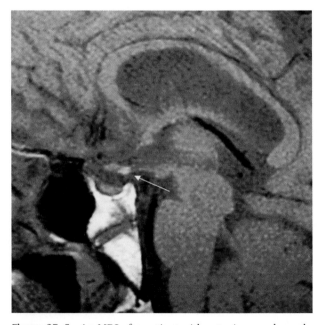

Figure 27–5 An MRI of a patient with ectopic neurohypophysis. This is a sagittal image showing that, when the pituitary stalk is unable to transmit releasing factors to the anterior pituitary, panhypopituitarism results. Note the hyperintense signal (*arrow*) arising from the secretory granules. (Courtesy of Dr. Leo J. Wolansky, Department of Radiology, New Jersey Medical School.)

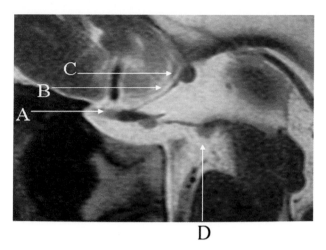

Figure 27-6 This MRI image shows the detailed anatomy of the suprasellar region including the chiasm (A), lamina terminalis (B), anterior commissure (C), and mammillary body (D). (Courtesy of Dr. Leo J. Wolansky, Department of Radiology, New Jersey Medical School.)

with an electron. This collision destroys both particles, and two gamma rays are emitted, which are then detected using special detectors. The areas of positron-electron collisions, representing the areas of high metabolic activity, can be imaged in this manner. It should be noted that PET scans taken in situations when the patient is hyperactive or shivering can give false-positive readings. Therefore, hyperactivity and shivering are controlled before the PET scanning procedure is carried out on the patient. This procedure is also used for detecting brain neoplasms because malignant cells have a relatively high glucose uptake.

SINGLE-PHOTON EMISSION COMPUTED TOMOGRAPHY

Single-photon emission computed tomography (SPECT) is less expensive and less complex than a PET scan. Gamma camera technology is used to determine regional cerebral blood flow after the injection of a specific radionuclide, such as hexamethyl-propyleneamineoxime (HMPAO). SPECT is useful as an adjunct to diagnosis in many neurologic conditions where there may be defects or alterations in blood flow to specific regions of the brain, such as a stroke.

ANGIOGRAPHY (ARTERIOGRAPHY)

Angiography usually involves introduction of a specially designed catheter into a femoral artery. The catheter is then advanced under fluoroscopic guidance until it reaches the aortic arch. The tip of the catheter is then steered towards the origin of the vessel under investigation (e.g., the internal carotid or vertebral artery). A radiopaque contrast material (e.g., an iodinated dye) is then injected via the catheter, and x-ray pictures are taken in rapid sequence as the contrast material flows through the artery (arterial phase), capillaries (capillary phase), and veins (venous phase). Photographic techniques are then used to visualize the blood vessels. Injection of the contrast material is contraindicated in patients who are allergic to the contrast-enhancing agents. Usually the contrast of the x-ray image prepared before the injection of the contrast material is reversed by making a positive image in which bones appear dark. The reverse-contrast image is superimposed on the x-ray image prepared after the injection of the contrast material. A print is then made of the two images together. More commonly, the x-ray images are processed digitally for clear visualization of blood vessels.

Angiography is used to identify structural abnormalities of vessels (e.g., stenosis [narrowing], occlusion, malformations, and aneurysms), displacement of the normal position of the cranial vessels, and changes in flow patterns (e.g., occlusion of a major vessel by a thrombus may promote collateral flow in a smaller branch).

Angiography is an invasive procedure and may cause stroke in some patients. Moreover, bleeding may occur sometimes at the arterial puncture site. Occasionally, occlusion of the femoral artery may develop at the puncture site, which may cause ischemia in the leg. Therefore, the arterial puncture site is carefully examined and observed for at least 24 hours after the procedure is completed. As mentioned earlier, in view of the invasive nature of conventional angiography, usually noninvasive procedures, such as magnetic resonance angiography (described earlier) or CT scanning, are used first for visualization of intracranial blood vessels. However, blood vessels are not imaged clearly in ordinary CT scans because the x-ray density of blood and CNS is similar. Therefore, a contrast material is usually injected intravenously before CT scanning to allow clear visualization of blood vessels. Computer processing of CT scans allows three-dimensional reconstruction of arteries and veins.

DEFICITS AFTER ARTERIAL OCCLUSION

The CNS areas supplied by different arteries are described in detail in Chapter 4. The areas supplied by the most commonly affected arteries and the deficits after their occlusion are described in the following sections.

Table 27–1 Deficits or Symptoms After the Interruption of Blood Flow in Major Branches of the Internal Carotid Artery

Occluded Artery	Deficits or Symptoms
Internal carotid branches	
Anterior cerebral	Contralateral hemiplegia and somatosensory loss, mainly of the leg
Middle cerebral	Contralateral hemiplegia and somatosensory loss of the upper limb and head region; aphasia

BRANCHES OF THE INTERNAL CAROTID ARTERY

Most prominent deficits after the interruption of blood flow in major intracranial branches of the internal carotid artery are summarized in Table 27-1.

Occlusion of the Anterior Cerebral Artery

The anterior cerebral artery and its branches supply blood to the medial and dorsal aspect of the frontal and parietal lobes of the cerebral hemisphere, including the postcentral gyrus (which is concerned with the processing of sensory information from the contralateral leg) and precentral gyrus (from which motor control of the contralateral leg originates). The region of the cerebral cortex supplied by the anterior cerebral artery is shown in Figure 27-7 (see also Fig. 4-2). Interruption of blood flow in the trunk of one of the anterior cerebral arteries damages the precentral gyrus and results in contralateral paralysis (contralateral hemiplegia) mainly of the leg. Occlusion of both anterior cerebral arteries produces bilateral paralysis, which is pronounced in the lower limbs. Ischemic damage to the postcentral gyrus results in impaired sensation mainly to the leg.

Occlusion of the Middle Cerebral Artery

The middle cerebral artery and its branches supply blood to the precentral gyrus (primary motor area), premotor region, the somesthetic and auditory areas, and the integrative association areas of the parietal lobe. The cerebral cortical areas supplied by the middle cerebral artery are shown in Figure 27-7 (see also Fig. 4-3). Interruption of blood flow in the main trunk of this artery results in contralateral hemiplegia predominantly in the upper extremities and face because the upper limb region is represented in a lateral position of the precentral gyrus. As described in Chapter 26, a contralateral sensory loss characterized by inability to discriminate between intensities of different stimuli may also occur. If the left hemisphere is involved, aphasia (disturbances in speech) may occur because the speech centers are located laterally in this hemisphere.

BRANCHES OF THE BASILAR ARTERY

The most prominent deficits after the occlusion of major branches of the basilar artery are summarized in Table 27-2.

Occlusion of the Posterior Cerebral Artery

The posterior cerebral artery supplies most of the midbrain, thalamus, and subthalamic nucleus (Fig. 27-7; see also Fig. 4-4). After this artery passes around the midbrain, three major branches arising from it (i.e., anterior and posterior temporal and parieto-occipital branches) supply the temporal and inferior occipital lobes of the cortex. The branch called the calcarine artery supplies the primary visual cortex.

Occlusion of branches of the posterior cerebral arteries that supply the midbrain results in midbrain infarction. Unilateral damage to the ventral region of midbrain causes **Weber's syndrome** (superior alternating hemiplegia), which is characterized by ipsilateral paresis of adduction and vertical gaze, pupillary dilation (due to damage to the ocu-

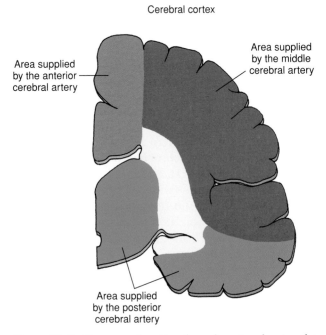

Figure 27–7 The coronal section through cortex showing the territories supplied by the anterior cerebral (blue), middle cerebral (red), and posterior cerebral (green) arteries.

Table 27–2 Deficits or Symptoms After the Interruption of Blood Flow in Major Branches of the Basilar Artery

Occluded Artery	Deficits or Symptoms
Posterior cerebral	Weber's syndrome (superior alternating hemiplegia) characterized by ipsilateral oculomotor malfunction (due to damage to the CN III) and contralateral hemiplegia (due to damage to descending corticospinal and corticobulbar tracts)
	Claude's syndrome, characterized by oculomotor paresis (due to damage to CN III) and contralateral ataxia and tremor (due to damage to the superior cerebellar peduncle)
	Parinaud's syndrome, characterized by impaired upward vertical gaze and loss of the pupillary light reflex (due to damage of the pretectal area)
	Benedikt's syndrome, characterized by oculomotor palsy (due to damage of CN III) and ataxia and tremor (due to damage to the region of the red nucleus and superior cerebellar peduncle)
	Hemianopsia (due to damage of the visual cortex)
Superior cerebellar	Ipsilateral analgesia and thermoanesthesia of the face (due to damage to the nucleus and spinal tract of the trigeminal nerve)
	Ipsilateral Horner's syndrome, characterized by constriction of ipsilateral pupil, drooping of upper eye lid, and sinking in of the eyeball due to unopposed parasympathetic effects on the eye. It is the result of injury of the descending sympathetic pathways that supply the eye.
	Contralateral loss of sensations of pain and temperature (due to damage to the spinothalamic tract)
	Ipsilateral limb and gait ataxia (due to damage to the superior cerebellar peduncle and adjoining cerebellar efferents)
Pontine paramedian	Contralateral upper motor neuron paralysis (hemiplegia due to involvement of the corticospinal tract), ipsilateral facial weakness (due to damage to the facial nucleus), and ipsilateral gaze paresis (due to damage to the pontine gaze center and abducens nucleus)
Short circumferential	Ipsilateral Horner's syndrome, due to damage to descending sympathetic fibers
	Cerebellar symptoms, due to probable damage of pontocerebellar fibers
	Contralateral hemianesthesia of the body, due to damage of the spinothalamic tract
Long circumferential	Paresis of conjugate eye movements, nystagmus, and contralateral hemianesthesia
Anterior inferior cerebellar	Ipsilateral loss of facial sensation, due to damage to CN V
	Ipsilateral Horner's syndrome
	Contralateral hemianesthesia, due to damage of the spinothalamic tract

Abbreviation: CN, cranial nerve.

lomotor nerve; see Chapters 12 and 14), and paresis of the contralateral face, arm, and leg (due to damage to the corticospinal and corticobulbar tracts).

Unilateral damage to the tegmental region of the midbrain causes **Claude's syndrome,** which is characterized by ipsilateral oculomotor paresis (due to the damage to the oculomotor nucleus) and contralateral ataxia and tremor (due to damage to the superior cerebellar peduncle).

Dorsal midbrain lesions cause **Parinaud's syndrome** (sylvian aqueduct syndrome or midbrain syndrome), which is characterized by impaired upward vertical gaze and loss of the pupillary light reflex (due to damage to the pretectal area).

Combined lesions of the ventral and tegmental midbrain cause **Benedikt's syndrome,** which is characterized by oculomotor paresis (due to damage to the rootlets of oculomotor nerve), ataxia,

and weakness (due to the damage to the region of the red nucleus and superior cerebellar peduncle).

Occlusion of the calcarine artery that supplies the primary visual cortex results in hemianopsia (see Chapter 16). CT scans taken 6 and 48 hours after the onset of a right homonymous hemianopsia, due to the embolization of the left posterior cerebral artery, are shown in Figure 27-2, A and B, respectively. A subtle loss of gray-white contrast and marked hypodensity of gray and white matter in the infarcted left visual cortex are visible after 6 and 48 hours of the onset of hemianopsia, respectively.

Occlusion of the Superior Cerebellar Artery

The superior cerebellar artery supplies the rostral pons, caudal midbrain, and the superior surface of the cerebellum (Fig. 27-8A; see also Fig. 4-1). Occlusion of this artery results in the following

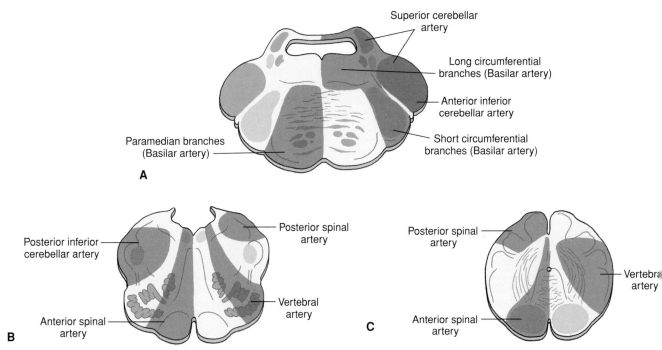

Figure 27–8 Blood supply to the pons and medulla. In all panels, the regions supplied by different arteries are shown as colored (orange) areas. (A) The regions in the pons supplied by the superior cerebellar and inferior cerebellar arteries and long and short circumferential and paramedian branches of the basilar artery are shown. (B) Medullary section through the inferior olivary nuclear complex; the regions supplied by the posterior and anterior spinal, vertebral, and posterior inferior cerebellar arteries are shown. (C) Medullary section through the posterior column nuclei; the territories supplied by the posterior and anterior spinal and vertebral arteries are shown. (Modified from Parent A: Carpenter's Human Neuroanatomy, 9th ed. Baltimore: Williams & Wilkins, 1996, p. 115.)

symptoms: (1) analgesia and thermoanesthesia on the ipsilateral side of the face due to damage to the nucleus and spinal tract of the trigeminal nerve; (2) ipsilateral Horner's syndrome, which is characterized by a triad of symptoms (constriction of ipsilateral pupil, drooping of upper eye lid, and sinking in of the eyeball); in this syndrome, there is a disruption of the descending sympathetic pathways that supply the eye, resulting in unopposed parasympathetic effects on the eye; (3) contralateral loss of sensations of pain and temperature due to damage to the spinothalamic tract; and (4) ipsilateral limb and gait ataxia due to damage to the superior cerebellar peduncle and adjoining cerebellar efferents, respectively.

Occlusion of the Pontine Paramedian Arteries

The pontine paramedian arteries arise from the basilar artery (see Fig. 4-1) and supply the medial portion of the lower and upper pons (Fig. 27-8A). Occlusion of the pontine paramedian arteries results in contralateral upper motor neuron paralysis (due to involvement of the corticospinal tract), ipsilateral facial weakness (due to damage to the fa-

cial nucleus), and ipsilateral gaze paresis (due to damage to the pontine gaze center and abducens nucleus).

Occlusion of the Short Circumferential Arteries

The short circumferential arteries supply a wedge-shaped area in the ventrolateral pons (Fig. 27-8A). Descending sympathetic fibers from the hypothalamus and portions of the trigeminal and facial nuclei and their fibers are located in the area supplied by these arteries. The most prominent effects of the occlusion of these arteries are: (1) ipsilateral Horner's syndrome (due to damage to descending sympathetic fibers); (2) cerebellar symptoms (due to probable damage of pontocerebellar fibers), and (3) contralateral hemianesthesia of the body (due to damage of the spinothalamic tract).

Occlusion of the Long Circumferential Arteries

The long circumferential arteries supply most of the tegmentum of the rostral and caudal pons (Fig. 27-8A) and lateral portions of the midbrain tegmentum. Occlusion of these arteries produces paresis of conjugate eye movements, nystagmus, and contralateral hemianesthesia.

Occlusion of the Anterior Inferior Cerebellar Artery

The anterior inferior cerebellar artery supplies the ventral surface of the cerebellum and lateral portions of the caudal pons (Fig. 27-8A). Prominent symptoms of the occlusion of this artery are: (1) ipsilateral loss of facial sensation (due to damage to cranial nerve [CN] V); (2) ipsilateral Horner's syndrome (due to disruption of descending sympathetic fibers); and (3) contralateral hemianesthesia (due to damage of the spinothalamic tract).

BRANCHES OF THE VERTEBRAL ARTERY

Prominent deficits after the interruption of blood supply in the vertebral artery and its branches are listed in Table 27-3.

Occlusion of the Anterior Spinal Artery

Two small arteries arise from the two vertebral arteries just caudal to their confluence and join to form one single anterior spinal artery (see Fig. 4-1), which supplies the medial structures of the medulla (Fig. 27-8, B and C). Occlusion of the anterior spinal artery results in the medial medullary syndrome. This syndrome is characterized by: (1)

contralateral loss of kinesthesia and discriminative touch sensation because of damage to the medial lemniscus; (2) upper motor neuron paralysis due to damage to the pyramidal tract; and (3) ipsilateral paralysis of tongue muscles, with the tongue deviating to the side of the lesion when it is protruded (due to damage to the hypoglossal nucleus). When the occlusion of the anterior spinal artery affects CN XII and the corticospinal tract, alternating hypoglossal hemiplegia results. Occlusion of the anterior spinal artery may affect fibers in the CN XII and the corticospinal tract because the two structures are juxtaposed in the medulla. This anatomic arrangement forms the basis of the inferior or hypoglossal alternating hemiplegia. This syndrome is characterized by a lower motor neuron paralysis of the ipsilateral half of the tongue and a contralateral hemiplegia.

Occlusion of the Posterior Spinal Artery

The posterior spinal artery arises from the vertebral or posterior inferior cerebellar artery (see Fig. 4-1) and supplies the fasciculus gracilis and cuneatus as well as gracile, cuneate, and spinal trigeminal nuclei, dorsal and caudal inferior cerebellar peduncles, and parts of the solitary tract and dorsal motor nucleus of vagus (Fig. 27-8, B and C). Occlusion of this artery results in loss of conscious proprioception of the ipsilateral body (due to damage of the nucleus cuneatus and gracilis).

Table 27–3 Deficits or Symptoms After the Interruption of Blood Flow in Major Branches of the Vertebral Artery

Occluded Artery	Deficits or Symptoms
Anterior spinal	Medial medullary syndrome characterized by: • Contralateral loss of conscious proprioception (due to damage of the medial lemniscus) • Upper motor neuron paralysis (due to damage to the pyramidal tract) • Deviation of the tongue to the side of the lesion when protruded, due to damage of CN XII
Posterior spinal	Loss of conscious proprioception of the ipsilateral body, due to damage of the nucleus cuneatus and gracilis
Posterior inferior cerebellar	Wallenberg's syndrome (lateral medullary syndrome) characterized by the following symptoms: • Dysphagia and dysarthria (due to damage of the nucleus ambiguus resulting in paralysis of laryngeal muscles) • Ipsilateral loss of pain and temperature of the face (due to damage of the nucleus and spinal tract of CN V) • Vertigo, nausea, vomiting, and nystagmus (due to damage of vestibular nuclei) • Ipsilateral Horner's syndrome (due to damage to descending sympathetic fibers) • Ipsilateral gait and limb ataxia (due to damage of the inferior cerebellar peduncle) • Contralateral loss of pain and temperature sensation (due to damage of the spinothalamic tract)

Abbreviation: CN, cranial nerve.

Occlusion of the Posterior Inferior Cerebellar Artery

The posterior inferior cerebellar artery arises from the vertebral artery (see Fig. 4-1) and supplies the regions of the lateral medulla (Fig. 27-8, B and C). Recall that these regions include the spinothalamic tract, dorsal and ventral spinocerebellar tracts, descending sympathetic fibers, descending tract of CN V, nucleus ambiguus, and portions of the vestibular nucleus.

Occlusion of this artery produces **Wallenberg's syndrome** (the lateral medullary syndrome; see Chapter 10). This syndrome is characterized by the following symptoms: (1) dysphagia (lack of coordination in speech), dysarthria (disturbance of articulation), and difficulty in swallowing (these symptoms are a result of the paralysis of the laryngeal muscles caused by the damage to the nucleus ambiguus, which innervates the laryngeal muscles); (2) analgesia and thermoanesthesia on the ipsilateral side of the face due to damage to the nucleus and spinal tract of the trigeminal nerve; (3) contralateral loss of pain and temperature due to damage to the spinothalamic tract; (4) vertigo, nausea, vomiting, and nystagmus due to damage to portions of the vestibular nuclei; (5) ipsilateral Horner's syndrome; and (6) ipsilateral gait and limb ataxia due to damage to the cerebellum.

STROKE

Diseases involving the blood vessels that supply the brain can cause stroke, which is characterized by an acute onset of neurologic deficit lasting for at least 24 hours. A stroke can be caused by blockage of blood vessels (occlusive stroke) or by bleeding from vessels (hemorrhagic stroke). Occlusive strokes are generally caused by atherosclerotic lesions or thrombosis in blood vessels supplying the brain. Neurologic deficits that result from occlusion of different arteries have already been described in this chapter. Hemorrhagic strokes are generally caused by long-standing high blood pressure or aneurysms in the vessels supplying the brain. When bleeding occurs at the surface of the brain, it is called an extraparenchymal hemorrhage. For example, some individuals are congenitally prone to have aneurysms at the circle of Willis that can rupture and cause subarachnoid hemorrhage. A blood clot (hematoma) is formed within the brain tissue when bleeding occurs intraparenchymally. The hematoma can obstruct blood flow to the adjacent brain tissue.

Insufficient blood flow to the brain is called **brain ischemia**; during brain ischemia, oxygen and glucose delivery to the brain tissue is reduced. In addition, toxic metabolites, such as lactic acid, cannot be removed efficiently due to reduced blood flow. Brief loss of consciousness caused by generalized cerebral ischemia due to insufficient flow of oxygenated blood to the brain is called **syncope**. Prolonged ischemia results in neuronal death, which is called **infarction**. The term "ischemia" should be distinguished from the condition known as "anoxia" in which the tissue is deprived of oxygen delivery. When the symptoms of ischemia last for short periods of time (usually 5-30 min, but less than 24 hours) and the ischemia is focal (as opposed to generalized ischemia), the term **transient ischemic attack** (TIA) is used. In a majority of cases, TIAs are caused by emboli dislodged from ulcerated atherosclerotic plaques located at the carotid bifurcation. Sometimes, reduction in the blood flow in the internal carotid artery due to atherosclerotic plaques can cause temporary interruption in the blood supply to the ipsilateral retina, which results in transient monocular blindness (fleeting blindness). There is a need for early recognition of TIAs because, if left untreated, 20% to 35% of these patients can develop permanent cerebral infarction.

Drugs that prevent or reduce platelet aggregation (e.g., aspirin) must be used for prophylaxis of stroke in patients with carotid stenosis. A vascular surgical procedure, called **carotid endarterectomy**, is beneficial in patients in whom marked stenosis (greater than 70%) of the carotid artery is present. In this surgical procedure, the common carotid artery and a portion of the external carotid artery are slit open by a longitudinal cut, and atherosclerotic plaques are removed. However, the procedure carries a risk of causing a stroke postoperatively due to dislodging of thrombi formed at the site where surgery is performed.

Drug treatment for TIAs and stroke include administration of agents that prevent or reduce platelet aggregation (e.g., aspirin, clopidogrel, and tirofiban), anticoagulants (e.g., heparin and warfarin), and thrombolytic agents (e.g., streptokinase, urokinase, and **tissue plasminogen activator [t-PA]**). The mechanism by which aspirin prevents or inhibits platelet aggregation can be summarized as follows. Normally, arachidonic acid (a 20-carbon fatty acid) is mobilized from membrane phospholipids by phospholipases. Arachidonic acid is then oxygenated by the enzyme cyclooxygenase (COX), and the prostaglandin, thromboxane A2, is formed. In pathological situations, thromboxane A2 released from the platelets promotes aggregation of platelets. Aspirin in low doses (81 mg) causes an irreversible acetylation of the enzyme cyclooxygenase and inhibits thromboxane synthesis in platelets. Reduction of thromboxane synthesis in platelets results in reduced release of this prostaglandin, leading to prevention or reduction of platelet aggregation. Adenosine diphosphate (ADP), another substance released from platelets in pathological situations, is also a platelet aggregator. Drugs like clopidogrel (Plavix) block ADP formation and thus prevent or attenuate platelet aggregation. Glycoprotein (GP) receptors (e.g., GP IIb/IIIa receptors), which are located on platelet membrane, bind fibrinogen and other molecules and promote clot formation. Activation of these GP receptors promotes platelet aggregation. Recently, drugs that block GP receptors on the platelets have been developed to prevent platelet aggregation. For example, tirofiban (Aggrastat) blocks GP IIb/IIIa receptors on the platelets and prevents their aggregation. As mentioned earlier, thrombolytic drugs (e.g., streptokinase, urokinase, and t-PA) lyse blood clots (thrombi) and are, therefore, useful in the treatment of stroke.

CLINICAL CASE

HISTORY

Joyce is a 76-year-old woman who has chronic hypertension. One morning, when she was walking in her house, she suddenly fell down and was taken to the emergency room. A CT scan and MRI of her head and an angiogram of the cerebral vasculature were taken. She was subsequently transferred to the Neurology Service.

EXAMINATION

The neurologic examination revealed that Joyce had myoclonus (rapid movements of her hands), dysarthria, nystagmus, Horner's syndrome, and some contralateral loss of pain and temperature. She also displayed a tremor of her right hand. The MRI scan of her head, angiogram of the cerebral vasculature, and neurologic evaluation revealed that Joyce had a stroke involving the right superior cerebellar artery.

EXPLANATION

Major symptoms of the superior cerebellar artery syndrome are ipsilateral intention tremor, limb ataxia, Horner's syndrome, some contralateral loss of pain and temperature, and nystagmus. The superior cerebellar artery supplies the superior cerebellar peduncle, dorsal surface of the cerebellum, the rostral part of the tegmentum of the pons, and parts of the midbrain, which include CN III and IV and the median longitudinal fasciculus.

CT scan and MRI of the head were performed to determine whether there was an existing subarachnoid or intracerebral bleed. The presence of an ongoing bleed would have required Joyce to be referred to a neurosurgeon. The angiogram was taken to rule out an aneurysm. In this case, there was a short-term bleed that affected the dorsal part of the cerebellum, superior cerebellar peduncle, and rostral pons. After some time in the Neurology ward, Joyce's condition stabilized, and she was sent to the Rehabilitation Service. Because the disorder was limited to the superior cerebellar artery, the patient showed considerable recovery within 6 months and was able to return home.

CHAPTER TEST

QUESTIONS

Choose the best answer for each question.

1. The diagram to the right represents a cross section of the cerebral cortex of a 65-year-old woman who suffered from a stroke and was admitted to an emergency room. The neurologist who examined her marked the infarcted region in her brain as a dark shaded area in the diagram. Occlusion of which one of the following arteries may have caused an infarction in the region represented by the shaded area in this diagram?

   a. Anterior cerebral artery
   b. Middle cerebral artery
   c. Posterior cerebral artery
   d. Anterior choroidal artery
   e. Superior cerebellar artery

Cerebral cortex

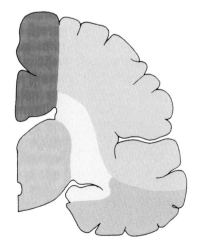

2. The figure shown below represents a cross section of the cerebral cortex of a 70-year-old stroke patient. The dark shaded region indicates a lesion resulting from an occlusion of which one of the following arteries?

a. Anterior cerebral artery
b. Middle cerebral artery
c. Posterior cerebral artery
d. Anterior choroidal artery
e. Superior cerebellar artery

Cerebral cortex

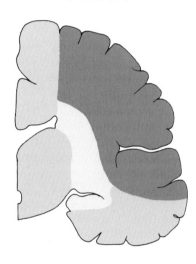

3. The diagram below represents a cross section of the medulla of a 55-year-old man who was admitted to the emergency room and was diagnosed as having had a stroke. Occlusion of which one of the following arteries may have caused an infarct in the dark shaded region of this diagram?

a. Posterior inferior cerebellar artery
b. Paramedian branches of the basilar artery
c. Posterior cerebral artery
d. Anterior cerebral artery
e. Superior cerebellar artery

Medulla

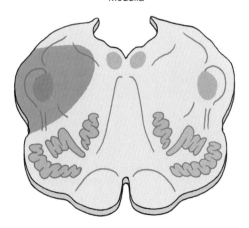

4. The diagram below represents a cross section of the lower pons of a stroke patient. The dark shaded region indicates a lesion resulting from an occlusion of which one of the following arteries?

a. Posterior inferior cerebellar artery
b. Anterior inferior cerebellar artery
c. Paramedian branches of the basilar artery
d. Anterior cerebral artery
e. Superior cerebellar artery

Lower pons

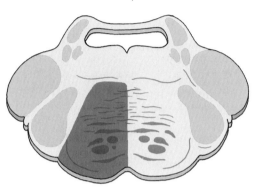

5. The diagram below represents a cross section of the upper pons of a 68-year-old stroke patient. The dark shaded region indicates an infarct resulting from an occlusion of which one of the following arteries?

a. Anterior cerebral artery
b. Middle cerebral artery
c. Posterior cerebral artery
d. Anterior choroidal artery
e. Superior cerebellar artery

Upper pons

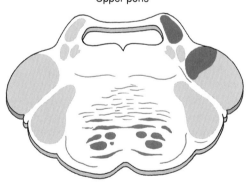

ANSWERS AND EXPLANATIONS

1. Answer: a

The dark shaded area represents the territory supplied by the anterior cerebral artery. It comprises dorsal and medial parts of the cerebral hemisphere, including parts of the frontal and parietal lobes and pre- and postcentral gyri. Symptoms due to occlusion of this artery include contralateral hemiplegia (more pronounced in the leg) and impaired sensation.

2. Answer: b

The dark shaded area represents the territory supplied by the middle cerebral artery. It includes the lateral convexity of the cerebral hemispheres, as well as parts of the temporal, frontal, parietal, and occipital lobes. Symptoms due to occlusion of this artery can be contralateral hemiplegia (more pronounced in the arm), contralateral sensory loss (inability to discriminate between intensities of different stimuli), or aphasia.

3. Answer: a

The dark shaded area represents the territory supplied by the posterior inferior cerebellar artery. It comprises the lateral structures of the medulla including the spinothalamic tract, rubrospinal tract, the spinal trigeminal nucleus and tract, dorsal motor nucleus of vagus, and parts of the cerebellar hemisphere. Some deficits that can occur after occlusion of this artery are: the lateral medullary syndrome of Wallenberg (characterized by ipsilateral facial thermoanesthesia and analgesia, vertigo, nausea, vomiting, and nystagmus), ipsilateral Horner's syndrome, ipsilateral gait and limb ataxia, and contralateral loss of pain and temperature sensation.

4. Answer: c

The dark shaded area represents the territory supplied by the paramedian branches of the basilar artery. It includes the medial part of the pons including the pontine nuclei and the corticopontine, corticospinal, and corticobulbar tracts.

5. Answer: e

The dark shaded area represents the territory supplied by the superior cerebellar artery. It includes the rostral pons and superior cerebellar peduncle. The deficits following occlusion of this artery may be sympathetic disturbances, nystagmus, paresis of conjugate eye movements, and contralateral hemianesthesia. See text for details.

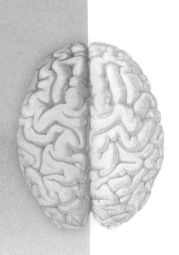

CHAPTER 28

BEHAVIORAL AND PSYCHIATRIC DISORDERS

OBJECTIVES

After reading this chapter, the student should understand and/or identify:

1. The behavioral and clinical characteristics of the major psychiatric and behavioral disorders (i.e., schizophrenia, depression, anxiety, and addiction)

2. The major transmitters that are thought to be linked to the expression of these disorders

3. The rationale for the pharmacological approaches applied to the treatment of these disorders

4. The brain regions that may be associated with these disorders

Over the past several decades, significant progress has been made concerning our understanding of the neural bases of the varied processes that comprise human behavior. Illustrations of such processes include sensation, perception, motor functions, learning, memory, and mood states. As a result of the explosion of knowledge of the neural bases of behavior, inroads have also been made in our understanding of the neural correlates of disorders of thought, mood, and **anxiety**. However, the acquisition of new knowledge is somewhat tempered by the lack of precise definitions of the different disorders, as well as difficulties in carrying out well-controlled studies in humans. For example, the term "schizophrenia" may not represent a unitary disorder but, instead, may encompass different disease states. As a result, studies may likely be conducted on a heterogenous rather than a homogenous population with respect to this disorder. Another major problem in conducting these studies is that it is difficult to dissociate the effects of long-term drug treatment from the behavioral disorder on neural and behavioral functions examined in the patient. Nevertheless, in this chapter, we attempt to identify and summarize the present state of knowledge of these behavioral disorders and the rationale for drug and related therapies used in the treatment of these disorders.

SCHIZOPHRENIA

BEHAVIORAL ASPECTS

Schizophrenia is a disorder characterized by psychosis, which is a dysfunction in the thought process in which the ability to correctly test reality is lacking. The general or primary criteria for schizophrenia include one or more of the following: delusional thought processes (i.e., false beliefs); disturbances in speech, appearance, and behavior; hallucinations (i.e., false perceptions: mostly auditory, such as hearing voices); apathy; a paucity of emotion; and the presence of a catatonic posture. Overall, there is an inability to perceive the world accurately.

MAJOR SUBTYPES

Paranoid Schizophrenia

Individuals suffering from paranoid schizophrenia are typically preoccupied with hallucinations (mainly auditory; i.e., hearing voices) or delusions, such as persecution, personal exaltation, or having a specific mission.

Disorganized (Hebephrenic) Schizophrenia

Disorganized schizophrenia is characterized by a flat affect, which is mostly inappropriate and incongruous. The consequent speech is often incoherent, disjointed, and rambling. Delusions and hallucinations play an insignificant role in this form of schizophrenia.

Catatonic Schizophrenia

Catatonic schizophrenia is characterized by one (or more) of the following: stupor, a decrease in reactivity to the environment, purposeless motor activity, rigidity of posture that may appear bizarre, resistance in responding to instructions, and placing of the body in externally imposed positions. Presently, this type of schizophrenia appears to be quite rare.

Undifferentiated Schizophrenia

In undifferentiated schizophrenia, the individual displays one or more of the general criteria listed for the other types of schizophrenia just described but cannot be clearly placed into one of these types.

COURSE OF DEVELOPMENT

In characterizing the development of schizophrenia, three phases may be identified. Prior to the first phase, premorbid signs appear suggesting the possibility of future onset of the disease. These signs could include schizoid behavior (characterized by passive and introverted behavior), where the patient withdraws from social contact. As the disorder evolves, the first phase includes **prodromal signs**, which typically precede the onset of the first psychotic episode. The patient initially expresses physical complaints, such as muscle pain and headaches, as well as an increased interest in religion, philosophy, and the occult. The patient may also display bizarre thoughts, distorted perception, and unusual speech. In the second or *psychotic stage*, the patient loses touch with reality. This loss is reflected by **positive symptoms**, which include hallucinations (such as hearing voices) and delusions (such as a feeling of persecution), and **negative symptoms**, which include disorganized thinking (expressed by the absence of normal association of thoughts, poor speech, and loss of affect). In the time between psychotic episodes, a **residual phase** takes place in which the patient is in touch with reality. However, even in the residual phase, the patient displays a flat affect, is withdrawn, and continues to have bizarre or eccentric (deviating from the normal pattern) thinking.

HEREDITARY FACTORS

In considering the etiology of schizophrenia, one of the most important discoveries has been the finding of a **genetic predisposition** to this disease. In a series of well-known studies conducted in the 1930s, the incidence of schizophrenia between identical (monozygotic) and fraternal (dizygotic) twins was compared. In identical twins, the genomes are virtually the same for both siblings, whereas approximately 50% of the genomes are shared by the fraternal twins. The most significant finding of this study was the concordance of the disease between the twins. If one identical twin had schizophrenia, then the occurrence of schizophrenia in the other twin ranged from 45% to 50%. In contrast, if one fraternal twin had schizophrenia, then the occurrence of this disease for the other twin was 10% to 15%.

While these findings provided support for the theory of a genetic core disposition, it did not necessarily exclude environmental factors because it was certainly possible that the environmental conditions for the identical twins studied could have been more similar than for fraternal twins. Consequently, other studies were conducted to further separate the environmental and genetic variables. This was achieved by investigators who demonstrated that: (1) the incidence of schizophrenia in twins reared by adoptive parents was similar to the rate for twin siblings reared by their biological parents, and (2) the incidence of schizophrenia was considerably higher in adopted children whose biological parents had schizophrenia.

Thus, the evidence clearly indicates that genetic factors play an important role in the etiology of schizophrenia. Recent studies have suggested that the genetic transmission of schizophrenia involves a combination of genes. Some reports have implicated the short arm of chromosome 19, the X chromosome, and the long arms of chromosomes 5, 11, and 18. Others have implicated chromosome 6 and the long arm of chromosome 22.

It should be pointed out that, while this evidence supports the notion of a genetic factor, psychosocial factors undoubtedly play a role as well. There is an extensive literature (which goes well beyond the scope of this book) involving psychoanalytic, psychodynamic, and learning theories that provide alternative interpretations of the etiology of this disease.

BRAIN ABNORMALITIES

Proponents of the view that schizophrenia results from brain dysfunction have suggested that neuropathological processes underlie neuronal loss in specific regions of the brain beginning *in utero* and continuing in the postnatal period. The rationale for this view is based on the observations that schizophrenics frequently exhibit cognitive and behavioral abnormalities during childhood or adolescence, and those elements of brain pathology have been identified in adults diagnosed with this disorder.

Attention has been given to the possible brain regions affected by maladaptive development in schizophrenics. One of the more impressive findings involved studies using magnetic resonance imaging (MRI) in twins. It was observed that if one twin was normal and the other was diagnosed with schizophrenia, then the lateral ventricles were enlarged only in the schizophrenic twin but not in the normal one. The enlargement of the ventricles results in damage to structures that lie proximal to the ventricle. These structures include the hippocampal formation, amygdala, cingulate gyrus, and parts of the ventral aspect of the pallidum. Postmortem examination of the brains of schizophrenics revealed decreases in the sizes of the hippocampal formation, amygdala, parahippocampal gyrus, and prefrontal cortex.

The involvement of limbic structures has been suspected because of their role in regulating emotional behavior. The association of the basal ganglia with schizophrenia is based on two factors: the first includes the extensive connections with the prefrontal cortex, and the second is that many schizophrenic patients exhibit movements characteristic of those associated with diseases of the basal ganglia, even in the absence of drug treatment. The prefrontal cortex has been linked with schizophrenia for a number of reasons. The first is that loss of neurons in the prefrontal cortex has been noted in schizophrenic patients. Second, the prefrontal cortex has been known to play an important, if not critical, role in cognitive functions, which are significantly affected in these patients. Third, a current leading neurochemical hypothesis, **the dopamine hypothesis**, focuses on the role of dopamine and its relationship to limbic and cortical structures, including the prefrontal cortex. This hypothesis is discussed in more detail in the next section. It should be pointed out, however, that the unequivocal evidence linking specific brain sites to this disorder have yet to be established. The available evidence suggests that, perhaps, schizophrenia results from dysfunction of different groups of neurons located mainly in the forebrain but that may also include brainstem monoaminergic groups as well.

NEUROCHEMICAL FACTORS

Extensive research concerning the neurochemistry of schizophrenia has provided evidence that a variety of transmitters may be implicated in this disorder.

Dopamine

The dopamine hypothesis of schizophrenia has prompted considerable research over the past two decades. The theory in its simplest form postulates that schizophrenia results from excess dopaminergic activity. The arguments in support of this hypothesis stem from the following lines of evidence. (1) Antipsychotic drugs, such as chlorpromazine, which have been used effectively for the treatment of schizophrenia by reducing hallucinations, delusions, and bizarre thinking, also block dopamine-D_2 receptors. Although five dopamine receptor subtypes (i.e., D_1, D_2, D_3, D_4, and D_5) have now been cloned, many antipsychotic drugs have a high affinity for D_2 receptors, suggesting that the D_2 receptor is a major site for the action of these drugs. (2) Chronic administration of high doses of amphetamine (which releases dopamine and other biogenic amines) produces schizophrenic-like symptoms. (3) Specific regions of the brain, such as the prefrontal cortex and limbic system, which have been linked to schizophrenia, receive significant dopaminergic inputs from the **mesocortical** and **mesolimbic** dopaminergic pathways, respectively.

Although the dopamine hypothesis still remains popular, there are some data that are not consistent with this hypothesis. These data include: (1) the absence of a relationship between schizophrenia and dopamine or its acidic metabolite, homovanillic acid, in relevant areas of the brain or in the cerebrospinal fluid (CSF); and (2) the inconsistencies in findings attempting to relate changes in dopamine D_2 receptor densities in nonmedicated schizophrenic patients relative to normal control subjects. In addition, there is also a lack of a clear understanding of the specific dopaminergic mechanism that serves to trigger schizophrenic behavior. As previously indicated, earlier views proposed that schizophrenia is associated with excess release of dopamine. Later views represented a modification of this hypothesis by suggesting the presence of any one or more of the following: (1) involvement of either D_3 or D_4 dopamine receptors, whose actions may be inhibitory rather than excitatory; (2) a reduction in dopamine receptor densities in schizophrenic patients; (3) hypoactivity of the mesocortical dopamine system with respect to the prefrontal cortex, rather than dopamine hyperactivity in this region as originally thought; or (4) an association of schizophrenia with an increase in activity of the mesolimbic dopamine system coupled with a decrease in the mesocortical system.

Serotonin

Although serotonin has been clearly associated with mood disorders (see discussion on pages 512–515), there is a body of literature that suggests that alterations in serotonin play a role in the development of cognitive impairment as well as positive and negative symptoms associated with schizophrenia. The hypothesis that the etiology of schizophrenia involves deficiencies in serotonin was based largely on studies using lysergic acid diethylamide (LSD), which was believed to antagonize 5-HT receptors and which caused visual hallucinations, a phenomenon remotely related to schizophrenia. Later studies indicated that LSD, instead, contained agonistic properties with respect to the 5-HT_{2A} receptor.

The more significant evidence in support of a serotonin hypothesis stems from drug studies. For example, clozapine, which is a potent 5-HT_{2A} and a weak dopamine D_2 receptor antagonist, has been shown to be effective in treating the positive symptoms associated with schizophrenia. However, because clozapine has also been shown to have a high affinity for histamine receptors and to cause increased extracellular concentrations of acetylcholine in the frontal cortex (of rats), it is likely that 5-HT interactions with other transmitter systems may account for the positive effects seen with this drug. Additional evidence in support of the serotonin hypothesis include such findings as a decrease in 5-HT_{2A} receptor binding in the prefrontal, cingulate, visual, and temporal cortices of schizophrenics and an increase in the density of 5-HT_{1A} receptors in the cortex and hippocampus in these patients. It is possible that the opposing effects on these receptor subtypes might have synergistic effects on processes associated with the development of schizophrenia. What is left unclear is whether the process of schizophrenia involves an increase or decrease in the release of serotonin. Only further research will help to clarify this issue.

Other Transmitters

Investigators have made attempts to implicate other neurotransmitters in schizophrenia. Studies examining the roles of γ-aminobutyric acid (GABA), acetylcholine, and excitatory amino acids have generally been conflicting and difficult to assess. Recent studies have attempted to implicate such neuropeptides as neurotensin and cholecystokinin (CCK) in the etiology of this disorder. The primary basis for studying these peptides is that they are frequently co-localized with dopamine in the midbrain and forebrain, including the cerebral cortex. However, the studies to date concerning these peptides have been incomplete and, at times, contradictory.

In summary, the studies conducted over the past few decades suggest that changes in the dopaminergic and perhaps serotoninergic systems play important roles in the etiology of schizophrenia. Because schizophrenia is such a complex disorder and these transmitter systems are known to interact with other transmitters, it is likely that a better characterization will be one that is not limited to a single neurotransmitter system.

DEPRESSION AND OTHER MOOD DISORDERS

Under ordinary conditions, individuals experience various emotions in which moods may vary from depressed to normal and elevated states. One of the basic differences between so-called "normal" individuals and those who experience a "mood disorder" is that the normal individual feels in control of his emotions, while one who is suffering from a mood disorder feels that he has lost control of his emotions. Disorders of mood states may take different forms, such as **unipolar** (depression or **dysthymia**), **bipolar**, or **cyclothymic** disorder. These disorders reflect disturbances in the emotional state of the patient, which is often highly distressful and results in difficulties in being able to function.

MAJOR DEPRESSIVE (UNIPOLAR) DISORDER

Because of the behavioral complexity of the disorder and the variations it may take in different individuals, it is probable that major depression reflects several (if not more) disease states. Nevertheless, there are features of major depression that appear, in general, to be common among individuals. The patient typically feels sad, helpless, guilty, and has low esteem. There is a lack of motivation, decreased appetite, and weight loss, and sleep patterns are poor. Feelings of anxiety are present, as well as suicidal ideation.

Major depression may include other characteristics. A few of these are identified here. Some patients express denial of the disorder and will seek out a general practitioner rather than a psychiatrist in response to physical symptoms that appear to be vague. This is called "masked depression." Depressive disorders may also be seasonal, called "seasonal affective disorder," which appears to occur more frequently during the winter months when there are fewer hours of sunlight. As indicated earlier, there is also an increased risk for

suicide. A variety of factors appear to contribute to suicidal tendencies. These include a previous serious suicide attempt, family history of depression, and, in particular, having a parent who committed suicide. Other factors include a serious medical condition such as cancer, substance abuse, a divorced person living alone, age (e.g., people over 65 years and adolescents), an individual at the initial stages of recovery from severe depression, impulsiveness, a feeling of hopelessness, and having psychotic symptoms or severe depression.

BIPOLAR DISORDER

Bipolar disorders are characterized by distinct episodes of both mania and depression and have been subdivided into *bipolar I* and *bipolar II* disorders. Bipolar I disorder is characterized by depression and clear-cut manic symptoms present during the course of the disease. Some of the manic symptoms include a tendency to be quick to anger and easily bothered (i.e., impulsive and irritable responses), a lack of modesty in dress, assaultive behavior, delusions of grandeur and power, and intense feelings of happiness and well-being. In bipolar II disorder, depression is coupled instead with hypomania. Some of the symptoms include a specific period of elevated, irritable, or expansive mood; a decreased need for sleep; inflated self-esteem; highly talkative; distracted behavior where attention is given to trivial stimuli; an increase in goal-directed behavior; and involvement in activities considered pleasurable but that can have significant negative consequences such as sexual indiscretions and buying sprees.

DYSTHYMIA AND CYCLOTHYMIA

The major feature of **dysthymic** disorder is the continued presence of a depressed state lasting most of the day and for most days, extending for a period of 2 years with no discrete episodes of the illness (as is the case with bipolar disorders). The patient may display irritability, anger, guilt, withdrawal from society, or a lack of both activity and productivity.

The major feature of **cyclothymic** disorder is that it basically reflects a mild form of bipolar II disorder in which there are episodes of mild depression and hypomania. However, in contrast to bipolar II disorder, there are no clear-cut discrete episodes associated with cyclothymia.

HEREDITARY FACTORS

Research studies suggest that genetic factors may play significant roles in both depression and bipolar disorders. One line of evidence is based on the observations that first-degree relatives of major depressive disorder probands (i.e., the patient or family member bringing a family under study) are much more likely to have this disorder than similar relationships obtained from a control population. Parallel findings have been reported with respect to individuals suffering from bipolar disorder. Moreover, with respect to depression, the concordance rate for monozygotic twins is much higher than for dizygotic twins. However, studies attempting to link specific chromosomal variations with this disorder have not yielded uniform results, and, accordingly, further studies are required to support a genetic factor as determined from chromosomal analysis.

BRAIN ABNORMALITIES

In general, the findings from studies attempting to identify specific regions of the brain linked to depression and related disorders have been inconclusive, but studies using positron emission tomography (PET) and MRI scans (see Chapter 27) have provided evidence of possible prefrontal cortical involvement. It should be pointed out that this region of the cortex has both direct and indirect projections to the hypothalamus, amygdala, and midbrain periaqueductal gray. These are areas of the brain that are significantly involved in the regulation of emotional behavior. That the prefrontal cortex is involved in depressive disorders is supported by studies showing that lesions of this region enhance aggression and disrupt thought processes and the making of rational decisions. It remains for future research to determine the extent to which dysfunctions involving other regions of the brain contribute to depressive disorders.

NEUROCHEMICAL FACTORS

Based, in part, on the known ubiquitous projections of the monoamine neurons to the forebrain (Figs. 28-1 and 28-2), most studies have focused on the role of *biogenic amines* in the etiology of depression and other mood disorders. In fact, one of the longest running theories of depression has been the *catecholamine hypothesis*, which states that a deficiency in catecholamines causes depression and that mania results from an excess of catecholamines, especially at key synaptic regions of the brain. While this theory is generally not followed in its original form, it has generated considerable research. Later studies expanded on this hypothesis to include serotonin as well.

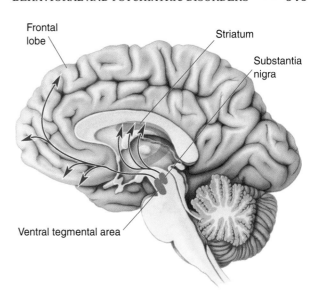

Figure 28–1 Dopaminergic pathways and depression. Schematic diagram indicating the distribution of the major dopaminergic pathways. (From Bear MF, et al.: Neuroscience: Exploring the Brain, 2nd ed. Philadelphia: Lippincott Williams & Wilkins, 2001, p. 697.)

Dopamine

The arguments in support of the view that dopamine is involved in depressive disorders comes from several sources. First is the finding that reserpine, which causes depletion of stores of monoamines and which was originally used to treat schizophrenia and hypertension, produced depressive-like symptoms. However, neuroleptics, which are used to treat psychotic disorders and which are known to block dopamine receptors, do not appear to cause depression. Second, Parkinsonism, which involves depletion of dopamine, is sometimes associated with depression (although there may be other factors involved). Third, drugs that increase concentrations of dopamine, such as tyrosine and amphetamine, tend to reduce the symptoms of depression as well as induce hypomania, which was observed after administration of the metabolic precursor of dopamine, levodopa (L-DOPA). Likewise, dopamine antagonists have been effective in treating hypomania (as it relates to bipolar disorder).

Norepinephrine

With respect to norepinephrine, several of the arguments presented earlier for dopamine involvement would also apply in implicating norepinephrine in depressive disorders because a number of the drugs that were used affected both dopamine and norepinephrine and others affected all of the monoamines. In addition, drugs such as venlafaxine hydrochloride (Effexor) (a potent re-uptake

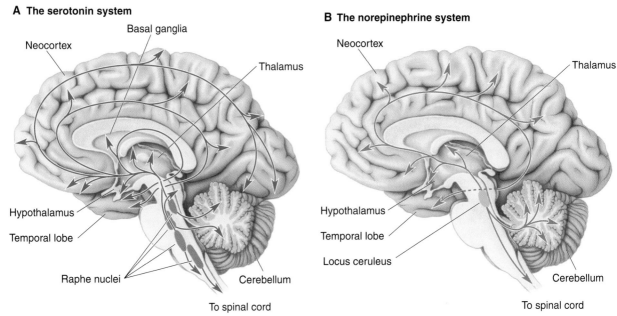

Figure 28–2 Serotonergic and noradrenergic pathways in depression. Schematic diagrams illustrating the distribution of the: (A) serotonergic pathways that arise from the raphe nuclei, and (B) noradrenergic pathways that arise from the nucleus locus ceruleus and other regions of the brainstem reticular formation. Both of these monoaminergic systems project to all parts of the central nervous system but, in particular, to the forebrain. (From Bear MF, et al.: Neuroscience: Exploring the Brain, 2nd ed. Philadelphia: Lippincott Williams & Wilkins, 2001, p. 697.)

inhibitor of norepinephrine and serotonin) have been shown to have antidepressant activity, and research studies have also shown a correlation between down-regulation of β-adrenergic receptors and antidepressant responses.

Serotonin

In recent years, considerable attention has been given to the role of serotonin in depressive disorders. Similar to dopamine and norepinephrine, serotonin has a ubiquitous distribution to wide areas of the forebrain, including regions normally associated with mood disorders. The most striking findings identifying serotonin as a key neurotransmitter involved in depression were the improved conditions of patients following administration of specific serotonin re-uptake inhibitors for the treatment of this disorder. Examples of these drugs include fluoxetine (Prozac) and sertraline (Zoloft). There are several other classes of antidepressant drugs that affect serotonin concentrations or serotonin receptors. One class includes **monoamine oxidase inhibitors**, such as iproniazid, which maintain or increase serotonin (and other monoamine) levels and which have been shown to be effective antidepressant drugs. Likewise, **tricyclic compounds**, such as amitriptyline, which also increase monoamine concentrations, help to diminish depressive states.

Other studies support a serotonin hypothesis of depression. These studies resulted in the observations that: (1) serotonin depletion has been correlated with the onset of depression; (2) in certain patients, low CSF levels of 5-hydroxy-indoleacetic acid (5-HIAA) have been associated with suicide; and (3) there are changes in 5-HT$_{1A}$ and 5-HT$_{2A}$ receptors in the prefrontal cortex of suicide victims.

THE ROLE OF LITHIUM FOR TREATMENT OF BIPOLAR DISORDER

For approximately three decades, **lithium** has been used for the treatment of bipolar disorder because it had been shown to reduce the intensity, recurrence, and length of the manic phase (and has been reported to have positive effects on the depressive phase as well). However, a specific mechanism by which lithium produces its positive effects has yet to be elucidated. Nevertheless, research studies have revealed that lithium generates a variety of effects on neural tissue. Several of these include: (1) changes in G-protein expression, adenylyl cyclase, and monoamine receptors; (2) effects on release and uptake of catecholamines; and (3) effects on brain phosphoinositide systems. It has been suggested that these changes might form the basis of the positive effects obtained from lithium for treatment of mania and depression.

NEUROENDOCRINE FUNCTION AND SLEEP

Patients with depressive disorders also experience neuroendocrine and sleep dysfunctions, which, in turn, can have serious effects on the psychiatric condition.

Concerning neuroendocrine function, significant changes in thyroid, reproductive, and adrenal hormonal activities have often been reported. Release of the anterior pituitary hormone, thyrotropin, and thyrotropin-releasing hormone in the hypothalamus are often reduced. For this reason, thyroid hormone treatment in patients with unipolar or bipolar disorder has been found to be helpful.

With respect to reproductive hormones, there is a decrease in the basal levels of follicle-stimulating hormone, luteinizing hormone, and testosterone (in males). It is possible that estrogen treatment may be effective for women suffering from premenstrual, menopausal, or postpartum depression. Likewise, the adrenal androgen, dehydroepiandrosterone, may also be helpful in treating depression in older men.

An established finding has been the correlation between the time of occurrence of a major depression and hypersecretion of cortisol (which is released from the adrenal cortex by the pituitary hormone, adrenocorticotropic hormone [ACTH], which in turn, is controlled by the paraventricular nucleus of the hypothalamus). Postmortem examination of depressed patients revealed higher levels of the corticotropin-releasing hormone in the hypothalamus as well as elevated levels of cortisol in the urine and blood. These observations suggest that administration of inhibitors of corticotropin-releasing hormone might reduce the symptoms of depression.

Sleep dysfunctions are also common in depressive disorders. Examples of sleep abnormalities include a shortened latency to rapid eye movement (REM) sleep (see Chapter 23), extended length of REM sleep and early morning awakening, delayed onset of sleep, and a lack of sleep.

ANXIETY DISORDERS

Anxiety, a normal response to a real or perceived dangerous situation that is present in our lives daily, is generally a practical, useful, and adaptive reaction for an individual. However, when anxiety reactions occur in response to environmental or perceived stimuli that, objectively, should not evoke such reactions or when anxiety reactions are elevated to levels that disrupt behavior, anxiety is said to be maladaptive and, thus, constitutes a form of behavioral disorder. In fact, of all the psychiatric illnesses, anxiety reactions are the most common, and additionally, they are symptoms in many other psychiatric disorders as well.

The *Diagnostic and Statistical Manual of Mental Disorders* (DSM-IV) lists different categories of anxiety disorders. Major categories of anxiety include panic attack, obsessive-compulsive disorder, posttraumatic stress disorder, and generalized anxiety disorder. A brief discussion of each of these disorders follows, together with their neurochemical correlates (where such information is available).

PANIC DISORDER

According to the DSM-IV classification, panic attack is defined as a "discrete period of intense fear or discomfort." During a given attack, which normally lasts for approximately 30 minutes or less, the patient typically exhibits symptoms such as shortness of breath, palpitations, sweating, trembling, and fear that he or she is going crazy or will die. Repeated episodes of panic attack are referred to as **panic disorder**. This disorder is sometimes accompanied by a condition called **agoraphobia**, which is a fear of leaving a familiar place. This kind of fear would require the patient to be escorted by a friend or family member into a crowded street or closed-in places such as a tunnel, elevator, or bridge.

From the results of various studies, there is some evidence suggesting that there may be a genetic component to this disorder. Such studies indicate that the risk of panic disorder is much higher if first-degree relatives have this disorder in contrast to first-degree relatives of patients with other psychiatric disorders. In addition, on the basis of co-twin studies, there is a higher concordance for panic disorder between monozygotic twins than dizygotic twins.

Panic attacks can be induced in some patients with this disorder by administering sodium lactate, a CCK agonist, or by inhaling carbon dioxide. Patients are also sensitive to caffeine and the α_2-adrenergic receptor antagonist, yohimbine. In normal individuals, these substances are not effective in inducing panic attacks. The neurobiology of panic disorders remains poorly understood, and we have little knowledge of the specific brain regions that mediate this form of anxiety disorder.

Several approaches have been used in treating panic disorder. One approach has been the application of cognitive and other behavior therapies. This approach has met with success, and individuals receiving such therapy have had long-lasting remission of their symptoms. The other successful approach involves pharmacotherapy. Some reports suggest that the most effective approach has been to combine pharmacotherapy with cognitive or other behavior therapies. Concerning pharmacotherapy, the most effective drugs for the treatment of panic disorders are considered to be serotonin-specific re-uptake inhibitors (SSRI). Although there have been wide, varying effects of these drugs, in general, drugs such as paroxetine (Paxil), sertraline, and flu-voxamine (Luvox) have been used in recent years with considerable success.

Other classes of drugs have also been used with varying degrees of success. One class includes **benzodiazepines**, such as lorazepam (Ativan), which work rapidly against panic. Benzodiazepines are used as a first drug in the treatment of panic disorder; the drug is later replaced by a drug-blocking serotonin re-uptake. However, a problem with the long-term use of benzodiazepines is that they could lead to drug abuse, drug dependence, and cognitive impairment. Tricyclic antidepressant drugs, such as **clomipramine**, and SSRIs, like paroxetine, have also been used successfully for the treatment of this disorder. Another class of drugs, the monoamine oxidase inhibitors (such as phenelzine [Nardil]), has also has been used but appears to require high doses to be effective.

OBSESSIVE-COMPULSIVE DISORDER

The DSM-IV defines obsessive-compulsive disorder as recurring obsessions or compulsions that are sufficiently severe to be time consuming or cause impairment and distress The **obsession** is a recurring sensation, thought, feeling, or idea that elevates anxiety levels; while the **compulsion** is a reaction that reduces anxiety levels (e.g., the need to wash ones's hands after touching any object). Because these responses are so irrational and disproportionate to reality, obsessive-compulsive disorders can be quite disabling and time consuming.

A number of brain imaging studies have been conducted to identify the possible brain regions associated with this disorder. Most, if not all, of the studies have identified the orbitofrontal cortex and adjoining regions of the dorsolateral and medial aspects of the prefrontal cortex as key areas (Fig. 28-3). Several other regions related to the orbitofrontal cortex, including the caudate nucleus (which receives many fibers from the prefrontal cortex), cingulate cortex, and parts of the dorsal thalamus, have also been linked with this disorder.

Neurochemical studies and clinical investigations have provided support for the view that serotonin plays some role in this disorder since serotonergic drugs have been more effective than other classes of drugs. In particular, the serotonin re-uptake inhibitors are effective in treating this disorder as is behavioral (conditioning) therapy.

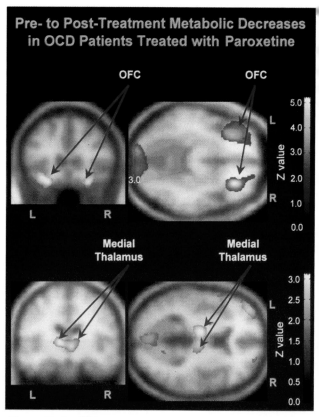

Figure 28–3 [^{18}F] Fluorodeoxyglucose PET scans of representative patients in the horizontal plane at a mid level of the caudate nucleus before and after successful drug treatment of obsessive-compulsive disorder (OCD). Scans are processed to reflect the ratio of glucose metabolic rate registered by each pixel element, divided by that of the whole brain. Abbreviations: Behav, behavioral; Tx, treatment. (Courtesy of Dr. L. Baxter.)

This would imply that dysregulation of the serotonin system in a "downward" direction contributes to the obsessive-compulsive disorder and that psychotherapy may serve to readjust the levels of serotonin to normal values.

POSTTRAUMATIC STRESS DISORDER

The DSM-IV defines posttraumatic stress disorder as a group of symptoms that develop after an individual experiences an event that is potentially life-threatening. As a result of this traumatic experience, the individual displays fear and helplessness and tries not to be reminded of the event but relives it anyway. To be classified as a posttraumatic stress disorder, the patient's symptoms must last for more than a month. The types of events that can produce this disorder are ones that would affect most people such as a tornado, hurricane, rape or other inappropriate sexual activity, war experience, assault, and a very serious accident. Although the patients re-experience the event in their thoughts and dreams, they do everything they can to prevent this from happening. As a result, the patient might display anxiety, depression, difficulties in cognitive functioning, hyperarousal, and a reduced responsiveness.

It has been suggested that a number of different neurotransmitter systems may be associated with this disorder. However, drug studies have implicated, in particular, the noradrenergic system. For example, administration of clonidine or propranolol, which decreases noradrenergic transmission, is effective in reducing some of the symptoms of posttraumatic stress disorder.

GENERALIZED ANXIETY DISORDER

The DSM-IV defines generalized anxiety disorder as a condition of worry or anxiety concerning several events for the larger part of a 6-month period. There is difficulty in controlling the anxiety, and it is accompanied by difficulties in sleeping, irritability, restlessness, and muscle tension. Because the anxiety is difficult to control, it can produce impairment in everyday living. Again, this form of anxiety differs from "normal" anxiety because generalized anxiety disorder is *pervasive* and *excessive*.

Although different classes of drugs have been used for the treatment of generalized anxiety, the drugs of choice are the benzodiazepines. Examples of these drugs include diazepam (Valium) and chlordiazepoxide (Librium). These drugs are effective because they interact with GABA$_A$ receptors, resulting in changes in membrane potential through the opening of Cl$^-$ channels (Fig. 28-4). The net effect is to hyperpolarize and ultimately inhibit the postsynaptic neurons. Benzodiazepines increase the affinity of the GABA$_A$ receptor for GABA, causing an increase in the frequency of opening of the Cl$^-$ channel, thus facilitating GABAergic transmission. Other support for the role of the GABAergic system regulating anxiety comes from studies using inverse agonists (such as those related to β-carbolines), which bind to the benzodiazepine site on the GABA receptor and reduce GABAergic transmission. In so doing, these drugs cause anxiety.

In considering other neurotransmitter systems that may relate to anxiety reactions, basic and clinical research has provided evidence that serotonin likely has a regulatory role as well. For example, buspirone (Buspar), a partial 5-HT$_{1A}$ agonist that has no direct effect on the GABA$_A$-benzodiazepine receptor and only a weak influence on dopamine receptors, has been effective in reducing, in particular, the cognitive symptoms of anxiety, as opposed to the somatic symptoms. In addition, acti-

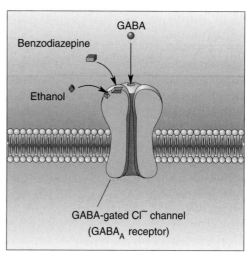

Figure 28-4 Benzodiazepines, ethanol, and GABA receptors. Benzodiazepines and ethanol act on the GABA$_A$ subunit of the GABA receptor. When GABA binds to GABA$_A$ receptors, the chloride channels open, and the influx of Cl$^-$ hyperpolarizes the cell. A benzodiazepine, such as diazepam, increases the affinity for the receptor for GABA and, consequently, increases Cl$^-$ conductance and the hyperpolarizing current. For this reason, this drug has been used successfully for the treatment of anxiety disorders. (From Bear MF, et al.: Neuroscience: Exploring the Brain, 2nd ed. Philadelphia: Lippincott Williams & Wilkins, 2001, p.685.)

vation of 5-HT$_2$ receptors by a selective agonist has been shown to have anxiogenic properties, suggesting a complex relationship of the serotonergic system in its regulation of anxiety reactions.

Several neuropeptides have recently been implicated in anxiety reactions. These include CCK (see earlier discussion on panic disorder), substance P, and opiates. It appears that both CCK and substance P have anxiogenic properties, whereas opiates have anxiolytic properties. The mechanisms by which their actions modulate anxiety have not yet been elucidated. In conclusion, it would seem that anxiety reactions are not regulated by a single transmitter system but, instead, require involvement of a variety of neurotransmitters.

SUBSTANCE ABUSE AND BRAIN FUNCTION

Substance abuse may be defined as the abnormal use of a substance that leads to impairment of physical, social, or occupational aspects of one's life. Closely related to the concept of substance abuse are the concepts of **dependence** and **tolerance**. Dependence involves not only substance abuse, but also withdrawal symptoms that occur after the individual stops or reduces the intake of the substance. Tolerance is experienced when a specific dose taken previously to generate a certain kind of psychological state is no longer effective when taken at a later time. The individual thus has to increase the dose of the substance to maintain the same psychological effect of the drug.

A wide range of substances of abuse have been identified. Substances that activate central nervous system functions, which may result in heightened alertness, agitation, mild improvement of mood, increased heart rate, loss of appetite, and aggression, are called **stimulants**. These include caffeine, amphetamines, cocaine, and nicotine. In contrast, agents that have a generally depressive effect on central nervous system functions, quite possibly by activating GABAergic inhibitory systems, are referred to as **sedatives**. Examples of this class of substance include alcohol, barbiturates, and benzodiazepines. They may produce a mild elevation of mood, sedation, sleep, behavioral disinhibition, and a decrease in anxiety. Other categories of substances of abuse include: (1) narcotics or opioid drugs (e.g., heroin and morphine), and (2) hallucinogens, such as LSD, phencyclidine (angel dust), bromocriptines (when used for treating Parkinson's disease), and **cannabis** (marijuana).

NEURAL MECHANISMS

To understand how drugs of abuse generate their addictive properties, two levels of analysis have been conducted. One approach has been to attempt to identify the molecular sites for the rewarding effects of different classes of drugs. A second approach has been to identify the neural circuits mediating the rewarding effects of these drugs.

MOLECULAR SITES

Considerable research has been carried out in attempting to identify the nature of the binding sites for opiate receptors. Details concerning this receptor and others described in this section are described in Chapter 8. In brief, the μ-receptor is considered to be the primary site for morphine reward, tolerance, and physical dependence. For example, in knockout transgenic mice lacking μ-receptors, the rewarding actions of morphine are absent. It is presumed that the μ-receptor activities are mediated through different classes of G-proteins, which may have different functions.

Another drug of abuse that has received considerable attention has been cocaine. Available evidence points to the link between cocaine and monoaminergic transporters and, in particular, dopamine. Lesions of dopaminergic neurons that express dopamine transporters also result in the loss of the rewarding properties of cocaine.

Because the effectiveness of the rewarding properties of cocaine (and also that of morphine) are associated with the rate at which they are administered, it is believed that dopamine transporter functions may be mediated through phosphorylation at specific brain sites.

The receptor mechanisms for other substances of abuse appear to be less well understood. Although different classes of cannabinoid receptors are found in the periphery and within the central nervous system, the precise regions and sites in the brain where marijuana interacts with cannabinoid receptors have yet to be elucidated. Likewise, concerning the actions of nicotine, it is believed that nicotine acts through presynaptic nicotinic acetylcholine receptors, but again, the precise sites in the brain where such interactions take place have not been clearly identified. With respect to barbiturates and benzodiazepines, it would appear that these classes of substances act through GABA$_A$ receptors, but the specific sites of interaction may relate more to the nature of the subunits of GABA rather than to the GABA receptor, per se. Concerning phencyclidine, it is known to bind with N-methyl-D-aspartate (NMDA) receptors of glutamate-gated ion channels, while LSD binds to serotonergic receptors. In contrast, alcohol's actions may be mediated through more diverse groups of receptors. A large number of studies have provided evidence that the side effects of alcohol (ethanol) are mediated through GABA (Fig. 28-4) and glutamate receptors. However, other researchers have also suggested that monoaminergic and neuropeptide receptors may be implicated as well. Complicating this picture is the fact that, once alcohol passes through the blood-brain barrier, it is presumably distributed in a diffuse manner through much of the brain, acting through a variety of receptors. For this reason, it is extremely difficult to identify specific anatomical sites in the brain associated with the rewarding properties of alcohol.

BRAIN CIRCUITS MEDIATING THE REWARDING EFFECTS OF DRUGS

Our knowledge of the brain sites associated with the rewarding properties (the positive, feel-good feedback that encourages use of these drugs) of different substances of abuse was facilitated by earlier studies that identified the sites that produced electrical self-stimulation in rodents. One of the most effective sites for generating electrical self-stimulation is the ventral tegmental area. Integral to the self-stimulation procedure is that the animal learns to press a bar for a reward. In this instance, the reward is a low-current stimulus applied to a specific site in the brain that is presumed to have pleasant, positive, reinforcing properties. Specifically, the neurons in the regions in question are, to a large extent, dopaminergic and project through the medial forebrain bundle to wide areas of the forebrain, including the nucleus accumbens, limbic structures, and the cerebral cortex. The following evidence implicates the ventral tegmental area as part of the brain circuit associated with rewarding drugs: (1) lesions of the medial forebrain bundle reduce the rewarding effects of drugs of abuse, such as cocaine and amphetamines; (2) these drugs potentiate the rate of electrical self-stimulation; and (3) intravenous injections of drugs of abuse, including morphine, cocaine, and amphetamines, enhance the release of dopamine at the terminals of ventral tegmental fibers, in particular, within the nucleus accumbens.

These findings suggest that different drugs of abuse may act through the same neural circuitry, although the precise mechanisms may differ. For example, certain drugs, such as cocaine, may raise the level of dopamine released at dopaminergic terminals in the nucleus accumbens by blocking the dopamine transporter, effectively extending the time for dopamine to remain in the synaptic cleft. In contrast, morphine may act on the same ventral tegmental circuit but by a different mechanism, namely, by inhibiting GABAergic neurons that normally suppress ventral tegmental dopaminergic neurons (Fig. 28-5). Why do these drugs of abuse appear to act on the same circuit? One possible answer is that, within the brains of different organisms, there exist selective brain circuits that become activated during certain hedonistic activities such as feeding, drinking, and sexual behavior. In so doing, the activation of the brain circuits provides positive and rewarding properties in association with these motivated activities, which helps to ensure the survival of the species. Thus, drugs of abuse may be able to generate their positively rewarding properties by engaging these very same circuits.

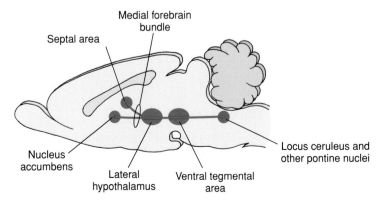

Figure 28–5 A key brain-reward circuit. Intracranial self-stimulation follows stimulation along the medial forebrain bundle, which links structures, such as the nucleus accumbens and septal area, with the lateral hypothalamus, ventral tegmental area, and brainstem monoaminergic cell groups. The sites where drug action is believed to occur include the nucleus accumbens, ventral tegmental area, and brainstem monoaminergic cell groups.

Moreover, treatment for this disorder with serotonergic drugs has been reasonably successful. The theory, in brief, suggests that lower levels of serotonin are associated with the onset and presence of depression (and up-regulation of 5-HT receptors), whereas higher levels of serotonin tend to be linked with remission of this disorder. In addition, treatment with antidepressant drugs has been shown to result in down-regulation of 5-HT$_2$ receptors.

Accordingly, Harry was administered a serotonin re-uptake inhibitor for a period of a month before he began to show signs of improvement. It has been suggested that the time course of improvement after treatment can be accounted for by the time required by G-proteins to affect signal transduction for modulating second messenger systems within the cell. The presumed regions of the brain where such effects may be most significant include limbic structures and, perhaps most importantly, the region of the prefrontal cortex. The effects of drug treatment are presumed to restore levels of serotonin and serotonin receptors to values typical of normal individuals.

After a period of 2 months, Harry resigned his position of interim Chairman and again returned to the laboratory and clinic. Because of the change in his work conditions, coupled with the aid of drugs such as a serotonin re-uptake inhibitor and valproic acid (both of which function as mood stabilizers), his mood and temperament improved and became more stable. Likewise, he began to perform at a level similar to that which he had been accustomed to before his illness. It was recommended that Harry remain on the same drug treatment regimen for the immediate future, stay away from chairmanships, and at a later date, consider a gradual lowering of the drug doses over time.

CHAPTER TEST

QUESTIONS

Choose the best answer for each question.

1. A 35-year-old man who has been working as an office manager for 9 years began to behave in a strange manner over the last 8 months. He said, on several occasions, that the people in the office were laughing at him and that others were watching him all the time. He experienced difficulties in interpersonal relationships, which led to a considerable number of arguments with fellow workers. He also reported that he heard voices of famous historical characters who were often speaking to him. He had always dressed quite sharply, but over the past several months, his appearance had become shabby. Lately, he rarely shaved and generally wore clothes that were unclean. Finally, his erratic behavior resulted in his being admitted to a hospital. Neurologic, general medical, and psychiatric evaluations were then carried out, including a brain MRI scan. Brain imaging analysis suggested dysfunction in the:

   a. Prefrontal cortex
   b. Occipital cortex
   c. Superior parietal cortex
   d. Thalamus
   e. Midbrain periaqueductal gray

2. A 29-year-old woman who recently received her Ph.D. in political science began a new job working for the State Department in Washington. After approximately 6 months, she began to lose interest in her job and other activities as well. When she would come to work, she would do little at the job, frequently stare out the window, feel sad, and begin to cry. She also showed the following additional symptoms: fatigue, loss of energy in performing tasks, refusal to exercise, difficulty in sleeping, loss of weight, and a reduced ability to concentrate. At the request of her employer, she was admitted to a hospital for evaluation. Research into the neurochemical correlates of this disorder have suggested that, within the brain, there is:

   a. An excess of dopamine
   b. A deficiency in excitatory amino acids
   c. An excess of GABA
   d. A deficiency of serotonin
   e. An excess of enkephalin

3. Lithium has been shown to be effective in the treatment of:

   a. Hypochondriasis
   b. Bipolar disorder
   c. Anxiety
   d. Schizophrenia
   e. Obsessive-compulsive disorder

4. Benzodiazepines are effective in treating anxiety reactions because they primarily interact with:

   a. GABA$_A$ receptors
   b. Cholecystokinin receptors
   c. Substance P
   d. Catecholamine receptors
   e. NMDA receptors

5. The pharmacodynamic action of cocaine involves:
   a. Blockade of glutamate re-uptake
   b. Blockade of GABA re-uptake
   c. Blockade of dopamine re-uptake
   d. Activation of acetylcholine receptors
   e. Activation of opioid receptors

ANSWERS AND EXPLANATIONS

1. Answer: a

The display of paranoid delusions and auditory hallucinations and poor dress habits are all features of schizophrenic behavior. Brain imaging and other approaches have provided evidence that schizophrenia is associated with dysfunctions of the prefrontal cortex. There is little evidence to support the notion that dysfunctions of other regions of the cortex, thalamus, or midbrain periaqueductal gray are linked with schizophrenia.

2. Answer: d

The patient was diagnosed as having depression. The pattern of behavior expressed by the patient (lack of interest in one's work, sitting around doing nothing, expressions of sadness, loss of weight, fatigue, and difficulty in sleeping) are all symptoms associated with major depression. These behavioral patterns are not characteristic of the other psychiatric and behavioral disorders listed in this question. Studies in recent years have focused on the role of several neurotransmitters in depression. While a variety of neurotransmitters are likely to play roles in the expression of this disorder, it is generally agreed that serotonin is the most significant of the neurotransmitters listed as options. These studies have suggested that reductions in monoamine levels are associated with depression. In particular, considerable attention has been given to the role of serotonin as evidenced by the effective results after administration of serotonin-specific re-uptake inhibitors. The amino acids and neuropeptides listed as other choices in this question have not been shown as yet to be linked experimentally or clinically with depression. Likewise, depressive disorders have never been associated with potentiated levels of dopamine.

3. Answer: b

Lithium has been used successfully in treating the manic and depressive phases of bipolar disorder and is not used for the other disorders listed in this question. For depression and obsessive-compulsive disorders, serotonin re-uptake inhibitors are considered the drugs of choice. For anxiety reactions, patients are often given antianxiety drugs such as benzodiazepines; for schizophrenia, antipsychotic drugs are often prescribed. For hypochondriasis, supportive psychotherapy is the strategy of choice.

4. Answer: a

Benzodiazepines interact with GABA$_A$ receptors, causing a change in membrane potential by the opening of chloride channels. This results in hyperpolarization of the membrane and inhibition of the postsynaptic neuron. Moreover, benzodiazepines increase the affinity of GABA$_A$ receptors, causing an increase in the frequency of opening of the chloride channel, which results in facilitation of GABAergic transmission. The other choices include receptors linked to excitatory neurotransmitters. Activation of these receptors would likely produce anxiogenic, rather than anxiolytic, reactions and, therefore, would not be useful in the treatment of anxiety disorders.

5. Answer: c

One major pharmacodynamic effect of cocaine is to block the re-uptake of dopamine. The net result is to increase dopamine levels in the brain, and the subsequent elevated levels of dopamine interact with specific circuits in the brain to produce the rewarding effects, which gives it the addictive properties. The other neurotransmitters listed in this question are not known to be affected in a specific manner by cocaine or account for its addictive properties.

GLOSSARY

abducens nucleus and nerve (cranial nerve [CN] VI) General somatic efferent nucleus of the lower pons whose axons innervate the lateral rectus muscle.

accessory cuneate nucleus Relay nucleus situated immediately lateral to the cuneate nucleus; mediates signals from muscle spindles and Golgi tendon organs from the ipsilateral upper limb to the cerebellum.

accommodation reaction (reflex) Reflex response associated with both somatomotor and parasympathetic components of CN III, resulting in constriction of the pupils, bulging of the lens (to allow for focusing at a near object), and medial deviation of the eyes, the overall effect of which is to allow an individual to correctly focus on an object when it is moved from a distant to a near position.

accommodation The change in refractive power of the lens of the eye.

acetylcholine (Ach) A small molecule neurotransmitter synthesized from choline in the presence of choline acetyltransferase. Ach serves as a neurotransmitter at the terminals of preganglionic neurons in the sympathetic as well as parasympathetic ganglia, at the terminals of parasympathetic postganglionic neurons, and at the neuromuscular junction. In the ganglia, its release results in the stimulation of postganglionic neurons; at the terminals of parasympathetic nerve terminals, it causes parasympathetic effects (e.g, decrease in heart rate, peristalsis in the gastrointestinal tract); and at the neuromuscular junction, its release results in contraction of the skeletal muscle.

acetylcholinesterase An enzyme, which is present at the synapses where Ach is released as a neurotransmitter, that inactivates released acetylcholine.

action potential Brief all-or-nothing reversal in membrane potential that is brought about by rapid changes in membrane permeability of Na^+ and K^+. During the *rising phase* of the action potential, there is a rapid depolarization of the membrane due to increased permeability of Na^+; the part of the action potential where the inside of the neuron is positive relative to the outside is called the *overshoot*. During the *falling phase* of the action potential, the neuron is repolarized by the opening of voltage-gated K^+ channels, which allow increased efflux of K^+. Hyperpolarization at the end of the falling phase is called *after-hyperpolarization* or *undershoot*. The period during which the voltage-gated Na^+ channels are in an inactivated state and an action potential cannot be generated is called the *absolute refractory period*. The *relative refractory period* follows immediately after the absolute refractory period; during this period, an action potential can be generated, but more depolarizing current is needed to shift the membrane potential to threshold level. See also *axon hillock*.

active transport The passage of ions or molecules across a cell membrane that is mediated by specific carrier proteins and requires coupling of the carrier protein to a source of metabolic energy (e.g., hydrolysis of ATP).

active zone Membrane associated with a pyramid-like structure consisting of proteins arising from the intracellular side of the presynaptic terminal membrane and projecting into the cytoplasm of the presynaptic terminal; possesses specialized release sites in the presynaptic terminal. Vesicles containing the neurotransmitter are aggregated near the active zones.

adenosine A purinergic neurotransmitter (a neurotransmitter containing a purine ring); at least three adenosine receptors (A1–A3) have been identified; all of them are metabotropic receptors.

Adie's pupil Disorder in which there is a prolonged and sluggish constriction of the pupil to light; after pupillary constriction, dilatation of the pupil is delayed. Patients with this disorder have pathological changes in the ciliary ganglion.

after-hyperpolarization See *action potential*.

ageusia Loss of taste sensation; total ageusia means loss of all taste sensation, partial ageusia refers to loss of a particular taste sensation, and hypogeusia means decreased sensation of taste.

agnosia Difficulty or inability to recognize objects. See also visual agnosia.

agoraphobia Fear of leaving a familiar place.

akinesia Lack of movement occurring in diseases of the basal ganglia.

alar plate Region of the developing nervous system situated dorsal to the sulcus limitans that will become sensory in function.

alpha rhythm electroencephalogram (EEG) Rhythm of 6–12 Hz associated with quiet and sometimes drowsy states.

alveus (of hippocampus) fiber layer of the hippocampus adjacent to the inferior horn of the lateral ventricle.

Alzheimer's disease Disorder of severe memory loss in aging individuals correlated with the presence of neurofibrillary tangles, extracellular deposition of the abnormal amyloid protein, and β-amyloid plaques in the cerebral cortex, coupled with cell loss in the basal nucleus of Meynert as well as reduced cholinergic content of cortical tissue.

AMPA α-amino-3-hydroxy-5-methyl-4-isoxazole-propionate; an agonist for a non—N-methyl-D-aspartic acid (NMDA) ionotropic glutamate receptor (AMPA receptor).

amphiphilic Substances that have a hydrophilic and a hydrophobic end.

amygdala Deep cortical structure situated in the medial temporal lobe just rostral to the hippocampal formation that is associated with regulation of emotional behavior and other hypothalamic functions.

amyotrophic lateral sclerosis (ALS) Disease characterized by degeneration of the motor neurons in the anterior horn of the spinal cord, brainstem, and cerebral cortex. Symptoms include widespread muscle fasciculations, flaccid weakness, and atrophy of the muscles. (Also known as Lou Gehrig's disease.)

anencephaly Partial or complete absence of the brain with associated defects of the cranial vault and scalp occurring during fetal development.

angiotensin II Peptide localized within the supraoptic and paraventricular hypothalamic neurons; plays an important role in the regulation of blood pressure and drinking behavior.

angular artery A branch of the middle cerebral artery that supplies the angular gyrus.

angular gyrus Situated in the inferior parietal lobule immediately posterior to the supramarginal gyrus and often associated with the posterior extent of the superior temporal sulcus.

anhidrosis Absence of sweating.

anosmia Loss of olfactory function; may result from damage to the olfactory mucosa caused by infections.

anosognosia See *sensory neglect*.

ansa lenticularis Major efferent pathway of the basal ganglia; exits from the ventral aspect of the medial pallidal segment and supplies ventrolateral and ventral anterior thalamic nuclei.

anterior (ventral) funiculus See *funiculus*.

anterior (ventral) white commissure Located ventral to the gray commissure; consists of decussating axons.

anterior Above the midbrain, anterior means "toward the front of the brain." Below the midbrain, anterior means "toward the ventral surface of the body."

anterior chamber Space between the lens and the cornea of the eye.

anterior commissure Fiber bundles connecting left and right olfactory and temporal lobes.

anterior communicating artery Connects the left and right anterior cerebral arteries.

anterior corticospinal tract See *corticospinal tract*.

anterior hypothalamus Region of the hypothalamus containing preoptic, suprachiasmatic, supraoptic, anterior, and paraventricular nuclei. Functions include temperature regulation, release of hormones into posterior pituitary, control of blood pressure, and related autonomic functions and associated emotional behavior. (See each type of nucleus individually.)

anterior inferior cerebellar artery Supplies the ventral and inferior surface of the cerebellum and parts of the pons.

anterior lobe of cerebellum One of the three lobes of the cerebellum situated in a rostral position; associated in part with the control of muscle tone.

anterior nucleus of thalamus Nucleus of thalamus situated in the dorsomedial aspect of the rostral thalamus; it projects its axons to cingulate gyrus and receives inputs from hippocampal formation and mammillary bodies.

anterior olfactory nucleus Located in the posterior aspect of each olfactory bulb; receives sensory signals from mitral and tufted cells and relays them to the contralateral olfactory bulb via the anterior commissure.

anterior spinal artery Courses along the midline of the ventral surface of the spinal cord and medulla.

anterograde amnesia Difficulty in generating new memories.

anterograde tracing techniques Involve microinjection of a marker (e.g., a fluorescent dye) at desired site in the central nervous system (CNS); marker is taken up by the neuronal cell bodies and transported anterogradely to their axon terminals; marker is then visualized under a microscope to ascertain the projections of the neuron.

anterolateral spinal vein See *spinal veins*.

anteromedian spinal vein See *spinal veins*.

antidiuretic hormone (ADH) See *vasopressin*.

antipyrogenic region Region of anterior hypothalamus that responds to actions of pyrogens (i.e., region contains vasopressin, which is capable of counteracting the actions of pyrogens, which are substances that increase body temperature).

aphasia Speech disorder in which the patient has difficulty in naming objects and repetition of words is impaired, while comprehension remains intact. See *Broca's motor speech area*.

apoptosis A genetically determined process of cell death; characterized by shrinkage of the cell, cellular fragmentation, and condensation of the chromatin; involves activation of a latent biochemical pathway in the cells.

apraxia Inability to produce a motor act correctly even though sensory and motor circuits are intact; disorder is associated with damage to the premotor cortex or the posterior parietal cortex.

aqueduct of Sylvius (cerebral aqueduct) Channel present in the midbrain that allows cerebrospinal fluid (CSF) to flow from the third ventricle to the fourth ventricle.

aqueous humor A watery fluid produced by the epithelial cells of the ciliary processes; fills the anterior chamber.

arachnoid granulations See *arachnoid villi*.

arachnoid mater Membrane covering the brain and spinal cord; lies between the dura and pia mater.

arachnoid trabeculae Fine strands of connective tissue that arise from the arachnoid, span the subarachnoid space, and then connect with the pia.

arachnoid villi Small tufts of arachnoidal tissue that project into the superior sagittal and other dural sinuses. They act as one-way valves, allowing flow of CSF into the sinuses but not in the reverse direction. Large aggregations of arachnoid villi are called arachnoid granulations.

arcuate nucleus Located in the extreme ventromedial aspect of the hypothalamus at the level of the median eminence; many of the neurons contain dopamine that may inhibit prolactin release (i.e., prolactin release-inhibiting hormone).

area postrema Rounded eminence located immediately rostral to the obex on each side of the fourth ventricle; contains arterioles, sinusoids, and a few unipolar neurons. Considered to be a chemoreceptor zone that triggers vomiting in response to emetic substances (e.g., digitalis glycosides, apomorphine) circulating in the blood.

Argyll Robertson pupil Disorder in which the pupil reacts to accommodation but not to light.

Arnold-Chiari malformation Disorder in which parts of the medulla and cerebellum are displaced and consequently pulled through the foramen magnum, blocking the flow of CSF that normally passes from the roof of the fourth ventricle to the cisterns and causing hydrocephalus.

association areas Areas of the cerebral cortex that do not comprise primary motor or sensory cortices but may be linked to them as secondary or tertiary regions. These areas mediate complex functions of the cerebral cortex.

association nuclei of the thalamus Receiving few, if any, afferents from ascending sensory pathways, these nuclei project to specific regions of cortex and, in turn, receive inputs from cerebral cortex, limbic nuclei, basal ganglia, and nonspecific thalamic nuclei.

astereognosia Disorder in which the patient cannot identify by touch the shape, size, or texture of an object in the hand contralateral to the side of a parietal cortical lesion.

astigmatism Disorder in which the shape of the cornea is oblong, causing the curvature of the cornea in one plane to be less than the curvature in the other plane. Because the light rays coming from an object are bent to a different extent in these two different planes, the light rays do not come to a single focal point, causing visual disturbances.

astrocyte Glial cell that supports neurons in the brain and regulates the chemical and extracellular environments.

asymmetrical synapse Postsynaptic membrane of the synapse is thicker than the presynaptic membrane; synapse is usually excitatory. (See *symmetrical synapse*.)

asynergy Loss of coordination.

ataxia Errors in the range, rate, force, and direction of movement that result in loss of muscle coordination.

athetosis Variant of choreiform movement involving slow, writhing movements of the extremities.

atrioventricular node Conductile tissue between the atria and the ventricles of the heart.

atrium One of the upper chambers of the heart.

auditory nuclei Nuclei associated with transmission of signals necessary for hearing.

autoinhibition A normal physiological mechanism in which a released neurotransmitter inhibits its own further release.

autonomic insufficiency Impaired function of the autonomic nervous system due to a defect in the central or peripheral nervous system.

autonomic nervous system Components of the peripheral and central nervous systems that regulate the functions of smooth muscle, glands, and heart.

axolemma The plasma membrane of the axon.

axon A single, long, cylindrical, and slender process arising from the soma of a neuron; conducts information from the cell body to different targets.

axon hillock A small conical elevation on the soma of a neuron that does not contain Nissl substance; the site of the generation of action potentials in a neuron.

axonal transport Movement of secretory and membrane products either from the cell body to the terminals or from the terminals to the cell body via the axon.

axoplasm The cytoplasm contained within an axon; devoid of the Nissl substance or Golgi apparatus but contains mitochondria, microtubules, and neurofilaments.

Babinski sign Characterized by an abnormal plantar response (extension of great toe while the other toes fan out) when the sole of a foot is stroked by a blunt instrument (normal plantar response consists of a brisk flexion of all toes); presence of this sign indicates damage of the corticospinal tract.

bacterial meningitis Inflammation of the membranes covering the brain and spinal cord; caused by bacteria (e.g., meningococcus); symptoms include nasopharyngeal catarrh, headache, convulsions, vomiting, and stiff neck.

baroflex See *baroreceptor reflex.*

baroreceptor reflex Mechanism by which fluctuations in systemic blood pressure and heart rate are adjusted; involves baroreceptor afferents, various CNS structures, and sympathetic and parasympathetic efferents. Also called baroreflex.

baroreceptors Stretch receptors located primarily in the carotid artery sinus and aortic arch that sense changes in blood pressure.

Barr body Represents one of the two X chromosomes in the female and is located at the inner surface of the nuclear membrane.

basal ganglia Region of the brain associated with the regulation of motor functions, consisting principally of the caudate nucleus, putamen, and globus pallidus.

basal nucleus of Meynert Large cholinergic cells found near the base of the rostral forebrain; axons project to wide regions of cerebral cortex and to limbic structures. Loss of these neurons is associated with Alzheimer's disease.

basal plate Region of the developing nervous system situated ventral to the sulcus limitans that will become motor in function.

basal vein of Rosenthal Receives blood from different regions of the cerebral cortex and corpus striatum and empties into the great cerebral vein of Galen.

basilar artery Formed by the union of two vertebral arteries at the caudal border of the pons and passes along in the midline on the ventral surface of brainstem.

basilar pons The ventral half of the pons containing pontine nuclei, transverse pontine fibers (that enter the middle cerebellar peduncle), and descending corticospinal and corticobulbar fibers.

basket cells Inhibitory neuron located in the molecular layer of cerebellar cortex; makes synaptic (axosomatic) contact with Purkinje cells.

basolateral amygdala Includes the lateral, central, and lateral anatomic aspects of the basal nuclei of the amygdala.

bed nucleus of the stria terminalis Nuclear structure situated immediately ventrolateral to the column of the fornix at the level of the anterior commissure. This structure (1) receives fibers from the amygdala via the stria terminalis and (2) regulates emotional and visceral processes related to hypothalamic functions.

Benedikt's syndrome Disorder affecting nerve fibers of CN III and neurons in the region of the red nucleus, causing an oculomotor paralysis, tremor of the contralateral limb, and possible somatosensory loss of the contralateral side of the body.

benzodiazepines Class of drugs used for the treatment of anxiety disorders such as panic attacks.

β-endorphin See *opioid peptides.*

beta rhythm Low-voltage, fast EEG rhythm associated with cortical desynchronization.

binocular visual field The central portion of the visual field of each eye that can be seen by both retinae.

biogenic amines A group of neurotransmitters including catecholamines (dopamine, norepinephrine, and epinephrine), serotonin, and histamine.

bipolar neurons Two processes, one on each end, arise from these neurons. One process ends in dendrites, and the other process, an axon, ends in terminals in the CNS. They are involved in sensory functions; information received by the dendrites on one end is transmitted to the CNS via the axon terminals on the other end.

blind spot Optic disc (contains no photoreceptors).

blob area Region of the visual cortex in which the mitochondrial enzyme, cytochrome oxidase, provides an intense staining pattern of small, ovoid areas (called blob); associated with color processing. See *interblob area.*

blood-brain barrier Prevents passage of large molecules from blood into the extracellular space between the neurons and neuroglia due to the close apposition of the endothelial cell membranes (tight junctions).

blood-cerebrospinal fluid (CSF) barrier Prevents passage of large molecules from blood into the CSF due to the presence of tight junctions in the outermost epithelial cell layer of the choroidal plexus.

bony labyrinth Complex series of cavities in the petrous portion of temporal bone in the ear; surrounds the inner membranous labyrinth.

Bötzinger complex Mostly expiratory neurons located rostral to the medullary rostral group of respiratory neurons. Located just caudal to the nucleus of the facial nerve (CN VII).

Bowman's gland Located in the olfactory mucosa; secretes olfactory-binding protein.

brachium of the inferior colliculus Fiber bundles that transmit auditory information from the inferior colliculus to the medial geniculate nucleus.

bradykinesia Slowness of movement characteristic of diseases of the basal ganglia.

brain anoxia Deprivation of oxygen delivery to the brain.

brain infarction Neuronal death caused by prolonged brain ischemia.

brain ischemia Insufficient blood flow to the brain during which oxygen as well as glucose delivery is reduced; in addition, toxic metabolites, such as lactic acid, cannot be removed efficiently due to reduced blood flow.

brainstem The part of the CNS situated between the forebrain, rostrally, and spinal cord, caudally, consisting of the medulla, pons, and midbrain.

branchial arches The arches where thickening of mesoderm occurs during development and from which various cranial nerves are derived.

Broca's motor speech area Region for the formulation of the motor components of speech situated in the ventrolateral aspect of the frontal lobe anterior to the precentral gyrus in the inferior frontal gyrus. Damage to this region produces a form of language impairment called aphasia.

Brodmann's areas Cytoarchitectural map of the cerebral cortex based on the distinctive histological appearance of the different areas of the cortex. Each number identifies a specific area of the cerebral cortex. Examples include primary visual cortex (area 17), primary motor cortex (area 4), and primary somatosensory cortex (areas 3, 1, and 2).

Brown-Séquard syndrome Results from hemisection of the spinal cord; loss of conscious proprioception and two-point discrimination occurs below the level of the lesion on the ipsilateral side and loss of pain and temperature sensation below the level of the lesion on the contralateral side; at the level of the lesion, there is bilateral loss of pain and temperature.

cacosmia Olfactory hallucinations of unpleasant smells; may be present in seizure activity involving parts of the temporal lobe; the neural structures affected in this condition are the uncus, parahippocampal gyrus, amygdala, and piriform (pyriform) and entorhinal cortices.

calcarine artery A branch of the posterior cerebral artery that supplies the primary visual cortex.

calcarine sulcus (calcarine fissure) A prominent sulcus formed on the medial surface that runs perpendicular into the parieto-occipital sulcus, which divides the occipital lobe from the parietal lobe.

caloric test Used to test disorders of the vestibulo-ocular pathways in patients complaining of dizziness or vertigo; cold water introduced into the external auditory canal produces nystagmus to the opposite side, while warm water produces nystagmus toward the same side.

canal of Schlemm A venous channel located at the junction of iris and cornea (the anterior chamber angle); the aqueous humor is reabsorbed through a specialized collection of cells (trabeculae) into this canal.

carbidopa Inhibitor of dopa-decarboxylase (an enzyme that converts dihydroxyphenyl alanine [DOPA] into dopamine); does not cross blood-brain barrier; used in the treatment of Parkinson's disease. See *Sinemet.*

cardiopulmonary receptors Located in the lungs and the heart; activated by noxious chemicals (e.g., capsaicin present in chili pepper).

cataplexy A condition involving loss of muscle tone; associated with narcolepsy. See *narcolepsy.*

catatonic schizophrenia Form of schizophrenia characterized by a decrease in reactivity to environment, purposeless motor activity, postural rigidity, and resistance in responding to instructions.

catecholamines Chemical compounds that contain a benzene ring with two adjacent hydroxyl groups (e.g., dopamine, norepinephrine, and epinephrine)

catechol-O-methyltransferase (COMT) An enzyme that destroys catecholamines.

cauda equina Consists of a bundle of nerve roots of all the spinal nerves caudal to the second lumbar vertebra.

caudal Above the midbrain, caudal means "toward the back of the brain." Below the midbrain, caudal means "toward the sacral end (or bottom) of the spinal cord."

caudal basal pontine syndrome Caused mainly by occlusion of paramedian branches of the basilar artery; affects corticospinal tract and sometimes root fibers of CN VI, resulting in contralateral hemiplegia and lateral gaze paralysis.

caudal tegmental pontine syndrome Caused by occlusion of circumferential branches of the basilar artery; affects caudal aspect of pontine tegmentum, resulting in facial nerve palsy, lateral gaze palsy, and Horner's syndrome.

caudal ventrolateral medullary depressor area (CVLM) A group of neurons located in the ventrolateral medulla; relay nucleus essential for mediating baroreflex. See *baroreflex* or *baroreceptor reflex.*

caudate nucleus Major component of the basal ganglia along with the putamen and globus pallidus.

causalgia Characterized by a burning sensation caused by increased sympathetic efferent activity after a peripheral nerve injury.

cavernous sinus A venous sinus found on each side of the sella turcica.

celiac ganglion Located in the abdomen; the axons of the greater, lesser, and least splanchnic nerves synapse on the postganglionic neurons in this ganglion; emerging postganglionic fibers innervate smooth muscle and glands in the stomach and small intestine, liver, pancreas, and kidney.

cell membrane Forms the external boundary of the neuronal cell body and its processes; consists of a double layer of lipids in which proteins, including ion channels, are embedded.

central canal Extends throughout the spinal cord; in the adult, it is patent only in the upper cervical segments.

central nervous system (CNS) The brain and spinal cord of vertebrates.

central tegmental area Region of the midbrain containing the reticular formation.

centromedian nucleus Intralaminar (and nonspecific) nucleus of the thalamus; receives inputs from the cerebral cortex and reticular formation; transmits information to the neostriatum and to widespread regions of the cerebral cortex.

cerebellar nystagmus See *postrotary nystagmus*, under *nystagmus.*

cerebellar peduncle See *inferior, middle,* and *superior cerebellar peduncles.*

cerebellum The region of the hindbrain associated with major motor functions; it is attached to the brainstem by three peduncles and contains an outer cortex and inner region composed of deep nuclei.

cerebral aqueduct See *aqueduct of Sylvius.*

cerebral arterial circle See *circle of Willis.*

cerebral dominance Refers to the fact that, for a given function, one side of the brain plays a more active role and has more neurons dedicated to that function than the other side.

cerebral hemispheres Comprises the cerebral cortex, which covers the surface of the brain, as well as deeper structures, including the corpus callosum, diencephalon, basal ganglia, limbic structures, and internal capsule.

cerebral peduncle Includes the crus cerebri and adjoining aspects of the tegmentum of the midbrain.

cerebrospinal fluid (CSF) Clear fluid present in ventricles of the CNS and secreted from the choroid plexus.

cerveau isolé Type of experimental preparation involving a transaction rostral to the trigeminal nerve (usually mid-collicular cut) resulting in an EEG pattern characteristic of a sleeping animal.

cervical cord The most rostral aspect of spinal cord containing eight pairs of cervical spinal nerves.

chemical transmission Communication between neurons via release of chemical substances (neurotransmitters) that are contained in synaptic vesicles in the presynaptic terminals.

chemoreceptor reflex Mechanism by which respiration is adjusted in order to correct changes in blood gases and pH; includes chemoreceptor afferents, various CNS structures, and efferents innervating different respiratory muscles.

chemoreceptor trigger zone See *area postrema.*

chemoreceptors Receptors that respond to changes in chemical environment.

cholinergic muscarinic receptor A metabotropic receptor activated by acetylcholine; located in the CNS, the heart, and smooth muscles.

cholinergic nicotinic receptors An ionotropic receptor activated by acetylcholine; located at the neuromuscular junction and the CNS.

chorea Hyperkinetic disorder associated with a loss of γ-aminobutyric acid (GABA) in the striatum and characterized by brisk involuntary movements of the extremities.

choroid plexus Specialized epithelial cells found mainly on the roofs of the ventricles that secrete CSF; tight junctions between cells prevent CSF from spreading to the adjacent tissue.

chromatin The genetic material of the nucleus consisting of DNA.

chromatolysis Degenerative changes in which the cell body swells up due to edema, becomes round in appearance, and the Nissl substance gets distributed throughout the cytoplasm and subsequently disappears; the nucleus moves from its central position to the periphery because of edema.

ciliary body Tissue that encircles the lens of the eye; consists of a muscle (ciliary muscle) that forms a ring around the lens and the ciliary processes that produce the aqueous humor.

ciliary muscles A smooth muscular ring around the lens of the eye; innervated by postganglionic parasympathetic neurons associated with the oculomotor nerve; constriction of the ciliary muscles causes a release of tension from the suspensory ligament of the lens, thus causing it to bulge (i.e., increase its curvature).

cingulate gyrus Region of cerebral cortex that lies rostral to the occipital lobe and immediately inferior to the precentral, postcentral, and premotor cortices; ventral border is the corpus callosum; considered part of limbic system (associated with the regulation of emotional behavior, visceral processes, and learning).

circle of Willis Formed by the anastomosis of the branches of the internal carotid artery and the terminal branches of the basilar artery; surrounds the optic chiasm and the infundibulum of the pituitary.

circumventricular organs Seven structures in the CNS that lack a blood-brain barrier, including the area postrema, pineal body, subcommissural organ, subfornical organ, organum vasculosum of lamina terminalis, neurohypophysis (the posterior pituitary gland), and the median eminence.

Claude's syndrome Characterized by ipsilateral oculomotor paresis of the oculomotor nucleus and contralateral ataxia and tremor due to damage to the tegmental region of the midbrain.

climbing fibers Axons that arise from the inferior olivary nucleus that project to the cerebellum and terminate on dendrites of Purkinje cell neurons.

closed medulla Caudal half of the medulla that does not contain the fourth ventricle.

coccygeal ligament See *filum terminale externum*.

coccygeal region Caudal end of the spinal cord containing one pair of spinal nerves.

cochlea One of the regions in the inner membranous labyrinth of the ear; shaped like a conical snail shell, it has a central tubular conical axis, called the modiolus, which is surrounded by a spiral cochlear canal of two- and three-quarter turns.

cochlear nerve Formed by the central processes of bipolar neurons in the spiral ganglion; projects to the cochlear nuclei.

cochlear nuclei Second-order relay neurons (i.e., dorsal and ventral cochlear nuclei); located at the medullopontine junction; associated with the transmission of auditory impulses.

color agnosia Disorder of a secondary visual area characterized by inability to name the color of an object or distinguish between colors.

coma State of unconsciousness in which the patient cannot be aroused; usually associated with a cerebrovascular accident involving the reticular formation.

coma vigil (akinetic mutism) A form of coma involving a pontine lesion in which the patient lies quietly and displays a variety of autonomic and somatomotor reflexes as well as normal eye movements.

combined systems disease Degenerative changes in the dorsal and lateral funiculi of the spinal cord causing defects in both sensory and motor function; results from a deficiency of enzymes necessary for vitamin B_{12} absorption.

commissure A bundle of nerve fibers connecting one side of the brain with the other.

communicating hydrocephalus Dilation of brain ventricles developed when the movement of the CSF into the dural venous sinuses is impeded or blocked by an obstruction at the arachnoid villi.

complex cell Found in the visual cortex (layers II, III, V, and VI) other than where simple cells are found; complex cells respond to a specific orientation of the beam of light, but the precise position of the image within the receptive field is not critical.

complex partial seizures Characterized by an impairment of consciousness, although not usually a loss of consciousness.

computed tomography (CT) Process by which a series of x-rays representing different slices of the tissue (tomograms) are obtained; these data are converted into images by a computer. Tomograms of different planes through the scanned body part are acquired; internal structures at any desired plane can be visualized.

cone-opsin A protein attached with a light-absorbing component similar to that present in rhodopsin.

confluence of sinuses The site where the superior sagittal, straight, transverse, and occipital sinuses converge.

connexin Subunits of identical proteins that form a connexon; each connexin consists of four membrane-spanning regions.

connexon Each hemichannel in a gap junction channel; the hemichannels located in presynaptic and postsynaptic neurons meet each other at the gap between the membranes of the two neurons and form a conducting channel.

conscious proprioception Perception of joint position, joint movements, and direction and velocity of joint movements or kinesthesia (perception of movement).

consensual light reflex Pupillary light reflex involving constriction of the pupil of the eye opposite to that which received the light.

contralateral homonymous hemianopia (homonymous hemianopsia) Characterized by blindness in the same half of the visual field of each eye as a result of damage to the contralateral optic tract.

contralateral inferior homonymous quadrantanopia Characterized by blindness in the lower quarter of the visual field of each eye resulting from damage to the contralateral geniculocalcarine tract. Also known as pie-in-the floor visual disorder.

contralateral On the opposite side with reference to a specific point.

contralateral superior homonymous quadrantanopia Characterized by blindness in the upper quarter of the visual field of each eye resulting from damage to the fibers contained in the temporal lobe (called Meyer's loop), which transmit information to the inferior bank of the calcarine sulcus. Also known as pie-in-the sky visual disorder.

conus medullaris The conical-shaped caudal end of the spinal cord; located at the caudal edge of vertebra at L1 or rostral edge of L2.

cordotomy Surgical interruption of fibers in the spinal cord; typically refers to the surgical interruption of the lateral spinothalamic tract to eliminate intractable pain.

corneal reflex Blinking in response to touching the cornea, which involves reflex connections between sensory afferent fibers in the ophthalmic nerve (CN V) that make synaptic connections with motor fibers of CN VII.

corpora cavernosa A spongy tissue consisting of cavernous spaces present in both male and female erectile tissue; these spaces are normally empty but become engorged with blood during erection.

corpora quadrigemina Superior and inferior colliculi.

corpus callosum A massive pathway of the cerebral cortex connecting homotypical regions of each side of the cortex.

corpus striatum Caudate nucleus and putamen.

cortical homunculus See *homunculus*.

corticobulbar fibers Descending corticofugal fibers arising from the lateral aspects of sensorimotor cortex that descend through the internal capsule, crus cerebri, and pyramid, terminating on cranial nerve and other brainstem nuclei.

corticomedial group of the amygdala Includes mainly the cortical, medial, and medial aspect of the basal nuclei of amygdala that lie within its dorsal and medial aspects.

corticoreticular fibers Axons that project from sensorimotor cortex to the reticular formation of the pons and medulla, enabling the cerebral cortex to regulate functions of the reticulospinal tracts.

corticospinal tract Major descending pathway from the cerebral cortex to the spinal cord that mediates voluntary control of motor activity. About 90% of the fibers in this tract cross to the contralateral side at the medullo-spinal junction, forming the *lateral corticospinal tract*, which descends to all levels of the spinal cord and terminates in the spinal gray matter of both the dorsal and ventral horns. Most of the uncrossed fibers constitute the *anterior corticospinal tract*; fibers in this tract descend through the spinal cord and ultimately cross over at different segmental levels to synapse with anterior horn cells on the contralateral side.

corticotropin-releasing hormone (CRH) Released from the paraventricular, supraoptic, and arcuate nuclei of hypothalamus; enters the portal system from axon terminals in the median eminence; CRH releases corticotropin (adrenocorticotropic hormone), which controls the release of steroid hormones in adrenal gland (e.g., cortisol) and stimulates release of β-endorphin from the anterior pituitary.

cranial epidural space Potential space located between the periosteal layer of the dura and the cranium that becomes filled with a fluid only in pathological conditions.

cribiform plate A thin sheet of ethmoid bone underlying the olfactory bulb.

crus cerebri Ventral aspect of the midbrain containing principally corticospinal, corticobulbar, and corticopontine tracts.

cuneocerebellar tract See *external arcuate fibers*.

cyclothymia Bipolar disorder characterized by distinct episodes of mania and depression.

cystic fibrosis A disorder believed to be due to a defect in the Cl^- channels that are involved in the production of secretions in the lungs.

cytoplasm Colloidal protoplasm in the cell containing various organelles.

cytoskeleton Cytoplasmic component of the neuron that is the main determinant of its shape; consists of fibrillar elements (e.g., neurofilaments and microfilaments) and their associated proteins.

Dandy-Walker syndrome Involves the congenital absence of the lateral apertures of Luschka and the median aperture of Magendie, which, through lack of communication with the remainder of the ventricular system, can be one cause of hydrocephalus.

decerebrate rigidity Hyperactivity of extensor muscles of all four limbs in experimental animals produced by intercollicular transection of the brain; traumatic injuries, vascular disease, or tumors in the midbrain can cause similar symptoms in humans.

decibel (dB) A logarithmic scale used to express the intensity of a sound relative to the threshold of human hearing. The lowest intensity of sound that we can hear is 0 dB, a soft whisper is about 20 dB, and a sound that produces hearing discomfort and even pain is usually above 120 dB.

declarative memory Refers to a form of memory in which the individual is conscious of the information that is remembered. Examples include the memory for such facts as an address, directions to get to a specific place, or a string of numbers such as a telephone number or a personal bank card code.

decomposition of movement Components of complex movements occurring as a series of simple individual movements; characteristic of a type of cerebellar dysfunction.

decussation of medial lemniscus A major decussation of the lower medulla situated immediately rostral to the pyramidal decussation; the decussation enables information from one side of the body to reach the contralateral ventral posterolateral thalamic nucleus, mediating conscious proprioception and tactile sensations.

decussation The crossing over of nerve fibers of a pathway from one side of the brain to the other.

deep cerebellar nuclei Efferent neurons of the cerebellum that project to the brainstem and thalamus.

deep pontine nuclei Neurons situated in the basilar pons that give rise to transverse pontine fibers that enter the middle cerebellar peduncle to reach the cerebellum.

deep tendon reflex See *myotatic reflex*.

defensive rage behavior Defensive aggression in cats; characterized by piloerection, marked vocalization, such as hissing and growling, retraction of the claws, significant pupillary dilation and other forms of sympathetic reactions, arching of the back, and striking out at a moving object within its visual field in response to a threatening object. An example of a human equivalent is "road rage."

Deiter's cells These cells surround the base of the outer hair cells and the nerve terminals associated with them; also called outer phalangeal cells.

delayed rectifiers Voltage-gated K^+ channels that open with a delay (about 1 msec) after the membrane depolarization. Rectifiers are channels that allow the flow of ions more readily in one direction than in the opposite direction.

delta rhythm Very slow, 1 to 3 Hz, synchronous waves, measured by EEG recordings, that occur under conditions of severe trauma to the brain.

dendrites Short processes arising from the cell body that branch distally; their primary function is to increase the surface area for receiving signals from axonal projections of other neurons.

dense-core vesicles Vesicles that appear dense under an electron microscope. Usually they contain peptide neurotransmitters.

dentate gyrus Region of hippocampal formation containing distinct cell layers, including the CA4 field; named for its tooth-like appearance.

dentate nucleus Largest of the deep cerebellar nuclei; axons project through the superior cerebellar peduncle to the ventrolateral nucleus of thalamus.

dentatothalamic fibers Fibers arising from the dentate nucleus of cerebellum that supply the ventrolateral thalamic nucleus, thus providing the circuitry by which the cerebellum communicates with the cerebral cortex.

depression Mood disorder characterized by difficulties in sleeping, in which the individual awakens very early or during the nighttime, excessive guilt, depressed mood and appetite, and difficulties concerning memory and concentrating on one's work.

dermatomes The area of skin supplied by the right and left dorsal roots of a single spinal segment.

descending tract of cranial nerve V Descending fibers of the trigeminal nerve that extend caudally as far as the second cervical segment and occupy a far lateral position within the medulla.

desensitization Reduction in the responsiveness of a receptor when subjected to a prolonged exposure to an endogenous or exogenous agonist.

diabetes insipidus Disease state resulting from damage to vasopressin neurons of the supraoptic or paraventricular nuclei; characterized by the flow of large amounts of urine coupled with the drinking of large quantities of fluids.

diagonal band of Broca Cells present within the ventral division of the septal area.

diencephalon The region of the forebrain that lies below the fornix and consists of two parts: (1) the thalamus, which is larger and responsible for relaying and integrating information to different regions of the cerebral cortex from a variety of structures associated with sensory, motor, autonomic, and emotional processes; and (2) the hypothalamus, which is smaller and lies ventral and slightly anterior to the thalamus and is involved in the regulation of a host of visceral functions, such as temperature, endocrine functions, and feeding, drinking, emotional, and sexual behaviors.

direct light reflex Pupillary light reflex involving constriction of the pupil in the same eye that received light.

direct pathway One of the two pathways comprising the internal circuitry governing the transmission of information through the basal ganglia; consists of a direct pathway from neostriatum to internal segment of globus pallidus; information is then transmitted to the cerebral cortex via the thalamus. See the opposite *indirect pathway*.

disfacilitation Reduction in facilitatory effects exerted on neuron A, which normally receives an excitatory input from neuron B; this is due to a subsequent inhibitory input exerted on neuron B by neuron C, thus reducing the excitation on neuron A.

disinhibition Reduction in inhibitory effects exerted on neuron A, which normally receives an inhibitory input from neuron B; this is due to a subsequent inhibitory input exerted on neuron B by neuron C, thus reducing the inhibition on neuron A.

disorganized (hebephrenic) type of schizophrenia Form of schizophrenia characterized by a flat affect that is mostly inappropriate; speech is incoherent, disjointed, and rambling. See also *schizophrenia*.

doll's eye maneuver Testing of the horizontal eye movement reflex by passively turning the head from side to side; if the reflex is intact, the eyes will move conjugately in the direction opposite to movement.

dopamine A small-molecule catecholamine neurotransmitter synthesized from tyrosine.

dopamine β-hydroxylase (DBH) An enzyme present in the storage vesicles that converts dopamine into norepinephrine.

dopamine hypothesis of schizophrenia A leading neurochemical theory postulating that schizophrenia results from an excess of dopaminergic activity.

dorsal Above the cephalic flexure (pontine-midbrain border), dorsal refers to the top of the brain; below the flexure, dorsal means toward the dorsal surface of the body.

dorsal medullary syndrome Overlaps with the lateral medullary syndrome and results from a vascular lesion of a medial branch of the posterior inferior cerebellar artery (PICA); symptoms include nystagmus, vomiting, and vertigo.

dorsal motor nucleus of vagus Preganglionic neurons located in the caudal aspect of the dorsal medulla; provide primarily parasympathetic innervation to the heart, lungs, pancreas, and gastrointestinal tract.

dorsal nucleus of Clarke Group of large neurons located at the base of the dorsal horn in all thoracic spinal segments C8–L3; receives muscle spindle and tendon afferents predominantly from the caudal aspect of the body and lower limbs; gives rise to dorsal spinocerebellar tract, which terminates in ipsilateral cerebellum.

dorsal respiratory group of neurons Group of respiratory neurons located in the ventrolateral subnucleus of the solitary tract.

dorsal root ganglia Cell bodies of the peripheral nervous system that form sensory ganglia of the spinal cord; these are first-order neurons mediating pain, temperature, and proprioceptive inputs to the CNS from the body.

dorsal root Nerve bundles emerging from the dorsal aspect of the spinal cord and associated with the transmission of sensory signals to the spinal cord.

dorsal spinocerebellar tract A tract arising from the dorsal nucleus of Clarke transmitting information from the muscle spindles and the Golgi tendon organs to the cerebellum.

dorsomedial nucleus Nucleus situated in the dorsomedial aspect of the middle third of the thalamus; receives inputs from limbic structures and is reciprocally connected with the prefrontal cortex.

down-regulation Reduction in the number of receptors; involves internalization and sequestration of receptors into the cell.

dura mater A tough, fibrous membrane covering the brain and spinal cord.

dural sinuses Channels for the passage of blood; created by separation of the periosteal and meningeal layers of the cranial dura.

dynorphins See *opioid peptides*.

dysarthria Disturbance in articulation.

dysdiadochokinesia Type of cerebellar disorder in which the patient may be unable to make rapid alternating rotational movements of the hand.

dyskinesia Diseases of the basal ganglia characterized by abnormal, involuntary movements at rest and by abnormal changes in muscle tone.

dysmetria Type of cerebellar disorder in which a patient, when asked to move one hand so a finger touches his nose, will either undershoot or overshoot the mark.

dysphagia Difficulty in ability to swallow.

dysphasia Lack of coordination in speech.

dysthymia Unipolar form of depression that lasts for most of a given day and that can extend for several years.

dystonia Sustained muscle contractions of the limb, axial, or cranial voluntary muscles, resulting in abnormal postures and repetitive or twisting movements.

Ecstasy A recreational drug of abuse; reported to induce sensory enhancement (a feeling that all is right with the world) and empathogenesis (a feeling of closeness with others and removal of barriers in communication, especially in intimate relationships).

ectoderm The surface layer of embryonic tissue.

Edinger-Westphal nucleus Group of preganglionic parasympathetic neurons whose axons form the parasympathetic component of CN III.

efflux Movement of substances (e.g., ions) from inside to outside of the cell.

electrochemical gradient Combination of the concentration and electrical potential gradients.

electroencephalogram (EEG) Measurement of electrical activity typically recorded from the scalp; represents brain activity consisting of a summation of excitatory postsynaptic potentials (EPSPs) and inhibitory postsynaptic potentials (IPSPs).

encephalé isolé Type of experimental preparation involving a high spinal transection that allows for a cortical arousal pattern to be maintained.

encephalitis Inflammation of the brain; usually caused by bacteria or viruses.

encephalocele Failure of portions of the anterior neuropore to close, manifested by the protrusion of a sac from the cranium consisting of portions of the meninges and CSF, glial tissue, and brain substance with or without the ventricles.

endocytosis The process by which materials (e.g., nerve growth factor, remnants of vesicular membranes) are taken back into the cytoplasm of the neuron.

endomorphins Tetrapeptides identified as endogenous μ-opioid receptor ligands; their effects are blocked by naloxone.

endoneurium Connective tissue layer that encloses individual nerve fibers.

endothelins Potent vasoconstrictor peptides; isolated initially from aortic endothelial cells.

end-plate potential (EPP) Electrical potential generated at the muscle end-plate; elicited by activation of nicotinic cholinergic receptors located at the end-plate by acetylcholine.

end-plate Specialized region on the muscle membrane; one of the components of the neuromuscular junction; axons of motor neurons innervating skeletal muscle are devoid of myelin sheath and give off several fine branches at the end-plate.

enkephalins See *opioid peptides*.

enophthalmos Sinking of the eyeball in the orbit; one of the symptoms of Horner's syndrome; caused by interruption of the sympathetic innervation to the orbital muscle of Müller.

enteric division of autonomic nervous system Consists of neurons in the wall of the gut that regulate gastrointestinal motility and secretion; includes the myenteric (Auerbach's) and submucosal (Meissner's) plexuses in the smooth muscle of the gut.

entorhinal cortex (paleopallium) Region of temporal cortex adjoining the hippocampal formation; receives inputs from various sensory regions and transmits this information to the hippocampal formation.

ependymal wall Pertaining to the walls of the ventricles of the brain.

ependymocytes Cuboidal or columnar cells forming a single layer of lining in the brain ventricles and the central canal of the spinal cord.

epidural space Space outside the dura mater.

epinephrine Small-molecule, catecholamine neurotransmitter synthesized from tyrosine in the CNS and adrenal medulla.

epineurium Connective tissue layer enclosing several bundles of nerve fibers.

epithalamus Group of structures forming the roof of the diencephalon; includes the habenular complex, stria medullaris, and pineal gland.

excitatory amino acid neurotransmitters Small-molecule neurotransmitters (e.g., glutamate and aspartate).

excitatory postsynaptic potential (EPSP) Depolarizing graded potential that drives the membrane potential towards the threshold and excites the neuron.

excitotoxicity Prolonged stimulation of neurons by excitatory amino acids resulting in neuronal death or injury; predominantly, postsynaptic neurons are lost due to excessive concentrations of intracellular Ca^{2+}.

exocytosis Process in which there is fusion of the neurotransmitter-containing vesicle with the presynaptic terminal membrane, resulting in an opening through which the neurotransmitter is released into the synaptic cleft.

external arcuate fibers Axons arising from the accessory cuneate nucleus that form the cuneocerebellar tract, which projects to the cerebellum; convey signals above the sixth thoracic segment (of the spinal cord) from individual muscles of the upper limb.

external plexiform layer Layer of hippocampus situated adjacent to the inferior horn of the lateral ventricle; contains axons of pyramidal cells that project outside the hippocampus as well as hippocampal afferent fibers from the entorhinal cortex.

external urethral sphincter Striated muscle innervated by alpha-motor neurons of Onuf's nucleus located in spinal sacral segments S2 to S4.

extrastriate area See *association area*.

facial colliculus A bulge found along the floor of the fourth ventricle formed from fibers of the facial nerve that pass over the dorsal aspect of the abducens nucleus.

facial nerve (CN VII) Mixed cranial nerve of the lower pons that contains autonomic fibers affecting salivary, lacrimal, and pterygopalatine glands; sensory impulses mediating taste signals from the anterior two thirds of the tongue; and special visceral efferent fibers that innervate muscles of facial expression.

falx cerebelli Sheet-like process (septum) extending from the meningeal layer of the dura; divides the cranium into two lateral compartments and partially separates the two cerebral hemispheres.

fasciculus cuneatus First-order sensory neurons contained in the dorsal funiculus that project to the nucleus cuneatus and that convey the modalities of conscious proprioception and tactile sensation from the ipsilateral side of the upper limb.

fasciculus gracilis First-order sensory neurons contained in the dorsal funiculus that project to the nucleus gracilis and that convey the modalities of conscious proprioception and tactile sensation from the ipsilateral side of the lower limb.

fasciculus retroflexus See *habenulopeduncular tract*.

fast anterograde axonal transport Orthograde (forward flowing) movement of peptide neurotransmitters, enzymes, and glycoproteins from the neuronal cell body to the terminals at a relatively fast rate (about 100 to 400 mm/day). For comparison, see *slow anterograde axonal transport*.

fast retrograde axonal transport Retrograde (backward flowing) movement of materials, such as remnants of vesicular membranes, from the nerve terminals to the neuronal cell body at a relatively fast rate (about 50 to 200 mm/day).

fastigial nucleus Deep cerebellar nucleus whose axons project to the reticular formation and vestibular nuclei.

feed-forward inhibition in the cerebellum Circuit in which a mossy fiber excites a Golgi cell, which, in turn, inhibits a granule cell; this type of inhibition is also present elsewhere in the CNS.

feedback inhibition in the cerebellum Circuit in which a mossy fiber excites a granule cell, which, in turn, excites a Golgi cell, which then inhibits the granule cell; this type of inhibition is also present elsewhere in the CNS.

fibrous astrocyte Glial cell found between nerve fibers in the white matter; functions to repair the damaged tissue; this process may result in scar formation.

filum terminale externum Caudal thin extension of the spinal dura that surrounds the filum terminale internum; also known as the coccygeal ligament.

filum terminale internum Thin filament emerging from the conus medullaris.

fixation point A point in the visual field with which the fovea of each retina is aligned.

fixed ions Negatively charged organic molecules (e.g., proteins, nucleic acids, carboxylic groups, and metabolites carrying phosphate) within the cell that are unable to cross the neuronal membrane; they render the cell inside the neuronal membrane negatively charged compared with the outside.

floaters Debris particles floating in the vitreous humor that cast shadows on the retina.

flocculonodular lobe Smallest lobe of the cerebellum situated in an inferior position; principally concerned with balance and eye movements.

floor plate Aspect of the developing nervous system whose cells lie along the midline of the ventral aspect of the neural canal.

fluoxetine (Prozac) A drug that selectively blocks reuptake of serotonin and enhances serotonin levels in the brain; produces beneficial effects in mental depression via enhancement of transmission through 5-HT receptors. See also *serotonin*.

foramen magnum Large opening at the base of the occipital bone through which the medulla is continuous with the spinal cord.

foramen of Magendie Median aperture of the fourth ventricle enabling CSF to flow into the cisterns.

foramina of Luschka Lateral apertures of the fourth ventricle enabling CSF to flow into the cisterns.

foramina of Monro (interventricular foramina) Apertures linking the lateral ventricles with the third ventricle.

forebrain The most rostral aspect of the brain that includes the diencephalon, basal ganglia, limbic system, and cerebral hemispheres.

fornix Major fiber system arising from the hippocampal formation that lies buried deep within the medial aspect of the temporal lobe; it emerges from the hippocampal formation posteriorly and passes dorsomedially around the thalamus to occupy a medial position inferior to the corpus callosum but immediately superior to the thalamus.

fourth ventricle Cavity containing CSF that extends from the rostral half of the medulla through the pons.

fovea Depression at the center of the macula; contains primarily cones; region of retina associated with the highest visual acuity.

Frey's syndrome Disorder in which parasympathetic fibers eliciting secretory responses in parotid glands grow erroneously into the overlying facial skin; parasympathetic stimulation causes sweating of this facial region instead of producing saliva.

frontal eye fields Region of the middle frontal gyrus (area 8) that coordinates voluntary control of eye movements through its projections to the horizontal gaze center and superior colliculus.

frontal gyri Region of cerebral cortex that lies immediately anterior to the premotor cortex and consists of superior, middle, and inferior gyri; involved in the integration of motor processes.

funiculus A bundle containing one or more tracts or fasciculi in the spinal cord.

GABA-transaminase (GABA-T) An enzyme that metabolizes GABA.

γ-aminobutyric acid (GABA) Small-molecule inhibitory neurotransmitter synthesized from glutamate by the enzyme, glutamic acid decarboxylase (GAD).

γ-motor neurons Neurons interspersed between alpha-motor neurons in the ventral horn of the spinal cord; regulate the sensitivity of muscle spindles.

ganglion (plural: ganglia) An aggregation of nerve cell bodies located in the peripheral nervous system.

gap junction Area where two neurons are apposed to each other at an electrical synapse.

gap junction channels Channels that connect neurons at gap junctions; formed by two hemichannels, one in the presynaptic neuron and the other in the postsynaptic neuron.

gaze palsy (Parinaud's syndrome) Disorder characterized by an upward gaze paralysis, possible nystagmus with downward gaze, large pupil, abnormal elevation of the upper lid, and paralysis of accommodation; results from a vascular lesion or a pineal tumor that damages the dorsal aspect of the midbrain, including the pretectal area and region of the posterior commissure.

general somatic afferent (GSA) neurons Components of afferent fibers of cranial nerves that are associated with transmission of somatosensory impulses mediating changes in temperature, noxious stimulation, touch, pressure, and proprioception from the periphery to the brain.

general somatic efferent fibers (GSE) Fibers that transmit signals from the CNS to skeletal muscle.

general visceral afferent fibers (GVA) Fibers that originate from visceral structures and provide the CNS with information concerning their status.

general visceral efferent fibers (GVE) Fibers that transmit autonomic signals from the CNS to smooth muscle and glands.

generalized seizures   Seizures that arise diffusely from the cerebral cortex and that reveal epileptic activity diffusely, often involving tonic-clonic phases.

geniculocalcarine tract   Axons emerging from the lateral geniculate nucleus that project to the primary visual cortex.

Gerstmann syndrome   Disorder of the parietal lobe that includes a finger agnosia (patient cannot recognize different fingers), agraphia (inability to write), acalculia (patient is deficient in performing calculations), and alexia (deficiency in reading).

glaucoma   Disease characterized by increased pressure within the anterior and posterior chambers of the eye; increase in intraocular pressure reduces blood supply to the eye, causing damage to the retina.

glial cells   Nonneural cells forming the interstitial tissue of the nervous system.

globus pallidus   Major component of the basal ganglia along with the caudate nucleus and putamen.

glossopharyngeal nerve (CN IX)   Consists of general (baroreceptor) and special (chemoreceptor) visceral afferent fibers, GSAs (from the external ear) and GVE (parasympathetic) fibers innervating the otic ganglion (which supplies the parotid gland), and special visceral efferent (SVE) fibers innervating the stylopharyngeus muscle.

glutamate   Major excitatory amino acid neurotransmitter in the CNS synthesized from glutamine in presence of the enzyme glutaminase.

glycine   Small-molecule, inhibitory neurotransmitter synthesized from serine.

glycolysis   The process in which glucose is split into two pyruvate (pyruvic acid) molecules with the concomitant production of a relatively small amount of ATP. It occurs in almost all cells including neurons. This process also serves as a source of raw materials for the synthesis of other compounds. For example, in a cholinergic neuron, pyruvate formed during glycolysis is transported into the mitochondria where it combines with coenzyme-A to form acetylcoenzyme-A, which is transported back into the cytoplasm and is used along with choline to synthesize acetylcholine in presence of the enzyme, choline acetyltransferase.

Golgi apparatus   Aggregations of flat vesicles of smooth endoplasmic reticulum; proteins are modified in this apparatus (by glycosylation or phosphorylation), packaged into vesicles, and transported to other intracellular locations (such as nerve terminals).

Golgi tendon organ   High-threshold receptor present in the tendon that responds to movement of the limb; information concerning changes in muscle tension is conveyed to the spinal cord and cerebellum.

gonadotropin-releasing hormone (GnRH)   Hormone released from wide areas of the hypothalamus and septal area; controls release of follicle-stimulating hormone (which facilitates growth of follicles and oocytes) and leuteinizing hormone (which governs induction of ovulation and formation of corpus luteum).

G-protein   A guanosine-5′-triphosphate (GTP)-binding protein; activation of a G-protein by binding of a neurotransmitter to its receptor results in activation of a second-messenger system that can either act directly on the ion channel to open it or activate an enzyme that opens the channel by phosphorylating the channel protein.

graded potentials   Brief local changes in membrane potential that occur in neuronal dendrites and cell bodies, but not in axons.

granule cell   Primary cell type comprising the deepest layer of the cerebellar cortex, called the granule cell layer; its axon is a parallel fiber that makes synaptic contact with both Purkinje and Golgi cell dendrites.

gray commissure   A band of gray matter extending onto both sides of the spinal cord.

gray matter   Brain and spinal cord tissue that appears gray with the naked eye; consists mainly of neuronal cell bodies (nuclei) and lacks myelinated axons.

great cerebral vein of Galen   A short vein, formed by the union of two internal cerebral veins at the level of the splenium of corpus callosum; courses caudally and joins the inferior sagittal sinus to form the straight sinus, which then empties into the confluence of sinuses.

growth hormone-inhibiting hormone   The peptide, somatostatin, that inhibits the release of growth hormone; also serves as a neurotransmitter or neuromodulator.

growth hormone-releasing hormone (GHrH)   Hormone released from the arcuate nucleus of hypothalamus that activates release of growth hormone for growth of the body and long bones.

Guillain-Barré syndrome   An autoimmune disease characterized by demyelination of peripheral nerves innervating the muscles and skin; conduction of action potentials along axons is slowed down or blocked, resulting in severe disturbances in motor and sensory functions.

gustation   Sensation of taste.

gyrus rectus   Medial aspect of the anterior prefrontal cortex.

H field of Forel   Region immediately rostral to the red nucleus where fibers of the lenticular fasciculus and ansa lenticularis merge and begin to course rostrally.

habenular commissure   Commissure connecting the habenular complex on both sides of the epithalamus.

habenular complex   Part of the epithalamus consisting of a lateral and medial nucleus; projects to the hypothalamus and related regions of the basal forebrain as well as to the interpeduncular nucleus of the midbrain.

habenulopeduncular tract (fasciculus retroflexus)   Pathway containing efferent fibers of the habenular complex that pass to the interpeduncular nucleus of the midbrain.

heat conservation center   Posterior lateral hypothalamus associated with heat conservation. A decrease in body temperature excites neurons in this region, causing autonomic neurons of the brainstem and spinal cord to activate heat-preserving mechanisms including vasoconstriction, tachycardia, piloerection, shivering, and elevations in basal metabolic rate.

heat loss center   Anterior hypothalamic neurons responsive to increases in body temperature, including pyrogens (i.e., substances that increase body temperature); activates heat loss mechanisms involving vasodilation and perspiration.

hematoma   Blood clot; can obstruct blood flow to the adjacent brain tissue.

hemiballism   Abnormal flailing movements of the arm and leg of the side of the body contralateral to the site of the lesion in the subthalamic nucleus.

Hertz (Hz)   Cycles per second; unit used to describe frequency of signals (e.g., sound waves).

heteronomous visual deficit   Loss of vision in different halves of the visual field for each eye.

heteronymous muscle   Antagonist muscle that controls the same joint but has an opposite mechanical function; e.g., an extensor has an antagonistic action to that of a flexor.

hippocampal formation   Deep cortical structure situated in the medial aspect of the temporal lobe, consisting of the hippocampus and subicular cortex; associated with short-term memory and regulation of emotional and autonomic functions.

Hirschsprung's disease   Disorder characterized by absence of peristalsis of the distal colon due to failure of development of myenteric plexus; the proximal part of the colon distends (megacolon) and is prone to impaction of feces.

histamine   Small-molecule neurotransmitter synthesized from histidine; also released from mast cells (a type of connective tissue cell).

histidine   A basic amino acid found in most proteins.

histogenesis   The process of formation of tissues from undifferentiated germinal cells in the embryo.

homotypical   Pertains to the same region or site on the opposite side of the brain.

homunculus   Somatotopic organization of sensory and motor regions of the cerebral cortex in which the cells of origin functionally associated with the head, arm, and leg are located in the ventrolateral, convexity, and medial wall of the hemisphere, respectively.

horizontal gaze center See *pontine gaze center*.

Horner's syndrome Characterized by drooping of the upper eyelid (pseudoptosis), constriction of the pupil (miosis), enophthalmos (sinking of eyeball in the orbit), dilation of arterioles of the skin, and anhidrosis (loss of sweating) at the face. It is caused by lesions of the brainstem and upper cervical cord that interrupt the sympathetic fibers descending from the hypothalamus to the intermediolateral cell column of the thoracolumbar cord.

horseradish peroxidase (HRP) Enzyme present in plant cells; used as a marker in anatomical tracing techniques.

Huntingtin Protein encoded by a gene associated with the short arm of chromosome 4, which, when mutated, is responsible for Huntington's disease.

Huntington's disease (chorea) Characterized by wild, uncontrolled movements of the distal musculature, which appear as abrupt and jerky; an inherited autosomal dominant illness with the genetic defect located on the short arm of chromosome 4; the gene encodes a protein referred to as huntingtin.

hydrocephalus Dilation of the ventricles occurring when CSF circulation is blocked or its absorption is impeded; results in an increase in ventricular pressure.

hydrophilic Water-soluble or polar substances.

hydrophobic Water-insoluble or nonpolar substances.

hyperalgesia Enhancement of pain sensation.

hyperglycinemia Neonatal disease characterized by lethargy and mental retardation due to high levels of glycine in the CNS; associated with mutations of genes coding for membrane transporters involved in removal of glycine.

hypermetropia (hyperopia, far-sightedness) Disorder resulting from shortening of or weakness in the lens system, causing light rays from an object to be focused behind the retina.

hypogastric (pelvic) plexus Neuronal network through which sympathetic postganglionic fibers are distributed to the urinary bladder, colon, rectum, and male (penis) and female (clitoris) erectile tissue.

hypoglossal nucleus Cell bodies of origin of CN XII.

hypokinetic disorders Disorders involving impaired initiation of movement characteristic of diseases of the basal ganglia.

hypophyseal portal vascular system Vessels that form a vascular link between the hypothalamus and anterior lobe of the pituitary.

hypophysis Pituitary gland.

hyposmia Reduction of olfactory function; may result from damage to the olfactory mucosa due to infections.

hypothalamohypophyseal portal vascular system Communication between the hypothalamus and anterior pituitary via a portal system of blood vessels.

hypothalamus Ventral aspect of the diencephalon; concerns a variety of cell groups associated with diverse visceral functions, including control of endocrine release of the pituitary, temperature regulation, feeding, drinking, sexual behavior, and aggression and rage behavior.

hypotonia Diminution of muscle tone.

ictal period Time of occurrence of a seizure.

ideational apraxia Inability to conceptualize and identify the sequences of movements that are necessary for carrying out a given response.

ideomotor apraxia Inability to execute a movement upon request.

immediate memory Recalling an event a few seconds after it occurs.

indirect pathway One of the two pathways comprising the internal circuitry governing the transmission of information through the basal ganglia; consists of an indirect pathway from the neostriatum to the internal segment of globus pallidus. This circuit includes an initial projection from the neostriatum to the external segment of globus pallidus, to a second neuron that passes to the subthalamic nucleus, and to a third neuron that projects back to the internal segment of globus

pallidus; information is then transmitted to the cerebral cortex via the thalamus. See *direct pathway*.

indirectly gated ion channels Type of channel in which the ion channel and recognition site for the transmitter (receptor) are separate.

infarction See *brain infarction*.

inferior At positions above and below the cephalic flexure, inferior means toward the bottom of the spinal cord.

inferior (nodose) ganglion of vagus (CN X) Consists of pseudounipolar neurons mediating the sensation of taste and baroreceptor and chemoreceptor functions.

inferior (petrosal) ganglion of the glossopharyngeal nerve (CN IX) Consists of pseudounipolar neurons mediating the sensation of taste and baroreceptor and chemoreceptor functions.

inferior anastomotic (Labbé's) vein This vein travels across the temporal lobe and connects the superficial middle cerebral vein with the transverse sinus.

inferior cerebellar peduncle Major afferent pathway to cerebellum from the medulla.

inferior colliculus Caudal aspect of the tectum of midbrain; part of the ascending auditory relay pathway to the medial geniculate nucleus of thalamus.

inferior oblique muscle An extraocular eye muscle innervated by the oculomotor nerve (CN III); stimulation of this nerve results in contraction in part of the inferior oblique muscle, causing the eye to be elevated when it is located in the medial position.

inferior olivary nucleus Large nuclear structure situated in the ventrolateral medulla serving as a relay for transmission of impulses from the spinal cord and red nucleus to the cerebellum.

inferior salivatory nucleus Consists of neurons whose axons form part of CN IX supplying the otic ganglion, which, in turn, innervates the parotid gland, thus contributing to the process of salivation.

inferior temporal gyrus Cortical structure situated on the ventral aspect of the temporal neocortex.

influx Movement of substances (e.g., ions) into the cell.

infundibular stalk (infundibulum) Connecting link between the hypothalamus and pituitary gland.

inhibitory amino acids Small-molecule neurotransmitters (e.g., GABA and glycine).

inhibitory postsynaptic potential (IPSP) Hyperpolarizing graded potential that drives the membrane potential away from the threshold and inhibits the neuron.

initial segment First 50 to 100 μm of the axon after it emerges from the axon hillock.

intention tremor Cerebellar disorder in which a patient displays a tremor when voluntarily attempting to move a limb.

interblob area Region around the blob areas staining less intensely with cytochrome oxidase; associated with orientation of lines having a spatial orientation. See *blob area*.

interictal period Time period between seizures.

intermediolateral cell column (IML) Lateral extension of spinal gray matter; present in thoracic (T1–L2) and sacral (S2–S4) cord; thoracic IML contains preganglionic sympathetic neurons; sacral IML contains parasympathetic preganglionic neurons.

internal arcuate fibers Fibers arising from dorsal column nuclei that pass ventrally for a short distance in an arc-like trajectory before crossing over to the contralateral side as the medial lemniscus.

internal capsule Contains descending fibers from the cerebral cortex to the brainstem and spinal cord as well as ascending fibers from the thalamus to the cerebral cortex.

internal carotid arteries Arteries arising at the carotid bifurcation that enter the cranium via the carotid canal in the petrous bone.

internal medullary lamina Band of myelinated fibers separating the medial from lateral thalamus.

internuclear ophthalmoplegia Disorder characterized by nystagmus; results from lesions that disrupt the mechanisms that regulate normal conjugate deviation of the eyes; lesion includes damage to the medial longitudinal fasciculus at levels rostral to the pontine gaze center.

interparietal sulcus Sulcus that separates the superior from the inferior parietal lobule.

interposed nuclei Deep cerebellar nuclei, consisting of the globose and emboliform nuclei; axons project through the superior cerebellar peduncle to the red nucleus.

interventricular foramen See *foramina of Monro.*

intracranial pressure Pressure within the cranial cavity. Usually lumbar cerebrospinal fluid pressure is used as a guide to assess intracranial pressure. Normal CSF pressure in adults is less than 200 mm of water.

intrinsic neurons (type II or Golgi type II neurons) Interneurons with very short axons; have inhibitory function.

inverse myotatic reflex Reduction of contraction of homonymous muscle elicited by stimulation of Golgi tendon organs.

ion channels Channels that allow some ions to cross the membrane in the direction of their concentration gradients.

ionotropic receptor Receptor in which 4 to 5 protein subunits are arranged in such a way that the recognition site for the neurotransmitter is part of the ion channel; a transmitter binds to its receptor and brings about a conformational change that results in the opening of the ion channel.

ipsilateral On the same side with reference to a specific point.

iris Colored portion of the eye that is visible through the cornea; has a central opening called the pupil.

ischemia See brain ischemia.

Jacksonian march Seizure activity, which begins locally over the cortex, causing either sensory motor activity directly corresponding to the homunculus of either the sensory or motor cortex; the patient experiences a "march" of sensory or motor activity from muscle to muscle in the same order as the homunculus.

juxtarestiform body Monosynaptic pathway from vestibular apparatus to cerebellum that courses along the medial side of the inferior cerebellar peduncle.

kainic acid (kainate) An agonist at kainite receptor (ionotropic glutamate receptor).

kinesin A microtubule associated with the enzyme ATPase (adenosine triphosphatase); involved in axonal transport.

Klüver-Bucy syndrome Constellation of behavioral response changes following amygdaloid lesions in the monkey consisting of hypersexuality, a change in dietary habits, a decrease in anxiety toward fear-producing objects, a tendency to explore and contact orally inedible objects, and visual agnosia. Rarely reported in humans.

Korsakoff's syndrome Memory disorder (usually associated with damage to the fornix or its projection targets) in which the patient displays amnesia (memory loss) of both anterograde and retrograde memory.

Lambert-Eaton (Eaton-Lambert) syndrome Disorder associated with muscle weakness; usually accompanied with small-cell carcinoma of the lung derived from primitive neuroendocrine precursor cells expressing voltage-gated calcium channels. An antibody produced against these calcium channels results in loss of voltage-gated Ca^{2+} channels in the presynaptic terminals at the neuromuscular junction; consequently, there is a reduction in the release of the transmitter (acetylcholine), causing muscle weakness.

lamina terminalis Wall forming the rostral limit of the third ventricle, rostral to which lies the telencephalon.

lateral Away from the midline.

lateral corticospinal tract See *corticospinal tract.*

lateral dorsal nucleus of pons Nucleus of the pons containing acetylcholine; associated with rapid eye movement (REM) sleep.

lateral dorsal thalamic nucleus Thalamic nucleus adjoining the dorsolateral aspect of the ventrolateral nucleus; projects to the medial aspect of the cerebral cortex immediately caudal to the postcentral gyrus.

lateral funiculus White matter of the lateral aspect of spinal cord; contains both ascending (spinothalamic, spinocerebellar) and descending (corticospinal, rubrospinal) fibers.

lateral geniculate nucleus Thalamic relay nucleus transmitting visual signals from the retina to the visual cortex.

lateral hypothalamic area (lateral hypothalamus) Lateral aspect of the hypothalamus extending rostrally from the preoptic region to the level of the mammillary bodies caudally. It contains both ascending and descending axons, including the medial forebrain bundle and cell groups, and is concerned with feeding, drinking, and predatory behavior.

lateral inhibition of photoreceptors Form of inhibition involved in processing of signals from photoreceptors; elicited when glutamate, released from photoreceptors, depolarizes horizontal cells, which, in turn, inhibit adjacent photoreceptors.

lateral lemniscus Axons constituting third-order auditory neurons from the superior olivary complex and nucleus of the trapezoid body that ascend bilaterally in the lateral lemniscus.

lateral medullary lamina Thin band of white matter separating the globus pallidus from the putamen.

lateral medullary syndrome (Wallenberg's syndrome) Syndrome resulting from a vascular lesion of the vertebral and inferior posterior cerebellar arteries (PICA), resulting in loss of pain and temperature to the ipsilateral face and contralateral body as well as Horner's syndrome, hoarseness, loss of gag reflex, and difficulties in swallowing.

lateral olfactory tract Large bundle of axons from the mitral and tufted cells that exit from the olfactory bulb to supply the pyriform lobe. See also *olfactory tract.*

lateral perforant pathway Fiber pathway passing from the lateral entorhinal cortex into the molecular layer of the hippocampus.

lateral posterior thalamic nucleus Nucleus adjoining the dorsolateral aspect of the ventrobasal complex of thalamus; projects to the superior parietal lobule.

lateral rectus muscle An extraocular muscle innervated by the abducens nerve (CN VI); contraction of this muscle causes the eye to be moved laterally.

lateral reticular nucleus Nucleus situated in the lateral aspect of the medulla; axons of these neurons project to the cerebellum.

lateral ventricle Cavity found throughout much of each cerebral hemisphere of the brain; consists of (1) an anterior horn, present at rostral levels deep in the frontal lobe; (2) a posterior horn, extending into the occipital lobe; and (3) an inferior horn, which extends in ventral and anterior directions deep into the temporal lobe, ending near the amygdaloid complex.

lateral vestibulospinal tract Motor pathway arising from the lateral vestibular nucleus that projects to all levels of spinal cord and powerfully facilitates extensor motor neurons.

L-DOPA (levodopa) Immediate metabolic precursor of dopamine; crosses blood-brain barrier; administered orally for the treatment of Parkinson's disease. See also *Sinemet.*

lenticular (lentiform) nucleus Putamen and globus pallidus.

lenticular fasciculus (H_2 field of Forel) Major efferent pathway of the basal ganglia; exits from the dorsal aspect of the medial pallidal segment and supplies ventrolateral and ventral anterior thalamic nuclei.

leptomeninges Collective term for the inner coverings of the brain (i.e., pia and arachnoid mater).

leuteinizing hormone-releasing hormone Neuroactive peptide synthesized in the hypothalamus affecting release of leuteinizing hormone of the anterior pituitary, which then stimulates testosterone production in males and follicle formation and ovulation in females.

levator palpebrae superior muscle A muscle innervated by the oculomotor nerve; stimulation of the oculomotor nerve results, in part, in contraction of this muscle, causing elevation of the upper eyelid.

L-glutamic acid-1-decarboxylase (GAD) An enzyme present

almost exclusively in GABAergic neurons; involved in the synthesis of GABA.

limbic structures (limbic system) Group of subcortical and cortical structures associated with emotional behavior and the control of other visceral processes normally linked to hypothalamic functions; includes the hippocampal formation, amygdala, septal area, prefrontal cortex, and cingulate gyrus.

lithium Drug used for the treatment of bipolar disorder.

locked-in syndrome Disorder characterized by paralysis of most motor functions, including the limbs (corticospinal loss), and functions associated with motor cranial nerves (corticobulbar loss) other than the ability to blink one's eyes and display vertical gaze. Results from a large infarct of the basilar pons affecting both the corticobulbar and corticospinal tracts; the patient can only communicate by blinking or moving his eyes.

long-term memory Events that are remembered weeks, months, or years after they have occurred.

long-term potentiation (LTP) An increase in synaptic strength as a manifestation of synaptic plasticity.

lordosis Increased curvature of the normally curved lumbar spine.

Lou Gehrig's disease See *amyotrophic lateral sclerosis*.

lower motor neuron Motor neuron located either in the brainstem or spinal cord whose axons innervate skeletal muscle.

lumbar cistern Cistern that extends from the caudal end of the spinal cord to the second sacral vertebra; because of the large subarachnoid space and relative absence of neural structures, this space is most suitable for the withdrawal of CSF by lumbar puncture.

lumbar cord Lower part of the spinal cord situated between the thoracic cord, rostrally, and sacral cord, caudally, containing 5 pairs of spinal nerves.

lysosomes Membrane-bound vesicles formed from the Golgi apparatus; contain hydrolytic enzymes and serve as scavengers in neurons.

macrocephaly A developmental abnormality characterized by an enlarged cranium.

macula lutea Circular portion near the lateral edge of the optic disc that appears yellowish due to the presence of a yellow pigment; this part of the retina is for central (as opposed to peripheral) vision.

magnetic resonance angiography (MRA) Macroscopic changes in spins (small magnetic fields) within the nuclei in blood that are detectable in magnetic resonance imaging (MRI); often used in stroke patients prior to conventional angiography.

magnetic resonance imaging (MRI) Imaging technique in which graded spatial variations in the magnetic field are generated by different sets of magnets oriented along different axes; when all the atomic nuclei are aligned by the magnetic field, a brief radiofrequency pulse is applied. The radiofrequencies emitted by the oscillating nuclei are monitored by sensitive detectors, and a computer converts signal intensities and magnetic gradient parameters into spatial locations; detailed images of the tissue under examination are then constructed. The brain and spinal cord can be imaged in three dimensions to reproduce the locations of specific structures and identify any abnormalities such as presence of tumors.

magnetic resonance spectroscopy Also known as nuclear magnetic resonance (NMR) spectroscopy; used in neuroscience research to identify specific neurotransmitters and other substances in specific regions of the brain.

magnocellular Pertains to a region containing large-sized cells.

mammillary bodies A large mass of neurons forming two bilateral prominences on the ventromedial surface of the most caudal aspect of the hypothalamus.

mammillotegmental tract Pathway from the mammillary bodies to the midbrain tegmentum.

mammillothalamic tract Pathway arising in the mammillary bodies that supplies the anterior nucleus of thalamus.

mantle layer The intermediate layer of the neural tube.

Marcus-Gunn pupil Condition in which one of the eyes has an optic nerve lesion; when light is shone on the normal eye, both pupils constrict (direct and consensual light reflexes); when the light is shone on the eye with the optic nerve lesion, a paradoxical dilation of both pupils occurs.

marginal layer Outer layer of the neural tube.

massa intermedia (interthalamic adhesion) Midline region of thalamus, above and below which lie components of the third ventricle.

matrix (of neostriatum) Compartment of neostriatum surrounding striosomes that receives inputs from sensory and motor regions of neocortex; many of the neurons in the matrix project to the globus pallidus.

medial Towards midline.

medial corticohypothalamic tract Pathway arising from subicular cortex that follows the fornix and supplies the ventromedial hypothalamus, including the region between the suprachiasmatic and arcuate nuclei.

medial forebrain bundle Principal pathway that traverses the rostral-caudal extent of the lateral hypothalamus. Many of the fibers constitute hypothalamic efferent projections to the brainstem; other fibers represent ascending monoaminergic projections from the brainstem that supply much of the forebrain, including the cerebral cortex; still others include fibers that arise from the septal area and diagonal band of Broca that project directly to the lateral and medial regions of hypothalamus, including the mammillary bodies.

medial geniculate nucleus Thalamic relay nucleus that transmits auditory information from inferior colliculus to the superior temporal gyrus.

medial hypothalamus Medial aspect of the hypothalamus containing varieties of cell groups concerned with control of pituitary-endocrine function, regulation of feeding behavior, and affective and visceral functions.

medial lemniscus Major ascending sensory pathway arising from the nucleus gracilis and nucleus cuneatus, mediating conscious proprioception and tactile sensations from the limbs to the contralateral ventral posterolateral thalamic nucleus.

medial longitudinal fasciculus (MLF) Located in a dorsomedial position within the medulla and pons; consists of both ascending and descending axons arising from vestibular nuclei. Ascending axons project to nuclei of CN VI, CN IV, and CN III, while descending axons project to the cervical cord.

medial medullary lamina Thin band of white matter separating medial and lateral pallidal segments.

medial medullary syndrome (Déjèrine's syndrome) Disorder resulting from a vascular lesion of the anterior spinal or paramedian branches of the vertebral arteries; characterized by (1) loss of conscious proprioception, touch, and pressure from the side of the body contralateral to the site of the lesion; (2) contralateral upper motor neuron paralysis; and (3) paralysis of the ipsilateral aspect of the tongue and deviation of the tongue upon protrusion to the side contralateral to the lesion.

medial olfactory tract Contains fibers from mitral and tufted cells; axons project ipsilaterally to basal limbic forebrain structures. See also *olfactory tract*.

medial perforant pathway Fiber pathway that enters the alveus of the hippocampus after passing through the white matter adjoining the subiculum.

medial tegmental syndrome Disorder resulting from a lesion restricted to the medial aspect of the pons, affecting the nucleus of the abducens nerve (CN VI), the fibers of the facial nerve (CN VII) that pass over the nucleus of CN VI, and possibly the medial lemniscus. Loss of functions include ipsilateral facial paralysis, loss of lateral gaze on the side ipsilateral to the lesion, and contralateral loss of conscious proprioception and discriminative touch if the lesion extends sufficiently ventral to involve the medial lemniscus.

medial vestibulospinal tract Pathway from the medial vestibular nucleus constituting the descending component of the MLF that projects to the cervical cord and serves to adjust changes in the position of the head in response to changes in vestibular inputs.

median eminence Ventral portion of the tuber cinereum (a narrow region of the ventral surface of hypothalamus caudal to the optic chiasm) where the axons of hypothalamic neurons containing hormone-releasing factors converge; ventrally, the median eminence is continuous with the infundibulum (the stalk connecting hypothalamus with the pituitary).

medulla Most caudal aspect of the brainstem extending from the pons to spinal cord.

medullary (lateral) reticulospinal tract See *reticulospinal tracts*.

megacolon See *Hirschsprung's disease*.

melanocytes Pigment-forming cells of the skin.

melatonin A neurohormone involved in regulating sleep patterns.

membrane potential Electrical potential difference across a membrane.

membrane transport proteins Proteins that mediate the influx of essential nutrients and ions and efflux of waste products and other ions across the cell membrane.

membranous labyrinth Includes the utricle and saccule (two small sacs occupying the bony vestibule), three semicircular canal ducts, and the cochlear duct located within the cavities of the bony labyrinth of the ear; contains endolymph (an intracellular-like fluid containing low Na^+ and high K^+).

Ménière's disease Disorder characterized by hearing loss, vertigo, nystagmus, and nausea; involves both auditory and vestibular systems.

meninges Connective tissue coverings of the brain and spinal cord.

meningocele Pertaining to a protrusion of the meninges.

meningomyelocele Pertaining to a protrusion of the meninges together with the spinal cord.

mesencephalic nucleus of CN V Sensory nucleus of CN V located in the upper pons that receives trigeminal inputs from muscle spindles of the face region.

mesenchymal cells Embryonic cells that will become highly vascular, become attached to the ependyma of the ventricles, and generate pia mater.

mesocortical pathway Ascending dopaminergic neurons from the ventral tegmentum that innervate the frontal and cingulate cortices.

mesolimbic pathway Ascending dopaminergic neurons from the ventral tegmentum that innervate limbic structures (amygdala, septal area, hippocampal formation).

mesothelium A single layer of flattened cells that lines serous cavities (e.g., peritoneum).

metabotropic receptors Receptor in which the ion channel and recognition site for the transmitter are separate; binding of a transmitter to the receptor results in the activation of a second-messenger system.

metencephalon Developing pons and cerebellum (from rhombencephalon).

Meyer's loop A loop in the inferior part of the temporal lobe formed by axons arising from the ventrolateral region of the lateral geniculate nucleus; axons travel toward the tip of the temporal horn of the lateral ventricle and pass further caudally to terminate in the inferior bank of the calcarine fissure of the visual cortex.

microfilaments Formed by two strands of polymerized globular actin monomers; arranged in a helix; play an important role in motility of growth cones during development and in the formation of presynaptic and postsynaptic specializations.

microglia Smallest glial cell in the brain and spinal cord that is responsible for repairing damage following injury by removing debris associated with dead neurons and glial cells.

microtubules Consist of helical cylinders made up of protofilaments; required in the development and maintenance of neuronal processes.

midbrain The most rostral aspect of the brainstem; situated between the forebrain and pons.

midbrain periaqueductal gray See *periaqueductal gray*.

midbrain syndrome See *Parinaud's syndrome*.

middle cerebellar peduncle Major afferent fiber bundle to the cerebellar cortex containing mainly transverse pontine fibers arising from deep cerebellar nuclei.

middle cerebral artery Arises from the internal carotid artery at the level just lateral to the optic chiasm; its branches supply blood to the lateral convexity of cerebral hemisphere.

middle meningeal artery Arises from the internal carotid artery and supplies the dura.

midsagittal plane Anatomical plane of the brain perpendicular to the ground that divides the left and right sides of the brain and spinal cord into two equal halves.

milk ejection reflex Contractions of the myoepithelial cells around the nipple of the mammary gland for ejection of milk.

mitochondria Spherical or rod-shaped structures consisting of a double membrane; present in soma, dendrites, and in the axon of the neuron; involved in the generation of energy for the neuron.

modiolus Central tubular conical axis in the cochlea.

monoamine oxidase (MAO) Enzyme that metabolizes catecholamines.

monoamine oxidase inhibitors Agents that inhibit monoamine oxidase; mechanism by which some antidepressant drugs maintain or increase monoamine levels in brain.

mossy fibers Primary type of axonal input to the cerebellum from the spinal cord and brainstem; axons terminate on granule cell neurons in cerebellar cortex.

motion sickness Nausea and vomiting usually experienced when traveling in a vehicle such as an airplane, car, train or ship; induced by activation of autonomic centers via afferents from the vestibular system projecting to the reticular formation of the pons and medulla.

motor end-plate See *end-plate*.

movement agnosia Disorder of the middle temporal cortex in which the patient cannot distinguish between objects that are stationary and those that are moving.

multiple sclerosis Autoimmune disease characterized by severe disturbances in motor and sensory functions; symptoms include muscle weakness, lack of coordination, and disturbances in speech and vision; caused by demyelination of axons in the CNS, resulting in the slowing of conduction along axons.

muscarinic acetylcholine receptor See *cholinergic muscarinic receptor*.

muscle spindle Present in skeletal (flexor as well as extensor) muscles; has a low threshold for activation; senses length of the muscle. See also *myotatic reflex*.

myasthenia gravis Autoimmune disease characterized by weakness of the eyelids, eye muscles, oropharyngeal muscles, and limb muscles; caused by an antibody against nicotinic acetylcholine receptors at the motor end-plate; associated with a reduction in the number of functional nicotinic acetylcholine receptors on the postsynaptic membrane at the motor end-plate.

myelencephalon Developing medulla (from rhombencephalon).

myelinated axons Largely lipid membranes that wrap around the axons that form the white matter of the brain and spinal cord.

myelination Process by which lipid membranes are formed and wrapped around axons in the central and peripheral nervous systems.

myelodysplasia A defect in the development of the vertebral column and lower aspect of the spinal cord.

myeloschisis See *spina bifida*.

myenteric (Auerbach's) plexus Neurons in the gut that control gastrointestinal motility.

myopia (near-sightedness) Disorder resulting from lengthening of eyeball or occasionally by increased power of the lens system, causing light rays from an object to be focused in front of the retina.

myotatic reflex (knee jerk response) Monosynaptic reflex whose primary involved receptor is the muscle spindle; afferent limb of the reflex includes a Ia fiber from the muscle spindle that makes synaptic contact with an alpha-motor neuron, which innervates the extrafusal muscle of the same muscle group containing the intrafusal muscle; also called stretch or deep tendon reflex.

Na⁺-K⁺ pump (Na⁺-K⁺ ATPase) Located in the membranes of neurons as well as other cells; consists of a small glycoprotein and a large multi-pass transmembrane catalytic subunit. The pump transfers Na^+ to the extracellular side and K^+ to the intracellular side; with each cycle, one molecule of ATP is hydrolyzed, and the energy generated is used to move Na^+ and K^+ ions across the neuronal membrane; three Na^+ ions are transferred out of the neuron for influx of two K^+ ions.

naloxone An opioid receptor antagonist.

nasal hemiretina Component of retina that lies medial to the fovea.

necrotic cell death Acute traumatic injury that involves rapid lysis of cell membranes.

negative feedback mechanisms Mechanism by which synthesis of a neurotransmitter (e.g., norepinephrine) is blocked at its rate-limiting step (e.g., conversion of tyrosine to dihydroxyphenylalanine by tyrosine hydroxylase).

neostriatum Caudate nucleus and putamen, which are the major afferent receiving areas of the basal ganglia.

nerve cell body (perikaryon or soma) Central component of the neuron; consists of a mass of cytoplasm bounded by an external membrane; contains the nucleus and various organelles.

neural crest Group of cells located in the lateral margin of the neural groove that separates and migrates to a dorsal position; this group develops into the dorsal root ganglion and other peripheral neurons.

neural folds Expanding and growing lateral edges of the plate that accumulate in a dorsal position.

neural groove Shallow groove formed along the longitudinal axis of the neural folds.

neural plate Thickened region of ectoderm formed by the third to fourth week of embryonic development, which develops into the neural tube.

neural tube Primal tissue of the CNS derived from ectoderm.

neuralgia Characterized by severe and persistent pain; mediated through a cranial or spinal nerve (e.g., trigeminal neuralgia).

neurites Processes arising from the neuronal cell body (e.g., axons, dendrites).

neurocytes Young or immature neurons that have yet to completely differentiate.

neurofilaments Composed of fibers that twist around each other to form coils; most abundant in the axon.

neuroglia (glial cells) Supporting cells located in the CNS; nonexcitable and more numerous than neurons.

neuron Anatomical and functional unit of the nervous system that consists of a nerve cell body, dendrites (which receive signals from other neurons), and an axon (which transmits the signal to another neuron).

neuropeptide Y Synthesized in the arcuate nucleus of hypothalamus; acts as a neuromodulator of neurons containing gonadotropin-releasing hormone and also stimulates feeding behavior.

neurosecretory Pertaining to neurons that secrete hormones or releasing factors into the circulating blood.

neurotransmitter Chemical substance that is synthesized in a neuron, released at a synapse following depolarization of the nerve terminal, and binds to receptors on the postsynaptic cell and/or presynaptic terminal to elicit a specific response.

nicotinic acetylcholine receptor See *cholinergic nicotinic receptor*.

night blindness (nyctalopia) Disorder in which a person cannot see in the dark; caused by vitamin A deficiency.

Nissl substance or bodies Material consisting of RNA granules (ribosomes); present in the entire cell body and proximal portions of the dendrites, but not in the axon hillock and axon.

nitric oxide (NO) A gaseous neurotransmitter; formed from L-arginine in the presence of nitric oxide synthase (NOS); stimulates soluble guanylate cyclase and increases cGMP (cyclic guanosine monophosphate) formation. The responses induced by NO are mediated by cGMP. These responses vary according to the target tissue. In the vascular tissue, NO acts as a naturally occurring vasodilator. In other tissues, the exact function of NO is not yet established.

N-methyl-D-aspartic acid (NMDA) Agonist at NMDA receptor (ionotropic glutamate receptor).

nociceptin Endogenous ligand for the ORL1 opioid receptor; naloxone does not block this receptor. See *opioid receptors*.

nociception Reception of signals from nociceptors by the CNS.

nociceptors Free nerve endings that sense noxious stimuli.

nodes of Ranvier Intervals between adjacent oligodendrocytes; devoid of myelin sheaths.

noncommunicating hydrocephalus Condition in which the movement of CSF out of the ventricular system is impeded (e.g., by blockage at the cerebral aqueduct or foramina of the fourth ventricle).

nonconscious (unconscious) proprioception Proprioception mediated by muscle spindles and Golgi tendon organs; impulses arising from proprioceptors mediating this type of sensation are relayed to the cerebellum.

nonhomonymous bitemporal hemianopia Disorder resulting from a lesion at the optic chiasm, which interrupts the axons from the nasal hemiretinae of both eyes, leaving the axons from the temporal retinae intact. Loss of vision occurs in the right half of the right visual field and left half of the left visual field.

nonhomonymous visual deficit See *nonhomonymous bitemporal hemianopia*.

nonrectifying synapse (bidirectional synapse) Synapse at which the current can pass equally well in both directions.

nonspecific thalamic nuclei Thalamic nuclei that modulate the activity of other major projection thalamic nuclei and also have wide-ranging effects on neurons throughout the cortex.

norepinephrine Small-molecule neurotransmitter synthesized from tyrosine.

notochord Cells of mesodermal origin that induce the development of the neural plate.

nucleus Round structure usually located in the center of the cell body; enclosed within a double-layered nuclear membrane with fine pores. The term also refers to groups of neurons located in a specific region of the brain or spinal cord that generally have a similar appearance, receive information from similar sources, project their axons to similar targets, and share similar functions.

nucleus accumbens Large cell group of the basal forebrain present at the level of the head of the caudate nucleus; located just lateral to the septal area and immediately ventral and medial to the neostriatum. It receives a large dopaminergic projection from the ventral tegmental area, which may be linked to addictive functions, and is also believed to integrate the sequencing of motor responses associated with affective processes.

nucleus ambiguus Contains cell bodies of origin of CN IX and CN X. The caudal half contains cell bodies of origin of CN X that innervate the muscles of the larynx and pharynx as well as the heart; rostral half contains cell bodies of origin of CN IX that innervate the stylopharyngeus muscle.

nucleus cuneatus Second-order neurons located in the lower medulla that receive conscious proprioceptive and tactile inputs from the fasciculus cuneatus; projects through the medial lemniscus to the ventral posterolateral nucleus of thalamus, conveying information from the upper limb.

nucleus dorsalis of Clarke See *dorsal nucleus of Clarke*.

nucleus gracilis Second-order neurons located in the lower medulla that receive conscious proprioceptive and tactile inputs from the fasciculus gracilis; projects through the medial lemniscus to the ventral posterolateral nucleus of thalamus, conveying information from the lower limb.

nucleus locus ceruleus (A6 neurons) Cells situated in the dorsolateral aspect of the upper pons; these cells contain norepinephrine, which projects to the thalamus, hypothalamus, limbic forebrain structures, and cerebral cortex, and modulate sleep and wakefulness, attention, feeding, and other behaviors.

nucleus of the solitary tract Located in the medulla; the rostral portion receives afferents mediating taste sensation (gustatory region); the medial and caudal portions receive afferents from cardiopulmonary receptors, peripheral chemoreceptors, and baroreceptors.

nucleus proprius Located in lamina II of the dorsal horn; neurons of this nucleus give rise to the neospinothalamic tract. Also known as proper sensory nucleus.

nucleus raphe magnus Located in the medulla, it contains serotonergic neurons and is involved in modulation of pain sensation.

nucleus reticularis gigantocellularis Large nucleus of the medial medulla that gives rise to the lateral reticulospinal tract.

nucleus reticularis pontis caudalis One of the principal nuclei of the pons giving rise to the medial reticulospinal tract.

nucleus reticularis pontis oralis One of the principal nuclei of the pons giving rise to the medial reticulospinal tract.

nystagmus (vestibulo-ocular reflex) Reflex response occurring under experimental conditions or spontaneously in patients with brainstem or cerebellar lesions; experimentally, it occurs as follows: as the head is rotated, the eyes show a smooth pursuit movement in the opposite direction in order to continue to fixate on a given object; continued rotation of the head will eventually bring the object out of the individual's visual field, and he will attempt to fixate on another object, resulting in a rapid (i.e., saccadic) movement of the eyes in the direction in which the head is turning; the process thus includes an initial slow movement of the eyes in the direction opposite of movement of the head, which is then followed by rapid rotation in the same direction in which the head is moving. Types of nystagmus are as follows: (1) *pendular* nystagmus is characterized by equal velocity of eye movement in both directions; (2) *jerk* nystagmus is characterized by a slow phase of movement that is followed by a fast phase in opposite direction; (3) *postrotary* nystagmus, which occurs following cessation of rotation induced experimentally, is characterized by a period of nystagmus in the direction opposite to that of movement and is due to the continued flow of endolymph (because of inertia) even after the individual has stopped moving.

obex Position at which the fourth ventricle empties into the central canal of the caudal medulla.

occipital eye field Region of occipital cortex that governs conjugate deviation of the eyes; this form of control is believed to be reflexive in nature and serves as a tracking mechanism.

occipital lobe Most caudal aspect of the cerebral cortex whose components lie on both the lateral and medial surfaces of the cortex; the primary visual receiving area is situated on the medial surface.

occipitotemporal gyrus Cortical structure that lies medial to the inferior temporal gyrus and is bounded medially by the collateral sulcus.

oculomotor nerve (CN III) Cranial nerve whose cell bodies lie in the midbrain at the level of the superior colliculus; somatomotor component supplies all extraocular muscles (except the superior oblique muscle); autonomic component supplies the ciliary and pupillary constrictor muscles.

Ohms law Refers to the relationship between electrical potential (V), conductance (g), and current (I); current equals the product of conductance and potential ($I = gV$).

olfaction Sense of smell; one of the chemical senses.

olfactory binding protein Protein secreted by the Bowman's glands; concentrated around the cilia of the olfactory sensory neurons; carries and/or concentrates the odorant around the cilia.

olfactory bulb Brain structure that appears as a primitive form of cortex consisting of neuronal cell bodies, axons, and synaptic connections; receives information from the first (olfactory) cranial nerve; consists of the following layers: (1) *glomerular layer*, which is located near the surface of the bulb and contains clusters of nerve terminals from olfactory sensory neurons, dendrites of the tufted and mitral cells, and GABAergic interneurons (periglomerular cells), (2) *external plexiform layer*, which contains tufted cells, (3) *inner plexiform layer*, which contains GABAergic interneurons called granule cells, and (4) *mitral cell layer*.

olfactory nerve (CN I) Special visceral afferent nerve supplying olfactory information to the olfactory bulb.

olfactory tracts Pathways arising from the olfactory bulb; include: (1) *lateral olfactory tract*, which is a large bundle of axons from the mitral and tufted cells that exits from the olfactory bulb and supplies the pyriform lobe, and (2) *medial olfactory tract*, which contains fibers from mitral and tufted cells that project ipsilaterally to basal limbic forebrain structures.

oligodendrocytes Supporting cells responsible for myelination of axons in the CNS.

one-and-a-half syndrome Disorder in which the patient cannot move the ipsilateral eye horizontally and the contralateral eye can only be abducted, usually resulting in nystagmus of that eye. In addition, the patient may also present with a combination of lateral gaze paralysis involving CN VI, coupled with an internuclear ophthalmoplegia (an inability to gaze to the side of the lesion); occurs as a result of a discrete lesion of the dorsomedial tegmentum involving the nucleus of CN VI, the pontine (lateral) gaze center of the paramedian pontine reticular formation, and the MLF.

Onuf's nucleus Circumscribed region in the ventral horn that innervates the external urethral sphincter.

open medulla Rostral half of medulla in which the fourth ventricle is present.

opioid peptides Endogenous opioid peptides including β-endorphin, enkephalins, and dynorphins.

opioid receptors Receptors activated by opioid peptides; include classical opioid receptors (mu, delta, and kappa receptors) and a new receptor (ORL1 receptor).

optic chiasm Convergence of the optic nerves of the two eyes when they reach the brain.

optic disc (optic nerve head) Pale circular region where the optic nerve exits the retina.

optic nerve Peripheral component of the axons of CN II originating in the retina prior to their entrance into the CNS.

optic radiations See *geniculocalcarine tract*.

optic tract CNS component of the axons of CN II originating in the retina that project to the lateral geniculate nucleus and superior colliculus.

orbital muscle of Müller Muscle in the orbit that maintains the normal forward position of the eyeball.

organ of Corti Sensory area of the cochlear duct located on the basilar membrane; contains hair cells that are the sensory receptors for sound stimuli.

organelles Subcellular units, including mitochondria; Golgi apparatus; nucleus; granular and agranular endoplasmic reticulum; microsomes; lysosomes; and certain fibrils.

organum vasculosum lamina terminalis (OVLT) See *lamina terminalis*.

orientation columns The interblob region containing vertically oriented columns that include neurons that respond to bars of lines having a specific spatial orientation.

orthostatic hypotension Disorder characterized by sudden dizziness, dimness in vision, and fainting; can be severe and prolonged.

ossicles Three small bones (the malleus, incus, and stapedius) suspended in the cavity of the middle ear; convert sound waves in the air to waves in the fluid located in the inner ear.

otic ganglia Autonomic ganglia from which postganglionic parasympathetic fibers innervating the parotid gland arise.

otolith organs Saccule and utricle located in the inner ear; detect linear acceleration.

otosclerosis Condition in which the bony outgrowth of the stapes impedes its movement against the oval window; ability for efficient conversion of airborne sound waves to pressure waves in the perilymph is lost.

outer phalangeal cells See *Deiter's cells*.

oxytocin Hormone synthesized from paraventricular and supraoptic hypothalamic neurons that is released from the posterior pituitary; instrumental in milk ejection reflex and stimulates uterine contractions (at birth).

panic disorder A form of anxiety disorder characterized by intense fear that lasts for a short period where the patient experiences shortness of breath, sweating, trembling, and fear of insanity or death.

Papez circuit A group of interconnecting neural structures, which include the cingulate gyrus, hippocampal formation, mammillary bodies, and anterior thalamic nucleus. Originally believed to be associated with the regulation of emotional behavior, this circuit is more likely related to the expression of short-term declarative memory.

papillae See *taste buds*.

papilledema Edema of the optic disk; may be caused by increased intracranial pressure.

parahippocampal gyrus Cortical structure that lies medial to the collateral sulcus on the ventral surface of the brain.

parallel fibers See *granule cell*.

paramedian arteries Branches of the basilar artery that supply the medial portion of the lower and upper pons.

paramedian reticular nucleus Nucleus situated in the medial aspect of the medulla whose axons project to the cerebellum.

paranoid schizophrenia Form of schizophrenia characterized by hallucinations or delusions of persecution, exaltation, or having a specific mission.

parasympathetic division of autonomic nervous system Component of the autonomic nervous system involved in producing decreased heart rate, increased digestive and reproductive functions, and decreases in energy metabolism. Parasympathetic outflow arises from preganglionic neurons located in the midbrain (CN III), pons (CN VII), medulla (CN IX and CN X), and the sacral region of the spinal cord (S2–S4); postganglionic neurons are located in or close to the organ innervated by this system; also referred to as craniosacral division.

paraventricular nucleus Hypothalamic nucleus located in the dorsomedial aspect of the anterior hypothalamus adjacent to the third ventricle; concerned with the release of vasopressin and oxytocin.

paravertebral ganglia Ganglia (25 pairs) present in the two sympathetic chains; represent one of the sites where sympathetic postganglionic neurons are located.

parieto-occipital sulcus Sulcus that divides the occipital lobe from the parietal lobe.

Parinaud's syndrome Disorder resulting from a lesion of the dorsal midbrain; characterized by impaired upward vertical gaze and loss of the pupillary light reflex. See *gaze palsy*, *Sylvian aqueduct syndrome*, and *midbrain syndrome*.

Parkinson's disease Involuntary movement disorder resulting from loss of dopamine neurons in the substantia nigra.

parotid gland Salivary gland that receives inputs from CN IX.

pars compacta See *substantia nigra*.

pars reticulata See *substantia nigra*.

parvocellular Pertains to region containing small-sized cells.

peduncles Massive fiber bundles; one group links the brainstem with the cerebellum (cerebellar peduncles) and another is present on the ventral aspect of the midbrain containing descending fibers from the cerebral cortex to the brainstem and spinal cord (cerebral peduncle).

peduncular region Component of the midbrain containing the crus cerebri and substantia nigra.

pedunculopontine nucleus Nucleus of the pons that contains acetylcholine; associated with REM sleep.

peptide bond Formed when an amino group of one amino acid is joined with the carboxyl group of another amino acid. The amino acids are connected by peptide bonds to form a chain. Protein molecules are made up of different combinations of 20 amino acids.

perforant fiber pathway Fibers from the entorhinal cortex that form excitatory connections with granule cells of the dentate gyrus.

periamygdaloid cortex The more posterior regions of the pyriform lobe underlying the amygdala.

periaqueductal gray (PAG) Gray matter surrounding the cerebral aqueduct of the midbrain.

perikaryon (soma) Nerve cell body.

perineurium Connective tissue sheath that encloses each bundle of nerve fibers.

peripheral nervous system Spinal and cranial nerves that are present outside the CNS.

perivascular space A small space around a blood vessel.

petrosal sinuses Small sinuses located on the superior and inferior regions of the petrous portion of the temporal bone (known as superior and inferior petrosal sinuses, respectively); a network of veins from the cerebellum and medulla empty into the great cerebral vein of Galen and superior and inferior petrosal sinuses.

phagocytosis Transport of solid material into the cells that remove debris (e.g., microglia).

phantom limb pain Perceived sensation of pain from an amputated limb; overactivity of the dorsal horn neurons on the side of the amputated limb may create a false feeling that the pain is emanating from the amputated limb.

phencyclidine (PCP; "angel dust") Drug of abuse taken for recreational purposes; blocks the NMDA receptor channel.

phenylethanolamine-N-methyl-transferase (PNMT) Enzyme present in the cytoplasm of a nerve terminal and in the adrenal medulla; catalyzes conversion of norepinephrine into epinephrine.

phospholipids Long nonpolar chains of carbon atoms that are bonded to hydrogen atoms; a polar phosphate group is attached to one end of the molecule; abundant in the neuronal membrane.

photoreceptors Rods and cones located in the retina.

phrenic motor nucleus Located in the ventral horn of the cervical spinal cord (C3–C5); driven predominantly by the inspiratory neurons located in the rostral group of respiratory neurons located in the ventrolateral medulla; provides innervation to the diaphragm (one of the muscles involved in inspiration).

pia mater The innermost layer of the meninges, which lies closest to the brain.

pie-in-the-floor visual disorder See *contralateral inferior homonymous quadrantanopia*.

pie-in-the-sky visual disorder See *contralateral superior homonymous quadrantanopia*.

pilomotor fibers Axons of postganglionic neurons located in the inferior and middle cervical paravertebral ganglia that innervate the erectile muscle of hairs.

pineal gland Conical-shaped structure attached to the roof of the posterior aspect of the third ventricle; displays a circadian rhythm to light with respect to the release of several hormones; contains biogenic amines, including melatonin.

pinealocytes Specialized secretory cells of the pineal gland.

pinna (external ear, auricle) Directs sound vibrations in the air to the external auditory canal.

pinocytosis Process that involves transport of liquid material into the cells that remove debris (e.g., microglia).

pitch Highness or lowness of the sound; dependent on the frequency of the pressure wave generated by the sound.

pneumotaxic center Group of respiratory neurons located in the dorsolateral pontine tegmentum, just caudal to the inferior colliculus; considered to be essential for maintaining a normal breathing pattern.

polypeptide A protein made of a single chain of amino acids.

pons Part of the brainstem extending from the midbrain to the medulla.

pontine (medial) reticulospinal tract Pathway arising from the nucleus reticularis pontis caudalis and nucleus reticularis pontis oralis. These neurons project ipsilaterally to the entire extent of the spinal cord, and their principal function is to facilitate extensor spinal reflexes.

pontine gaze center Region of the pons adjacent to the abducens nucleus that integrates inputs from the cerebral cortex and vestibular nuclei in order to regulate horizontal eye movements.

positron emission tomography (PET) Imaging technique involving injection of a radiolabeled substance into the circulation. Excess protons are converted into neutrons by radioactive decay, and a positron (a positively charged electron) is emitted; the positron collides with an electron, releasing two photons that are sensed by detectors. Blood flow and glucose utilization in the desired region of the body are then monitored.

postcentral gyrus Region of cerebral cortex that has the central sulcus as its anterior border and the postcentral sulcus as its posterior border. It is the primary receiving area for kinesthetic and tactile information from the periphery (trunk and extremities).

postcommissural fornix Component of the fornix that is distributed to the diencephalon.

posterior Above the midbrain, posterior means "toward the back of the brain," and below the midbrain, posterior means "toward the dorsal surface of the body."

posterior cerebral arteries Arteries that arise at the terminal bifurcation of the basilar artery and supply the occipital lobe and most of the midbrain, thalamus, and subthalamic nucleus.

posterior chamber Space between the lens and the iris in the eye.

posterior commissure Commissure of the brain located on the border of the diencephalon and midbrain; associated with functions of the oculomotor complex.

posterior communicating arteries Arteries that arise from the internal carotid arteries at the level of the optic chiasm; travel posteriorly to join the posterior cerebral arteries.

posterior lobe Largest lobe of the cerebellum associated, in part, with regulation of coordinated movements of the distal musculature.

posterior neuropore A temporary opening of part of the neural tube of the early embryo extending from the central canal to its posterior aspect.

posterior parietal cortex Region of the superior aspect of the parietal cortex that integrates different modalities of sensory inputs and projects its axons to area 6 of the frontal lobe. This region is essential for programming and sequencing of motor responses, and damage to this region results in apraxia and sensory neglect.

posterior spinal arteries These arteries typically arise from the posterior inferior cerebellar artery (PICA) and descend on the dorsolateral surface of the spinal cord slightly medial to the dorsal roots.

posterolateral fissure Major fissure of the cerebellum separating the flocculonodular from posterior lobes.

posteromarginal nucleus Located in the lamina I of the spinal cord. Terminals of dorsal root fibers mediating pain and temperature sensations synapse on these cells; axons of these cells cross to the opposite side and ascend as the lateral spinothalamic tract.

postganglionic parasympathetic fibers Fibers arising from ganglia that lie close to their target organs and that receive inputs from preganglionic parasympathetic fibers.

postictal period The time following a seizure.

postrotary nystagmus See *nystagmus*.

post-traumatic stress disorder Psychiatric disorder resulting from a life-threatening event in the distant past of the individual; such an event reappears in the patient's memory during the daytime or in the evening in dreams and may relate to the disruption of mechanisms that control REM sleep.

postural hypotension See *orthostatic hypotension*.

pre-Bötzinger complex An area just caudal to the Bötzinger complex in the medulla implicated as the site of respiratory rhythm generation.

precentral gyrus Region of the cerebral cortex bounded posteriorly and anteriorly by the central and precentral sulci, respectively. Integrates motor signals from different regions of the brain and serves as the primary motor cortex for control of contralateral voluntary movements; neurons within the precentral gyrus are somatotopically organized.

precommissural fornix Component of the fornix that passes rostral to the anterior commissure and that is distributed to the septal area.

prefrontal cortex Region of the far rostral cerebral cortex, which includes inferior (orbital gyri), medial, and lateral aspects of the frontal lobe; this region plays an important role in the processing of intellectual and emotional events.

prefrontal lobotomy A neurosurgical procedure (not used anymore) involving the undercutting of the afferent and efferent connections of the prefrontal cortex in order to control manifestations of hostility, anger, and violent behavior.

preganglionic parasympathetic fibers See *parasympathetic division of autonomic nervous system*.

premotor area (premotor cortex) Region of cerebral cortex immediately rostral to the precentral gyrus and immediately ventral to the supplemental motor area (area 6 of Brodmann); this region regulates movements associated with the contralateral side of the body by playing an important role in the initiation and sequencing of movements.

preoptic region Anterior aspect of the basal forebrain containing lateral and medial preoptic nuclei; concerned with endocrine functions and temperature regulation.

prepyriform area Region of cortex extending from the lateral olfactory stria to the rostral aspect of the amygdala.

prestriate area An association area related to functions of the visual system.

pretectal area Most rostral region of midbrain bordering on the diencephalon; it comprises a component of the pathway mediating visual reflexes.

prevertebral ganglia Sympathetic ganglia, separate from the sympathetic chain ganglia. Neurons in these ganglia receive preganglionic axons that pass uninterrupted through the paravertebral ganglia.

primary somatosensory cortex Postcentral gyrus (areas 3, 1, and 2 of Brodmann).

primary visual cortex Located on both sides of the calcarine sulcus; receives visual signals from the temporal half of the ipsilateral retina and nasal half of the contralateral retina; concerned with perception of signals from the contralateral half of the visual field.

principal neurons (projecting, type I or Golgi type I neurons) Possess axons that form long fiber tracts in the brain and spinal cord.

procedural memory Refers to a form of memory that differs from declarative memory in that the individual may not be consciously aware of the procedures involved in carrying out a task (e.g., shooting a basketball, skiing, hitting a baseball).

prolactin Pituitary hormone essential for milk production from the lactating mammary gland.

proper sensory nucleus See *nucleus proprius*.

proprioceptors Sensory receptors associated with the stretch of a muscle, tendon, or bodily position.

prosencephalon Developing forebrain that will become the diencephalon and telencephalon.

prosopagnosia Disorder of the inferotemporal cortex in which there is a loss of the ability to recognize familiar faces even though the patient is able to describe the physical features of such individuals.

protoplasmic astrocytes Present in the gray matter in close association with neurons; serve as metabolic intermediaries for neurons; give out thicker and shorter processes that terminate in expansions called end-feet.

Prozac See *fluoxetine*.

pseudobulbar palsy Mild form of weakness in muscles that regulate breathing, swallowing, speech, and chewing after damage to corticobulbar fibers.

pseudo-unipolar neuron Neuron from which a single process arises that divides into two branches; one branch projects to the periphery, and the other projects to the CNS. Information collected from the peripheral end is transmitted to the CNS via the axonal terminals (e.g., sensory cells in the dorsal root ganglion).

ptosis Drooping of the eyelid resulting from damage to the nerves innervating the levator palpebrae superior muscle.

pulmonary stretch receptors Located in the smooth muscles of the lung; activated during inspiration.

pulvinar Large nucleus of the posterior thalamus that projects to the inferior parietal lobule and is believed to be concerned with mediating complex auditory and visual discriminations.

pupil Central circular opening in the iris of the eye.

pupillary constriction The result of shining light into the eye, causing a reflex (pupillary light reflex) mediated through the parasympathetic component of CN III, resulting in contraction of the pupillary constrictor muscles with a reduction in the size of the pupil.

pupillary constrictor muscles See *pupillary constriction*.

pupillary light reflex See *pupillary constriction*.

Purkinje cells Large inhibitory neurons of the gray matter of the cerebellar cortex that project to deep cerebellar nuclei.

putamen Major component of the basal ganglia, along with the caudate nucleus and globus pallidus.

pyramid Protuberance on the ventromedial aspect of the lower brainstem containing corticospinal and corticobulbar fibers.

pyramidal cell layer Layer of hippocampus containing pyramidal cells; major source of output neurons of the hippocampus.

pyramidal cells Prominent cells of the cerebral cortex and hippocampal formation that form the main output neurons of these regions.

pyramidal decussation Region of the caudal medulla where the corticospinal tract crosses from one side of the brainstem to the other.

pyriform cortices (paleopallium) Region of temporal cortex adjoining the amygdala; receives olfactory information and transmits it to amygdaloid nuclei.

quarternary polypeptide Formed when different polypeptide chains assemble to become a large protein molecule; each polypeptide is called a subunit.

quiet biting (predatory) attack A form of aggressive behavior (premeditated murder and hunting behavior in humans) in which an animal will stalk and then bite the back of the neck of the prey object, ultimately killing it; lacks autonomic signs characteristic of defensive rage and, in nature, constitutes a form of hunting behavior.

radionuclide A natural or artificial nuclear (atomic) species that exhibits radioactivity.

raphe nuclei Midline nuclei situated in the brainstem that give rise to serotonin neurons that supply the brain and spinal cord.

Rathke's pouch An ectodermal diverticulum from which the anterior lobe of the pituitary is derived.

Raynaud's disease Characterized by spasmodic vasoconstriction of arteries in the fingers and toes of upper and lower limbs, respectively; precipitated by the activation of sympathetic nervous system in response to cold or emotional stress; the digits appear cyanosed periodically due to the deoxygenation of stagnant blood.

receptive field of a bipolar cell A circular area of the retina that, when stimulated by a light stimulus, changes the membrane potential of the bipolar cell; consists of "the receptive field center," which provides a direct input from the photoreceptors to the bipolar cells, and "receptive field surround," which provides an indirect input from the photoreceptors to the bipolar cells via horizontal cells; changes in membrane potential of bipolar cells in the receptive field center and surround are opposite.

receptors Membrane-spanning proteins that serve as recognition sites for the binding of a neurotransmitter.

recurrent inhibition Type of inhibition resulting from activation of an alpha-motor neuron in spinal cord; mechanism involves excitation of a Renshaw cell (interneuron) via excitatory (cholinergic) collaterals of the alpha-motor neuron; Renshaw cells, in turn, inhibit (via glycinergic synapses) the activity of the same alpha-motor neuron.

red nucleus See *rubrospinal tract*.

referred pain Pain arising from deep visceral structures that is perceived as coming from a site different from its true origin. The phenomenon can be explained by the fact that the same dorsal horn neuron receives afferent signals from deep visceral, cutaneous, and skeletal muscle nociceptors; higher centers incorrectly ascribe the pain stimuli to the skin or skeletal muscle instead of coming from a deeper visceral structure

regeneration Recovery of neuronal injury.

releasing hormones Hypothalamic peptides that regulate the release of pituitary hormones.

REM (paradoxical) sleep Phase of sleep characterized by a beta-type EEG rhythm (i.e., low voltage, fast frequency) and rapid eye movements.

Renshaw cells See *recurrent inhibition*.

resting membrane potential Potential difference across the cell membrane during the resting state.

reticular activating system Pertains to the region of the tegmentum of the brainstem (i.e., the reticular formation), which, when stimulated from sensory or other inputs, can cause arousal (and modulate sleep and wakefulness) by exciting neurons in the cerebral cortex.

reticular formation Central core of the brainstem extending from the medulla through the midbrain; consists of the numerous cell groups and ascending and descending axons; functions include: control of sensory, motor, and visceral processes, as well as states of consciousness.

reticular nucleus Nucleus situated in the lateral margin of the thalamus containing GABAergic neurons that project to other thalamic nuclei.

reticulospinal tracts Pathways arising from the medulla (lateral tract) and pons (medial tract) that pass to different levels of the spinal cord and modulate muscle tone.

reticulotegmental nucleus Nucleus situated in the tegmentum of the pons whose axons project to the cerebellum.

retina Innermost layer of the eye. Consists of the following layers: (1) *the pigment epithelium layer*, which is the outermost layer consisting of melanin-containing cells that provide nutrition (glucose and essential ions) to photoreceptors and other cells associated with them; (2) *the layer of rods and cones* (photoreceptors); (3) *the external limiting membrane*, which contains the processes of rods and cones and *Müller cells* (homologous to the glial cells of the central nervous system); (4) *the outer nuclear layer*, which contains the cell bodies of rods and cones; (5) *the outer plexiform layer*, which contains the axonal processes of rods and cones, processes of horizontal cells, and dendrites of bipolar cells (synaptic interaction between photoreceptors and horizontal and bipolar cells takes place in this layer); (6) *the inner nuclear layer*, which contains the cell bodies of amacrine cells, horizontal cells, and bipolar cells (amacrine and horizontal cells, sometimes called *association cells*, function as interneurons); (7) *the inner plexiform layer*, which contains the axons of bipolar cells, processes of amacrine cells, and dendrites of ganglion cells (synaptic interaction between different retinal cells takes place in this layer); (8) *the layer of ganglion cells*, which contains the cell bodies of multipolar ganglion cells (the final output from the retina following visual stimulation is transmitted to the CNS by the ganglion cells via their axons in the optic nerve); and (9) *the optic nerve layer*, which contains the axons of ganglion cells that form the optic nerve exiting from the eye. Neural retina is concerned with sensing and processing of light stimulus and includes the layer of rods and cones, external limiting membrane, outer nuclear layer, outer plexiform layer, inner nuclear layer, inner plexiform layer, layer of ganglion cells, and optic nerve layer. The retina is supplied by the *central artery of the retina*, which arises from the ophthalmic artery.

retinal detachment Disorder in which the pigment epithelium layer becomes detached from the neural retina; this occurs because the contact between the pigmented epithelium layer and the neural retina is mechanically unstable; the photoreceptors can be damaged in this disorder because they may not receive nutrition that is normally provided by the pigment epithelium layer.

retrograde amnesia Refers to difficulty in retrieving old memories.

etrograde degeneration Degenerative changes in the cell body and proximal part of the axon after damage to the axon.

etrograde messenger A substance (e.g., the neurotransmitter NO) that diffuses from the postsynaptic neuron into the presynaptic terminal and elicits further release of the neurotransmitter.

etrograde tracing technique Involves microinjection of a marker (e.g., horseradish peroxidase, fluorescent dyes, cholera toxin, or viruses) at the predicted terminal region of neurons whose cell bodies are to be determined. The marker is taken up by axon terminals and transported retrogradely into the neuronal cell bodies; the neurons labeled with the marker are visualized.

euptake A mechanism in which the neurotransmitter (e.g., dopamine, norepinephrine) released in the synaptic cleft is actively transported back into the neuronal terminal where it is recycled for release or destroyed.

hodopsin A photoreceptor pigment present in the rods; consists of a protein called opsin that is attached with a light-absorbing component, called retinal (an aldehyde form of vitamin A).

ibosomes Cell organelles where amino acids assemble to form proteins according to instructions provided by messenger RNA; the amino acids are connected by peptide bonds to form a chain.

Rinne's test Compares hearing by air conduction versus bone conduction. A vibrating tuning fork is held in the air near the affected ear and then the base of the tuning fork is placed on the mastoid process. If the sound perceived by the patient is louder when the tuning fork is placed on the mastoid process, when compared to the sound of the tuning fork held in the air, the patient is diagnosed as suffering from conductive hearing loss. If the sound perceived by the patient is louder when the tuning fork is placed in the air near the affected ear, the patient is diagnosed as suffering from sensorineural hearing loss.

roof plate Aspect of the developing nervous system whose cells lie along the dorsal midline of the neural canal.

rostral Above the midbrain, rostral means "toward the front of the brain," and below the midbrain, rostral means "toward the cerebral cortex."

rostral basal pontine syndrome Disorder characterized by contralateral hemiplegia, loss of facial sensation, and loss of ability to chew; caused mainly by occlusion of paramedian branches of the basilar artery, affecting the corticospinal tract and sensory and motor components of CN V.

rostral interstitial nucleus Region for vertical gaze movements situated in the ventrolateral aspect of the rostral midbrain PAG.

rostral pontine tegmental syndrome Characterized by ipsilateral loss of sensation to the face and ability to chew; contralateral loss of pain, temperature, and conscious proprioception from the body; as well as possible ataxia of movement; associated mainly with occlusion of the long circumferential branches of the basilar artery affecting sensory and motor nuclei of CN V, medial lemniscus, spinothalamic tracts, and possibly cerebellar afferent fibers contained in the middle cerebellar peduncle.

rostral ventrolateral medullary pressor area (RVLM) Located caudal to the facial nucleus; involved in the maintenance of sympathetic tone of arteries.

rough endoplasmic reticulum Endoplasmic reticulum with ribosomes attached to its membrane.

rubrospinal tract Pathway from the red nucleus of midbrain to spinal cord, which facilitates spinal cord flexor motor neuron activity.

saccadic movements Horizontal eye movements that occur quite rapidly, the duration of which is less than 50 milliseconds.

saccule An ovoid sac-like structure in the ear that is connected to the cochlea and the utricle; detects linear acceleration.

sacral cord Most caudal aspect of spinal cord situated between the thoracic cord rostrally and cauda equina caudally, containing five pairs of spinal nerves (S1–S5).

sacral sparing Phenomenon in which damage to the spinothalamic tracts leaves pain, temperature, and simple tactile sensations intact in sacral dermatomes.

saltatory conduction Rapid conduction of an action potential along the axon when the action potential jumps from one node of Ranvier to another; the action potential becomes regenerated at the nodes of Ranvier, which are uninsulated, have a lower resistance, and are rich in Na^+ channels.

Scarpa's ganglion Consists of two ganglia; neurons located in these ganglia innervate receptors (hair cells) in the vestibular labyrinth in the ear.

Schaffer collaterals Collaterals of axons arising from CA3 hippocampal pyramidal cells, which project back to the CA1 field of the hippocampus.

schizophrenia Disorder characterized by a dysfunction in the thought process in which the ability to correctly test reality is lacking; includes delusional thought processes (i.e., false beliefs); disturbances in speech, appearance, and behavior; hallucinations (i.e., false perceptions, which are mostly auditory such as hearing voices); apathy, or a paucity of emotion; and the presence of a catatonic posture. There is an overall inability to perceive the world accurately. See also *disorganized (hebephrenic) type of schizophrenia*.

Schwann cells Supporting cells of the peripheral nervous system responsible for the formation of myelin.

secondary visual cortex Brodmann's area 18.

sella turcica A saddle-like bony prominence on the upper surface of the sphenoid bone; with its dural covering, it forms the hypophyseal fossa in which the pituitary gland (hypophysis) is located.

semicircular canals Three canals (anterior or superior, posterior and lateral or horizontal semicircular canals) in the labyrinth of the ear that lie in different planes and are perpendicular to each other; they detect angular acceleration.

sensorineural deafness Result of pathological lesions in the cochlea, cochlear nerve, or central auditory pathways.

sensory neglect (anosognosia) Disorder in which the patient denies having a disease condition or is unaware of it. It is caused by damage to the right posterior parietal cortex and can be demonstrated when the patient is asked to draw a clock and the numbers on the clock are all drawn on the right side of the clock.

septal area Limbic structure representing a major relay nucleus of the hippocampal formation.

septal rage Intensified aggressive response following lesions placed in the septal area of rats. Lesions of the region of the septal area and septum pellucidum in humans have also been reported to be associated with aggressive behavior as well.

septum pellucidum A structure that lies immediately ventral to the corpus callosum, is most prominent anteriorly, and consists of two thin-walled membranes separated by a narrow cleft, forming a small cavity (cavum of septum pellucidum).

serine One of the amino acids present in proteins.

serotonin (5-hydroxytryptamine; 5-HT) A small-molecule neurotransmitter synthesized from tryptophan (a nutritionally essential amino acid present in proteins).

sexually dimorphic nucleus Nucleus in preoptic region of rodents which is larger in males than in females.

short circumferential arteries Pontine arteries that travel a short distance around the pons and supply substantia nigra and lateral portions of the midbrain tegmentum.

short-term memory disorder A disorder of memory that selectively affects memory of recent events (i.e., those occurring within seconds to minutes of the time of testing).

simple cell Cell type located near the region of sublayer 4Cβ of the visual cortex; has circular receptive field and receives inputs from the lateral geniculate nucleus. The cell responds to a bar of light presented in a specific position (i.e., in a given receptive field).

simple partial (psychomotor) seizures Form of seizure that does not cause a change in consciousness, but the patient experiences various sensory and motor symptoms, usually not lasting for more than 1 to 2 minutes.

Sinemet A combination of L-DOPA and carbidopa used for the treatment of Parkinson's disease. See also *carbidopa*.

single-photon emission computed tomography (SPECT) Imaging technique used to determine regional cerebral blood flow after the injection of a specific radionuclide; useful in diagnosis of many neurological conditions where there may be alterations in blood flow to specific regions of the brain, such as stroke.

sinoatrial node Region of the heart where pacemaker cells regulating heart rate are located.

sleep apnea Condition characterized by an interruption of breathing in which there is a decline in the oxygen content of the blood; interruption of breathing leads to arousal from sleep or results in lighter stages of non-REM sleep so that breathing can be maintained.

slow anterograde axonal transport Transport of materials (e.g., neurofilaments, microtubules, soluble proteins) from the cell body to the terminals at a slow rate (0.25–5 mm/day). See also *fast anterograde axonal transport*.

somatic nervous system Component of the nervous system that innervates musculoskeletal structures and the sense organs of skin.

somatosensory Somatic sensation involving touch, pressure, temperature, and pain.

somatostatin Neuroactive peptide synthesized in hypothalamic paraventricular neurons (and other regions of the forebrain).

somatotopic Refers to different parts of a given region associated with distinct parts of the body, both functionally and anatomically.

somesthetic Pertains to kinesthetic and tactile information from the periphery.

somites Mesodermal cells located alongside the neural tube that will develop into skeletal muscle, vertebrae, and dermal layer of the skin.

Sommer's sector Region of CA1 field of the hippocampus highly susceptible to anoxia, especially during temporal lobe epilepsy.

spatial summation Superimposition (summation) of multiple signals that arrive at the trigger zone (axon hillock in efferent neurons) simultaneously.

special sensory afferent (SSA) neurons Afferent components of cranial nerves associated with the transmission of visual, auditory, and vestibular impulses.

special visceral afferent (SVA) neurons Components of afferent fibers of cranial nerves that are associated with transmission of chemical sensation.

special visceral efferent (SVE) neurons Cell groups that are derived from mesenchyme of the branchial arches.

specific thalamic nuclei Thalamic nuclei that relay specific sensory information originating in the periphery to specific regions of the neocortex.

sphincter vesicae Sphincter located at the neck of the bladder; activation of sympathetic nervous system contracts this sphincter during ejaculation and prevents seminal fluid from entering the bladder.

spina bifida (myeloschisis) Failure of the closure of the posterior neuropore during development of the nervous system.

spina bifida aperta A disorder involving the protrusion of either the meninges alone or spinal cord and the meninges.

spina bifida occulta A disorder of mesodermal origin in which one or more vertebrae fail to close.

spinal accessory nerve (CN XI) Motor (SVE) cranial nerve arising from ventral horn cells of the first 5 to 6 cervical segments that supply the trapezius and sternomastoid muscles and that mediate contralateral turning and lifting of the head.

spinal medullary and radicular arteries Arteries that arise from segmental arteries and communicate with the posterior and anterior spinal arteries; they provide blood supply to the thoracic, lumbar, and sacral regions of the spinal cord.

spinal nucleus of the trigeminal nerve Receives inputs from the descending tract of CN V and mediates second-order sensory signals from the head region to the contralateral ventral posteromedial thalamic nucleus; present throughout the entire length of the medulla and extends into the lower pons.

spinal veins On the ventral side of the spinal cord, the *anteromedian spinal vein* is located in the midline, and two *anterolateral spinal veins* are located along the line of attachment of the ventral roots. On the dorsal side, the *posteromedian spinal vein* is located in the midline, and two *posterolateral spinal veins* are located along the line of attachment of the dorsal roots. The posteromedian and posterolateral vein are drained by *posterior spinal medullary* and *radicular veins*. The anterior median and anterolateral spinal veins are drained by *anterior spinal medullary* and *radicular veins*.

spinocerebellar pathway Pathway from spinal cord to cerebellum mediating unconscious proprioception.

spinocerebellum (paleocerebellum) See *anterior lobe of cerebellum*.

spino-olivary fibers Fibers originating in spinal cord that project to the inferior olivary nucleus.

spinothalamic pathway Pathway from the spinal cord to the thalamus that mediates pain, temperature, and tactile sensation.

spiral (cochlear) ganglion Located within the spiral canal of the bony modiolus; contains bipolar neurons whose peripheral processes innervate the hair cells and whose central processes form the cochlear division of CN VIII.

splanchnic nerves Axons of the sympathetic preganglionic neurons located in the IML at T5-T9, T10-T11, and T12; they pass through the sympathetic chain without synapsing and emerge as greater, lesser, and least splanchnic nerves, respectively. These axons synapse on neurons in the celiac ganglion; the postganglionic fibers emerging from the celiac ganglion innervate smooth muscle and glands of the stomach and small intestine.

split brain Cerebral commissures that have been divided in the midline (the practice is carried out in patients to stop the spread of seizures).

stellate ganglion Fusion of the last two cervical and first two thoracic ganglia to form this star-shaped ganglion; sympathetic postganglionic fibers arising from this ganglion (when it is present) innervate all regions of the heart (sinoatrial node, atria, atrioventricular node, and ventricles).

stem cells Undifferentiated cells from which neurons (as well as other types of cells) may be formed.

stereognosis Appreciation of shape, size, or texture of objects by means of touch.

strabismic amblyopia A disorder present in some infants; the visual axes of the two eyes are not parallel.

stratum oriens Layer of hippocampus containing basal dendrites and basket cells.

stratum radiatum-lacunosum-moleculare Two layers of the hippocampus that contain the apical dendrites of pyramidal cells and hippocampal afferents from the entorhinal cortex.

stretch reflex See *myotatic reflex*.

stria Refers to fiber bundle in the CNS.

stria medullaris Pathway passing along the roof of the thalamus conveying afferent and efferent signals in relation to the habenular nuclei.

stria terminalis Major efferent pathway of the amygdala, the primary projections of which supply the medial hypothalamus and bed nucleus of the stria terminalis.

striosomes Inputs to the neostriatum that end in patches surrounded by a larger compartment referred to as a matrix; contain acetylcholinesterase, somatostatin, substance P, and enkephalin; receive inputs mainly from limbic regions of cortex, and neurons from this region preferentially project to the substantia nigra.

stroke Characterized by an acute onset of a neurological deficit lasting for at least 24 hours; can be caused by blockage of blood vessels (occlusive stroke) or by bleeding from vessels (hemorrhagic stroke).

subarachnoid space Space between the arachnoid and pial membranes filled with CSF.

subfornical organ A small neuronal structure in the third ventricle consisting of fenestrated capillaries that lack a blood-brain barrier and allow passage of blood-borne molecules.

sublenticular component of internal capsule Components of internal capsule fibers that originate in the temporal lobe or posterior parts of the thalamus.

submucosal (Meissner's) plexuses Neurons in the gut that control water and ion movement across the intestinal epithelium.

substance P An undecapeptide (composed of 11 amino acids); a neurotransmitter or neuromodulator.

substantia gelatinosa Region of gray matter of the dorsal horn of spinal cord that receives mainly pain and temperature inputs from the periphery.

substantia innominata Region of the basal forebrain situated immediately lateral to the preoptic region; linked anatomically with the amygdala and projects to widespread regions of the cerebral cortex.

substantia nigra Structure found in the ventral aspect of the midbrain associated with functions of the basal ganglia; one group of cells (pars compacta) produces dopamine and supplies the neostriatum, while a second group (pars reticulata) produces GABA and supplies the ventrolateral and ventral anterior thalamic nuclei.

subthalamic nucleus Structure found in the ventral aspect of diencephalon associated with functions of the basal ganglia; receives inputs from neostriatum and projects to the globus pallidus.

sudomotor fibers Axons of postganglionic neurons located in the inferior and middle cervical paravertebral ganglia that innervate the sweat glands.

sulcus limitans Landmark in the developing nervous system that separates sensory from motor regions.

sumatriptan (Imitrex) A 5-HT$_{1D}$ receptor agonist; a vasoconstrictor found useful in treating migraine headaches.

superficial middle cerebral vein Passes along the lateral sulcus, drains the temporal lobe, and empties into the cavernous sinus.

superior At positions above and below the cephalic flexure, superior means toward the dorsal surface of the cerebral cortex.

superior anastomotic vein of Trolard Largest superficial vein; travels across the parietal lobe and drains into the superior sagittal sinus.

superior cerebellar peduncle One of the three cerebellar peduncles constituting the major output pathway of the cerebellum.

superior colliculus Rostral aspect of the tectum of midbrain associated with visual reflexes and tracking movements of the eyes.

superior medullary velum Roof of the fourth ventricle attached to the superior cerebellar peduncle on each side.

superior oblique muscle An extraocular muscle innervated by the trochlear nerve; stimulation of this nerve results in contraction of the superior oblique muscle, causing the eye to be moved downward when it is located in a medial position.

superior olivary nucleus Auditory relay nucleus of the lower pons.

superior salivatory nucleus of the facial nerve Nucleus of CN VII; located in the lower pons; provides parasympathetic innervation to the lacrimal, sublingual, and submandibular salivary glands.

superior temporal gyrus The most superior aspect of the temporal lobe containing transverse gyri of Heschl, which constitute the primary auditory receiving area.

supplemental motor area Region of cortex immediately rostral to the precentral gyrus (area 6 of Brodmann).

suprachiasmatic nucleus Nucleus found in the ventromedial aspect of the anterior hypothalamus. It receives inputs from the retina, which affect circadian rhythms for release of several hormones.

supramarginal gyrus Situated in the inferior parietal lobule just superior to the posterior extent of the lateral sulcus.

supranuclear paralysis Paralysis resulting from a cortical lesion affecting corticobulbar fibers normally directed to motor nuclei of cranial nerves.

supraoptic nucleus Hypothalamic nucleus located near the lateral edge of the optic chiasm concerned with the release of vasopressin and oxytocin.

suspensory ligaments of the lens Ligaments attached to the lens of the eye; relaxation or stretching of these ligaments causes the lens to become more convex (suitable for near vision) or less convex (suitable for distant vision), respectively.

Sylvian aqueduct syndrome See *Parinaud's syndrome*.

symmetrical synapse Synaptic arrangement in which postsynaptic and presynaptic membranes are similar in thickness; this type of synapse is usually inhibitory. See also *asymmetrical synapse*.

sympathetic chains Consist of nerve trunks (one on each side of the vertebral column) connecting paravertebral ganglia (25 pairs); each ganglion represents one of the sites where sympathetic postganglionic neurons are located.

sympathetic division of autonomic nervous system Division of the autonomic nervous system associated with the thoracolumbar cord; regulates heart rate, blood pressure, energy metabolism, and digestive functions.

sympathetic dystrophy syndrome See *causalgia* (another name for this syndrome).

sympathetic postganglionic neurons Located in the paravertebral and prevertebral ganglia.

sympathetic trunks See *sympathetic chains*.

sympatholytic drugs Agents that attenuate or block the effects of sympathetic nervous system.

synapse A special zone of contact where one neuron communicates with another one.

synaptic transmission Mechanism by which neurons communicate with each other.

syringomyelia A developmental abnormality. It is characterized by an expansion of the central canal of the spinal cord; there is a segmental loss of pain and thermal sensation because of the interruption of crossing fibers of the spinothalamic tracts in the same and adjoining segments at the level of the lesion; tactile sensation is preserved.

tabes dorsalis (tertiary or neurosyphilis) Disorder characterized by loss of vibration sensation, two-point discrimination, and conscious proprioception, and presence of ataxia; represents late consequences of syphilitic infection of the nervous system. Large-diameter central processes of the dorsal root ganglion neurons (primary afferent sensors) degenerate in the lower thoracic and lumbosacral segments.

tachykinins A group of polypeptides including substance P.

tactile sensations Sensations of touch, pressure, and vibration.

tanycytes Specialized ependymal cells found in the floor of the third ventricle; their processes extend into the brain tissue, where they are juxtaposed to blood vessels and neurons. They are implicated in the transport of hormones from the CSF to capillaries of the portal system and from hypothalamic neurons to the CSF.

tardive dyskinesia Characterized by involuntary movements of the tongue and face, such as repetitive chewing movements and irregular movement of the tongue in and out of the mouth; associated with depletion in GABA and its synthesizing enzyme, glutamic acid decarboxylase.

taste bud Sensory organ for taste; located in different types of papillae (protrusions on the surface of the tongue); sense salty, sour, sweet, and bitter tastes.

tectospinal tract Pathway from the superior colliculus to cervical cord, which follows the MLF and mediates postural movements in response to visual stimuli reaching the superior colliculus.

tegmentum Dorsal aspect of the pons and midbrain containing the reticular formation and a variety of nuclear groups.

telencephalon Developing cerebral cortex and basal forebrain (derived from prosencephalon).

temporal hemiretina Component of retina located lateral to the fovea.

temporal summation Superimposition (summation) of multiple signals that arrive at the trigger zone (axon hillock in neurons) at different times; arriving signals drive the axon hillock to threshold membrane potential so that an action potential is generated; threshold refers to a membrane potential at the trigger zone at which action potentials automatically trigger the adjacent membrane regions into producing an action potential.

tentorial notch   Notch through which the midbrain traverses; rostral free edge of the tentorium cerebelli forms the boundary of this notch.

tentorium cerebelli   A septum that forms a tent-like roof over the posterior cranial fossa; occipital lobes lie on the dorsal surface of this tentorium.

teratogen   An agent that causes an abnormality in development during early pregnancy.

tertiary visual cortex   (V3 and V5; Brodmann's area 19)   Located adjacent to the primary visual cortex.

tethered cord   A malformation involving the anchoring of the lowest part of the spinal cord to the sacrum; results in sensory and motor deficits of the lower extremities as well as bladder emptying difficulties, back pain, and scoliosis.

thalamic fasciculus (H₁ field of Forel)   Collective grouping of the ansa lenticularis, lenticular fasciculus, and dentatothalamic fibers as they pass into and through the posterior thalamus to the ventral anterior and ventrolateral thalamic nuclei.

thalamic pain syndrome   Syndrome resulting from a thalamic infarct, frequently involving its posterior aspect; the patient feels a very painful and unpleasant sensation that persists generally as a burning sensation.

thalamostriate fibers   Projections from the centremedian nucleus of thalamus to the putamen.

thalamus   Dorsal and largest part of the diencephalon; consists of varieties of nuclei that project mainly to the cerebral cortex.

theta rhythm   A slow EEG wave of 4–7 Hz recorded over the temporal lobes or within the hippocampal formation; in humans, this type of EEG typically indicates dysfunction of hippocampal tissue.

third ventricle   One of the brain cavities; connected rostrally to the lateral ventricles (via the foramina of Monro) and caudally to the fourth ventricle (via the aqueduct of Sylvius); forms the medial surface of the thalamus and hypothalamus.

thoracic cord   The part of the spinal cord situated between the cervical cord rostrally and lumbar cord caudally; contains 12 pairs of spinal nerves.

threshold potential   A membrane potential at the trigger zone at which action potentials become self-propagating (an action potential automatically triggers the adjacent membrane regions into producing an action potential).

thyrotropin-releasing hormone (TRH)   Hypothalamic releasing hormone affecting release of the pituitary hormones, thyrotropin, and prolactin.

tic douloureux   Trigeminal neuralgia (severe pain of the face).

tight junctions   An anatomic arrangement in which adjacent capillary endothelial cells are in close apposition to each other; this arrangement prevents movement of ions and molecules from the capillaries to the surrounding tissue.

tinnitus   A condition characterized by a "ringing" noise in the ears.

tissue plasminogen activator (t-PA)   Thrombolytic agent (a substance that lyses blood clots).

tolerance   Phenomenon in which repeated administration of a drug elicits weaker responses.

torsion tremor   Movements producing severe torsion of the neck or shoulder girdle, resulting in rhythmic shaking of the head.

tract   Many axons grouped together that typically pass from a given nucleus to a common target region or to several regions.

transducin   A G-protein present in rods in the eye. See also *G-protein*.

transient ischemic attack   (TIA) Refers to symptoms of ischemia that last for short periods of time (about 30 minutes).

transverse gyrus of Heshl   See *superior temporal gyrus*.

transverse pontine fibers   Fibers that arise from deep pontine nuclei and pass horizontally to the opposite side where they enter the middle cerebellar peduncle.

trapezoid body   Commissure comprising fibers from th cochlear nuclei and superior olivary nucleus that pass to th inferior colliculus via the lateral lemniscus.

tricyclic compounds   A class of antidepressant drugs (such a amitriptyline and clomipramine) that increases monoamir concentrations in brain.

trigeminal (Gasserian) ganglion   Ganglion for CN V.

trigeminal nuclei and nerve (CN V)   Includes sensory ar motor nuclei associated with CN V. Sensory nuclei, which re ceive somatosensory inputs from the head, include (1) th spinal nucleus, which is located mainly in medulla and me diates pain and temperature; (2) the main sensory nucleus which is located in the middle pons and mediates consciou proprioception; and (3) the mesencephalic nucleus which i located in the upper pons and mediates signals associate with muscle spindles. The motor nucleus, which is situated i the middle pons, controls muscles of mastication.

trigger zone   The site where action potentials are generatec the axon hillock is the trigger zone in neurons.

trochlear nerve (CN IV)   Motor nerve whose cell bodies lie i the midbrain at the level of the inferior colliculus and whos axons supply the superior oblique muscle.

tuber cinereum   See *median eminence*.

tuberal nuclei   Hypothalamic nuclei adjoining the third ven tricle; concerned with release of releasing and release-in hibiting hormones transmitted through the portal system t the anterior pituitary gland, the net effect of which is to reg ulate the release of hormones from this region.

two-point discrimination (Weber two-point discrimination   A technique for measuring the minimal distance between twc stimuli applied by a two-point caliper to two adjacent area of skin simultaneously to determine the minimal distanc where the two stimuli can be distinguished. The principle i that the closer the distance between the two stimuli that ca be perceived, the denser the innervation of the receptors sub serving tactile discrimination; used as a test of somatosen sory function when the minimal distance for two-point dis crimination is compared between the identical regions of th two sides of the body.

tympanic membrane   Membrane located at the end of the au ditory canal.

tyrosine hydroxylase   Enzyme involved in the synthesis o catecholamine neurotransmitters; catalyzes conversion of ty rosine to dihydroxyphenylalanine (rate-limiting step in th synthesis of catecholamine neurotransmitters).

uncinate fasciculus   Fibers arising from the fastigial nucleu of cerebellum that lie in a position just dorsal to the superio cerebellar peduncle and that project bilaterally to the reticu lar formation.

uncinate fits   See *cacosmia*.

uncus   Medial extension of the anterior end of the parahip pocampal gyrus.

undershoot of the action potential   See *action potential*.

unipolar neuron   Neuron in which there is only a single neu rite (axon), of which different segments serve as receptors or axon terminals; found in invertebrates.

upper motor neuron   Neurons of the brain that innervate, ei ther directly or through an interneuron, lower motor neurons of the spinal cord and brainstem.

upper motor neuron syndrome   A form of paralysis associ ated with damage to the motor cortex or its descending path ways; in addition to paralysis, the affected limb(s) display hy pertonia, spasticity, hyperreflexia, and a positive Babinski sign.

utricle   An ovoid sac-like structure in the vestibular labyrinth; detects linear acceleration.

vagus nerve (CN X)   Consists of general (baroreceptor) and special visceral afferent (chemoreceptor) fibers, general so matic afferent (from the back of the ear) and general visceral efferent (parasympathetic) fibers innervating thoracic and abdominal viscera, and special visceral efferent fibers inner vating the larynx and pharynx.

vasoconstrictor fibers Axons of postganglionic neurons that innervate the arterioles.

vasodilation Dilation of blood vessels.

vasopressin (antidiuretic hormone) Hormone synthesized in paraventricular and supraoptic hypothalamic neurons; released from the posterior pituitary; causes water retention (decrease in urine production of the kidney).

ventral Above the cephalic flexure, ventral refers to the bottom of the brain, and below the flexure, it refers to the ventral surface of the body.

ventral amygdalofugal pathway Fiber bundle arising chiefly from the basolateral amygdala and parts of the adjoining pyriform cortex that course medially from the amygdala into the lateral hypothalamus where many fibers terminate.

ventral anterior nucleus Thalamic nucleus situated at approximately the same level as the anterior nucleus, which receives inputs from the globus pallidus and substantia nigra; projects mainly to the premotor cortex and to widespread regions of other parts of the frontal lobe.

ventral basal complex Region of thalamus consisting of the ventral posterolateral and ventral posteromedial nuclei.

ventral lateral nucleus Thalamic nucleus situated posterior to the ventral anterior nucleus; receives inputs from the globus pallidus, substantia nigra, and cerebellum and projects to the primary motor cortex.

ventral posterolateral nucleus Nucleus situated in the ventrolateral aspect of the posterior thalamus; receives inputs from the medial lemniscus and spinothalamic tract and projects to the postcentral gyrus.

ventral posteromedial nucleus Nucleus situated in the ventrolateral aspect of the posterior thalamus just medial to the ventral posterolateral nucleus; receives inputs from secondary trigeminal fibers and projects to the lateral aspect of the postcentral gyrus.

ventral respiratory group of neurons Group of respiratory neurons located in the ventrolateral medulla.

ventral tegmental area Region of the ventral midbrain adjoining the pars compacta of the substantia nigra; contains dopamine neurons that supply much of the forebrain except the neostriatum.

ventral tegmental decussation Refers to the crossing of axons of the red nucleus in the ventral midbrain tegmentum.

ventricles Cavities present within the brain that contain CSF.

ventricular layer Inner layer of the neural tube that is in contact with the cavity of the neural tube.

ventromedial nucleus of the hypothalamus Prominent nucleus of the ventromedial aspect of the hypothalamus; concerned with inhibition of feeding, endocrine regulation, and expression of rage behavior.

vermis Midline region of the cerebellar cortex associated with the control of balance and eye movements.

vertebral artery First branch arising from the subclavian artery in the chest; ascends through foramina in the cervical vertebrae and enters the cranium through the foramen magnum.

vertical gaze center Region of the midbrain that coordinates the up and down movements of the eyes.

vertigo Sensation of turning or rotation in space; usually, debris from the otolithic membrane accumulates at the ampulla of the posterior semicircular canal and adheres to the cupula, making it more sensitive to angular movement.

vestibular nuclei Pertaining to lateral, medial, inferior, and superior vestibular nuclei, which are associated with transmission of signals necessary for balance; receive direct inputs from the vestibular apparatus; many of the neurons project through the MLF to cranial nerve nuclei of extraocular muscles, cerebellum, and spinal cord.

vestibulocerebellum See flocculonodular lobe.

vestibulocochlear nerve (CN VIII) Special sensory afferent nerves mediating auditory and vestibular inputs through separate receptors and neural pathways.

vestibulo-ocular reflex (nystagmus) See *nystagmus*.

viscerotopy Topographic association of positional arrangement of neurons in the sympathetic chain ganglia innervating the viscera; e.g., preganglionic neurons innervating the eye are located most rostrally, whereas those innervating the genitals lie most caudally.

visual agnosia Disorder of a secondary visual area in which there is failure to understand the meaning or use of an object.

visual field of an eye Region of space that the eye can see while looking straight ahead without movement of the head.

vitreous body (vitreous humor) Thick, gelatinous material filling the space between the lens and retina; contains phagocytes that remove blood and debris in the eye under normal circumstances.

Wallenberg's syndrome See *lateral medullary syndrome*.

Wallerian degeneration Changes that occur in the axon distal to the site of axonal damage; the axon swells up and becomes irregular; eventually, the axon and the terminals are broken down into fragments that are phagocytosed by adjacent macrophages and Schwann cells.

Weber's syndrome (superior alternating hemiplegia) Disorder affecting the ventromedial midbrain, damaging oculomotor nerve fibers and axons of the crus cerebri and thus causing an ipsilateral oculomotor paralysis and contralateral upper motor neuron paralysis of the limbs.

Weber's test Used to ascertain if a person's deafness is due to conduction disturbance or sensorineural loss. The base of a vibrating tuning fork is placed at the top of the head in the midline. If the person's deafness is due to conduction disturbance in the right ear, the sound from a vibrating tuning fork will be heard louder in the same (right) ear. If the person's deafness is due to sensorineural loss in the right ear, the sound will be louder in the left ear.

Wernicke's area Region of the ventral aspect of the angular and supramarginal gyrus, extending onto the adjoining part of the superior temporal gyrus; essential for comprehension of spoken language; lesions of this region produce a form of aphasia characterized by impairment of comprehension and repetition, although speech remains fluent.

white matter Brain and spinal cord tissue that appear white with the naked eye due to the presence of a large number of myelinated axons.

working memory Form of short-term memory requiring recall of a sequence of events for a few minutes in order to complete a task.

xanthochromia Process by which red blood cells undergo lysis and release hemoglobin, which is broken down into bilirubin that imparts a yellow color to the CSF after subarachnoid hemorrhage.

zona incerta Thin band of forebrain cells separating the lenticular fasciculus from the thalamic fasciculus.

zone of Lissauer (dorsolateral tract or fasciculus) Refers to the tract formed by central axons of sensory neurons mediating pain that branch into ascending and descending collaterals.

zonule fibers Radially arranged connective tissue bands that are attached to the ciliary muscle and hold the lens in place in the eye.

INDEX

Page numbers in *italic* designate figures; page numbers followed by the letter "t" designate tables; page numbers preceded by a "G" designate glossary entries; (*see also*) designates related topics or more detailed subtopic lists.